# ADVANCES IN

# Ophthalmology and Optometry

**Editor-in-Chief**
**Myron Yanoff, MD**

Chair Emeritus, Department of Ophthalmology, Drexel University, Adjunct Professor, Department of Ophthalmology, University of Pennsylvania, Philadelphia, Pennsylvania

ELSEVIER

PHILADELPHIA LONDON TORONTO MONTREAL SYDNEY TOKYO

# ADVANCES IN
Ophthalmology and Optometry

VOLUMES 1 to 5 (OUT OF PRINT)

## VOLUME 6

Editor: Megan Ashdown
Developmental Editor: Jessica Cañaberal



Editorial Office:
Elsevier
1600 John F. Kennedy Blvd,
Suite 1800
Philadelphia, PA 19103-2899

International Standard Serial Number: 2452-1760
International Standard Book Number: 13: 978-0-323-96187-5

# ADVANCES IN
## Ophthalmology and Optometry

STEPHEN E. ORLIN, MD – Cornea and External Diseases
Associate Professor, Scheie Eye Institute, University of Pennsylvania, Perelman School of Medicine, Philadelphia, Pennsylvania

JOSEPH M. ORTIZ, MD, FRCOphth – Glaucoma
Consultant in Ophthalmology, Sacred Heart Hospital, Allentown, Pennsylvania; Consultant in Ophthalmology, Abington Memorial Hospital, Abington, Pennsylvania; Formerly Assistant Professor of Ophthalmology, Hahnemann University Hospital, Drexel University School of Medicine, Philadelphia, Pennsylvania

LEONARD J. PRESS, OD, FAAO, FCOVD – Optometry
Press Consulting, P.C, Lakewood, New Jersey; Adjunct Professor, Southern College of Optometry, Memphis, Tennessee

APARNA RAMASUBRAMANIAN, MD – Pediatric Ophthalmology
Director of Retinoblasma and Ocular Oncology, Phoenix Children's Hospital, Phoenix, Arizona

## CONTRIBUTORS

REDDIN AHMAD, BMBS, iBSC, Foundation Year 2 Doctor, Bradford Teaching Hospitals NHS Foundation Trust, Bradford, West Yorkshire, United Kingdom

MARIB AKANDA, MD, Resident Physician, Department of Ophthalmology, Northwell Health Eye Institute, Great Neck, New York, USA

TOMAS ANDERSEN, MD, MPH, Scheie Eye Institute, Perelman School of Medicine, University of Pennsylvania, Philadelphia, Pennsylvania, USA

SHAHZAN ANJUM, MSc, Ocular Pathology Services, Dr. Rajendra Prasad Centre for Ophthalmic Sciences, All India Institute of Medical Sciences, New Delhi, Delhi, India

RAMESH AYYALA, MD, Department of Ophthalmology, University of South Florida College of Medicine, Tampa, Florida, USA

NOORAN BADEEB, MBBS, Department of Ophthalmology, School of Medicine, University of Jeddah, Jeddah, Saudi Arabia

ALIREZA BARADARAN-RAFII, MD, Department of Ophthalmology, University of South Florida College of Medicine, Tampa, Florida, USA

SUZANNAH BELL, MBChB, DTMH, MSc, Queen Alexandra Hospital, Portsmouth, United Kingdom

RUPAK BHUYAN, MD, Department of Ophthalmology, Icahn School of Medicine at Mount Sinai Hospital, New York, New York, USA

KASTURI BHATTACHARJEE, MS, FRCSEd, Head, Department of Ophthalmic Plastic and Reconstructive Surgery and Oculofacial Aesthetics, Sri Sankaradeva Nethralaya, Guwahati, Assam, India

ELENA Z. BIFFI, OD, MS, FAAO, Associate Professor of Optometry, New England College of Optometry, Boston, Massachusetts, USA

MARIE I. BODACK, OD, FAAO, Diplomate, Binocular Vision, Perception and Pediatrics Optometry; Professor, Department of Pediatric Primary Care, Southern College of Optometry, Memphis, Tennessee, USA

JEFFREY BROWN, MD, Department of Ophthalmology, Icahn School of Medicine at Mount Sinai Hospital, New York, New York, USA

MEHAR CHAND SHARMA, MD, Department of Pathology, All India Institute of Medical Sciences, New Delhi, Delhi, India

EMILY CHANG, MD, Resident, Department of Ophthalmology, Kellogg Eye Center, University of Michigan, Ann Arbor, Michigan, USA

BHAVNA CHAWLA, MD, Professor of Ophthalmology, Ocular Oncology Service, RP Centre for Ophthalmic Sciences, All India Institute of Medical Sciences, New Delhi, India

BENSON S. CHEN, MBChB, MSc, FRACP, Department of Clinical Neurosciences, University of Cambridge, Cambridge, United Kingdom; Cambridge Eye Unit, Addenbrooke's Hospital, CUH-NHS, Cambridge, United Kingdom; Gonville and Caius College, University of Cambridge, Cambridge, United Kingdom

RAO V. CHUNDURY, MD, Truhlsen Eye Institute, University of Nebraska Medical Center, Omaha, Nebraska, USA

CAROLINE W. CHUNG, MD, Resident Physician, Scheie Eye Institute, Philadelphia, Pennsylvania, USA

Y. GRACE CHUNG, BS, Emory University School of Medicine, Atlanta, Georgia, USA

DEVIN COHEN, MD, Scheie Eye Institute, Perelman School of Medicine, University of Pennsylvania, Philadelphia, Pennsylvania, USA

STUART COUPLAND, PhD, Department of Ophthalmology, Faculty of Medicine, University of Ottawa, Ottawa Hospital Research Institute, The Ottawa Hospital, Ottawa, Ontario, Canada

KEVIN J. EVERETT, MD, Director of Refractive Surgery, Henry Ford Hospital Department of Ophthalmology, Detroit, Michigan, USA; Henry Ford OptimEyes Super Vision Center - Sterling Heights, Sterling Heights, Michigan, USA

SHAILESH GAIKWAD, MD, FNAMS, CCST, Professor, Department of Neuroimaging and Interventional Neuroradiology, All India Institute of Medical Sciences, New Delhi, India

SAMUEL GELNICK, MD, Northwell Health Eye Institute, Great Neck, New York, USA

ROBIN GINSBURG, MD, Director of the Vitreoretinal Service, Assistant Professor, Department of Ophthalmology, Icahn School of Medicine at Mount Sinai Hospital, Department of Ophthalmology, New York Eye and Ear Infirmary at Mount Sinai, New York, New York, USA

CHLOE GOTTLIEB, MD, Department of Ophthalmology, Faculty of Medicine, University of Ottawa, Ottawa Hospital Research Institute, The Ottawa Hospital, Ottawa, Ontario, Canada

ANGELA GUPTA, MD, PhD, Resident Physician, Scheie Eye Institute, Philadelphia, Pennsylvania, USA

MARIAM S. HAMID, MD, Chief Ophthalmology Resident, Henry Ford Hospital Department of Ophthalmology, Detroit, Michigan, USA

GEORGE JIAO, MD, Resident Physician, Department of Ophthalmology, Northwell Health Eye Institute, Great Neck, New York, USA

MAN LI JIN, MD, Chief Ophthalmology Resident, Henry Ford Hospital Department of Ophthalmology, Detroit, Michigan, USA

PRIYA KALYAM, MD, Oculo Facial Plastic and Reconstructive Surgeon, Legacy Eyelids & Cosmetic Surgery, Plano, Texas, USA

PUSHPINDER KANDA, MD, PhD, Department of Ophthalmology, Faculty of Medicine, University of Ottawa, Ottawa, Ontario, Canada

JOSEPH EDWARD KANE Jr, OD, FAAO, Attending Optometrist, Veterans Affairs Boston Healthcare System

LYNCA KANTUNGANE, COMT, Department of Ophthalmology, Faculty of Medicine, University of Ottawa, Ottawa, Ontario, Canada

RUSTUM KARANJIA, MD, PhD, Department of Ophthalmology, Faculty of Medicine, University of Ottawa, Ottawa Hospital Research Institute, The Ottawa Hospital, Ottawa, Ontario, Canada; Doheny Eye Institute, Doheny Eye Centers UCLA, Department of Ophthalmology, David Geffen School of Medicine at UCLA, Los Angeles, California, USA

JAMIE A. KEEN, MD, Department of Ophthalmology and Visual Sciences, University of Iowa, Iowa City, Iowa, USA

SERENA LI, BA, Department of Clinical Neurosciences, University of Cambridge, Cambridge, United Kingdom; Gonville and Caius College, University of Cambridge, Cambridge, United Kingdom

RONNI M. LIEBERMAN, MD, Assistant Professor, Department of Ophthalmology, Mount Sinai Medical Center, Ichan School of Medicine, Mount Sinai Health Systems, New York, New York, USA

JACOB LIECHTY, MD, Department of Ophthalmology, University of South Florida College of Medicine, Tampa, Florida, USA

TIANYU LIU, MD, Ophthalmology Resident, Scheie Eye Institute, University of Pennsylvania, Philadelphia, Pennsylvania, USA

STEPHANIE M. LLOP, MD, Bascom Palmer Eye Institute, University of Miami Miller School of Medicine, Miami, Florida, USA

SAMANTHA L. MAREK, MD, Ophthalmology Resident, Scheie Eye Institute, University of Pennsylvania, Philadelphia, Pennsylvania, USA

KERRI MCINNIS-SMITH, BA, Mayo Clinic Alix School of Medicine, Scottsdale, Arizona, USA

ADITI MEHTA, MD, Fellow, Department of Ophthalmic Plastic and Reconstructive Surgery and Oculofacial Aesthetics, Sri Sankaradeva Nethralaya, Guwahati, Assam, India

HOLLY K. MILLER, DO, Phoenix Children's Hospital, Phoenix, Arizona, USA; Mayo Clinic, Scottsdale, Arizona, USA

MARIYA MOOSAJEE, MBBS, BSc, PhD, FRCOphth, Professor, Moorfields Eye Hospital NHS Foundation Trust, University College London Institute of Ophthalmology, The Francis Crick Institute, London, United Kingdom

JENNIFER B. NADELMANN, MD, Resident Physician, Scheie Eye Institute, Philadelphia, Pennsylvania, USA

MEHDI NAJAFI, MD, PhD, Vitreoretinal Surgeon, Boston Vision, Beth Israel Deaconess Medical Center, Boston, Massachusetts, USA

BRIAN J. NGUYEN, MD, Ophthalmology Resident, Scheie Eye Institute, University of Pennsylvania, Philadelphia, Pennsylvania, USA

JACQUELYN O'BANION, MD, MSc, Emory Eye Center, Atlanta, Georgia, USA; Department of Ophthalmology, Emory University School of Medicine

STEPHEN E. ORLIN, MD, Associate Professor of Ophthalmology, Chief of Cornea Service, Scheie Eye Institute, Perelman School of Medicine, University of Pennsylvania, Philadelphia, Pennsylvania, USA

CHRISTIE M. PERSON, OD, FAAO, Grady Health System, Eye Clinic, Atlanta, Georgia, USA

SUSAN A. PRIMO, OD, MPH, FAAO, Emory Eye Center, Atlanta, Georgia, USA; Department of Ophthalmology, Emory University School of Medicine

VIVIAN L. QIN, MD, Scheie Eye Institute, Perelman School of Medicine, University of Pennsylvania, Philadelphia, Pennsylvania, USA

APARNA RAMASUBRAMANIAN, MD, Phoenix Children's Hospital, Phoenix, Arizona, USA

ERICK RIVERA-GRANA, MD, Assistant Professor of Clinical Ophthalmology, Department of Ophthalmology, University of Puerto Rico School of Medicine, San Juan, Puerto Rico, USA

CHRISTINE RYU, MD, Truhlsen Eye Institute, University of Nebraska Medical Center, Omaha, Nebraska, USA

SEEMA SEN, MD, Ocular Pathology Services, Dr. Rajendra Prasad Centre for Ophthalmic Sciences, All India Institute of Medical Sciences, New Delhi, Delhi, India

RAHUL A. SHARMA, MD, MPH, FRCSC, Department of Ophthalmology and Vision Sciences, University of Toronto, Toronto, Ontario, Canada; Prism Eye Institute, Oakville, Ontario, Canada

ERIN M. SHRIVER, MD, Department of Ophthalmology and Visual Sciences, University of Iowa, Iowa City, Iowa, USA

NAVNEET SIDHU, MD, Senior Resident, Ophthalmology, RP Centre for Ophthalmic Sciences, All India Institute of Medical Sciences, New Delhi, India

MINH TRINH, MD, Northwell Health Eye Institute, Great Neck, New York, USA

SRAVANTHI VEGUNTA, MD, Pediatric Ophthalmology and Adult Strabismus Fellow, Department of Ophthalmology, Indiana University School of Medicine, Indianapolis, Indiana, USA; Assistant Professor, Department of Ophthalmology and Visual Sciences, University of Utah School of Medicine, Salt Lake City, Utah, USA

VATSALYA VENKATRAMAN, MD, Fellow, Department of Ophthalmic Plastic and Reconstructive Surgery and Oculofacial Aesthetics, Sri Sankaradeva Nethralaya, Guwahati, Assam, India

LAURA WINDSOR, OD, FAAO, Low Vision Centers of Indiana, Division of the Eye Associates Group, LLC, Indianapolis, Indiana, USA

RICHARD WINDSOR, OD, FAAO, DPNAP, Low Vision Centers of Indiana, Division of the Eye Associates Group, LLC, Indianapolis, Indiana, USA

BENJAMIN YOUNG, OD, FAAO, Assistant Professor of Optometry, New England College of Optometry, Boston, Massachusetts, USA

CAROLINE Y. YU, MD, Department of Ophthalmology and Visual Sciences, University of Iowa, Iowa City, Iowa, USA

AMY ZHANG, MD, Assistant Clinical Professor, Department of Ophthalmology, Kellogg Eye Center, University of Michigan, Ann Arbor, Michigan, USA

**CONTENTS** VOLUME 7 • 2022

threatening pathologies may be identified and assessed using this procedure. A thorough understanding of the principles and practical applications of B-scan ultrasonography is essential to maximize use of this technique in patient management.



## Nonsurgical Treatment of Strabismus

Marie I. Bodack

Nonsurgical treatment options for esotropia and exotropia may be indicated for some patients to improve outcomes presurgery or postsurgery or in lieu of surgery. The ideal outcome is for a patient to have binocularity and excellent alignment. Current nonsurgical treatment options for patients with esotropia and exotropia include lenses, prisms, occlusion, and vision therapy.

## Pediatric

### Update on Pediatric Optic Neuritis

Sravanthi Vegunta

Pediatric optic neuritis (ON) is a condition with a broad differential including demyelinating syndromes, astrocytopathies, and infectious processes. Many retrospective studies have been published on the similarities and differences between pediatric ON secondary to clinically isolated syndrome, multiple sclerosis, myelin oligodendrocyte glycoprotein, and neuro-myelitis optica spectrum disorder. The presentations, visual outcomes, and laboratory testing, and imaging findings have significant overlap but important differences. This article details how to distinguish between various causes of autoimmune ON to provide the appropriate acute and chronic therapies to patients. Gaps in our current knowledge and suggestions for future studies are discussed.



### Genetics of Congenital Cataract

Reddin Ahmad, Suzannah Bell, and Mariya Moosajee

Up to 40,000 children are born with cataracts annually worldwide. In the UK, children presenting with bilateral cataract most commonly have a genetic basis. Mutations in genes involved in lens-specific proteins or regulation of eye development can cause isolated cataract, those associated with more complex ocular defects and/or syndromic features. Early surgery and frequent follow-up are vital to avoid amblyopia and optimize visual potential. Routine genetic testing is important to allow accurate diagnosis and personalized management of patients including tailored genetic counseling. Multidisciplinary care is vital, including clinical genetic and ophthalmic teams, pediatricians, school, and local pediatric visual support services.



**Pediatric Graft-Versus-Host Disease**

Kerri McInnis-Smith, Holly K. Miller, and Aparna Ramasubramanian

Even with the support of evidence-based medicine available, the proper diagnosis and treatment of graft-versus-host disease (GVHD) and its ophthalmologic manifestations, especially in the pediatric population, is quite nuanced. The wide array of disease presentations, the existence of confounding factors such as underlying disease and concurrent treatment, and the challenge of children accurately conveying their symptoms can further contribute to the difficulty in effectively managing young patients with chronic GVHD. Clinicians must consider the expert recommendations for management while choosing diagnostic approaches and therapeutic regimens according to the individual patient.



## Ophthalmic Pathology & Ocular Oncology

### Fluorescence In Situ Hybridization in Ocular Oncology

Seema Sen, Shahzan Anjum, and Mehar Chand Sharma

Fluorescence in situ hybridization is a useful tool to visualize and map the genetic material in an individual's cells, including specific genes or portions of genes. This technique has diagnostic and prognostic implications for a variety of ocular malignant tumors because genetic mutations detected by FISH provide useful information for better management including targeted therapy. Chromosomal abnormalities including t(14;18) translocation in lymphoma, monosomy of chromosome 3 in uveal melanoma, and t(6;9) translocation in adenoid cystic carcinoma of lacrimal gland are some of the common genetic hallmarks of these malignancies.

**Intra-arterial Chemotherapy for Retinoblastoma: An Update**
Bhavna Chawla, Navneet Sidhu, and Shailesh Gaikwad

Retinoblastoma is the most common primary intraocular tumor in children. It also is one of the most successfully treated tumors using various treatment strategies. Conventional globe salvage treatments include the use of focal therapies in combination with systemic chemotherapy. Intra-arterial chemotherapy (IAC) is a comparatively newer treatment modality used primarily for globe salvage in refractory retinoblastoma. It involves the direct administration of chemotherapy drugs into the ophthalmic artery to achieve a high local intraocular concentration. IAC has been found to successfully treat retinoblastoma, and a few newer modifications are being tried. Our article discusses the significance of IAC, technique employed, drugs used, and newer advances in its administration.



**Advances in Pediatric Periocular Vascular Neoplasms**
Kasturi Bhattacharjee, Aditi Mehta, and Vatsalya Venkatraman

Pediatric periocular vascular neoplasms originate from transformed endothelial cells showing increased proliferation. Commonest of these is infantile hemangioma, which presents in the first year of life. The lesion exhibits initial rapid growth followed by spontaneous regression. Locally infiltrative and malignant tumors, although rare, may exhibit metastatic potential. Neoplasms need to be differentiated from congenital vascular malformations, which are noninvoluting, exhibit growth commensurately with age, and do not demonstrate endothelial proliferation. Timely treatment of periocular lesions obscuring the visual axis helps prevent amblyopia. Systemic involvement or presence of large lesions (>5 cm) warrants assessment of cardiac function as the high-flow lesions may produce high-output cardiac failure. Mass effect of extensive perioral/nasal/subglottic lesions may compromise the airway. A multidisciplinary approach is important for optimizing treatment outcomes. Propranolol has gained FDA approval in 2017 as the first-line therapy for infantile hemangioma. In contrast, malformations are difficult to treat, and therapy mostly is symptomatic.



## Cataract & Refractive Surgery

### Femtosecond Laser-Assisted Cataract Surgery

Emily Chang and Amy Zhang

Since femtosecond laser-assisted cataract surgery (FLACS) first became commercially available approximately a decade ago, it has continued to provoke much interest as well as controversy. As femtosecond laser technology continues to evolve, FLACS has shown to be a safe alternative to the conventional phacoemulsification surgery. However, the successful adoption of a new technology requires both cost efficiency and significant improvement over conventional techniques. This article summarizes the utilization of femtosecond laser technology in certain steps of cataract surgery and reviews its safety and efficacy in each step.

## Advanced Technology Intraocular Lenses

Mariam S. Hamid, Man Li Jin, and Kevin J. Everett

Recently developed advanced technology intraocular lenses (IOLs) aim to provide patients with the ability to see in-focus images at multiple distances to mimic the natural accommodative function of the eye. Multifocal IOLs use diffractive, refractive, or hybrid technologies to allow images from multiple focal points to be simultaneously focused on the retina. This inadvertently causes photic side effects including glare or haloes and reduced contrast sensitivity, and therefore, careful patient selection and consent are indicated. Extended depth-of-focus IOLs use a single, elongated focal point to reduce photic side effects, though often at the expense of near vision compared with multifocal IOLs. This article will review recent developments in advanced technology IOLs such as multifocal, accommodative, and extended depth-of-focus IOLs and discuss their visual outcomes and side effects.



## Vitreoretinal Disease

## Diagnostic and Treatment Considerations for Macular Holes

Rupak Bhuyan, Jeffrey Brown, and Robin Ginsburg

Video content accompanies this article at http://www.advancesinophthalmology.com

Macular holes are foveal neurosensory disruptions that can impair vision and cause symptoms such as metamorphopsia and scotomas. Stages 1A and 1B should be observed. Stage 2 can be treated with multiple modalities including topical dehydration agents, pneumatic vitreolysis, and surgery. Surgery remains the most used treatment, because it can prevent additional vision loss from progression to stages 3 and 4. Surgery is also the recommended treatment of stages 3 and 4. Inverted internal limiting membrane flaps, human amniotic membrane plugs, mesenchymal stem cell injections, and autologous retinal transplants are newer adjunctive treatments that offer encouraging results.



## Peripheral Retinal Degenerations and Treatment Options

George Jiao, Marib Akanda, and Ronni M. Lieberman

There are numerous pathologies that can be found in the peripheral retina, including degenerative disease. Involvement of the vitreoretinal interface and certain intraretinal degenerations can lead to retinal tears or detachments. The standard of care for diagnosing and monitoring these peripheral retinal degenerations is dilated fundus examination, but current technologies may aid us when the diagnosis is unclear. Prophylactic treatments may be warranted in many cases of predisposing lesions. Definite treatments for retinal tears are important in preventing retinal detachments.

## Update on Retinal and Ocular Imaging

Samuel Gelnick, Minh Trinh, and Ronni M. Lieberman

Retinal imaging has experienced rapid growth over the past decades. An increase in resolution, field of view, and accessibility has led to an increase in the use of retinal imaging in clinical practice across all specialties of ophthalmology. Understanding the advantages and disadvantages of these retinal imaging modalities is crucial to obtaining the appropriate studies to diagnose and monitor retinal pathologies. In this article, we review common imaging modalities, including their evolution and clinical applications.

## Glaucoma

### 30-Gauge Needle in Glaucoma/Anterior Segment Management

Ramesh Ayyala, Alireza Baradaran-Rafii, and Jacob Liechty

Video content accompanies this article at http://www.advancesinophthalmology.com

Many clinical presentations and complications of glaucoma, whether acute or chronic, including bleb fibrosis, encapsulation, and so forth along with anterior segment surgeries can be managed at the slit lamp with the help of a 30 gauge (G) needle. This article presents the indications and techniques involved in the use of 30G needle at the slit lamp in the management of a myriad of ophthalmologic presentations and complications.

## Neuro-ophthalmology

### Screening for Plaquenil

Pushpinder Kanda, Stuart Coupland, Chloe Gottlieb, Lynca Kantungane, and Rustum Karanjia

Hydroxychloroquine use needs to be carefully monitored for retinal toxicity that can lead to significant visual impairment. This review summarizes the current screening guidelines and imaging modalities recommended by the American Academy of Ophthalmology and highlights future research trends for improving test sensitivity. It also discusses the utility of using mfERG for detecting early retinopathy and research supporting its use as a primary screening tool.



### Update on Optic Neuritis in Adults: Multiple Sclerosis, Neuromyelitis Optica Spectrum Disorder, and Myelin Oligodendrocyte Glycoprotein Antibody–Associated Disease

Serena Li, Rahul A. Sharma, and Benson S. Chen

This review provides an update on the diagnosis and management of inflammatory optic neuritis in adults, focusing on presentations associated with multiple sclerosis, neuromyelitis optica spectrum disorder, and myelin oligodendrocyte glycoprotein antibody–associated disease. Clinical clues that enable early recognition of these distinct disorders are discussed, including patient demographics, clinical features, and radiologic findings. The use of corticosteroids, plasmapheresis, and other acute management treatment strategies for optic neuritis are appraised, followed by an overview of long-term management, specifically strategies for immunosuppression including when to initiate and with which therapies. Finally, prognosis and future avenues are considered.

**Efficacy and Safety of Tocilizumab in the Treatment of Ocular Manifestations in Giant Cell Arteritis**

Nooran Badeeb and Rustum Karanjia

Vision loss in GCA is an ophthalmic emergency that requires prompt medical intervention. The goal of the treatment is to preserve the remaining vision and prevent further systemic complications. Corticosteroids are the first-line treatment for GCA but are prone to cause iatrogenic side effects. In this review, we discuss the role of other immunosuppressant medications, especially Tocilizumab in controlling cases of GCA with ocular involvement and review the literature on the indication, guidelines of administration, and safety of Tocilizumab.



**Coronavirus Disease 2019–Related Health Disparities in Ophthalmology with a Retrospective Analysis at a Large Academic Public Hospital**

Y. Grace Chung, Christie M. Person, Jacquelyn O'Banion, and Susan A. Primo

The coronavirus disease 2019 pandemic has disproportionately affected racial and ethnic minorities in the United States. Although recent meta-analyses have identified the prevalence of ocular manifestations in severe acute respiratory syndrome coronavirus 2 infection, no studies with these potential findings have been implemented in examining ophthalmic disparities in racial and ethnic minorities. It is additionally clear that patient access to eye care from coronavirus disease 2019 has been disproportionate in underserved communities. Large public hospitals and urban academic medical centers provide a unique opportunity to further study ocular disease presentation and health disparities from coronavirus disease 2019 in these populations.



## Cornea and External Diseases

### Stepwise Approach to the Diagnosis and Management of Dry Eye and Ocular Surface Disease

Jennifer B. Nadelmann, Angela Gupta, Caroline W. Chung, and Stephen E. Orlin

Dry eye disease (DED) is a multifactorial disorder caused by abnormalities of the tear film that causes damage to the ocular surface. Screening tools are helpful in making the diagnosis and in determining disease severity. It is important to take a careful history and to evaluate meibomian gland physiology, tear film quality, meibomian gland status, and tear production. Clinicians should take a stepwise approach in treating DED. Treatments vary for evaporative dry eye, aqueous deficiency, and/or inflammatory DED. For patients with symptoms that have not improved following conservative measures, prescription medications, blood products, procedures or devices can be considered.

**Update on the Classification and Management of Corneal Dystrophies**

Vivian L. Qin, Devin Cohen, Tomas Andersen, and Stephen E. Orlin

The most recent IC3D classification (2015) categorizes the corneal dystrophies based on genetic, clinical, and histologic characteristics. Here we review the classification of the corneal dystrophies as epithelial and subepithelial, epithelial-stromal *TGFB1*, stromal, and endothelial. We discuss the variety of available medical and surgical treatment modalities based on symptomatology and anatomic area of the cornea affected. We explore the recent advancements in the area of corneal regeneration without the use of donor grafts, including injection of cultured endothelial cells and gene therapy.



**Surgical Management of the Aphakic Eye**

Tianyu Liu, Brian J. Nguyen, Samantha L. Marek, and Stephen E. Orlin

Current approaches to the surgical correction of aphakia include anterior chamber intraocular lenses (IOLs), iris-fixated IOLs, sulcus IOLs, and scleral-fixated IOLs with or without sutures. Anterior chamber and iris-fixated IOLs are technically easier to place but are associated with risks including corneal decompensation, uveitis, and glaucoma. Sulcus placement of IOLs can achieve physiologic positioning of the lens but requires adequate capsular support. Overall, current approaches to correction of aphakia have comparable efficacy and safety outcomes, and the advantages and disadvantages of each technique should be considered in light of patient and surgeon factors in surgical planning.



## Oculoplastics

### Teprotumumab: A Major Advance in the Treatment of Thyroid Eye Disease Management

Caroline Y. Yu, Jamie A. Keen, and Erin M. Shriver

Thyroid eye disease (TED) is an uncommon orbital inflammatory disease that can lead to disfigurement and permanent vision loss. Traditional therapies such as glucocorticoids and orbital radiation primarily were used to treat inflammation during the active phase of the disease. Teprotumumab, the first Food and Drug Administration-approved medication for TED, targets the insulin-like growth factor-1 receptor and has been shown to decrease proptosis, diplopia, and clinical activity score. In this review, the pathophysiology and treatment landscape of TED are summarized, and the mechanism, clinical data, and associated adverse events of teprotumumab are described in detail.

Uveitic glaucoma is a complex disease whose pathogenesis and treatment differ greatly from other glaucoma syndromes. Intraocular pressure elevation can be due to open-angle, closed-angle, or mixed mechanisms and steroid-induced processes. Up to 20% of patients with uveitis develop glaucoma. It is important to adequately recognize the differences in the treatment of this disease to accurately manage both glaucoma and ocular inflammation. We provide a review of the most common inflammatory etiologies that cause glaucoma and different treatment modalities used to manage it, both medical and surgical.



## Solo Private Practice Journey

Priya Kalyam

On completing medical training, physicians have little to no experience with choosing their future job. Much of their experience has been tied up with choosing a career and then competing for the best training experience. This article provides the author's insight into the path of entering solo practice.

Advances in Ophthalmology and Optometry 7 (2022) xxxv

ADVANCES IN OPHTHALMOLOGY AND OPTOMETRY

# PREFACE

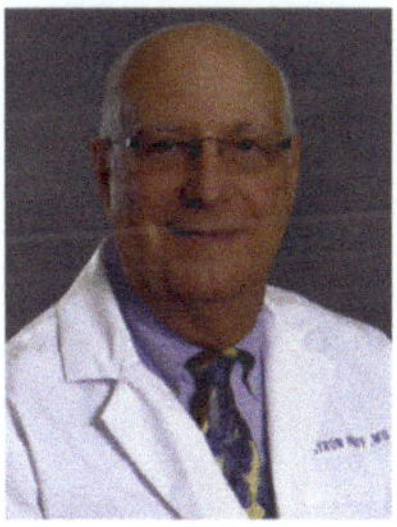

Myron Yanoff, MD
*Editor*

## LOOKING BACKWARD AND FORWARD

In Volume 7 of *Advances in Ophthalmology and Optometry*, we again have asked experts in each of the pertinent fields to sift through the current literature to give us insights on the latest developments, such as bioptic driving in the United States; the use of B-scan ultrasound in primary eye care; nonsurgical treatment of strabismus; an update on pediatric optic neuritis; genetics of congenital cataract; intra-arterial chemotherapy for retinoblastoma: an update; screening for plaquenil; femtosecond laser-assisted cataract surgery; COVID-19-related health disparities in ophthalmology with a retrospective analysis at a large academic public hospital; a stepwise approach to the diagnosis and management of dry eye and ocular surface disease; teprotumumab: a major advance in the treatment of thyroid eye disease management; and much more.

We continue to explore the new ideas, new treatments, and new ways of doing things to give us a fresh frame of reference to sort through the crush of data and to make sense in a real way of how to proceed.

Myron Yanoff, MD
Department of Ophthalmology
University of Pennsylvania
Department of Ophthalmology
Drexel University
219 North Broad Street, 3rd Floor
Philadelphia, PA 19107, USA

*E-mail address:* myanoff4@gmail.com

https://doi.org/10.1016/j.yaoo.2022.05.002

# Optometry

Advances in Ophthalmology and Optometry 7 (2022) 1–29

ADVANCES IN OPHTHALMOLOGY AND OPTOMETRY

# Biopic Driving in the United States

Laura Windsor, OD*, Richard Windsor, OD

Low Vision Centers of Indiana, Division of the Eye Associates Group, LLC, 9002 North Meridian Street, Indianapolis, IN 46260, USA

**Keywords**

• Bioptic telescope • Bioptic driving • Vision impairment • Low vision
• Behind-the-wheel training • Driver's training

**Key points**

- Bioptic driving, using a telescope mounted into the top of eyewear, allows the patient with a mild to moderate visual impairment the opportunity to drive in most states.
- Proper candidate selection and the fitting of the bioptic system is a crucial step in the process of becoming a bioptic driver.
- A multi-disciplinary approach to training in the use of the system and behind-the-wheel will increase the success and safety of the bioptic driver.

## INTRODUCTION

Bioptic driving began in 1971 when California licensed the first bioptic driver. For patients with visual impairments, as with all licensed drivers, the ability to drive is a privilege, giving them the independence that is life-altering. In the United States, the ability to drive is key to employment opportunities, maintaining independence, enjoying social events, improved mental health, and accessing health care [1]. Driving cessation has been attributed to an increase in depression and social isolation in seniors [2]. In some states, patients with mild visual impairments usually can drive with minimal restrictions like daytime only, a limited radius from their home, and/or a speed restriction. For those with moderate visual impairments, they may be able to become bioptic drivers which lead to a higher quality of life [3].

*Corresponding author. *E-mail address:* drlaura@eyeassociates.com

https://doi.org/10.1016/j.yaoo.2022.03.020
2452-1760/22/

A bioptic system has 2 components consisting of carrier lenses with the patient's prescription in a frame and a telescope mounted in or at the superior portion of the carrier lens(es). Most of the driving is conducted viewing through the carrier lenses and the telescope is used to quickly identify signs, traffic lights, and hazards in the distance [2] (Fig. 1).

## HISTORY OF BIOPTICS AND DRIVING IN THE UNITED STATES

Dr. William Feinbloom pioneered the field of optometric low vision rehabilitation in the United States. Out of frustration in helping a patient in 1938, he used a small astronomer's 3X telescope and mounted it into his patient's lenses and frame. He then began to work on his design and in 1958 in a session on Contact Lenses and Subnormal Vision at the American Academy of Optometry, Dr. Feinbloom introduced his concept of a bioptic telescopic system (BTS) that combined a small Galilean telescope mounted superiorly through prescription lenses in a frame [3]. In 1961, he founded Designs for Vision which began producing not only bioptics and microscopes for patients with low vision but also surgical and dental telescopes based on his bioptic concept, which still are used by doctors throughout the world today.

Dr. Feinbloom dramatically demonstrated his bioptic driving concept by artificially blurring his vision to 20/200 and had his son film him as he drove the streets of New York City. He was able to easily drive but could not read the signs. He then, while still blurred, drove through the city with a bioptic system

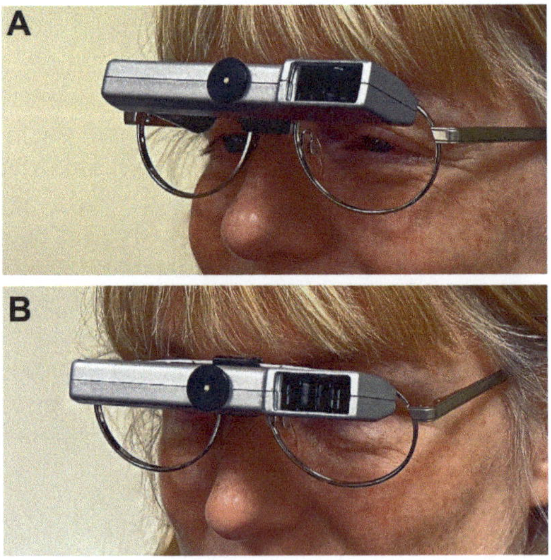


**Fig. 1.** On the top picture (*A*) with the head is the straight-ahead position, the patient views through the carrier lenses of the frame. In the bottom photo (*B*), the driver demonstrates switching from the carrier lenses to a view through the bioptic telescope by tilting their head downward 10 to 15°.

and demonstrated how he could read traffic signs with the use of the bioptic. The first study on bioptic driving was published in 1970 by Dr. Donald Korb, a previous intern of Dr. Feinbloom [4]. In 1977, Feinbloom published a study of 300 bioptic drivers showing there were no accidents causing bodily injury or significant property damage [5]. (Fig. 2).

During the 1970s and 1980s, bioptic driving emerged as a viable option to aid a select group of visually impaired individuals to become licensed bioptic drivers. California began issuing bioptic driver's licenses in 1971. The first licensed bioptic driver in the US was Dennis Kelleher, a graduate student at the University of California at Berkley. He was fit with his BTS by Dr. Edwin Mehr and received his license on March 8, 1971. He went on to publish numerous articles on bioptic driving to help others. Then in 1975, Korb, Jose, and Butler published articles laying a framework for a multidisciplinary approach to training the bioptic driver [6,7].

## A legal pathway for bioptic driving

In 1974, Section 5004 of the Rehabilitation Act was passed barring the discrimination of an individual with a disability [8]. In 1984, the US Department of Transportation (DOT) issued a statement indicating that a visually impaired individual should not be discriminated against in obtaining a driver's license. The DOT's action, though of limited power, did lead to more states looking at the option of bioptic driving. This led to the adoption of bioptic driving programs in some states in the 1980s, including Indiana's development of a model program which began in 1987.

In 1991, the Americans with Disabilities Act (ADA) was passed into law. Title II of the ADA law states that a governmental licensing agency cannot discriminate against a person with a documented disability and must allow for an "individual assessment" of the person before denying licensing privileges. The evolution of this legislation, through court cases, was the catalyst for more states to develop their own bioptic programs (Fig. 3).

The US has been the model for other countries including the Netherlands and some provinces of Canada to implement bioptic driving programs [9]. Australia is now allowing bioptic drivers on a case-by-case basis. Table 1 lists the timeline of bioptics in driving in the US.

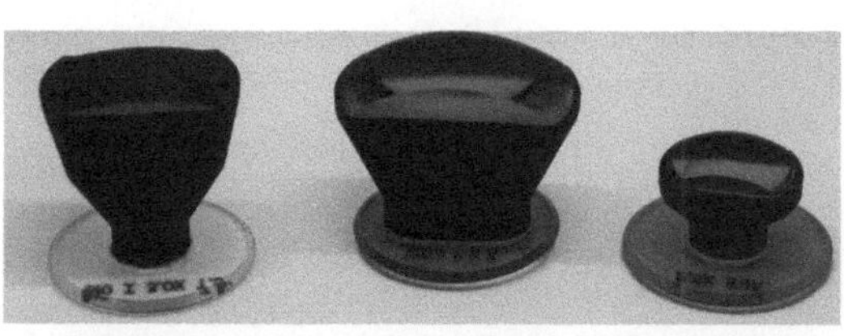

**Fig. 2.** Dr William Feinbloom developed a series of bioptic telescopes evolving from his original bioptic design.

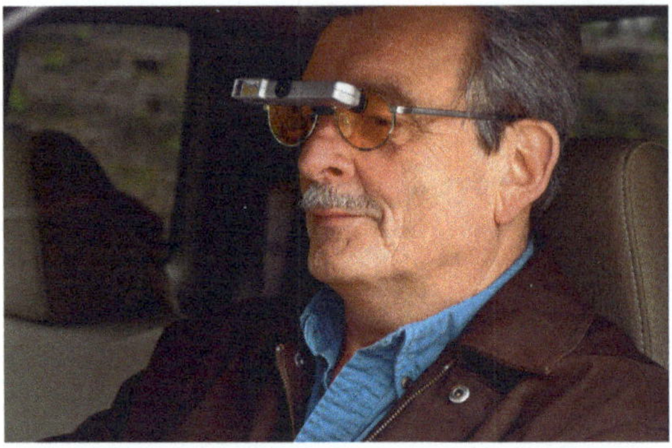

**Fig. 3.** This 78-year-old patient uses an Ocutech Sport system to drive and has been a bioptic driver for 23 years.

## CONTROVERSIES AND RESEARCH IN BIOPTIC DRIVING

The concept of allowing the visually impaired individual to drive was quite revolutionary when it was introduced. The safety of the visually impaired driver, bioptic usage, and issues of the BTS making a ring scotoma has all been debated.

### Wearing the bioptic only to obtain licensure

Some researchers have suggested that drivers only wear and use the bioptic until they are licensed drivers and then discontinue its use [13,14]. A survey of 58 bioptic drivers published in 2005 by Bowers and colleagues reported that 62% of drivers surveyed said they always wore their bioptic with only 10% saying they never wore it [15]. Also, 74% of the drivers reported they found the bioptic very helpful in driving, with an additional 17% saying it was moderately

**Table 1**
Timeline of bioptic development and use in driving

| | |
|---|---|
| 1958 | Feinbloom introduces bioptic telescopic system |
| 1961 | Feinbloom founds Designs for Vision |
| 1970 | Korb publishes first paper on bioptic driving |
| 1971 | California licenses the first bioptic driver |
| 1973 | Section 504 of the Rehabilitation Act passed barring discrimination due to disability |
| 1975 | Korb, Jose, and Butler published multiple papers on training a bioptic driver |
| 1977 | Feinbloom publishes paper on 300 bioptic drivers and New York adopts bioptic driving |
| 1983 | 13 states allow bioptic driving |
| 1984 | US Department of Transportation issues antidiscrimination statement |
| 1991 | Americans with Disabilities Act is passed by Congress |
| 2007 | The Netherlands adopt bioptic driving for the visually impaired |
| 2017 | Australia's National Transport Commission allows bioptics on a case-by-case basis |
| 2022 | To date, most states and the District of Columbia allow bioptic driving |

*Data from* Refs [10–12].

helpful. Moreover, 90% of the bioptic drivers in that survey responded that they would continue to use the system for driving even if it were not required for licensure. Studies have shown most drivers found the telescope useful for seeing traffic lights, pedestrians, and other roadway obstacles [15,16]. Newer naturalistic driving studies, which involve monitoring the patient's driving in the car by cameras and data collected from sensors, have shown that many bioptic drivers do rely on their systems while driving [17].

### Ring scotoma of the telescope

Another concern has been that the BTS causes a ring scotoma, which may impair the detection of hazards on the road. A recent study by Tang, and colleagues showed that the bioptic driver's other eye can compensate, in part, for the ring scotoma created by the telescope when mounted monocularly [18]. Binocular systems and monocular systems that are mounted across the top of the eyewear may have a scotoma, but it is important to note that a properly trained driver is looking through these telescope(s) for only 1 to 2 seconds in moving traffic [6,7]. Jung and colleagues took photographs through a BTS to depict the ring scotomas from the telescope [19]. They demonstrated that a 3X Keplerian telescope's ring scotoma did not pose any major impairment when viewing through the telescope and it did not interfere with the view through the carrier lenses when in its superior position (Figs. 4 and 5).

### Bioptic driving safety

In the early days, some individuals like Gerald Fonda, MD, argued with the concept of bioptic driving [14]. However, little scientific data were available at the time to make a judgment for or against bioptic driving. In a review of studies on driving in 2010, Owsley and colleagues found that visual acuity, at best, is very weakly linked to driver safety (ie, collision involvement). [20] Swain and colleagues in 2021 published a study that showed associations between contrast sensitivity loss, slowed visual processing speed, and impaired motion perception as greater indicators of at-fault accidents and near crashes in a group of older drivers with visual impairments [21].

In 2015, a license review of 237 Ohio bioptic drivers showed no increase in motor vehicle collision rates between patients of varying best-corrected spectacle acuities from 20/50 to 20/250 [22]. Dougherty and colleagues reported that new drivers, with no prior experience, did have a higher collision rate per year in the first few years of bioptic licensure [22]. They pointed out this is consistent with increased collision rates by new drivers in the general population. For previous drivers, they reported no significant effect on collision rate by being a bioptic driver. Additionally, a 2016 study of age-related macular degeneration patients showed that these patients did well with a BTS for driving and, for the most part, did not alter their normal driving habits after becoming a bioptic driver [23]. In 2020, Moharrer and colleagues published a study looking at bioptic drivers in a naturalistic setting [17]. They did not find that bioptic drivers were prone to more near collisions than fully sighted individuals.

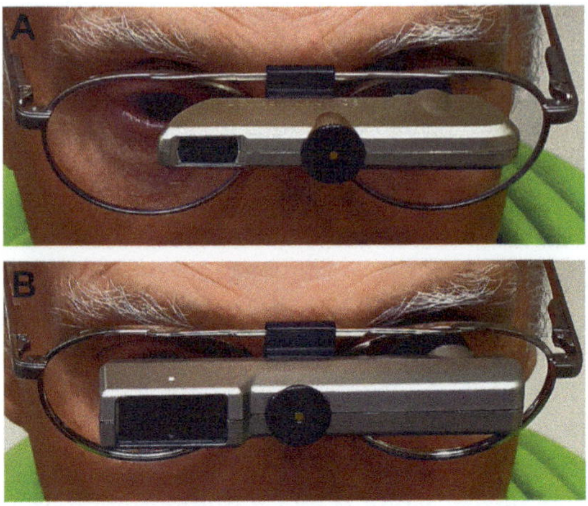


**Fig. 4.** The top image (*A*) shows the recently designed Ocutech Explorer. It is narrower and thinner with less potential scotoma for the driver. The bottom image (*B*) shows the Ocutech Sport which has worked well in bioptic driving, but its bigger and wider profile had the potential for more scotoma creation.

## BIOPTICS IN THE UNITED STATES

Each state has been responsible for the design of its own bioptic driving program. These programs began in the 1970s and have continued today with Pennsylvania and Washington, DC, adopting their programs in 2021. As of

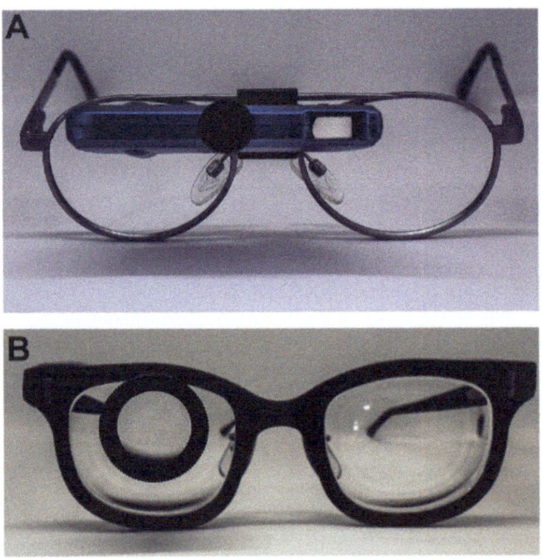


**Fig. 5.** Two types of monocular bioptics are shown. The top picture (*A*) is an Ocutech Explorer, a Keplerian bioptic. The lower picture (*B*) shows a traditional Galilean Designs for Vision monocular bioptic.

this publication, all states except for Connecticut, Iowa, and Utah allow for bioptic driving in some capacity. These 3 states do not allow bioptics but do have restricted driver's licenses for some with visual impairments. Some states, like Florida and Hawaii, allow for bioptics to be used while driving, but do not allow for the bioptic to be used to pass the vision test for licensure with the department of motor vehicles (Fig. 6).

## Visual acuities

Most states use the visual acuity of 20/40 as their cut-off for an unrestricted driver's license. However, little evidence exists that a person with visual acuity worse than 20/40 is at an increased risk of having a motor vehicle accident [9,24].

State minimum visual acuity requirements through the carrier lenses range from 20/40 to 20/400 with 20/100 to 20/200 being the most common range. Some states list the minimum carrier lens acuity needed and others only specify that the bioptic can or cannot be used to pass the vision examination. Table 2 lists the state maximum visual acuities for bioptic driving. Patients with Monocular, with one eye severely impaired or a prosthetic, can become a bioptic driver in many states if visual acuity and visual field in the functioning eye is adequate. Visual acuity requirements through the bioptic telescope have a broad range as well, with a minimum visual acuity from 20/40 to 20/70 depending on the state.

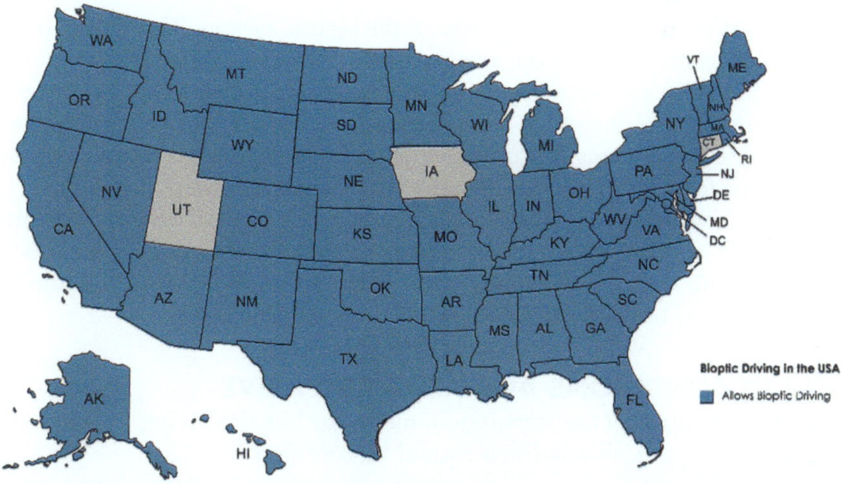


**Fig. 6.** Currently, all the states in the US, except Utah, Iowa, and Connecticut, allow for bioptic driving. However, each state has its own regulations for licensure. (Created with mapchart.net.)

### Visual fields

Visual field regulations in the United States vary by state, ranging from no documented visual field requirement to a minimum of 105 to 140° binocularly. Some states list generalities for binocular fields and others have very specific requirements for fields both temporally and nasally. Also, some states define visual field requirements for patients with monocular vision.

### Bioptic training

Formalized training of the bioptic driver is variable by state. Seventeen states specify what training must be conducted, while many do not. Some states recommend behind-the-wheel training with a certified driver rehabilitation specialist (CDRS). The CDRS is an instructor who specializes in driver rehabilitation for those with disabilities and can be located through this website: https://www.aded.net/. When the state requires training, the amount of bioptic behind-the-wheel training ranges from 10 to 60 hours depending on the state. Previously licensed drivers may require less behind-the-wheel training.

### Nighttime driving

Daylight driving only is the most common restriction on bioptic drivers. Some states do not have regulations, and they rely on the patient's vision through the bioptic telescope to justify if they can drive at night. Other states may allow nighttime driving after 1 to 3 years of daytime bioptic driving and/or an evaluation of their driving abilities at night. If the doctor recommends a nighttime driving evaluation, the CDRS will test the patient before sunrise or just after sunset.

### Bioptic telescope requirements

Many states do not dictate the power of the bioptic system. The power can be as high as needed to meet the requirements. However, telescopic powers no higher than 3-4X are the most common restrictions. A few states even specify that they cannot be focusable telescopes and/or require monocular telescopes versus binocular systems. Focusing is not an issue, because the patient adjusts and sets the focus to optical infinity and never focuses it while driving (Fig. 7).

Table 2 lists the current guidelines by the state for bioptic driving. States may change their regulations at any time and may require other requirements for bioptic driving that are not published here. The most up-to-date guidelines can be found at http://www.biopticdrivingusa.com/state-laws.

## OCULAR CONDITIONS AND ABILITY TO DRIVE

In addition to meeting the state requirements for bioptic driving, other characteristics of the patient's condition should be considered.

- How stable are the visual acuities and visual fields?
- Are there other ocular problems that need to be addressed first, such as cataracts?
- Is there severe ptosis or dermatochalasis that could be surgically corrected?

**Table 2**
Bioptic driving regulations by state

| State | Bioptics Allowed | Visual Acuity Minimums | Visual Fields Minimums | Training Required | Other Requirements |
|---|---|---|---|---|---|
| Alabama | Yes | Carrier: 20/200<br>BTS: 20/40 | 110° horizontally<br>80° vertically | Yes | BTS to 4X only |
| Alaska | Yes | Carrier: NA<br>BTS: 20/100 | 60% | Yes | |
| Arizona | Yes | Carrier: NA<br>BTS: 20/60 | 70° temporally and 35° nasally, in at least one eye | No | BTS to 4X only |
| Arkansas | Yes | Carrier: NA<br>BTS:<br>20/40 Unrestricted<br>20/50 Restricted<br>20/60 Daytime Only | Binoc: 140°<br>Mono: 105° | No | |
| California | Yes | Carrier: 20/200<br>BTS: 20/40 | Not specified | Yes | Daytime Only with Bioptic |
| Colorado | Yes | Carrier: Up to 20/200<br>BTS: 20/40 if carrier VA is less than 20/200 in worse eye; 20/70 if carrier VA is 20/200 or better | Not Specified | No | |
| Connecticut | No | Regular Licensure Only (No Bioptics):<br>Up to 20/199 with Restrictions | When VA Under 20/70: Binoc: 100°<br>Mono: 70° | | |

(*continued on next page*)

**Table 2**
***(continued)***

| State | Bioptics Allowed | Visual Acuity Minimums | Visual Fields Minimums | Training Required | Other Requirements |
|---|---|---|---|---|---|
| Delaware | Yes | Carrier: NA<br>BTS: 20/50 | Not Specified | No | |
| District of Columbia | Yes | Carrier: NA<br>BTS: 20/70 | 110-130° | | |
| Florida | Yes | Carrier: 20/70<br>BTS: Can't use to pass vision test | 130° | No | |
| Georgia | Yes | Carrier: 20/200<br>BTS: 20/60 | Binoc: 140°<br>Mono:<br>70° temporally and 50° nasally | No | |
| Hawaii | Yes | Carrier: 20/40<br>BTS: Can't use to pass vision test | Binoc: 140°<br>Mono: 70° | No | |
| Idaho | Yes | Carrier: 20/200<br>BTS: 20/40 | Not Specified | No | Daytime Only |
| Illinois | Yes | Carrier: 20/100<br>BTS: 20/40 | Binoc: 140°<br>Mono:<br>70° temporally and 35° nasally | No | BTS to 3X only |
| Indiana | Yes | Carrier: 20/200<br>BTS: 20/40 | 120° | Yes | BTS to 4X only |
| Iowa | No | Regular Licensure Only (No Bioptics):<br>20/40 unrestricted<br>20/50 in the better eye- daylight only | 140° degrees- no restrictions.<br>115° to 140° -restrictions | | |

| | | | | | |
|---|---|---|---|---|---|
| | | 20/70 in the better eye- daylight only and up to 35 mph. | | | |
| Kansas | Yes | Carrier: 20/400<br>BTS: Not Specified | 110° | Yes | 20/60-20/400 requires special review |
| Kentucky | Yes | Carrier: 20/200<br>BTS: 20/60 | 120° horizontally and 80° vertically | Yes | |
| Louisiana | Yes | Carrier: 20/200<br>BTS: 20/60 | 110° | Yes | |
| Maine | Yes | Carrier: 20/100<br>BTS: 20/60 | Binocular 110-140° | No | |
| Maryland | Yes | Carrier: 20/100<br>BTS: Not Specified | 110° with at least 35 degrees temporal to the midline of each side | No | |
| Massachusetts | Yes | Carrier: 20/100<br>BTS: Not Specified | 120° | No | Monocular BTS up to 3X non-focusable only |
| Michigan | Yes | Carrier: 20/200<br>BTS: 20/40-70 | 140° unrestricted<br>90°-140°- restrictions | Yes | |
| Minnesota | Yes | Carrier: 20/100<br>BTS: Not Specified | 105° | No | |
| Mississippi | Yes | Carrier: 20/200<br>BTS: 20/50 | 150° | Yes | BTS to 4X only |
| Missouri | Yes | Carrier: 20/160<br>BTS: 20/40-70 | Binoc: 55° in each eye<br>Mono: 85° | No | |
| Montana | Yes | Carrier: 20/100<br>BTS: Not specified | Not specified | No | |
| Nebraska | Yes | Carrier: Not Specified<br>BTS: 20/40-20/70 | 140°- unrestricted<br>101-140- restrictions | No | |
| Nevada | Yes | Carrier: 20/120<br>BTS: 20/40 | 130° | No | |

(*continued on next page*)

**Table 2**
***(continued)***

| State | Bioptics Allowed | Visual Acuity Minimums | Visual Fields Minimums | Training Required | Other Requirements |
|---|---|---|---|---|---|
| New Hampshire | Yes | Carrier: NA<br>BTS: 20/70 | Not specified | No | |
| New Jersey | Yes | Carrier: NA<br>BTS: 20/50 | Not specified | No | |
| New Mexico | Yes | Carrier: 20/80<br>BTS: Can't use to pass vision test | 120° horizontal with minimum of 30°nasal in one eye | No | |
| New York | Yes | Carrier: 20/100<br>BTS: 20/40 | 140° | Yes | |
| North Carolina | Yes | Carrier: 20/200<br>BTS: 20/70 | Binoc: 70° horizontally<br>Mono: 40° temporal and 30° nasally | Yes | |
| North Dakota | Yes | Carrier: 20/130<br>BTS: 20/40 | 105° | No | |
| Ohio | Yes | Carrier: NA<br>BTS: 20/30-70 | Binoc: 70° in each eye<br>Mono: 70°in better eye and 40° in the other | Yes | |
| Oklahoma | Yes | Carrier: NA<br>BTS: 20/60-20/100 | Binoc: 70°<br>Mono: 75° | Yes | BTS to 4X only |
| Oregon | Yes | Carrier: 20/200<br>BTS: Not Specified | 120° horizontally<br>80° vertically | Yes | |
| Pennsylvania | Yes | Carrier: 20/200<br>BTS: Not Specified | Binoc: 120° | Yes | |
| Rhode Island | Yes | Carrier: 20/100<br>BTS: 20/40 | Binoc: 115°<br>Mono: 75° temporally and 40° nasally | No | Monocular BTS up to 3X non-focusable only |
| South Carolina | Yes | Carrier: 20/120<br>BTS: 20/40 | Binoc:<br>120° horizontally and | Yes | |

| | | | | | |
|---|---|---|---|---|---|
| | | | 80° vertically<br>Mono: 70° horizontally<br>and 70° vertically | | |
| South Dakota | Yes | Carrier: NA<br>BTS: 20/40 | Not specified | No | |
| Tennessee | Yes | Carrier: 20/200<br>BTS: 20/60 | 150° | No | BTS to 4X only |
| Texas | Yes | Carrier: NA<br>BTS: Up to 20/70 | Not specified | No | |
| Utah | No | Regular Licensure Only (No Bioptics):<br>Up to 20/100 with Restrictions | 120° horizontally<br>20° vertically | | |
| Vermont | Yes | Carrier: NA<br>BTS: 20/40 | Binoc:<br>60° in each eye<br>Mono: 60° temporally<br>and 60° nasally | No | |
| Virginia | Yes | Carrier: 20/200<br>BTS: 20/70 | Binoc: 70°<br>Mono: 40 temporally<br>and 30° nasally | No | |
| Washington | Yes | Carrier: NA<br>BTS: 20/100 | 110° | No | |
| West Virginia | Yes | Carrier: 20/200<br>BTS: 20/40 | 120° horizontally<br>70° vertically | Yes | BTS to 4X only |
| Wisconsin | Yes | Carrier: 20/100<br>BTS: Can't use to pass vision test | 70° | No | |
| Wyoming | Yes | Carrier: NA<br>BTS: 20/100 | 120° horizontally | No | |

These requirements are based on information posted from each state and can change at any time. There may be states that have some variances in their rules that are not published to the public and may not be accounted for in this table.

*Data from* Bioptic Driving USA. State Laws. www.biopticdrivingUSA.com/state-laws. Accessed February 14, 2022.

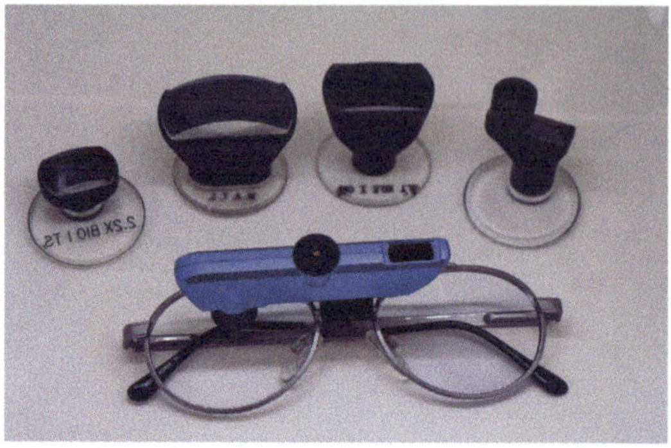

**Fig. 7.** An assortment of both Keplerian and Galilean bioptic systems from Ocutech and Designs for Vision.

- In an aniridia patient, would an artificial iris implant or a contact lens aid the patient? In rapid high amplitude nystagmus, would surgery slow the nystagmus?
- If active wet age-related macular degeneration (AMD) is present, it should be stabilized first. Additionally, due to the age demographic of patients with AMD, cognitive and physical issues should be considered and screened before pursuing bioptic driving [22].

Bioptic driving always is discussed as a window of driving. It might be a few years or many decades. In conditions like Stargardt's macular dystrophy, some patients may be able to drive for several decades or more. It is important to advise the patient that we are unable to predict when their vision may drop below licensure levels. However, even a decade of driving can be life-altering for these patients.

Table 3 categorizes patients with ocular conditions and generalized candidacy for bioptic driving. Each patient should be addressed on an individual case-by-case basis, but some conditions present obvious red flags. Many patients have conditions that cannot be aided by a BTS for driving such as retinitis pigmentosa, advanced glaucoma, severe ischemic optic neuropathies, and other conditions that cause major losses of peripheral vision.

## OTHER FACTORS IN PATIENT SELECTION FOR BIOPTIC DRIVING

Selecting candidates for bioptic driving is not only based on visual acuity, telescope acuity, and visual field status, but also on other pertinent factors. The low-vision specialist should consider each individual patient for the following before prescribing a bioptic for driving.

### Visual processing skills and cognitive abilities

Patients with cognitive or visual processing issues are not good candidates for bioptic driving. Cognitive impairments have been shown to have a greater

**Table 3**
Ocular conditions and candidacy for bioptic driving

| Good candidate | On a case-by-case basis | Not a candidate |
|---|---|---|
| • Albinism (ocular and oculocutaneous)<br>• Mild Macular Dystrophies<br>• Mild Optic Atrophies<br>• Congenital Nystagmus<br>• Mild Dry Macular Degeneration<br>• Macular Hole<br>• Mild Diabetic Retinopathy | • Moderate Cone Dystrophies<br>• Moderate Macular Degeneration<br>• Moderate Optic Atrophy<br>• Aniridia<br>• Achromatopsia<br>• Toxoplasmosis<br>• Histoplasmosis<br>• Coloboma<br>• Myopic Degeneration<br>• Retinopathy of Prematurity<br>• Moderate Diabetic Retinopathy | • Retinitis pigmentosa<br>• Other rod-cone dystrophies<br>• Advanced Macular Degeneration<br>• Advanced Glaucoma<br>• Severe Diabetic Retinopathy<br>• Other conditions with significant peripheral vision loss or large central scotomas |

correlation to crash risk than visual impairment [1,3,23–25]. Tests like the Useful Field of View and Trails Making A and B tests are used to screen for cognitive difficulties.

### Motor skills and functioning

Does this patient have any other physical disabilities affecting their legs, neck, or arms that would limit their proficiency in operating a motor vehicle?

### Age and maturity

How motivated is the patient to drive? In young patients, does the patient have the maturity to go through the bioptic driving training process? Has the patient been a licensed driver previously?

### Medical and medication history

Does the patient take medications for pain, neurologic conditions, etc.? Could the medications affect the ability to safely operate a motor vehicle? Does any history of a seizure disorder, addiction, DUIs, or brain injury exist?

### Emotional/mental status

Does the patient suffer from anxiety attacks or other mental health diagnoses that could cause an issue with bioptic driving?

### Family support

Is the family supportive of the decision to pursue bioptic driving? Does the patient have family support to help with training? Is the family more motivated than the patient for bioptic driving?

## DESIGNING THE BIOPTIC SYSTEM

A well-designed BTS is imperative for the patient to be successful. Approximately 95% to 98% of the driving is conducted while viewing through the carrier lenses of the system [25]. The BTS needs to be angled upward properly for quick head movements in and out of the telescope while driving. The driver will look through the telescope for only 1 to 2 seconds to quickly identify a sign, traffic light, or an object down the road [6,7]. Several important things should be considered when prescribing and fitting a BTS.

### Power and position of the telescope

The power of the BTS must be appropriate to meet the state's vision requirements. Too low a power makes sign recognition more difficult, forcing the driver to be in the telescope longer than 1 to 2 seconds. Too high a power will decrease the field of view through the telescope making it more difficult to locate what they are trying to see. The visual acuity through the telescope should be a minimum of 20/40 or better. The telescope should be positioned high in the frame, leaving at least half or more of the carrier lens underneath it for viewing. Picking too small a frame will impede the patient's driving vision through the carrier lenses (Fig. 8).

The angle of the BTS should be 10° to 15° up from the horizon to allow for a slight head tilt downward to view through the telescope. The pupillary distance should be carefully measured so that the telescope lines up perfectly with the pupil. Bioptic telescope systems are either Galilean or Keplerian optics and vary greatly in cosmetic appearance. The sensitivity of the patient to the appearance of the BTS should not be underestimated.

If the patient has a high ametropia (+/−6.00D sphere or 3.00D cylinder), this prescription should be incorporated into the eyepiece of the telescope to afford maximum clarity. Fitting patients with high prescriptions into contact lenses can be beneficial.

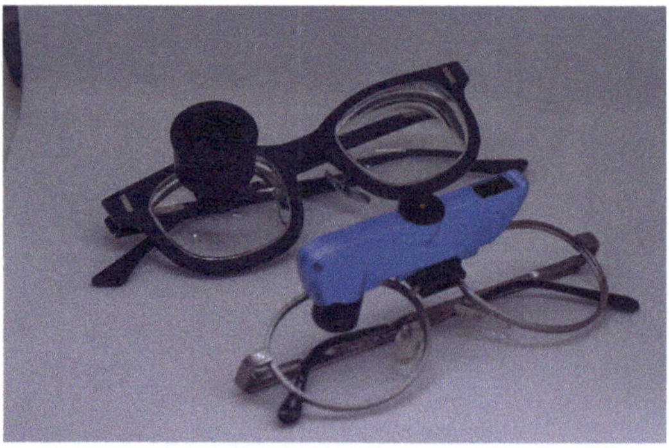

**Fig. 8.** The Designs for Vision Monocular Galilean bioptic (upper system) is compared with an Ocutech Sport Keplerian Telescope (lower system). Both are effective monocular systems for bioptic driving.

## Field of view through the telescope

Deciding which telescope is needed should be based not only on the power but also on the field of view provided. The difference in Galilean versus Keplerian optics comes into play when discussing the field of view [26,27].

A traditional Galilean telescope has a smaller field of view when compared with a Keplerian telescope of the same power. Galilean telescopes have a simple design, are small and lightweight, and have the brightest image [26]. Wide-angle Galilean telescopes, with larger fields of view, are available in a range of powers and can be focusable. The most common Galilean powers used in bioptic driving are 1.7X, 2.2X, 3X, and 4X (Fig. 9).

Keplerian telescopes are larger and focusable. They have a wider field of view than Galilean telescopes of the same power [26]. A Keplerian telescope has a slightly dimmer image than the Galilean telescope because they require mirrors or prisms to reverse the inverted image. This may be compensated for by having a larger objective lens, allowing more light through the telescope. These telescopes currently are fabricated in 2 styles. The first is a telescope mounted directly outward protruding from the lens, and the second is mounted horizontally at the top of the frame. The most common Keplerian powers used for bioptic driving are 3X, 4X, 5X, 5.5X, and 6X. Table 4 shows the relationship of magnification to the field of view of commonly used bioptic systems. Experience in our clinics has shown that a field of view of 9° or more is desirable for bioptic driving.

## Adaptability of the bioptic for light and glare issues

The ability to adapt the bioptic system to weather and sunlight conditions is imperative in selecting a system. Visually impaired patients may suffer from photophobia, poor glare recovery, and some suffer from hemeralopia as in achromatopsia. In Owsley's study, more than 60% of the bioptic drivers surveyed stated that driving into bright light caused either moderate or severe difficulty

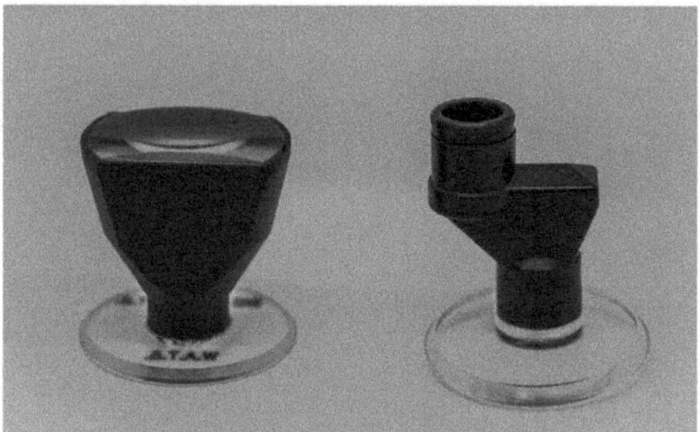

**Fig. 9.** This photo demonstrated the field of view advantage of the Keplerian bioptic as the power increases. On the left is a 3X Galilean Wide-Angle by Designs for Vision. Although wider in its physical appearance, it has a field of view of 11° compared with the 15° field of view of the Ocutech Mini 3X Keplerian on the right side.

**Table 4**
Field of view by power of common bioptic telescopes

| Name | 1.7X | 2.2X | 3.0X | 3.5X | 4.0X | 4.5X | 5.0X | 5.5X | 6.0X |
|---|---|---|---|---|---|---|---|---|---|
| Designs for Vision | | | | | | | | | |
| Galilean | 18° | 12° | 8° | | 6° | | | | |
| Galilean Wide Angle | 28° | 16° | 11° | | | | | | |
| Micro Spiral Galilean | | 7° | 5° | | 4° | | | | |
| Politzer Galilean Bioptic I | 18° | 12° | 8° | | | | | | |
| Spiral Galilean | 20° | 11° | 8° | | 5° | | | | |
| Keplerian Expanded Field | | | | 14° | | 9° | | | |
| Spiral Expanded Field (Keplerian) | | | 14° | | 9° | | 8° | | 6.5° |
| Ocutech | | | | | | | | | |
| Sightscope (Galilean) | 26° | 18° | | | | | | | |
| VES Mini | | | 15° | | | | | | |
| VES Explorer | | | 14° | | 12.5° | | | | |
| Sport | | | | | 12.5° | | 10.5° | | 9.6° |

*Data from* Refs.28,29

[24]. Because of this, adaptability of their systems for driving during the day is needed. The use of slip-in or custom fit over sun filters of various colors is needed for most drivers. Filter caps placed over the bioptic telescopic objective lenses can be used as well. Custom filters in contact lenses are used in tandem with the bioptic system for severely photophobic patients as with achromatopsia patients (Fig. 10).

## TRAINING THE BIOPTIC DRIVER

As previously mentioned, states vary greatly in the requirements for bioptic training. Research on how to train a bioptic driver and the amount of training needed has been limited [9]. Early articles detailed how to train a bioptic driver but did not have scientific studies showing safety and effectiveness. A bioptic

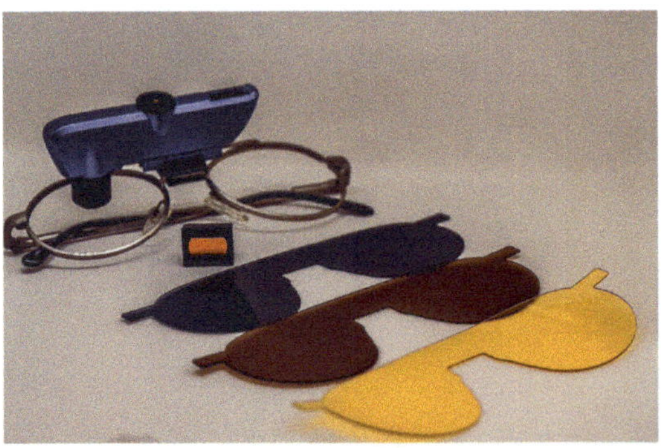

**Fig. 10.** Light and glare can be controlled by the selection of the appropriate slip-in filter for this Ocutech Explorer. Additionally, a cap with the appropriate filter can be placed over the objective lens.

training study by Szlyk and colleagues compared a 3-month training period on how to use the bioptic versus no training at all [30]. The group of drivers with the training in the use of the bioptic had greater improvements in task performance versus the nontrained group. The tasks that showed improvements were peripheral identification, recognition, and scanning.

### Training to use the bioptic

The first step in training begins with instructing the patient in using the bioptic system. This training usually is performed by the low vision optometrist or ophthalmologist, orientation and mobility specialist, occupational therapist, or other allied professionals' familiar with bioptics. Box 1 highlights the initial training goals for the bioptic driver [12,31,32]. The goal is for the patient to be successful in spotting targets and the quick recognition of signs using the bioptic. We use a series of exercises for patients to work on at home between training visits. This includes spotting objects in various situations, learning signs by flashcards (especially important for new drivers), and descriptive driving as a passenger with a friend or family member. Jose in 1983 and Nowakowski in 1994 introduced the bioptic training concepts in their respective books on low vision [12,31]. Additionally in 2001, Chapman laid out a rationale and framework for training the bioptic driver [32].

Those who have never driven before usually have not paid much attention to the traffic signs around them, so learning to identify these types of signs by shape and color helps them recognize them quicker. Practicing with family or friends by riding as a passenger and spotting signs, traffic lights, and hazards on the road helps the patient prepare for the next phase: behind-the-wheel training. Making sure the patient has the proper sun filters for the various weather conditions is important during this training time. These issues can be addressed by the low vision optometrist or ophthalmologist before beginning behind-the-wheel training.

### Training with the certified driver rehabilitation specialist

Once the patient has satisfactorily learned spotting techniques and has become proficient in the use of the BTS, they are referred to the CDRS which specializes in behind-the-wheel training [9]. The CDRS has had specialized instruction

**Box 1: Training goals for using the bioptic system**

- Spotting Stationary Objects while Stationary
- Spotting Stationary Objects while Moving
- Spotting Moving Objects while Stationary
- Spotting Moving Objects while Moving
- Rapid Sign Recognition
- Address Issues of BTS Alignment or Usage
- Address Any Light/Glare Issues when Using the BTS

*Data from* Refs [12,31,32].

and has been certified by the Association for Driver's Rehabilitation Specialists (ADED), as cited previously (www.aded.net/). However, not all CDRSs specialize in bioptic driver's training. In Indiana, for example, CDRSs also do cognitive, reaction time, and motor functioning screenings before the evaluation with the patient as a passenger in the car. After their evaluation, the bioptic user will apply for a bioptic permit with the state before beginning the behind-the-wheel training (Fig. 11).

The patient works with the CDRS as a passenger first and then progresses over time to low traffic volume areas for initial driving. They then progress to higher traffic volume areas as the driver gains experience and confidence. Some states require classroom training as well before getting behind the wheel. New drivers will be taught the basic driving skills and when to use their bioptic for driving. This training provides extended practice to gain the skills needed for licensure with the bioptic system. Box 2 lists the common training goals each driver must attain behind-the-wheel.

The training process is usually much easier for patients who have had previous driving experience. In fact, previous driving experience has been shown to lessen a bioptic driver's crash risk [8,22]. Once the patient has finished training with the CDRS, they must pass an extended driver's test by the state for licensure.

## After bioptic licensure

After the bioptic patient is licensed, most states require annual or biannual reviews of the license with their low vision optometrist or ophthalmologist. This is to verify that the patient still meets the state's visual bioptic guidelines.

Driving habits of bioptic drivers vary, but most start out very conservatively. Many limits the radius in which they can drive and the routes they take daily, which has been confirmed by several surveys of bioptic drivers [22,24]. They plan routes ahead of time and may even practice the route with family. As with all drivers, once they gain experience and confidence, they start to expand their driving radius.

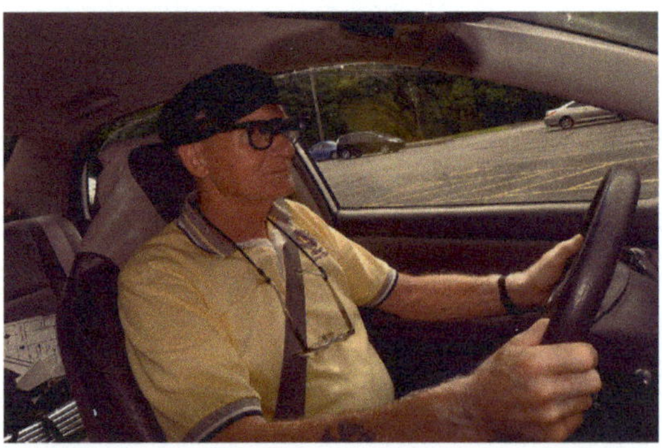

**Fig. 11.** Here a bioptic driver with retinal dystrophy uses binocular 3X Wide-Angle Galilean bioptics from Designs for Vision. He has driven for more than 2 decades.

**Box 2: Training goals with the CDRS**

Use the bioptic correctly in all presented traffic situations:

- Independently identify critical information on signs and potential hazards.
- Identify and use filters in different lighting conditions.
- Perform proper procedures for right and left turns.
- Independently complete lane changes including entering and exiting lanes and ramps correctly.
- Complete basic and parallel parking maneuvers independently.
- Complete a nighttime evaluation if allowed by low vision specialist and state rules.

*Data from* Chapman, B. Chapter 35: Driving with Telescopic Glasses: A Training Program. *Coping With Vision Loss: Maximizing What You Can See and Do.* Hunter House, Inc.; 2001.

## VEHICLE MODIFICATIONS FOR BIOPTIC DRIVERS

Technology has evolved rapidly in the automotive industry, leading to innovations that can help the visually impaired when driving.

### Vehicle selection

When selecting a vehicle, we sometimes recommend an SUV, pickup truck, or minivan, as it sits higher than a traditional car. This allows the bioptic driver to see over traffic and to be able to see lights and traffic signs farther away. Also, selecting a car with special features like adaptive cruise control, lane departure warnings, lane control, automatic braking, and backup sensors can help with daily driving tasks.

### Global positioning systems

Global positioning systems (GPS) like a Garmin device, in-car GPS, or using the GPS app on the smartphone allow for greater safety when driving [9,33]. GPS provides 2 main advantages for all drivers because it audibly tells the driver what to do. First, it prevents the need to be searching for and reading street signs. Second, it facilitates safer lane changes by warning the patient in advance when and whereby they need to turn.

### Speedometer

Portable large print speedometers are available and can be mounted on the dashboard for visually impaired patient. Some smartphones have large font speedometer apps and can be used in a holder on the dash as well.

### Windshield and dash glare

Excessive glare from the windshield and dashboard can be minimized with a few car adaptations. For the windshield, after thoroughly cleaning it inside and out, applying white vinegar can prevent dirt build up and glare. As for the dashboard, using black felt material, cut to the dashboard's size with holes for vents, will absorb the reflected light, cutting down on glare coming off the dash (Fig. 12).

## THE INDIANA PROGRAM FOR VISUALLY IMPAIRED DRIVERS

Our practice has been prescribing for and training bioptic drivers in Indiana since 1987. Indiana has a two-step program for visually impaired drivers, which has served as a model for other states. This process was designed through a series of meetings with low vision specialists, CDRSs, and representatives from the Bureau of Motor Vehicles (BMV).

### Part 1: waivered drivers

The Indiana BMV allows for the mildly impaired driver (up to 20/80 vision in one eye with an adequate visual field) to drive daytime only with a waivered license. This waiver allows many seniors and other experienced drivers with mild visual impairments, who have usually driven for many decades, to continue their limited driving without requiring the time, cost, and complexity of bioptic driving. This driver's license is issued by the BMV after careful testing by the doctor and an initial behind-the-wheel evaluation with a CDRS and requires annual reviews of the license.

### Part 2: bioptic drivers

With visual acuities up to 20/200 in one eye, patients can be a candidate for bioptic driving. However, a potential new driver, for example, with 20/70 from retinal dystrophy, may be better served to become a bioptic driver, as their vision loss may slowly progress, and the patient will benefit from the additional training. The doctor makes the decision if a patient can be a waivered or bioptic driver on a case-by-case basis.

If pursuing bioptic driving, the patient must do a minimum of 30 hours of behind-the-wheel training with a CDRS. Indiana also specifies additional guidelines for those less than 21 years old. The ability to drive at night, if applicable, is assessed during the 30 hours of training. Although the amount of training may be more than needed for a previously licensed driver, the training requirement allows for adequate training of the new bioptic driver. Every bioptic driver is

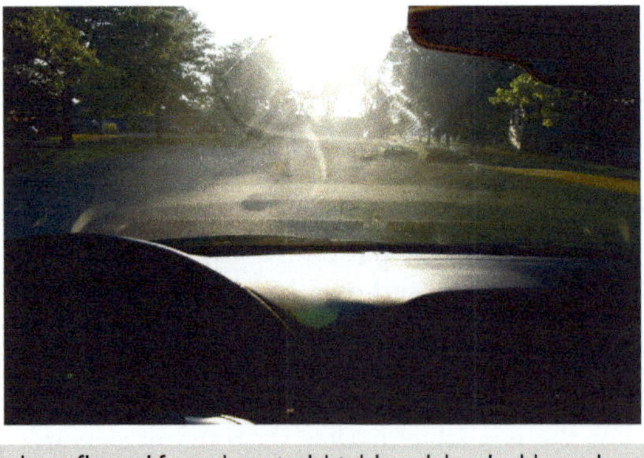

**Fig. 12.** Glare can be reflected from the windshield and the dashboard as seen here. A piece of black felt cut to the dashboard can help alleviate some of the glare bioptic drivers' experience.

required to have a vision examination annually or biannually, and the results are sent to the BMV for review. The Indiana program has been highly successful in allowing mild to moderately visually impaired patients to drive.

## THE FACES OF BIOPTIC DRIVING

Providing opportunities to drive for the mildly visually impaired allows them to live more independently and be productive citizens in our society. Examples of the patients we see daily in our clinics are discussed in the following.

Case 1: TM is an 82-year-old man with a history of moderate visual impairment from blue cone monochromatism. He has been a bioptic driver for more than 30 years using binocular 3X Designs for Visions bioptic system. Despite his visual impairment and age, TM currently works 2 part-time jobs and drives daily to work (Fig. 13).

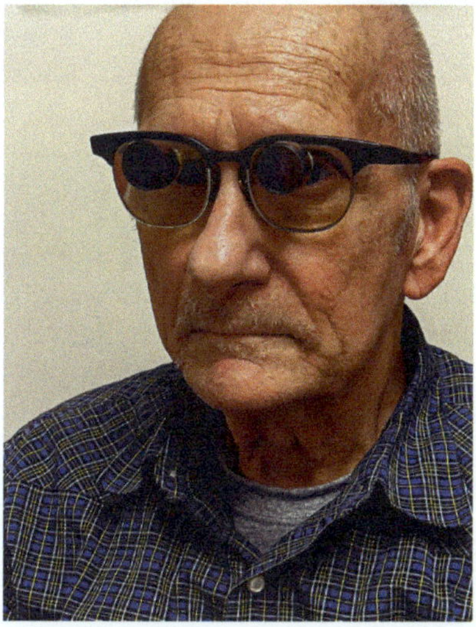

**Fig. 13.** Case 1: TM

Case 2: JK is a 51-year-old woman and works as a Director's Assistant for a developmental preschool. She has a history of retinopathy of prematurity with best-corrected acuities of 20/120 right eye and light perception only left eye. She has a full right visual field on a Zeiss Humphrey 120 field test. She has driven with biopics for 19 years and currently wears a 4X Ocutech Sport bioptic system (Fig. 14).

Case 3: MO is a 36-year-old man with oculocutaneous albinism. He presented with best-corrected visual acuities of the right eye 20/150 and left eye 20/200. He has pendular nystagmus and debilitating photophobia in bright light. He was initially fit with a 4X Ocutech Sport but found his photophobia could not be controlled with standard slip-in sun filters. His photophobia was much more debilitating than most patients with albinism. He was then fitted

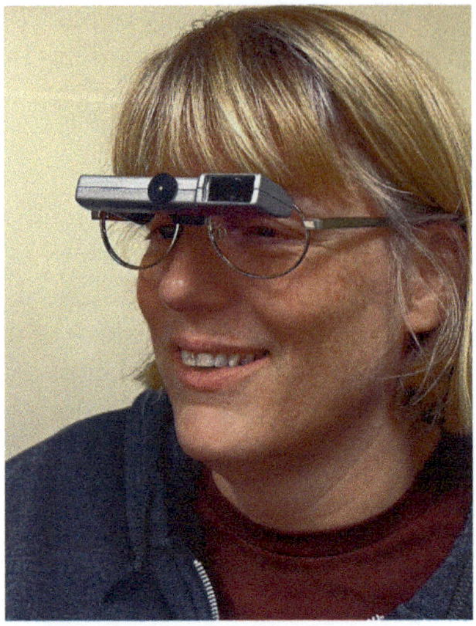

**Fig. 14.** Case 2: JK

with a 3X Pulitzer by Designs for Vision mounted in a dark tinted lens within a Wiley X frame which has a cushion seal around the frame to prevent light leak. This system allows him to drive in bright daytime. At night and in lower daytime lighting, he switches to the Ocutech system. He has been a licensed bioptic driver day and night for more than 9 years and works full-time as an accountant. Most patients with albinism do not require this approach, but without it, he would have been unable to drive (Fig. 15).

Case 4: RH is a 35-year-old physician's assistant with a history of retinopathy of prematurity. Her visual acuities are right eye 20/100 and left eye 20/120. Her Esterman monocular visual fields were full. She has driven with a

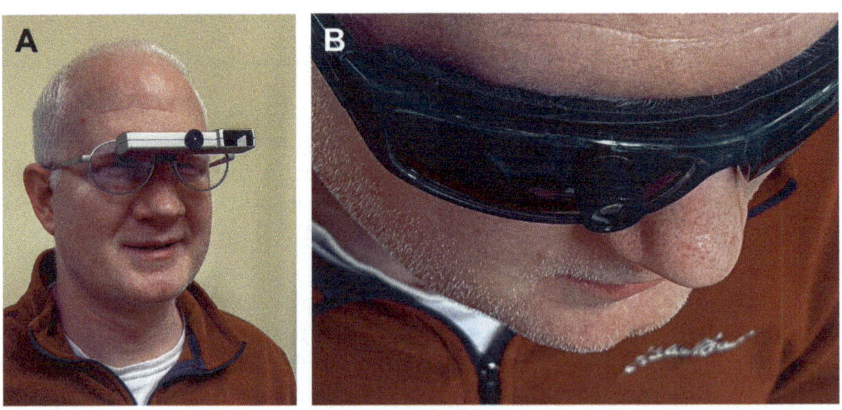


**Fig. 15.** Case 3: MO

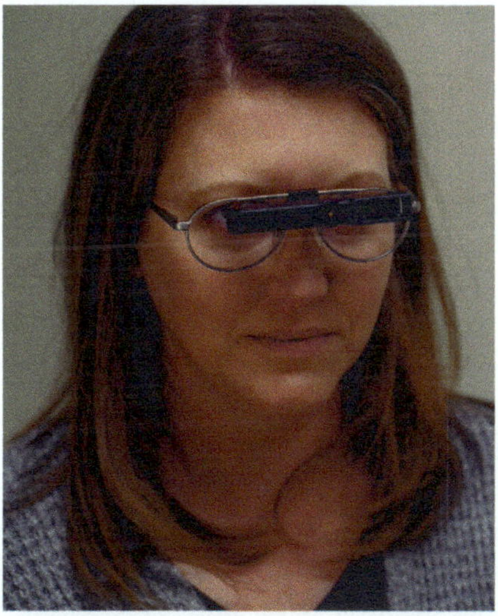

**Fig. 16.** Case 4: RH

bioptic for 15 years and is currently using a 4X Ocutech Explorer. She has been granted night driving privileges (Fig. 16).

Case 5: AD is a 44-year-old woman with a history of autosomal dominant Stargardt's dystrophy. Her visual acuities were right eye 20/150 and left eye 20/150. She uses an 4X Ocutech Explorer and has been driving with a BTS for 10 years. She is a homemaker and spends much of her driving time shuttling her daughters to school, activities, and to appointments (Fig. 17).

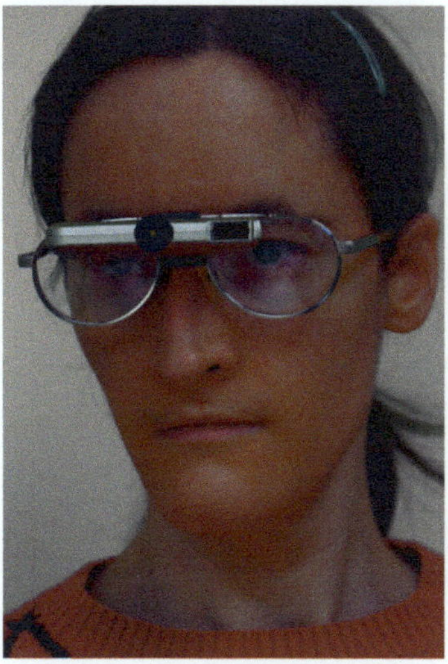

**Fig. 17.** Case 5: AD

### Dr. Dennis Kelleher: first legally licensed bioptic driver in the United States

Dr. Kelleher was the first bioptic driver to be legally licensed in the United States in 1971. He has a stable retinal condition, which has allowed him to continue to drive for more than 50 years. He has a Doctorate of Education and has spent his career working the field of Special Education with the California Department of Education. Dr. Kelleher was instrumental at the beginning of bioptic driving and published 14 papers on the subject. He reports that he has had no accidents and only 3 speeding tickets in 50 years of being a bioptic driver (Fig. 18).

## FUTURE RESEARCH IN BIOPTIC DRIVING

Many studies have been published on bioptic driving dating back to 1970. Research on bioptic driving has proven to be difficult because each patient is different [9]. These studies recruit patients with many different ocular conditions, ranges of visual acuities, ages, and experiences with driving. People with better acuities may use the bioptic telescope less than those with worse acuity. Drivers with previous experience before becoming a bioptic driver are not the same as drivers with little or no driving experience. Different ocular conditions may make glare and light sensitivity issues for some patients. Some of the studies have been limited by small sample sizes where the issues listed above can skew the results. Additionally, each state has different regulations, so comparisons between states is complicated.

In the past several years, new studies are looking at ways to assess bioptic driving in a more naturalistic setting behind-the-wheel. This includes dash-mounted in-car cameras and sensors in the patient's car to evaluate the bioptic use over a length of time [17,25]. This is a significant improvement in assessing how bioptics are used by patients in real day-to-day life. Continued naturalistic

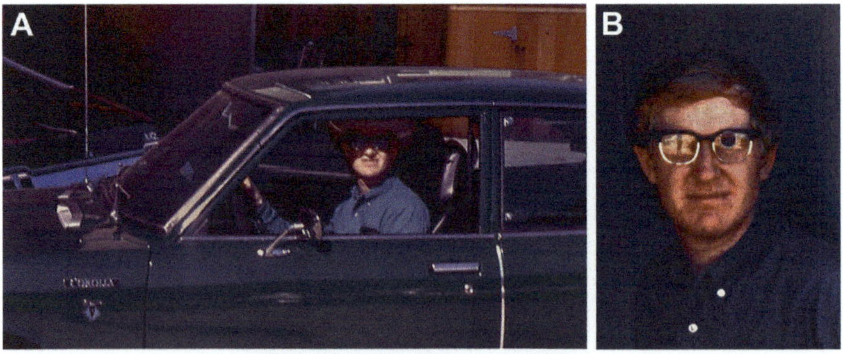


**Fig. 18.** (*A, B*). Pictures provided by Dennis Kelleher. Here is Dr Kelleher in 1971 after receiving the first legal bioptic license in the US. He continues to be a bioptic driver to this day. (*Courtesy of* Dennis Kelleher, EdD.)

bioptic research still is needed to further elucidate the level of visual impairment that one can drive with or without a bioptic. Also, research in areas of training the bioptic driver are needed.

## SUMMARY

Despite early concerns about the safety of driving with a visual impairment, today 47 states and the District of Columbia have recognized bioptic driving. The ability to drive has been life changing for thousands of patients, both personally and professionally. Bioptic drivers can drive to work, go to the grocery store, pursue educational opportunities, or simply take their child to the doctor.

Thus, today after 50 years of bioptic driving, the real question should not be simply whether bioptic driving is safe, but rather which drivers, visual conditions, and bioptic systems are the safest. Also, how do we continue to reduce the risk with bioptic driving? Driving always is a matter of risk for any driver. We must constantly strive to reduce these risks in all populations, especially bioptic drivers. New naturalistic research methods may help us reduce these risks and define the best practices for safe bioptic driving.

## CLINICS CARE POINTS

- Each mildly to moderately impaired patient should be assessed on an individual case-by-case basis to determine if they are a candidate for driving.
- An extensive driving history should be conducted for each candidate including previous driving experience, annual mileage, accidents, or tickets in the past, and new difficulties in driving.
- New inexperienced, visually impaired drivers, especially ocular albinism patients with nystagmus, often do better as a bioptic driver even when they qualify for a regular restricted license due to fluctuations in visual functioning resulting from lighting conditions or nystagmus.
- The Humphrey 120 Full Field or the Esterman monocular and binocular visual field tests are the quickest way to test visual fields for driving.
- When designing the bioptic system, one should consider if it should be a monocular or binocular system, the maximum power of the telescope needed, and a system that can be adapted to control glare and light issues.
- A multi-disciplinary approach to training is ideal in making sure the patient has the skills needed for bioptic driving.

### Disclosure

The authors have nothing to disclose.

### References

[1] Owsley C. Vision and driving in the elderly. Optom Vis Sci 1994;71:727–35.

[2] Ragland DR, Satariano WA, MacLeod KE. Driving cessation and increased depressive symptoms. J Gerontol A Biol Sci Med Sci 2005;60(3):399–403.
[3] Feinbloom W. The training and after care of the partially blind patient. J Am Optom Assn 1958;29:724.
[4] Korb DR. Preparing the visually handicapped person for motor vehicle operation. Am J Optom Arch Am Acad Optom 1970;47(8):619–28.
[5] Feinbloom W. Driving with bioptic telescopic spectacles (BTS). Am J Optom Physiol Opt 1977;54:35–42.
[6] Jose RT, Butler JH. Driver's training for partially sighted persons: An interdisciplinary approach. New Outlook for the Blind 1975;69(7):305–11.
[7] Jose RT, Butler JH. Training a patient to drive with telescopic lenses. Am J Optom Physiol Opt 1975;52(5):343–6.
[8] Zhou AM, Flom RE, Raasch TW, et al. Vision, Driving Exposure, and Collisions in Bioptic Drivers. Optom Vis Sci 2022;99(2):121–6.
[9] Owsley C. Driving with bioptic telescopes: organizing a research agenda. Optom Vis Sci 2012;89:1249–56.
[10] Chun R, Cucuras M, Jay WM. Current perspectives of bioptic driving in low vision. Neuro-ophthalmology 2016;40(2):53–8.
[11] Huss C, Corn A. Low vision driving with bioptics: an overview. J Vis Impair Blind 2004;98:641–53.
[12] Jose R. Understanding low vision. American Foundation for T.H.E. Blind Press; 1983. p. 278.
[13] Keeney AH. Field loss versus central magnification. Arch Ophthalmol 1974;92:273.
[14] Fonda G. Training in use of the bioptic telescopic spectacle (BTS) for driving is unreasonable. Trans Pa Acad Ophthalmol Otolaryngol 1988;40:716–8.
[15] Bowers AR, Apfelbaum DH, Peli E. Bioptic telescopes meet the needs of drivers with moderate visual acuity loss. Invest Ophthalmol Vis Sci 2005;46(1):66–74.
[16] Wood JM, McGwin G, Elgin J, et al. Characteristics of on-road driving performance of persons with central vision loss who use bioptic telescopes. Invest Ophthalmol Vis Sci 2013;54:3790–7.
[17] Moharrer M, Wang S, Dougherty BE, et al. Evaluation of the driving safety of visually impaired bioptic drivers based on critical events in naturalistic driving. Transl Vis Sci Technol 2020;9(8):14.
[18] Tang X, Bronstad PM, Doherty AL, et al. Hazard detection with monocular bioptic telescopes in a driving simulator. Transl Vis Sci Technol 2020;9(4):26.
[19] Jung JH, Kurukuti NM, Peli E. Photographic depiction of the field of view with spectacles-mounted low vision aids. Optom Vis Sci 2021;98(10):1210–26.
[20] Owsley C, McGwin G Jr. Vision and driving. Vis Res 2010;50(23):2348–61.
[21] Swain TA, McGwin G Jr, Wood JM, et al. Naturalistic Driving Techniques and Association of Visual Risk Factors With At-Fault Crashes and Near Crashes by Older Drivers With Vision Impairment. JAMA Ophthalmol 2021;139(6):639–45.
[22] Dougherty BE, Flom RE, Bullimore MA, et al. Previous driving experience, but not vision, is associated with motor vehicle collision rate in bioptic drivers. Invest Ophthalmol Vis Sci 2015;56(11):6326–32.
[23] Bowers AR, Sheldon SS, DeCarlo DK, et al. Bioptic telescope use and driving patterns of drivers with age-related macular degeneration. Transl Vis Sci Technol 2016;5(5):5.
[24] Owsley C, McGwin G Jr, Elgin J, et al. Visually impaired drivers who use bioptic telescopes: self-assessed driving skills and agreement with on-road driving evaluation. Invest Ophthalmol Vis Sci 2014;55(1):330–6.
[25] Wang S, Moharrer M, Baliutaviciute V, et al. Bioptic telescope use in naturalistic driving by people with visual impairment. Transl Vis Sci Technol 2020;9:11.
[26] Greene H, Schuldiner R. Telescopic spectacles: under prescribed, misunderstood, but very helpful. Optom Management. Low Vision Newsletter; 2021. https://www.optometricmanagement.com/newsletters/managing-low-vision/july-2021.

[27] Designs for Vision. Low Vision Telescopes. Available at: www.designsforvision.com. Accessed February 14, 2022.
[28] Ocutech. Ocutech Products Overview. Available at: www.ocutech.com. Accessed February 14, 2022.
[29] Bioptic Driving USA. State Laws. Available at: www.biopticdrivingUSA.com/state-laws. Accessed February 14, 2022.
[30] Szlyk JP, Seiple W, Laderman DJ, et al. Measuring the effectiveness of bioptic telescopes for persons with central vision loss. J Rehabil Res Dev 2000;37(1):101–8.
[31] Nowakowski R. Primary low vision care. 1st edition. Alameda (CA): Appleton & Lange; 1994. p. 277–9.
[32] Chapman B. Chapter 35: driving with telescopic Glasses: a training program. Coping with vision loss: maximizing what You can see and do. Hunter House, Inc; 2001.
[33] Cucuras M, Chun R, Lee P, et al. GPS usage in a population of low-vision drivers. Semin Ophthalmol 2017;32(4):438–42.

Advances in Ophthalmology and Optometry 7 (2022) 31–49

ADVANCES IN OPHTHALMOLOGY AND OPTOMETRY

# The Use of B-Scan Ultrasound in Primary Eye Care

Elena Z. Biffi, OD, MS[a,*], Benjamin Young, OD[a], Joseph Edward Kane Jr, OD[b], Mehdi Najafi, MD, PhD[c]

[a]New England College of Optometry, Boston, MA, USA; [b]Veterans Affairs Boston Healthcare System; [c]Boston Vision, Beth Israel Deaconess Medical Center, Boston, MA, USA

**Keywords**

• B-Scan ultrasound • Ocular ultrasound • Ophthalmic ultrasound • Ophthalmic ultrasonography • Vitreous pathology • Retinal diseases • Posterior segment ocular diseases • Choroidal diseases

**Key points**

- Ocular B-scan ultrasonography is a rapid, portable, and noninvasive diagnostic tool that can be performed safely as an adjunct procedure in both pediatric and adult populations.
- B-scan ultrasonography can objectively image lens, vitreous, retina, choroid, sclera, and orbit, even when the posterior ocular surface is obscured by media opacity.
- Performing reliable ocular B-scan diagnostics requires a thorough understanding of what part of the globe the acoustic wavefront is directed toward in relation to the patient's gaze.
- Recent advancements in ultrasound technology demonstrate significant potential for a wide range of clinical applications.

## INTRODUCTION

Ocular imaging technologies have revolutionized our approach to ocular disease identification, diagnosis, and decision-making. The superior imaging capability of modern ophthalmic imaging devices allows for the detailed visualization of ocular structures, aiding in a deeper understanding of disease pathophysiology and progression. B-scan ophthalmic ultrasonography has

*Corresponding author. 424 Beacon Street, Boston, MA 02115. *E-mail address:* BiffiE@neco.edu

https://doi.org/10.1016/j.yaoo.2022.04.004

the unique ability to evaluate the posterior ocular segment in cases when view of the retina is otherwise obscured by anterior segment or vitreous pathology. As distinct from A-scan ultrasound examination, which measures axial length in conjunction with refractive concerns, B-scan ultrasound examination is used to aid the detection and management of ocular disease. In a quick and noninvasive approach, B-scan allows clinicians to perform reproducible, real-time analysis of the lens, vitreous, retina, choroid, sclera, and orbit. Posterior segment diseases can be identified and differentiated from each other based on the B-scan ultrasonography appearance and their specific ocular localization.

As an adjunct to clinical examination, ocular B-scan ultrasonography has been used in eyecare since 1956 [1,2]. Standard B-scan ultrasonography uses focused short-wavelength acoustic waves with frequencies of approximately 10 million oscillations per second (10 MHz) [1,3], even though higher frequencies of up to a 20- to 30-MHz range have been explored for imaging of the posterior pole [4]. The depth of acoustic wave penetration into the tissue directly relates to its wavelength: the longer the wavelength (shorter frequency), the deeper the penetration. Conventional B-scan ultrasound examination with a frequency of approximately 7 to 10 MHz has a penetration of approximately 30 to 40 mm [5], which is ideal for visualization of the ocular posterior segment, retina, and choroid. In contrast, ultrasound biomicroscopy, which uses much higher frequencies of 50 to 100 MHz, can only penetrate a few millimeters, and, thus, is typically used for anterior segment analysis, cornea, and ciliary body evaluation [6].

Advances in instrumentation and the use of higher frequencies to improve image resolution have resulted in a continuous improvement in B-scan image quality. The goal of this article is to describe the principles and indications for the use of B-scan ocular ultrasonography to aid in the diagnosis and management of posterior segment diseases.

## INDICATIONS AND CONTRAINDICATIONS

B-scan ultrasonography is a rapid, portable, and noninvasive diagnostic tool. Therefore, it can be performed safely in both pediatric and adult populations, including in critically ill patients as part of a bedside ocular evaluation [7]. B-scan ultrasonography allows the penetration of acoustic waves through optical opacities, and, thus, it is particularly useful when light-based ocular imaging and visualization (ophthalmoscopy, optical coherence tomography [OCT], etc) is not possible. Acoustic waves can bypass pathology and provide information on intraocular structures when direct assessment via funduscopic exam is difficult owing to media opacity [8]. In addition, B-scan ultrasonography can be used to obtain topographic information (location and configuration) for a variety of ocular lesions, ranging from the anterior segment to the posterior segment of an eye, even when the view of the posterior segment is not compromised. In fact, B-scan ultrasonography is considered a diagnostic test for a variety of conditions, including optic disc drusen (ODD), choroidal melanoma, and retinal detachment (RD) [8–11]. High-frequency B-scan ultrasound examination also can be used to localize an intraocular foreign body to obtain information on the nature of the foreign body (metallic, etc), as well as its size and location [9].

B-scan ocular ultrasonography generally is a safe procedure with few contraindications. It can be performed through both open or closed eyelids. However, owing to the absorption of acoustic waves by ocular structures, B-scan ultrasonography has greater resolution when done on an eye with an open lid. Instilling a topical anesthetic would be necessary to perform examination on an open eye. In this case, caution should be taken because the procedure may lead to minor corneal abrasions. Important contraindications to B-scan ultrasonography include scleral laceration and suspected ocular globe rupture (open globe) in patients with trauma or recent ocular surgery, because the procedure may result in the extrusion of ocular contents [11–14].

## PRINCIPLES OF B-SCAN ULTRASOUND EXAMINATION

### B-scan description

#### *Echogram*

B-scan ocular ultrasound examination uses an echographic probe with an internal piezoelectric crystal near its tip. The function of the probe is to convert electrical energy into mechanical energy to emit acoustic signals into the eye. When sound waves reach an ocular surface, the tissues reflect the signal back toward the probe. The signal then gets amplified and displayed on the video screen as 1 dot with its brightness indicating its strength. The stronger the reflection (echo), the brighter the projected dot [3]. Collection of these dots forms a 2-dimensional image of approximately 2 to 3 mm in width [14] and is called an echogram (Fig. 1A). Typical individual scans encompass between 4 and 6 clock-hours. The angle of incidence of the probe is critical in obtaining strong echo signals. The probe should be held perpendicular to the area of interest, so acoustic waves are reflected directly back to the probe. An oblique probe angle results in weaker return signals, thus compromising the quality of the B-scan display.

#### *Coupling gel*

Various other factors play a role in obtaining a high-quality B-scan image, namely, velocity, reflectivity, and absorption of sound waves. Sound waves travel faster through solids than liquids, so the velocity of the sound wave depends on the density of the medium. When performing a B-scan ultrasound study, it is important to use a coupling gel. The purpose of the gel is to focus the acoustic energy (soundwaves) from the probe to the ocular surface without crossing the air, thus, enhancing reflectivity of the signal. The denser the medium, the greater the absorption of the acoustic waves, and subsequently the lesser the scan quality. As was mentioned elsewhere in this article, to optimize the quality of the B-scan, it is recommended to perform ocular ultrasonography on an eye with an open lid [1,2].

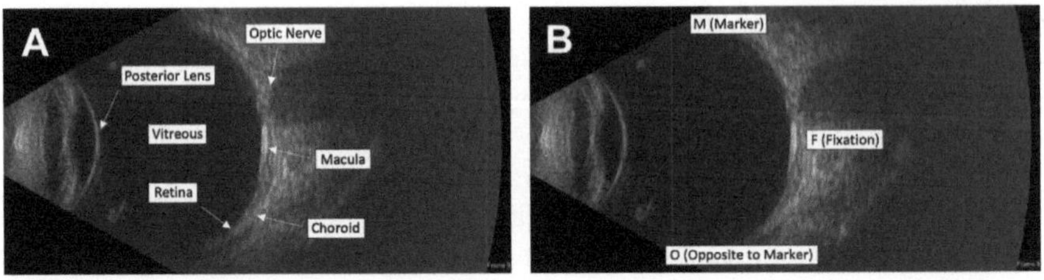


**Fig. 1.** B-scan echogram of a normal eye. (*A*) The horizontal axis represents ocular tissue depth, and the vertical axis shows the scanned segment of the globe. Horizontal axial probe position allows visualization of multiple ocular structures, including macula and optic nerve. (*B*) Image of the retina in the M-F-O orientation, where Marker (M) is always at the top of echogram, patient's fixation (F) is in the middle (horizontal axis) and (O) is the opposite end of the fan of acoustic waves.

*Gain*

Another important factor when performing B-scan ultrasound examination is the ability to adjust the gain. Gain, which is measured in decibels (dB), adjusts amplification of the returning echo, changing the sensitivity of the instrument's display screen [3]. A high gain level allows for capture of weaker signals (such as vitreous opacities). A low gain level causes the weaker signals to disappear and only the stronger ones remain displayed on the screen. Typically, an ultrasonography study begins on higher gain settings, and then gain can be lowered or adjusted as indicated [1,2].

## Probe positions and image interpretation

Performing a reliable and well-executed ocular B-scan requires training and a thorough understanding of where in the globe sounds waves are being projected to. A probe has a line or a dot (marker), which is a reference point that always indicates the upper portion of the echogram. There are 3 parameters that determine what part of the tissue is projected (scanned) on the echogram (see Fig. 1B).

- Probe (P): where the probe is positioned on the eye
- Marker (M): the orientation of the marker, which indicates the top of the echogram
- Fixation (F): where patient is looking, which is the middle portion of the echogram

It is critically important to know the orientation of the marker and what area of the globe the acoustic wavefront is directed toward in relation to the patient's gaze. The 2-dimensional echogram will image the retina in the M–F–O orientation. The marker (M) always represents the top portion of the echogram. The patient's fixation (F) usually is seen in the middle portion of the echogram. The lower portion of the echogram shows the opposite end (O) of the fanlike sound wave projection (see Fig. 1B).

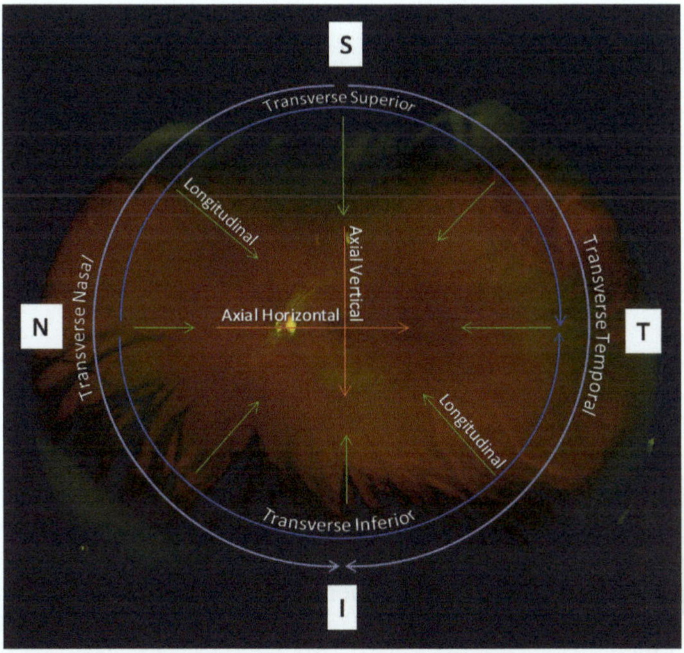


**Fig. 2.** Schematic of the transverse, longitudinal, and axial probe positions and how these relate to the specific part of the retina being scanned, left eye.

B-scan ultrasonography can be performed in 3 different orientations (Fig. 2 and Table 1).

1. *Transverse scan* (see Fig. 2; Fig. 3): this determines the presence of a peripheral lesion in various positions of gaze. This scan shows the lateral extent of a lesion, encompassing circumferentially between 4 and 6 clock-hours of the globe. To perform this scan, the patient is asked to look in one of the 4 primary meridians (12:00, 3:00, 6:00, and 9:00). The probe is oriented tangentially to the limbus and placed on the opposite (to the gaze) conjunctival surface with the marker being oriented perpendicular to the patient's gaze (Table 1).
2. *Longitudinal scan* (see Fig. 2; Fig. 4): this examines the fundus in a radial pattern extending from anterior (periphery) to posterior (posterior pole) at a specific clock-hour position. To perform the longitudinal scan, the patient is asked to look in the direction of the lesion. The probe is oriented perpendicular to the limbus and placed on the opposite (to the gaze) conjunctival surface with marker pointing to the cornea (see Table 1).
3. *Axial scan* (see Fig. 2; Fig. 5): this is a posterior pole assessment. Acoustic waves are projected straight into the eye through the cornea and lens in either vertical or horizontal directions. A horizontal axial scan is the scan of choice to visualize both the macula and the optic nerve on the same B-scan echogram. To perform an axial scan, the patient is asked to look straight ahead. The probe is placed on the center of the cornea with the marker pointing superiorly (for an axial vertical scan) or nasally (for an axial horizontal scan) (see Table 1).

**Table 1**
Summary of probe position, patent's fixation, and marker orientation for 3 types of B-scans

| Scan orientation | Probe position | Marker position | Patient fixation |
|---|---|---|---|
| Transverse | | | |
| Superior | Inferior conjunctiva | Nasally | Up |
| Inferior | Superior conjunctiva | Nasally | Down |
| Nasal | Temporal conjunctiva | Superiorly | Nasally |
| Temporal | Nasal conjunctiva | Superiorly | Temporally |
| Longitudinal | | | |
| Specific clock-hour | Opposite side to patient's fixation | Toward the cornea | Toward the direction of the lesion |
| Axial | | | |
| Vertical | Inferior conjunctiva | Center of the cornea | Straight |
| Horizontal | Nasal conjunctiva | Center of the cornea | Straight |

## Clinical examination principles

*Basic screening protocol*

The basic B-scan ultrasound evaluation is performed when a media opacity obscures the view of the posterior portion of the globe. This technique should include performing transverse scans in the 4 main quadrants (12:00, 3:00, 6:00, and 9:00). The posterior pole should be assessed by doing a horizontal axial scan to view the posterior lens surface, optic nerve, and macula simultaneously.

*Topographic evaluation of the lesion*

For lesions identified via a basic screening protocol, topographic evaluation of the lesion needs to be performed. This is accomplished by determining the clock hour of a lesion, then examining the lateral (transverse scan) and radial extent (longitudinal scan) of the lesion.

*Limbus to fornix*

B-scan ultrasonography is a dynamic study of the globe, as opposed to a static photographic image. The operator needs to continuously move the probe and rotate the marker with the goal of obtaining real-time visualization of the entire globe. For transverse and longitudinal scans, the limbus-to-fornix technique will allow scanning for lesions from the posterior pole to the periphery of the eye. It is recommended to initially position the probe closer to the limbus (to allow visualization of lesions from the posterior pole to The mid-periphery) and gradually move the probe to the fornix (to allow visualization of peripheral lesions).

# B-SCAN APPLICATIONS IN CLINICAL CARE

## Vitreous diseases

On B-scan ultrasonography, the normal vitreous is an anechoic region posterior to the crystalline lens with a composition that changes with age [8].

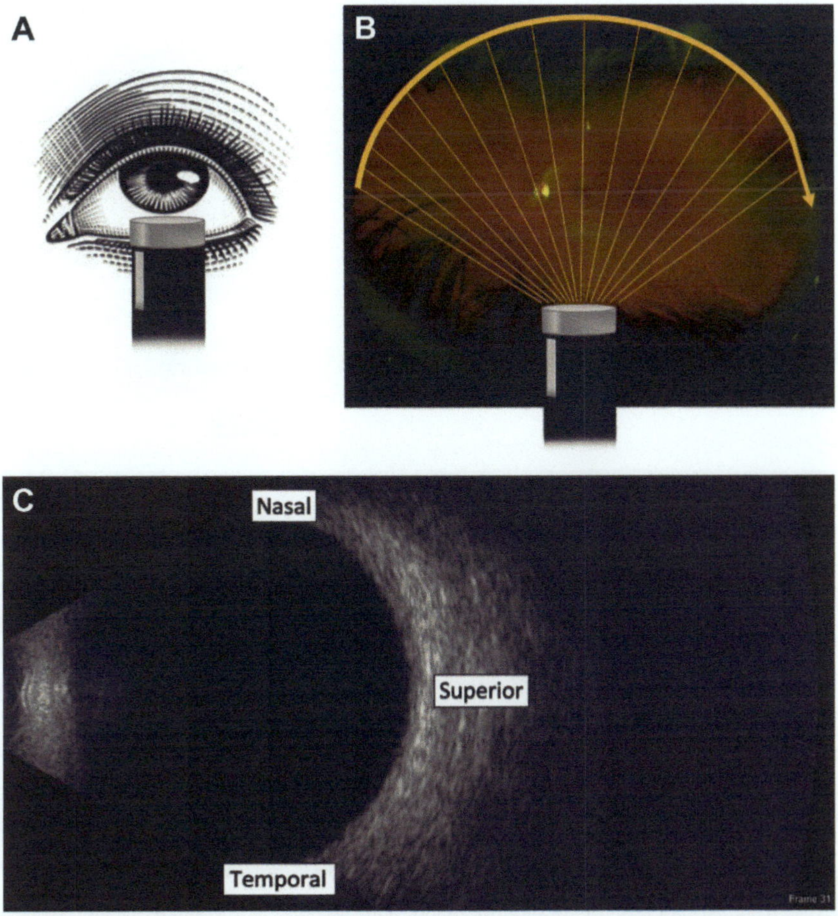


**Fig. 3.** Transverse scan of the superior retina of the left eye. (*A*) Schematic of the probe position, marker orientation, and patient's gaze. (*B*) Schematic of sound waves traveling through the superior retina circumferentially from nasal to the temporal side of the eye. (*C*) Corresponding B-scan echogram showing superior peripheral retina.

Visualization of anomalies and degenerations of the vitreous body can be assessed using B-scan ultrasound examination. Table 2 summarizes common indications for B-scan ultrasound examination in patients with vitreous abnormalities. Relatively benign age-related phenomena including vitreous syneresis may be demonstrated as small, dotlike reflections on B-scan ultrasound examination [15]. Fig. 6 shows an example of a patient with vitreous syneresis. Vitreous strands are visible with high gain and disappear when the gain is decreased (Fig. 6). Calcium-laden bodies appear as highly reflective crystals suspended within (asteroid hyalosis) or freely floating (synchysis scintillans) in the vitreous body [15]. The developmental anomaly persistent hyperplastic

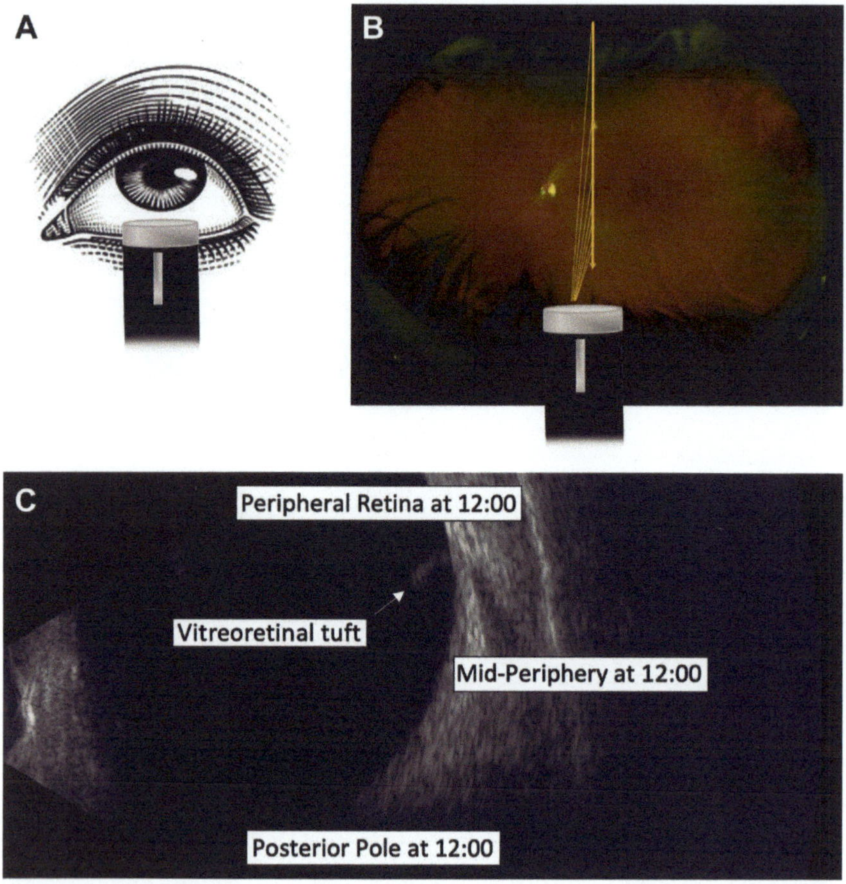


**Fig. 4.** Longitudinal scan of the superior retina of the left eye. (*A*) Schematic of the probe position, marker orientation, and patient's gaze. (*B*) Schematic of sound waves traveling radially along the 12:00 meridian. (*C*) Corresponding B-scan echogram of a patient with vitreoretinal tuft located mid-peripherally along the 12:00 meridian.

primary vitreous has 2 characteristic features on B-scan ultrasound examination: (1) hyperechoic membranous structure extending from the posterior lens toward the optic nerve head, and (2) microphthalmos [8,15].

Vitreous hemorrhage, regardless of the etiology, may be identified via B-scan ultrasound examination both within the vitreal cavity and in the retrovitreal space. The appearance of a vitreous hemorrhage on B-scan depends on the extent of and phase of the bleeding [8]. Of note, a high fluid exchange rate is thought to exist in the retrovitreal space, so a hemorrhage may clear from this area (become echo free) within days or weeks after an acute vitreous hemorrhage [15]. Patients with Terson syndrome (intraocular hemorrhage in the setting of acutely elevated intracranial pressure typically from intracranial or

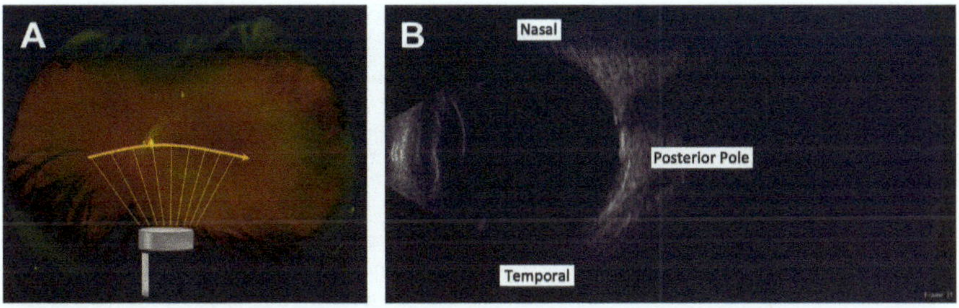


**Fig. 5.** Axial horizontal scan of the left eye. (*A*) Schematic of sound waves traveling through the posterior pole horizontally from the nasal to the temporal side of the eye. (*B*) Corresponding B-scan echogram showing normal macula just below the optic nerve.

subarachnoid hemorrhage) may present with hemorrhage into the vitreous that obscures retinal visualization [15–17]. It often is difficult to distinguish between vitreous inflammation and hemorrhage via B-scan ultrasound imaging alone, and other clinical features often aid in the diagnosis [14].

## Retinal diseases

On B-scan ultrasound examination, the retina is normally seen as a part of the retina–choroid–sclera, complex forming the posterior ocular wall [8].

Assessment of retinal integrity via B-scan ultrasonography is of paramount importance, particularly when media opacification (ie, corneal scarring or haze, hyphema, dense lenticular haze or cataract, vitreous hemorrhage) precludes a direct assessment using standard funduscopic examination techniques [15]. In emergency settings, cases of ocular or periocular trauma with coexisting eyelid swelling or edema, or if the patient is unable to tolerate a retinal examination, clinicians may evaluate the retinal structure via an ultrasound examination [15]. It should be emphasized that a B-scan ultrasound examination is contraindicated in cases of suspected open globe injury [14].

Retinal breaks (ie, holes, tears) and RD (ie, rhegmatogenous, exudative, serous) all may be identified via B-scan ultrasound examination [15]. The retina's strongest points of attachment are at the optic nerve and ora serrata, so identifying these structures on the B-scan aids the examiner in assessing retinal integrity [15]. The so-called funnel RD may result from the retina folding centrally into itself within the globe, because the optic nerve pierces the retina (and, therefore, cannot detach from it) [10,13,15].

Prior data from a 2009 study by Lorenzo-Carrero and colleagues [18] demonstrated that B-scan ultrasound examination may play an adjunct role in the identification of retinal tears in patients with acute symptomatic posterior vitreous detachment. Their study found that B-scan ultrasound examination using a 105-dB gain setting demonstrated a sensitivity of 96% and specificity of 98% in detecting retinal tears in their cohort of 234 patients [18]. The authors noted that a B-scan may detect retinal tears that could go overlooked on a

**Table 2**
B-Scan ultrasound features for various conditions involving the vitreous

| Ophthalmologic conditions involving the vitreous | B-scan findings |
|---|---|
| Asteroid hyalosis/synchysis scintillans | Highly reflective crystals suspended within or freely floating in vitreous body |
| Endophthalmitis | Widening of the ocular wall may indicate presence of choroidal inflammation or infiltrates, vitreous abscess may be present |
| Intraocular foreign body | Variable reflectivity pattern depending on the foreign object (ie, a metallic foreign body has a strong reflectance signal), may have a comet's tail artifact if a spherical foreign body is embedded in the ocular wall |
| Persistent hyperplastic primary vitreous | Hyperechoic membranous structure extending from the posterior lens surface toward the optic nerve head, microphthalmos, with or without congenital cataract |
| Proliferative vitreoretinopathy | Multiple membranes within the vitreous, may mimic RD |
| Terson syndrome (intraocular hemorrhage with intracranial or subarachnoid hemorrhage) | Vitreous hemorrhage may be present, a variable layer retinal hemorrhage (including preretinal) may be present, often near the optic disc and posterior pole |
| Vitreous degeneration or syneresis | Small dotlike reflections, no retinal abnormalities associated |
| Vitreous hemorrhage | Small particles with hazy hyperechoic signal within the vitreous cavity, snow globe effect, erythrocytes may gravitate toward vitreous strands, neovascularization of the retina or retinal break or detachment may be evident, use high gain setting to better visualize |
| Vitritis or posterior uveitis | Dotlike reflections, may be difficult to differentiate from hemorrhage |

*Data from* Refs [8,13,14].

dilated funduscopic examination alone, but may also result in false positives; the study authors concluded that B-scan ultrasound examination "is an accurate diagnostic test for detection of retinal tears in symptomatic patients" [18].

A total RD has characteristic features on B-scan ultrasound examination, depending on the plane of the imaging. The total RD may adopt an ultrasound appearance similar to an isosceles triangle (open toward the anterior segment, converging toward the optic disc) [15]. With the ultrasound probe placed at the temporal canthus and globe in the adducted position, the total RD will instead appear circular or oval owing to the conical shape of the detachment [15].

The ability of B-scan ultrasound examination to image the eye in a dynamic fashion allows the clinician to better characterize retinal and vitreous findings on examination. A potentially helpful feature in acute rhegmatogenous RD is

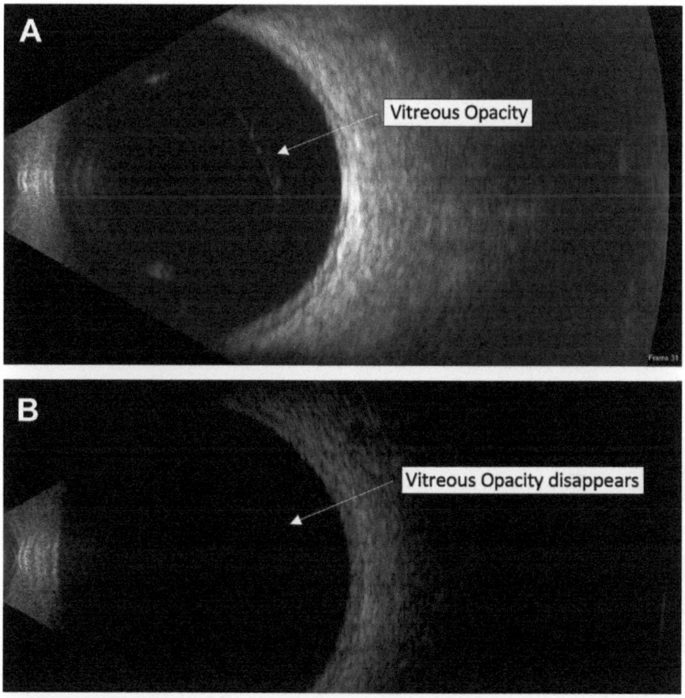


**Fig. 6.** B-scan echogram of patient with vitreous opacities. (*A*) High gain. (*B*) Low gain.

the whiplash effect, which is evident on B-scan ultrasound examination following quick eye movements [15]. An acute RD shows relatively short aftermovements with a whiplash effect at the point of attachment, whereas patients with vitreous hemorrhage or asteroid hyalosis exhibit smaller, less extensive aftermovements; the retina moves more slowly than the vitreous [15]. In cases of chronic RD (Fig. 7), the thickness of the retina increases, cysts may develop within the detached retina, and the aftermovements may become altered and slowed compared with acute RD [10,15]. Retinoschisis, a splitting within the neurosensory retinal layers, also may be identified on B-scan ultrasound examination [15]. Important B-scan features of retinoschisis that allow differentiation from RD include less apparent or absent aftermovements on ultrasound examination following eye movements and a lack of prominent vitreous adhesions [15].

Retinoblastoma is another critical diagnosis that may be facilitated by B-scan ultrasound examination. These life-threatening lesions often present in childhood with leukokoria, lenticular opacification, vitreous seeding, and other findings that may hinder funduscopic examination [15]. Characteristic calcium deposits within retinoblastoma lesions result in an extremely high sound reflection and acoustic shadowing, but as many as one-third of cases may not exhibit significant calcification [14,15]. Reducing the amplification during ultrasound imaging to the point where only the calcified areas of the tumor are visible

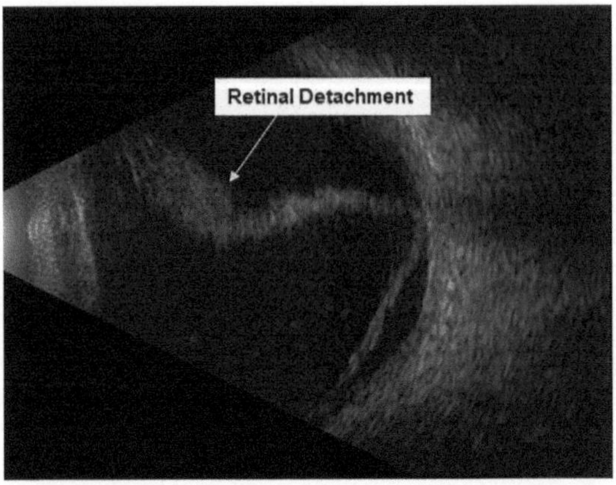


**Fig. 7.** B-scan echogram of a patient with a chronic retinal detachment demonstrating retinal thickening.

may be helpful in some cases [15]. Ultrasound examination also may identify extraocular tumor extension (ie, optic nerve, orbit), which impacts management decisions, although these features may be more optimally visualized by other imaging modalities [15].

Many other posterior segment diseases may be visualized with B-scan ultrasonography, a full list of which is beyond the scope of this report. Reported indications for B-scan ultrasound imaging of the macula or retina include vitreomacular traction, macular edema, Coats disease, and age-related macular degeneration [14,15]. However, macular diseases more commonly are assessed via OCT and other modalities in modern clinical practice [14].

## Choroidal diseases

B-scan ultrasonography has several utilities in evaluation and management of choroidal disorders. Using ultrasonography, it is possible to probe intraocular or extraocular areas, such as the pars plana or ciliary body, which are challenging to visualize on direct examination or using other imaging modalities. B-scan plays a critical role in evaluation and management of choroidal tumors by characterizing their size and shape. One of the most important criteria in differentiating a choroidal melanoma from a choroidal nevus is the measured thickness on B-scan [15]. Occasionally, the pathognomonic shape of a choroidal tumor on B-scan leads to a final diagnosis of a mushroom-shaped choroidal melanoma (Fig. 8). The ultrasonography also provides important information about the interval echogenicity of choroidal lesions. Although vascular tumors such as choroidal hemangiomas tend to demonstrate a high internal reflectivity, choroidal melanomas usually possess low to medium reflectivity with occasional acoustic hollowing [15]. Other important utilities of B-scan examination include evaluation for possible extraocular extension of a malignant choroidal tumor or performing serial B-scans to confirm stability versus growth of a suspicious choroidal mass.

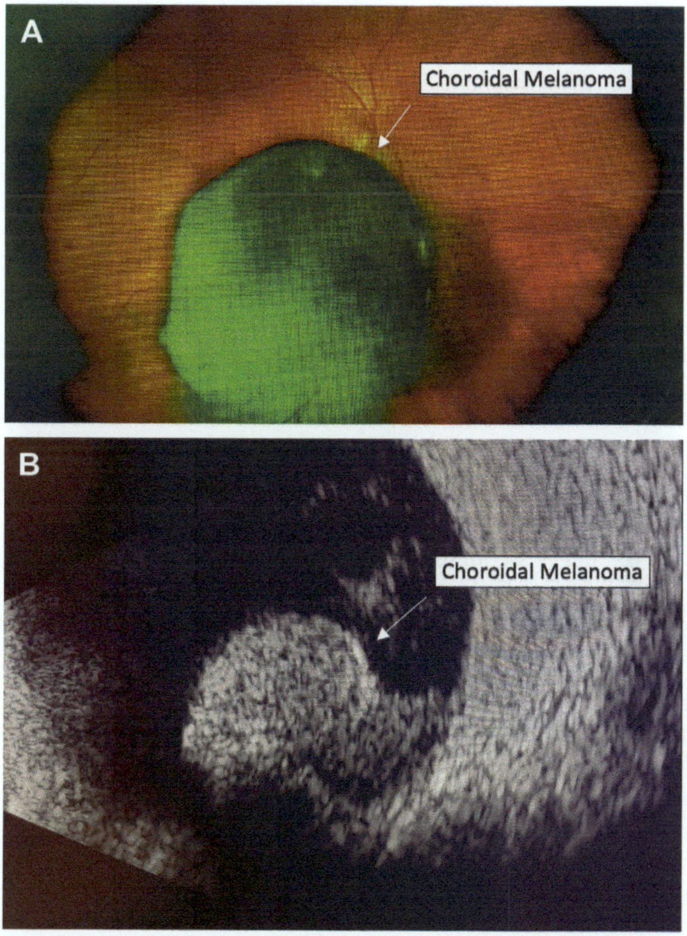


**Fig. 8.** Patient with choroidal melanoma. (*A*) Fundus photography. (*B*) B-scan echogram.

The role of B-scan imaging in the diagnosis and management of choroidal disorders is not limited to tumors. B-scan examination can be used to differentiate choroidal effusions from choroidal hemorrhages. Although a choroidal effusion appears as a hollow dome-shaped mass with occasional bridging vessels, ultrasound examination of a choroidal hemorrhage reveals higher echogenicity of a hemorrhage [15,16]. This differentiation is important, because choroidal effusions almost always are managed medically, whereas choroidal hemorrhages may need surgical intervention. Finally, B-scan ultrasonography can assist in diagnosis of select inflammatory disorders of choroid and sclera. A prominent example is posterior scleritis where choroidal inflammation along with episcleral fluid creates the classic T-sign on B-scan ultrasonography [15].

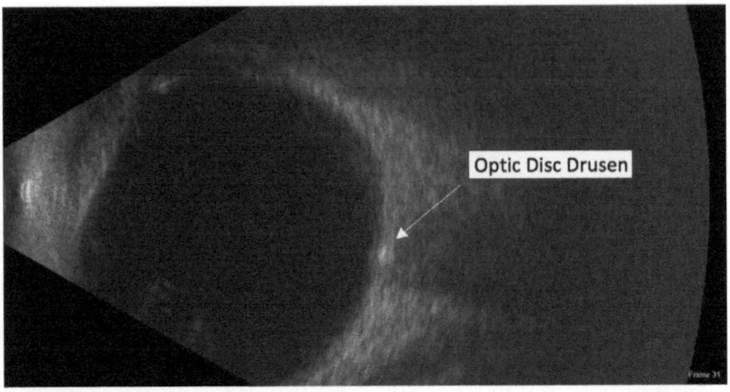


**Fig. 9.** B-scan echogram of patient with ODD.

## Optic nerve diseases

Normal B-scan ultrasonography of the optic nerve demonstrates low reflectivity through the nerve's course, which is behind the globe in a tubular appearance, surrounded by a high reflectivity signal owing to the optic nerve sheath [14]. Various optic nerve abnormalities have characteristic patterns on B-scan imaging.

### *Optic disc drusen*

B-scan ultrasound examination is a part of a battery of testing that contributes to the diagnosis of ODD, which are acellular deposits composed of calcium, amino acids, and other constituents found at varying levels of the optic disc [19]. In addition to traditional dilated fundus examination, other ancillary test modalities that aid in diagnosis of ODD include enhanced depth imaging OCT, fundus autofluorescence, computed tomography scans, and intravenous fluorescein angiography [19]. Historically, B-scan ultrasound examination has been considered the gold standard in the diagnosis of ODD [20]. Calcified ODD adopts a characteristic hyperechoic and highly reflective appearance on B-scan ultrasound examination (Fig. 9) [19], which helps to solidify the diagnosis. Importantly, clinicians should turn down the B-scan gain setting to help visualize ODD that may otherwise be masked by the high reflectivity orbital tissue [14]. Deeper (buried) or less calcified ODD may go undetected via B-scan ultrasound examination, and enhanced depth imaging OCT may be necessary to identify deeper or smaller ODD [19]. Recent data from various groups including the Optic Disc Drusen Studies (ODDS) Consortium have suggested that enhanced depth imaging OCT is more reliable in diagnosis of ODD [19,21]. The ODDS Consortium defines ODD as "hyporeflective structures with a full or partial hyperreflective margin" [22].

### *Peripapillary hyperreflective ovoid mass-like structures*

Peripapillary hyperreflective ovoid mass-like structures (PHOMS) have more recently been described in patients with ODD. PHOMS may represent a herniation of optic nerve axons into the peripapillary retinal space [22]. Although it has been posited that PHOMS may represent either a precursor to or variant of ODD, there are a number of factors that help to differentiate the 2 entities [22]. Features that may be helpful in distinguishing PHOMS from ODD include following: PHOMS are not visible via B-scan ultrasound examination, do not autofluoresce, and appear hyper-reflective via OCT imaging [21].

*Papilledema*

In clinical practice, differentiating papilledema and pseudopapilledema (ie, from ODD) represents a critical decision in patient management. It is believed that an increase in intracranial pressure results in a pressure gradient that is transmitted through the subarachnoid space to the region surrounding the optic nerve, resulting in clinically apparent optic disc edema and also an increase in optic nerve sheath diameter (ONSD) [23]. Because the optic nerve sheath is contiguous with the intracranial dural tissue, the optic nerve sheath may widen during periods of increased intracranial pressure [14].

Emerging data regarding the usefulness of B-scan ultrasound examination suggests that the ONSD may be a valuable, noninvasive technique that may aid in the diagnosis of papilledema and/or intracranial hypertension in select populations, particularly for children [23] and bedside patients [24] where traditional clinical examination may not be possible.

A recent study that compared 36 eyes in children with papilledema to 145 eyes in children with pseudopapilledema suggested that optic nerve sheath widening greater than 4.5 mm on B-scan ultrasound examination was both sensitive (86%; 95% confidence interval, 64%–96%) and specific (88%; 95% confidence interval, 79%–94%) for diagnosing papilledema [25]. Other groups have used ONSD greater than 3.3 mm as a cut-off for papilledema and reported a sensitivity of 68% [26]. A review of the literature surrounding ONSD pointed out that normal reference values for this diagnostic criterion are quite challenging and variable in reported studies [27]. Additionally, various ultrasound protocols are reported in the literature, and some have proposed greater than 5.0 mm as the cut-off for increased ONSD; the results also could be subject to interobserver variability [26,27]. It should be noted that the presence of ODD does not exclude the possibility of coexisting papilledema, and currently no gold standard test exists to differentiate true papilledema from pseudopapilledema [26].

The ONSD may be measured by the so-called 30° test during ultrasonography: the ONSD is measured in primary gaze and then again at 30° laterally [14]. Normally, the ONSD remains constant with different gaze positions [14]. If increased intracranial pressure occurs, the ONSD may increase; however, any increase in ONSD may be reduced in lateral gaze owing to stretching of the optic nerve or sheath as a result of redistribution of cerebrospinal fluid over a larger area [14]. A decrease in the ONSD by 10% or more in lateral gaze compared with the primary gaze position is considered a positive 30° test

[14]. Further studies evaluating ONSD criteria may be helpful in clarifying the role of this parameter in the evaluation of patients suspected to have papilledema and/or intracranial hypertension or hypotension. At this time, ONSD alone should not be used as the sole measure to indicate the presence or absence of papilledema [26].

*Optic nerve tumors*

Optic nerve gliomas may demonstrate a relatively small echo height with low to medium reflectivity on ultrasonography (owing to the uniform nature of the tumor constituents), whereas optic nerve sheath meningiomas' irregular surface can result in jagged surface echoes with medium to high internal reflectivity patterns [14]. However, these lesions may be better visualized with other imaging modalities (ie, MRI).

## ADVANCES IN ULTRASONOGRAPHY

B-scan plays an important role in the evaluation and management of lesions related to ocular diseases by characterizing their size and shape. Some ultrasound devices are equipped with measurement calipers to obtain information about the lesion's size and depth. Other newer models have the ability to zoom in and out on a lesion, to change image contrast, to display a recorded video, or to reconstruct a 3-dimensional analysis of an eye [28]. Most recently, the B-scan ultrasonography industry developed various enhancements to make it easier and more intuitive to use this imaging technology. Newer models are equipped with a position sensor that can provide real-time essential information on the location of the probe on the eye and the direction of the ultrasound beam, to help the operator identify the area of examination more rapidly.

Other advances in instrumentation include the use of higher frequencies to improve image resolution. New annular arrays at high frequencies (20–40 MHz) allow for increased depth of field and increased lateral resolution, while maintaining high axial resolution of a B-scan image [4,6]. This technology makes it possible to simultaneously examine pathologies of the vitreous, retina, and orbit without compromising image quality.

Color Doppler imaging technologies permit gray-scale ultrasound imaging of tissue structure to be combined with Doppler measurement of blood flow velocities. A color Doppler imaging analysis focuses primarily on diagnosis and management of orbital vascular lesions and ocular ischemic syndrome, adding color to the B-scan gray-scale image of the eye to represent the motion of blood through the arteries behind the globe [29]. Coupled with advanced signal processing methods (eg, swept source), these novel technologies promise to revolutionize ocular clinical practice, allowing for diagnostic investigation of perfusion physiology and disease with previously unachievable temporal and spatial resolution [6].

One of the most recent developments in the field is the use of ultrasound examination to enhance the delivery of various therapeutics. New research in this field demonstrated a significant potential for ultrasound-mediated ocular drug delivery with the potential for a wide range of clinical applications including glaucoma, age-related macular degeneration, and diabetic retinopathy [30].

## SUMMARY

Ocular ultrasonography is extremely helpful in imaging, measuring, and defining a variety of ocular conditions ranging from the anterior segment (cornea and ciliary body) to the posterior segment and choroid. B-scan imaging is a safe procedure that provides a real-time kinetic assessment of ocular lesions, even when the view of the posterior segment is obscured. B-scan ultrasonography serves a critical role in assessment of ODD, as well as tumors of the optic nerve, retina, and choroid. The capability of B-scan to identify potentially cancerous lesions in situations where other examination techniques fail underscores its vital role in eye care. With proper training and thorough understanding of ultrasonography principles and image interpretation, B-scan ultrasound examination is an excellent tool for the imaging-driven diagnostic approach to common and rare ocular diseases. The use of higher frequencies, improved sensitivity, and increased resolution have resulted in continuous optimization of image quality. Novel applications in the field have potential to revolutionize ocular clinical care.

## CLINICS CARE POINTS

- When performing ocular B-scan ultrasonography, start on higher gain settings and then adjust or lower the gain, as indicated.
- A basic screening protocol is done when a media opacity obscures the view of the posterior portion of the globe. It includes performing transverse scans in the 4 main quadrants (12:00, 3:00, 6:00, and 9:00), as well as doing a horizontal axial scan to obtain view of the macula and optic nerve.
- Use limbus-to-fornix technique to scan lesions from the mid-periphery to the periphery.
- For topographic evaluation of a lesion, examine the lateral (transverse scan) and radial (longitudinal scan) extent of the lesion at the specific clock-hour where the lesion is located.

## DISCLOSURE

The authors have nothing to disclose.

## References

[1] Byrne SF, Green RL. Ultrasound of the eye and orbit. 2nd edition. Philadelphia (PA): Mosby; 2002.

[2] Richard L, Hart LJ. Ultrasound Diagnosis of the eye and orbit. Principle Pract Ophthalmol 1997;5:98.

[3] Casser L, Fingeret M, Woodcome TH. Atlas of primary eyecare procedures. Stamford, CT: Appleton & Lange; 1997.
[4] Coleman DJ, Silverman RH, Chabi A, et al. High-resolution ultrasonic imaging of the posterior segment. Ophthalmol 2004;111(7):1344–51.
[5] Silverman RH. High-resolution ultrasound imaging of the eye – a review. Clin Experiment. Ophthalmol 2009;37(1):54–67.
[6] Coleman DJ, Silverman RH, Rondeau MJ, et al. Explaining The Current Role Of High Frequency Ultrasound In Ophthalmic Diagnosis (Ophthalmic Ultrasound). Expert Rev. Ophthalmol 2006;1(1):63–76.
[7] Cornetta P, Marotta G, De Bernardo M, et al. Ultrasound and optic neuritis. Am J Emerg Med 2019;37:1598.
[8] De La Hoz Polo M, Torramilans Lluís A, Pozuelo Segura O, et al. Ocular ultrasonography focused on the posterior eye segment: what radiologists should know. Insights Imaging 2016;7(3):351–64.
[9] Bengal SV, Bhandari AJ, Siddhiqui F. Pattern of ocular pathologies diagnosed with B-scan ultrasonography in a hospital in rural India. Niger J Ophthalmol 2016;24:71–5.
[10] Uduma FU, Iquo-Abasi AS, Rosemary NN. B-scan ophthalmic ultrasonography: a review corroborated with echograms. New Front Ophthalmol 2019;5:1–5.
[11] Pavlin CJ, Sherar H, et al. Clinical use of ultrasound biomicroscopy. Ophthalmol 1991;98: 287–95.
[12] Lorente-Ramos RM, Armán JA, Muñoz-Hernández A, et al. US of the eye made easy: a comprehensive how-to review with ophthalmoscopic correlation. Radiographics 2012;32(5):E175–200.
[13] Dessì G, Lahuerta EF, Puce FG, et al. Role of B-scan ocular ultrasound as an adjuvant for the clinical assessment of eyeball diseases: a pictorial essay. J Ultrasound 2015;18(3): 265–77.
[14] Kendall CJ, et al. Diagnostic ophthalmic ultrasound for radiologists. Neuroimaging Clin N Am 2015;3:327–65.
[15] Andrew P, Sadda SR, Hinton DR, et al. Diagnostic ophthalmic ultrasound. In: Schachat AP, editor. Ryan's retina, vol. 1, 6th edition. Elsevier; 2018. p. 273–324.
[16] Schrieber C, Liu Y. Choroidal effusions after glaucoma surgery. Curr Opin Ophthalmol 2015;26:134–42.
[17] Gauntt CD. Sherry RG. Kannan C. Terson syndrome with bilateral optic nerve sheath hemorrhage. J Neuro-Ophthalmology. 27(3):193-194.
[18] Lorenzo-Carrero J, Perez-Flores I, Cid-Galano M, et al. B-Scan Ultrasonography to Screen for Retinal Tears in Acute Symptomatic Age-Related Posterior Vitreous Detachment. Ophthalmology 2009;116(1):94–9.
[19] Silverman AL, Tatham AJ, Medeiros FA, et al. Assessment of Optic Nerve Head Drusen Using Enhanced Depth Imaging and Swept Source Optical Coherence Tomography. J Neuroophthalmol 2014;34:198–205.
[20] Kurz-Levin M, Landau K. A Comparison of Imaging Techniques for Diagnosing Drusen of the Optic Nerve Head. Arch Ophthalmol 1999;117(8):1045–9.
[21] Costello F, Rothenbuehler SP, Sibony PA, et al. Optic Disc Drusen Studies Consortium. Diagnosing optic disc drusen in the modern imaging era: a practical approach. Neuro Ophthalmol 2020;45(1):1–16.
[22] Malmqvist L, Bursztyn L, Costello F, et al. The Optic Disc Drusen Studies Consortium recommendations for diagnosis of optic disc drusen using optical coherence tomography. J Neuroophthalmol 2018;38(3):299–307.
[23] Fontanel L, Pensiero S, Ronfani L, et al. Optic nerve sheath diameter ultrasound: optic nerve growth curve and its application to detect intracranial hypertension in children. Am J Ophthalmol 2019;208:421–8.
[24] Wang L-J, Zhang Y, Li C, et al. Ultrasonographic optic nerve sheath diameter as a noninvasive marker for intracranial hypotension. Ther Adv Neurol Disord 2022;15:1–9.

[25] Farazdaghi MK, Trimboli-Heidler C, Liu GT, et al. Utility of ultrasound and optical coherence tomography in differentiating between papilledema and pseudopapilledema in children. J Neuroophthalmol 2021;41:488–95.
[26] Kohli AA, Pistilli M, Alfaro C, et al. Role of ocular ultrasonography to distinguish papilledema from pseudopapilledema. J Neuroophthalmol 2021;41:206–11.
[27] Vitiello L, De Bernardo M, Capasso L, et al. Optic nerve ultrasound evaluation in animals and normal subjects. Front Med 2022;8:797018.
[28] Muldoon TO, Garcia JPS, Garcia PTM, et al. Surface rendering of 3D ultrasound images in ophthalmology. Invest Ophthalmol Vis Sci 2005;46:2579.
[29] Keane PA, Ruiz-Garcia H, Sadda SR. Advanced imaging technologies. In: Retina, vol. 1, 5th edition. Elsevier; 2013. p. 133–50.
[30] Lafond M, Aptel F, Jean-Louis Mestas J, et al. Ultrasound-mediated ocular delivery of therapeutic agents: a review. Expert Opin Drug Deliv 2017;14(4):539–50.

Advances in Ophthalmology and Optometry 7 (2022) 51–70

ADVANCES IN OPHTHALMOLOGY AND OPTOMETRY

# Nonsurgical Treatment of Strabismus

Marie I. Bodack, OD

Department of Pediatric Primary Care, Southern College of Optometry, 1245 Madison Avenue, Memphis, TN 38104, USA

**Keywords**

• Esotropia • Exotropia • Observation • Occlusion • Orthoptics • Prism • Strabismus • Vision therapy

**Key points**

- A functional cure for the treatment of strabismus is one where the patient has a high level of binocularity; this should be the goal of strabismus treatment.
- Surgical treatment not always is indicated or desired and practitioners should be aware of nonsurgical treatment options.
- A hyperopic prescription may lead to good alignment and fusion in some patients with esotropia.
- Decompensation is rare for patients with intermittent exotropia. Observation is an acceptable option.

## INTRODUCTION

When treating strabismus, the principal goal is establishing or restoring binocular vision; this usually is judged by the extent of improvement in ocular alignment and stereopsis. In 1958, Flom described the concept of "functional" cure, which is the restoration of binocular vision [1]. In order to achieve a functional cure, good alignment is needed. However, even with good alignment, good binocularity is not always is possible; the patient may have only a "cosmetic" cure. Later, Duckman expanded on Flom's concept of cure [2]. Unfortunately, even today, no consistent definition exists of success that combines structural and functional outcomes for strabismus treatment. Flom and Duckman provide stringent, but helpful goals, that should be considered by practitioners (Table 1: Strabismus Cure).

*E-mail address:* mbodack@sco.edu

https://doi.org/10.1016/j.yaoo.2022.03.019

**Table 1**
Strabismus cure types

| | Flom's Criteria [1] | Duckman's Criteria [2] | |
|---|---|---|---|
| Functional Cure | • Clear, comfortable, single binocular vision at all distances<br>• Stereopsis and normal ranges of motor fusion<br>• Deviation may be present up to 1% of the time[a]<br>• Prism up to 5 prism diopters can be worn | • Comfortable without asthenopic symptoms<br>• Phoria for distance and near in primary and reading positions<br>• Absolute convergence not <20 for distance and near<br>• Relative convergence not < 15 for distance and near<br>• Unlimited near point of convergence (NPC)<br>• No suppression<br>• Excellent awareness of diplopia during testing | Excellent |

[a]Patient must experience diplopia when this happens.

The initial treatment of patients with strabismus is an appropriate prescription, if indicated, to give the patient clear vision, which also may help with alignment. If amblyopia is present, it should be treated before restoring binocularity. In some cases, surgical treatment may be indicated. In other cases, due to the magnitude of the deviation, patient age, or desire to avoid or delay surgery, nonsurgical treatments might be necessary. Practitioners should be aware of these nonsurgical options, which can be divided into the following categories: observation, lens or prism correction, occlusion, or vision therapy/orthoptics.

## SIGNIFICANCE/PRESENT RELEVANCE

### Esotropia

Esotropia can be divided into accommodative and nonaccommodative types (Table 2).

### Observation

Observation traditionally is not considered for patients with unilateral esotropia due to the risk of developing amblyopia if left untreated. However, the Pediatric Eye Disease Investigator Group (PEDIG) conducted the Congenital Esotropia Observation Study (CEOS) to determine the likelihood of spontaneous resolution of esotropia (defined as a deviation of <8Δ) in infants [4]. Investigators looked at infants between 4 and less than 20 weeks of age with at least a 20Δ esotropia. An outcome visit was conducted between 28 and 32 weeks of age. The esotropia resolved in 27% of patients, 8.7% of whom were treated with spectacles [4]. An additional 4% of patients experienced resolution after the end of the study but before the age of 1 year [4]. Resolution was more likely in patients who presented at less than 20 weeks of age, had a deviation less than 40Δ, or had an intermittent or variable deviation [4].

**Table 2**
Classification of esotropia

| Type of Esotropia | | Magnitude of Refractive Error |
|---|---|---|
| Accommodative | | |
| Refractive/fully | Corrected to 10Δ of orthophoria with full prescription | +2.00 to +6.00 [3] |
| Partially refractive | A residual deviation > 10Δ remains with full prescription | +2.00 to +6.00 |
| Nonrefractive/high AC/A | Deviation at near > distance by 10Δ+ | Minimal hyperopia at distance |
| Nonaccommodative | | |
| Infantile/congenital | — | Minimal hyperopia |
| Acquired | — | Minimal hyperopia/myopia |

Δ = prism diopter.

## Lens correction

Patients with nonaccommodative esotropia typically have a refractive error of +1.50 diopters or less [5]. In these patients, full plus likely will not result in improved alignment, but may be indicated for acuity, poor accommodation, or other concerns.

In infantile esotropia, correcting hyperopia is advocated, although disagreement occurs on how much to correct. Maples advocates a "conservative and symmetric spherical lens prescription based on dynamic retinoscopy." [6] For patients younger than 24 months, Christenson advocates full plus correction based on a cycloplegic refraction with an extra diopter to correct for a possible latent hyperopic component and to account for near visual demands [7]. For patients older than 24 months, a decrease in hyperopia from the cycloplegic refraction of 0.50 to 1.00 is considered to allow for tonic accommodation [7].

In accommodative esotropia, refractive correction is based on a cycloplegic refraction. Generally, full plus is prescribed [8,9]. The rationale for prescribing full plus is to eliminate the need for accommodation during distance viewing so that the eyes will stay aligned [9]. One study found that not prescribing full plus can result in a worsening of the esotropia [10]. Reducing plus by 1 diopter from the full cycloplegic retinoscopy in the final prescription resulted in a decompensation of the esotropia in 20% of patients, whereas decreasing by 2 diopters of plus resulted in a decompensation in 67% of patients [10].

However, some disagreement still occurs on whether a full plus correction is necessary. Park and Oh found that undercorrection by a maximum of +1.50 diopters did not lead to reduced visual acuity, stereopsis, fusional ability, or alignment [11]. Black also reported that approximately two-thirds of patients with satisfactory alignment were able to have their hyperopia prescription gradually undercorrected [12]. In cases where prescribing full plus blurs distance vision, the correction can be reduced by 0.50 or 1.00 diopter [8].

If a residual near esotropia of 8Δ or more with single vision correction occurs, some practitioners prescribe a bifocal [9]. The magnitude of the bifocal generally is +2.50 or +3.00 [13]. Instead of prescribing a set add power, some practitioners advocate increasing the plus add until the deviation is minimal [14]. Studies have found that 43.6% to 79% of children with accommodative esotropia given full plus achieved satisfactory alignment, whereas 24.5% to 34% still had a residual near deviation and required a bifocal [5,8,13,15]. One study found that only 35% achieved satisfactory alignment at near with the bifocal [13].

Risk factors for poor alignment with single vision lenses include a larger esotropia (>35Δ) at distance, lower amounts of hyperopia, age less than 3 years at the time of diagnosis, the presence of amblyopia, and a longer time from the appearance of the esotropia until correction [5,13,16].

In addition to normal changes in refractive error over time [12,17–22], patients with accommodative esotropia and good alignment may be able to be weaned from their spectacles over time even if the refractive error does not change. Many practitioners will wean by −0.25 to 1 diopter increments, provided the alignment remains stable [9,21,23,24]. Lambert and colleagues [24] found that 91% of patients with an initial refractive error of less than +3.00 were able to be weaned from glasses, whereas only 22% of patients with a refractive error of +3.00 to +5.00 were able to be successfully weaned. Black found that 13% of patients were able to discontinue glasses because of adequate alignment [12]. In contrast, Swan found that of 39 adults first treated for accommodative esotropia as children, only one was able to discontinue glasses [16].

Changes in alignment over time have been reported, with some patients developing a consecutive exotropia and others a decompensation of the esotropia after treatment. Consecutive exotropia has been reported in 3% to 18.4% of patients [8,15,19,23,25]. The average time for the development of consecutive exotropia is after 4 to 6.7 years of treatment [8,19,23,25]. Risk factors reported include amblyopia, onset when younger than 2 ½ years, a higher refractive error, a larger difference between the distance and near deviation, a larger decrease in hyperopia/year, no binocular vision, and the presence of a dissociated vertical deviation or inferior oblique overaction [15,23,25–27]. Other studies found that variables such as amblyopia or a younger age were not risk factors [23,25]. In patients who show a consecutive exotropia, treatment first involves decreasing the plus correction [23]. Decompensation has been reported in 5% to 24.5% of patients [8,12,15]. Risk factors include a younger age, oblique muscle dysfunction, and an abnormal accommodative-convergence (AC) over accommodation (A) (AC/A) ratio [12].

Stereopsis of any level has been reported in 43.6% to 67% of patients [5,19]. Stereopsis development did not seem to be influenced by age of onset of esotropia or onset of treatment [19]. Compliance with spectacle wear has been linked to more favorable sensory and motor outcomes [28]. Patients who wore their glasses less than 75% of the time were more likely to have no measurable stereopsis and an esotropia greater than 10Δ [28].

Treatment options for patients with high AC/A esotropia generally include a bifocal prescription. When fitting bifocals for these patients, the add is placed higher than for a presbyopic patient to ensure the child uses it. On average, +2.50 or +3.00 diopter adds are prescribed, but some recommend the lowest add that results in a phoria [29]. Raab advocates a near add (+2.50) if the deviation is 10 to 12Δ greater at near than distance [30]. An add is not indicated if the near deviation cannot be corrected to 8Δ, as that is the limit of binocular vision or monofixation at near [30].

Bifocal use is controversial in high AC/A esotropia as limited data exist on their effectiveness [31]. Prior studies have found neither a reduction in the magnitude of esotropia nor an improvement in sensory status, whereas others have found a greater increase in the magnitude of distance esotropia from baseline in patients who were treated with bifocals compared with single vision lenses. [32–34].

Because of cosmetic concerns about children wearing glasses with a visible line, some have advocated for progressive addition lenses (PALs) with accommodative esotropia, but studies are limited [35,36]. A benefit, however, is the ability to correct for intermediate viewing distances [36]. Mezer and colleagues [36] found good alignment and stereopsis in children treated with either PALs or bifocals for high AC/A esotropia. When fitting PALs, the investigators recommend adding +0.50 to the add [36].

Single vision contact lenses may be a viable treatment of patients with accommodative esotropia, but data are limited. Abdi and colleagues [37] looked at fully correcting patients' noncycloplegic, hyperopic refractive error with contact lenses and then adding increased plus over time. Patients experienced a decrease in the magnitude of their esotropia at distance and near with the addition of +0.60 diopters, which the investigators suggested acts as a near add [37]. In contrast, Gonzalez found that soft contact lenses provided poorer stability of alignment than glasses [38].

Monovision and bifocal contact lenses also have been studied as treatment options [39–41]. A study of monovision contact lenses for these patients found excellent alignment but data on binocularity were limited [39]. Bifiocal soft and rigid gas permeable (RGP) lenses have shown varied results, with some studies finding larger deviations with contacts than glasses and others finding the opposite [40,41].

*Occlusion*

Although not used as frequently as other treatments, binasal occlusion (only covering the nasal portion of the spectacle lens) using opaque or translucent tape may be an option for esotropes [6,42–44]. The goal of binasal occlusion is to stimulate alternation of the eyes to inhibit sensory adaptations (anomalous correspondence [AC]) and to encourage divergence [42,43]. Rutstein and Daum recommend this treatment be reserved for patients with a nonalternating fixation pattern or residual amblyopia [44]. Although no consensus exists on the width of the strip or how much temporal retina remains stimulated,

Greenwald provides fitting guidelines [42,45]. Disadvantages of binasal occlusion include possible reinforcement of anomalous processing and the development of head turns [42]. Limited studies occur on their efficacy.

Recently, a randomized clinical trial using binasal occlusion for 6 months on children age 3 to 10 years was conducted [46]. Patients had an esotropia of 20Δ or more after 6 to 9 months of wearing a full hyperopic prescription. Pretreatment, the average magnitude of the esotropia was 33Δ, which reduced to 18Δ after treatment; this was statistically significant [46].

*Prism correction*

Patients with pure nonaccommodative forms of esotropia or with a residual nonaccommodative component can also be treated with prism. Most of the studies recommend prism for magnitudes less than 20Δ [7,47,48]. Although Fresnel prisms are an option before prism is ground into glasses, Fresnel prisms at magnitudes greater than 12Δ can blur distance vision and affect cosmesis, and powers greater than 15Δ can blur near vision [49,50]. Higher prism powers can reduce fusion and stereopsis [49].

Practitioners should be aware of the possibility of prism adaptation (when a patient shows an increase in the magnitude of the deviation after prism placement). The theories for the cause of prism adaptation include "an avoidance response to avoid bifoveal stimulation" as well as a "vergence response to the motor stimulation." [50,51] To assess for prism adaptation, base-out prism, in a magnitude slightly higher than the deviation, is placed before the eyes [52]. The patient wears the prism for up to 1 hour, and the alignment is remeasured [52]. Favorable responses include orthophoria or a small exotropia with the prism. If residual esotropia occurs with the prism, the patient has adapted to the prism, which may indicate AC or poor sensory-motor fusion [7,52].

One study found that only 30.6% of patients with partially accommodative esotropia and a residual deviation of 20Δ or less, treated with prism glasses for 3 years, had good alignment and fusion ("success group") [47]. Prism adaptation was common, especially in the first 3 months; patients were corrected for the full deviation at each visit. Sixty-eight percent of the successful patients had less than a 6Δ increase in esotropia after 3 months [47]. Only 23.7% of the successful patients, or 7.3% of all enrolled patients, were able to be weaned off prism [47]. Randot stereopsis improved in 60.5% of the success group and 27.9% of the failure group [47].

Patients with acquired comitant esotropia are unlike patients with accommodative esotropia in that their strabismus is not due to uncorrected hyperopia. These patients typically have normal binocularity and then develop a sudden onset esotropia with symptoms of diplopia. Treatment often is designed to eliminate the diplopia and improve fusion. Chang treated 30 patients with the minimum amount of prism to alleviate diplopia [48]. Diplopia was alleviated in 27/30 patients, all of whom regained fusion [48]. Unlike with the other forms of esotropia discussed, the average refractive error in these patients was −5.25 diopters [48].

*Vision therapy/orthoptics*

Vision therapy can be incorporated in isolation, concurrent with spectacle or prism treatment or prestrabismus and/or poststrabismus surgery. Good prognostic indicators for the treatment of patients with esotropia include purely accommodative esotropia, later onset, intermittent deviation, no AC, bifoveal fusion, or stereopsis of 67 seconds or better [53–56].

Patients with esotropia are more difficult than patients with exotropia to treat with vision therapy, especially if amblyopia, suppression, or AC is present [57]. Using Flom's cure criteria, only 23% of patients with esotropia and AC (compared with 62% of patients with exotropia and AC) were "cured" after vision therapy [58].

For patients with infantile esotropia, after lens correction, treatment options include binasal or sectoral occlusion to help promote alternate fixation and then monocular and binocular fixation activities especially in abduction, followed by eye-hand coordination activities [6,7]. In addition, work with gingham patterns to stimulate binocular cortical cell development is advocated [7,56]. Patients should be followed-up every 2 to 4 weeks to check for improvement. For patients older than 24 months, abduction work still is important, but therapy should focus on treatment of AC, and in patients with normal correspondence, the establishment of second-degree fusion at the angle of deviation [7].

FitzGerald recommends a similar treatment of infants and toddlers: working first on eye movements with attention to the z axis and incorporation of reach, grasp, and release while the infant fixates a target. In addition, crib placement should be varied, and infants should be fed from alternate sides, both of which help stimulate each eye. He then recommends gross motor activities [56].

Even with equal acuity, monocular skills may not be equal [59]. Therapy for preschool children should include monocular eye-hand activities and then anti-suppression activities, if needed, progressing to monocular fixation in a binocular field task, followed by motor and sensory fusion work–moving from flat fusion to stereopsis [59].

Wick treated 54 patients with intermittent or constant esotropia without AC with prism, bifocal adds, and home therapy, when indicated [60]. Total success (defined as no strabismus, stereopsis of at least 100 seconds, equal acuity, no symptoms, no amblyopia or eccentric fixation) was achieved by 92.6% of patients, whereas partial success (defined as amblyopia up to 20/40 or central suppression, reduced or absent stereopsis, but no strabismus) by 7.4% [60].

Although small angle esotropia with anomalous correspondence has a less favorable prognosis, Wick outlines a treatment plan using the Flom divergence technique [61].

Table 3 provides a summary of treatment options for patients with esotropia.

Fig. 1 shows a flowchart of esotropia treatment based on examination findings.

**Table 3**
Treatment options for patients with strabismus

| | Nonaccommodative Esotropia | Accommodative Esotropia | Treatment | Exotropia | |
|---|---|---|---|---|---|
| **Concerns** | **Indications/ Guidelines** | **Indications/ Guidelines** | — | **Indications/ Guidelines** | **Concerns** |
| | Infantile: 29% resolution | Not recommended | *Observation* | Option for any age, before other treatments | Decompensation. Assess with control score recommended |
| Decompensation<br>Consecutive Exotropia | Cycloplegia<br>Plus considered especially if > +1.50 | Cycloplegia for maximum plus.<br>Residual deviation at near *may* require BF<br>Near deviation only may require BF | *Lenses* | 2–4 diopters overminus over cycloplegia<br>Option before/in lieu of other treatments | Avoid/caution in myopes |
| Some do not recommend as first option. | Binasal | Binasal for residual deviation | *Occlusion* | 3–6 h/d (range 2 h to full time)<br>Alternate eyes or dominant eye<br>Option for > 3 y | Cosmesis<br>Does not seem to benefit toddlers |
| Cosmesis and blur especially with larger amounts | May consider if symptoms of diplopia<br>Consider for deviations < 20Δ split between the eyes<br>Consider Fresnel trial | May consider if deviation at distance = near<br>Consider for deviations <20Δ<br>Split evenly between the eyes<br>Consider Fresnel trial | *Prism* | Different fitting types<br>Magnitude varies: one-third distance, 40% large angle<br>May taper | Same as for esotropia |
| Magnitude of deviation, frequency of deviation may be a factor in success AC more difficult | May be helpful for symptoms. May be more successful due to normal binocularity previously | Consider for residual deviation, poor binocularity, accommodation | *Vision Therapy* | In lieu or surgery or as an adjunct pre-/postsurgery | Same as exotropia |

*Abbreviation:* BF, bifocal

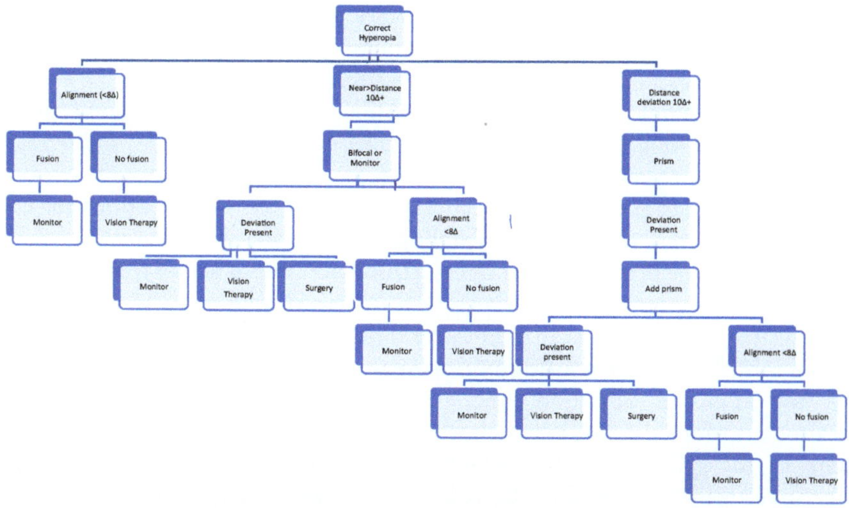


**Fig. 1.** Flow chart for patients with esotropia and hyperopia.

## Exotropia

Many studies on exotropia treatment divide patients by Duane's classification: convergence insufficiency, basic, and divergence excess [62,63]. Most of the treatments focus on intermittent exotropia.

In a 1992 review of 59 studies on the treatment of intermittent exotropia, Coffee and colleagues [64] found the following success rates: overminus lenses 28%, prism 28%, occlusion 37%, surgery 46%, and vision therapy 59%. The investigators noted flaws in the studies including small sample size, poorly defined treatment and success criteria, limited statistical analysis, or sample bias [64]. Subsequent to that, some randomized clinical trials, addressing the aforementioned flaws, have been developed looking at some, but not all, of the treatment options.

## Observation

In a retrospective study of pediatric and adult patients followed-up for at least 4 years, Rutstein and Corliss found that intermittent exotropia "improved for many patients quantitatively and qualitatively over time," even without treatment [65]. Most of the patients (71%) had basic exotropia, followed by divergence excess (15%) and convergence insufficiency (14%). Overall, 36% of patients converted to orthophoria or exophoria at the last visit. Nonsurgical treatment options included observation (18%), overminus lenses (27%), prism (34%), vision therapy (49%), or multiple modalities (33%). The investigators noted that improvement was not related to whether or not patients were prescribed treatment [65].

Another retrospective study looked at pediatric patients with intermittent exotropia, seen over the course of a 20-year period for 2 or more visits [66].

Approximately 4% of patients spontaneously resolved over a mean follow-up of 9.2 years. Twenty-one percent received nonsurgical treatment (11% each orthoptics and overminus, 2.8% prism, 8.3% alternate patching, and 63.9% dominant eye patching). The investigators estimated that the likelihood of the deviation increasing by 10Δ or more was 23.1% at 5 years, 29.2% at 10 years, and 52.8% at 20 years [66].

Buck and colleagues [67] prospectively looked at treatment options for children with intermittent exotropia including observation (53%), glasses, patching, orthoptics and/or prism (13%), surgery (16%), and visual acuity treatment only (17%). Patients undergoing surgery were assessed at 6 months postsurgery, whereas patients with nonsurgical interventions were assessed at 2 years. Outcomes included the Newcastle Control Score (NCS) [68], changes in visual acuity, the angle of deviation, and stereopsis. Children in the nonsurgical treatment groups did not experience a significant change in the angle of deviation or the NCS but did have some improvement in near stereopsis [67]. The investigators noted that the risk of conversion from intermittent to constant exotropia is minimal [67].

Holmes and colleagues [69] reviewed pediatric patients treated with surgery or no surgery seen for 5 years of follow-up. There was no statistically significant difference in cure rate between both groups; 30% of the surgical cohort and 12% of the nonsurgical cohort achieved cure, defined as motor and sensory [69]. In the surgical cohort, patients who received an additional surgery in the 5-year period could not be considered cured. Treatment options in the nonsurgical cohort included observation (58%), part time occlusion (39%), and "convergence exercises" (3%). One patient in the part-time occlusion cohort also received treatment with overminus lenses. The investigators noted that "conservative management, including watchful waiting, can sometimes result in an excellent outcome." [69].

Prospectively, PEDIG looked at the course of intermittent exotropia in children aged 3 to 10 years over 3 years [70]. Outcome measures included deterioration: loss of motor control (a constant deviation ≥ 10Δ at distance or near) or a drop in near stereopsis (greater than 2 octaves from the maximum). The cumulative probability of deterioration over 3 years was 15%. The investigators noted that the 15% was likely an overestimation due to misclassifications; 12/25 patients started treatment without meeting either motor or sensory criterion [70].

## LENSES

### Overminus lenses

Overminus lenses are used primarily in younger patients and those with small angle deviations [71]. The goal of these lenses is to stimulate accommodative convergence to reduce the exotropic angle to fall within the range of motor fusion [64]. However, a consensus of the strength for the overcorrecting lenses does not exist. Values have ranged from −1.00 to −6.50 diopters [72–77].

One of the earliest reports on overminus lenses describes the investigator's approach to determining the optimal overminus prescription, evaluating acuity and accommodation [74]. He reported results as "eyes straight no fusion" (28%), "eyes straight with fusion" (54%), and "eyes straight, constant fusion" (18%) [74].

A retrospective study by Caltrider and Jampolsky found that 72% of children overminused by 2 to 4 diopters for a median time of 18 months showed increased control ("qualitative change") (46%) or increased control and a decrease in the magnitude of the deviation by 15Δ or more ("quantitative change") (26%) [72]. Treatment gains were maintained in 70% of the successful patients for 1 year after treatment ended [72].

More recently, a retrospective study by Bayramlar and colleagues [73] looked at children who were prescribed 2 to 4 diopters of overminus correction for a median time of 18 months. Success was measured by Caltrider and Jampolsky's qualitative and quantitative definitions and the NCS. Eighty four percent of children showed success: 47% qualitative, 37% quantitative. The investigators did not look specifically at myopia progression but noted that significant myopic progression was not observed [73].

In a prospective study, Watts and colleagues [76] found that 72% of children showed an improvement in control of their intermittent exotropia with overminus lenses of 2 to 4 diopters. The duration of the study was only 4 months so refractive error changes were not recorded [76].

Kushner treated children with 1 to 2 diopters of overminus correction for 6 months, with a subset continuing for 5 years [77]. At the 5-year follow-up, no difference occurred between the progression of myopia between the treatment and control groups for both myopic and hyperopic patients [77].

PEDIG recently conducted a multicenter, randomized clinical trial of overminus lenses for children with intermittent exotropia [78]. Subjects were overminused by 2.5 diopters for 1 year and then by 1.25 diopters for 3 months, after which time they were treated with nonoverminus lenses for an additional 3 months. The primary outcome was distance control, using the IXT Office Control Score at 12 and 18 months [78,79] (Table 4). At the 18-month visit, a significant difference in the control scores between both groups did not occur. During the course of the study, it was noted that myopia progression was greater in the overminus group than the control group [78]. For this reason, the overminus treatment ended early [78].

## Occlusion

Another treatment option for patients with intermittent or constant exotropia is occlusion. The mechanism of occlusion therapy is that of passive antisuppression [80]. Additional benefits include improving control of the deviation and decreasing the magnitude of the strabismus [75]. Studies have looked at occlusion of the nondeviating eye or alternate eyes [80–82]. As with overminus lenses, no consensus exists on the recommended hours per day of treatment. Treatment times range from 2 hours a day to full time [80–84].

Spoor and Hiles prospectively looked at the effects of 3 to 6 hours of daily occlusion on the preferred eye of children for an average of 15 months [82].

**Table 4**
Intermittent exotropia control score

| Score | Findings | Notes |
|---|---|---|
| 5 | Constant exotropia | Patient is observed for 30 s |
| 4 | Exotropia > 50% of the time before dissociation | |
| 3 | Exotropia < 50% of the time before dissociation | |
| 2 | No exotropia unless dissociated; recovers in > 5 s | 1. Occlude OD 10 s. Note the time taken to reestablish fusion |
| 1 | No exotropia unless dissociated; recovers in < 5 s | 2. Occlude OS same as earlier<br>3. Same as 1. |
| 0 | No exotropia unless dissociated. Recovers in < 1 s | Use the worst score of the 3 measurements. |

*Abbreviations:* OD, right eye, OS left eye.

Assessed at 6 m and 33 cm. In PEDIG studies, control is assessed at 3 different times during the examination. Distance done before near.

*Adapted from* Mohney BG, Holmes JM. An office-based scale for assessing control in intermittent exotropia. Strabismus. 2006;14 (3):147 - 150.

Pretreatment, at distance, 26% of patients had latent deviations. After treatment, latent deviations were seen in 65%. Fifty-eight percent of patients no longer required surgery [82]. In a follow-up study, 3 years after treatment ended, 80% of the cohort was reevaluated and 78% maintained their improvements [85].

Freeman and Isenberg also patched the preferred eye of patients aged 9 months to 5 years for 4 to 6 hours a day, with tapering as patients showed improvement [80]. During treatment, all patients became orthophoric "at least temporarily" [80]. After 22 months of patient follow-up, 27% became orthotropic, whereas 27% became unresponsive to treatment [80].

The PEDIG group conducted 2 prospective randomized clinical trials on part-time patching; one looking at children age 3 to 10 years and the other children younger than 3 years [83,84]. Patients were assigned to observation or patching 3 hours a day for 5 months followed by a 1-month washout period. Deterioration was defined as described previously in the observation study [83,84]. Patients were assessed at 3 and 6 months. Both studies found that deterioration was not common in either group [83,84]. From these studies insufficient evidence exists to recommend part-time patching for toddlers, but that patching and observation are both acceptable for children aged 3 years and older [83,84].

Others have conducted studies similar to the PEDIG group but extended treatment for 1 year [86]. In a study of 3- to 10-year-old previously untreated patients with intermittent exotropia, Choi and colleagues found an overall improvement in 31.6% of patients. They found the following factors were associated with higher success: female gender, myopic refractive error, convergence insufficiency type exotropia, poor distance stereopsis, and a larger magnitude of the deviation at distance [86].

Akbari and colleagues [81] looked at 2 hours a day of alternate patching in patients aged 3 to 8 for 9 months. Outcomes included 3- and 6-point scale. After treatment, patients showed improvements in control at distance and near on the 6-point scale [81].

## Prism

Concerns about prism are the same as mentioned in the esotropia section.

Three types of prism designs can be used for exotropia: relieving, neutralizing, or overcorrecting. Relieving prism compensates for some of the magnitude of deviation to reduce demand on fusional vergence and allow for greater fusion stability. Neutralizing prism corrects the entire magnitude of the deviation, whereas overcorrecting prism corrects for a greater magnitude than the deviation, causing the patient to converge [64,87]. Another treatment option, inverse prism, uses base-out prism to increase fusional vergence ability [88,89]. Although relieving prism is the most common treatment option, with all approaches, practitioners will usually reduce the magnitude of prism power as the stability improves [64].

As with the other approaches, no consensus exists to the most effective magnitude of prism or treatment duration. For neutralizing prism power, Hardesty recommended a value between the distance and near deviation or a different prismatic value for distance and near viewing to be worn for at least 6 months [90].

When comparing inverse prism with relieving prism in patients aged 5 to 7 years, researchers did not find statistically significant differences in the distance angle of deviation, the NCS, or tolerance [88]. The investigators chose to fit Fresnel prism in the magnitude of one-third the distance angle of deviation for 3 months, then to cut the prism magnitude in half for 3 months, and eliminate the prism for the final 3 months.

Other researchers have looked at combining treatment methods. Feng and colleagues [91] looked at overminus spectacles with relieving prism in the treatment of intermittent exotropia in children aged 3 to 6 years. Patients were treated with −2.50 diopters over their distance cycloplegic refraction and 2$\Delta$ base in for each eye for 12 months. The treatment group showed a significant reduction in the angle of deviation especially at near and an improvement in stereopsis. The refractive error change was similar between the 2 groups [91].

## Vision therapy/orthoptics

A review by Duckman found a success rate of 43% to 100% in studies using vision therapy as a treatment of intermittent exotropia. In the cases of purely active vision therapy, 61% of studies had success of good or better, based on his criteria (see Table 1) [2]. Subsequently, Coffee and colleagues [64] reviewed studies.

To date, much of the literature involving vision therapy as a treatment of exotropia is in the form of case reports [92–96]. In addition, many case reports include multiple forms of treatment, not solely vision therapy [93–96].

Many investigators have used combinations of treatment including home- or office-based therapy, occlusion, base-in prism, overminus lenses, either presurgery or postsurgery or presurgery and postsurgery [93–96].

In addition to case reports, investigators have written on their exotropia therapy approaches, sometimes offering different strategies [97,98]. As with esotropia, vision therapy for exotropia includes equalizing monocular skills, including accommodation [96]. Therapy emphasizes gross convergence and incorporates fusional vergence techniques [92,95,96]. Work on antisuppression and diplopia awareness often is incorporated, in either early or later phases, depending on the practitioner [92,96–98]. Therapy often begins at near and progresses to distance [92]. Unlike with esotropia, fusion work progresses from third degree to simultaneous perception (first degree) [92,96].

In a retrospective review of 149 patients with strabismus treated with vision therapy, Ludlam found that patients with exotropia required fewer therapy visits than patients with esotropia. In addition, exotropes with an anomalous response on one or more tests were more likely to be "cured" than were esotropes; 62% versus 23% [58].

A retrospective review looking at patients age 5 to 22 years with intermittent exotropia found that vergence and accommodative therapy resulted in a significant improvement in the distance and near control scores [99]. Another retrospective study using pencil push-ups, occlusion, prism, and "3D activities" found success rates of 88% in patients with basic and divergence excess and 100% in those with convergence insufficiency [100].

A prospective study looked at patients with intermittent exotropia treated with a combination of occlusion, antisuppression, convergence, and fusion activities. Vision therapy was effective for angles less than 25Δ [101]. Although the magnitude of the deviation did not significantly change in many patients, 64% to 85.7% experienced an improvement in function and/or symptoms [101].

A pilot study randomized clinical trial looked at 12 weeks of office-based vergence/accommodative therapy with home reinforcement in patients aged 6 to 18 years with intermittent exotropia, excluding convergence insufficiency [102]. The researchers found that after treatment, patients experienced a significant improvement in the distance control score, the near magnitude of the deviation, and positive fusional vergence at distance [102].Table 3 provides a summary of the treatment options for patients with exotropia

## SUMMARY

When treating patients with strabismus, the ultimate goal should continue to be the improvement of cosmesis and binocularity. As such, practitioners who are primarily surgical should be cognizant of nonsurgical treatments either in lieu of or as an adjunct to surgery. Similarly, practitioners who are solely nonsurgical should be aware of indications for surgery (which is beyond the scope of this article) as well as the various nonsurgical treatment options.

Unfortunately, no consensus exists on what constitutes treatment success for either esotropia or exotropia. Motor success is generally recognized as a deviation of 10Δ or less, but that magnitude is not consistent in the literature. In addition, assessments of sensory fusion and binocularity are wide-ranging from the appreciation of basic fusion (Worth 4 Dot) to the highest level of binocularity (stereopsis). It would be helpful, if a more consistent recognition of the clinical assessment of binocularity was available.

Limited randomized clinical trials or even prospective studies exist, especially with esotropia. For esotropia treatment there is general agreement that patients should have maximum plus to best alignment, but in some cases, still disagreement occurs on how much plus can be cut. Recently, the use of bifocals in patients with high AC/A esotropia has been challenged, and currently conflicting data exist to support one treatment over another. Even in cases where surgery is indicated, researchers do not know why some children have better sensory outcomes than others. Is there more that we can do presurgically or postsurgically for these children?

For intermittent exotropia, more randomized clinical trials exist, which are helping to change the standard of care, particularly in the areas of patching and overminus treatment. However, still questions need to be answered, especially what are the optimal durations for treatment with overminus lenses, occlusion, or vision therapy? And, what is the appropriate magnitude for overminus or number of hours for occlusion?

The biggest discrepancies continue to be in the area of vision therapy/orthoptics primarily because there is such a difference in management approaches for the same condition. Many case reports, including others not included in this review, show success, but are vague in terms of specific procedures. Randomized clinical trials, using more specific treatment protocols, will provide data showing the most effective treatments for both esotropia and exotropia and would support the validity of this treatment option.

Despite all the areas that still need improvement, a solid foundation exists for the treatment of both esotropia and exotropia with considerations for both a cosmetic and functional cure. The flowcharts and treatment table in this article serve to provide a starting point for the treatment of these patients.

## CLINICS CARE POINTS

- When correcting accommodative esotropia, it is important to monitor accommodation and binocularity.
- Prism can be an effective treatment option for esotropia and exotropia.
- In intermittent exotropia, if no fixation preference is present, alternate patching may be an option. If a fixation preference exists, patching the dominant eye is an option.
- If prescribing overminus lenses, it is important to monitor for myopia progression or development. Remember that average progression of myopia is −0.50 diopters/y. Vision therapy has higher success rates for patients with intermittent exotropia than for patients with esotropia.

## DISCLOSURE

Nothing to disclose.


### References

[1] Flom MC. The prognosis in strabismus. Am J Optom Arch Am Acad Optom 1958;35: 509–14.

[2] Duckman RH. Management of binocular anomalies: efficacy of vision therapy, exotropia. Am J Optom Physiol Opt 1987;64:421–9.

[3] Rutstein RP, Daum K. Anomalies of binocular vision: diagnosis and management. St. Louis: Mosby; 1998. p. 205–46, Esotropia Chapter 8.

[4] Pediatric Eye Disease Investigator Group. Spontaneous resolution of early-onset esotropia: experience of the congenital esotropia observational study. Am J Ophthalmol 2002;133: 109–18.

[5] Brennan R, McCance P, Yeong JL, et al. Esotropia outcomes and the influence of delay to wearing full hypermetropic correction. J Pediatr Ophthalmol Strabismus 2020;57:85–9.

[6] Maples WC, Bither M. Treating the trinity of infantile vision development: infantile esotropia, amblyopia, anisometropia. Optom Vis Dev 2006;37:123–30.

[7] Christenson GN, Rouse MW, Adkins DA. Management of infantile-onset esotropia. J Am Optom Assoc 1990;61:559–72.

[8] Mohan K, Sharma A. Long-term treatment results of accommodative esotropia. JAAPOS 2014;18:261–5.

[9] Rubin SE. Bringing the management of accommodative esotropia into sharp focus. Am J Opthalmol 2006;141:914–5.

[10] MacEwen CJ, Lymburn EG, Ho WO. Is the maximum hypermetropic correction necessary in children with fully accommodative esotropia? Br J Ophthalmol 2006;92:1329–32.

[11] Park KA, Oh SY. The effect of reducing hyperopic correction in patients with accommodative esotropia. JAAPOS 2013;17:363–6.

[12] Black BC. The influence of refractive error management on the natural history and treatment outcome of accommodative esotropia. Trans Am Ophthalmol Soc 2006;104: 303–21.

[13] Reddy AK, Freeman CH, Paysee EA, et al. A data-driven approach to the management of accommodative esotropia. Am J Ophthalmol 2009;148:466–70.

[14] Liang SLH, Friske TR. Diagnosis and management of accommodative esotropia. Clin Exp Optom 2006;89:325–31.

[15] Watanabe-Numata K, Hayasaka S, Watanabe K, et al. Changes in deviation following correction of hyperopia in children with fully refractive accommodative esotropia. Ophthalmologica 2000;214:309–11.

[16] Swan KC. Accommodative esotropia long range follow-up. Ophthalmology 1983;90: 1141–5.

[17] Bonafede L, Bender L, Shaffer J, et al. Refractive change in children with accommodative esotropia. Br J Ophthalmol 2020;104:1283–7.

[18] Repka MX, Wellish K, Wisnicki HJ, et al. Changes in the refractive error of 94 spectacle-treated patients with acquired accommodative esotropia. Binoc Vis 1989;4:15–21.

[19] Berk AT, Kocak N, Ellidokuz H. Treatment outcomes in refractive accommodative esotropia. JAAPOS 2004;8:384–8.

[20] Raab EL, Spierer A. Persisting accommodative esotropia. Arch Ophthalmol 1986;104: 1777–9.

[21] Hutcheson KA, Ellish NJ, Lambert SR. Weaning children with accommodative esotropia out of spectacles: a pilot study. Br J Ophthalmol 2003;87:4–7.

[22] Rutstein RP, Marsh-Tootle W. Clinical course of accommodative esotropia. Optom Vis Sci 1998;75:97–102.

[23] Shin DH, Choi CY, Han SY. Risk factors for spontaneous consecutive exotropia in children with refractive and nonrefractive accommodative esotropia. Jpn J Ophthalmol 2020;64: 292–7.
[24] Lambert SR, Sramek J, Hutcheson KA. Clinical features predictive of successfully weaning from spectacles those children with accommodative esotropia. JAAPOS 2003;7:7–13.
[25] Senior JD, Chandna A, O'Connor AR. Spontaneous consecutive exotropia in childhood. Strabismus 2009;17:33–6.
[26] Stager DR, Weakley DR, Everett M, Birch EE. Delayed consecutive exotropia following 7mm bilateral medial recuts recession for congential esotropia. J Pediatr Ophthalmol Strabismus 1994;31:147–50.
[27] Ludwig IH, Imberman SP, Thompson HW, et al. Long-term study of accommodative esotropia. J AAPOS 2005;9:522–6.
[28] Hussein MA, Weakley D, Wirazka T, et al. The long-term outcomes in children who are not compliant with spectacle treatment for accommodative esotropia. JAAPOS 2015;19: 169–71.
[29] Parks MM. Management of acquired esotropia. Br J Ophthalmol 1974;58:240–7.
[30] Raab EL. Accommodative ET-high AC/A ratio esotropia: the case for glasses. Am Orthopt J 2016;66:1–4.
[31] Olitsky SE. High AC/A ratio esotropia: do we really need to be using bifocals? Am Orthoptic J 2016;66:5–9.
[32] Albert DG, Lederman ME. Abnormal distance:near esotropia. Doc Ophthalmol 1973;34: 27–36.
[33] Pratt-Johnnson JA, Tillson G. The management of esotropia with high AC/A ratio (convergence excess). J Pediatr Ophthalmol Strabismus 1985;22:238–42.
[34] Whitman MC, MacNeill K, Hunter D. Bifocals fail to improve stereopsis outcomes in high AC/A accommodative esotropia. Ophthalmology 2016;123:690–6.
[35] Jacob J-L, Beaulieu Y, Brumet G. Progressive-addition lenses in the management of esotropia with a high accommodative/convergence ratio. Can J Ophthalmol 1980;15:166–9.
[36] Mezer E, Wygnanski -Jaffe T, Stolovich C. Progressive-addition lenses for accommodative esotropia with a high accommodative element. Strabismus 2015;23:170–5.
[37] Abdi S, Thunholm-henriksson I, Pansell T. Stepwise increase of hypermetropic correction using contact lenses in intermittent partially accommodative esotropia. Clin Exp Optom 2016;99:258–63.
[38] Gonzalez E, Barra F, Sanchez I, et al. High AC/A accommodative esotropia strabismus treatment with contact lenses: a single case design (N=1) study. Binocul Vis Strabismus Q 2007;22:90–5.
[39] Eustis HM, Mungan NK. Monovision for treatment of accommodative esotropia with a high AC/A ratio. JAAPOS 1999;3:87–90.
[40] Morton GV, Kushner BJ, Lucchese NJ, et al. The efficacy of SimulVue and Unilens RGP aspheric bifocal contact lenses in the treatment of esotropia associated with a high accommodative convergence/accommodation ratio. JAAPOS 1998;2:108–12.
[41] Moore B. Treatment of accommodatie esotropia with unilens RGP aspheric multifocal contact lenses 1994. Available at: https://www.aaopt.org/detail/knowledge-base-article/treatment-accommodative-esotropia-unilens-rgp-aspheric-multifocal-contact-lenses Last accessed January 21, 2022.
[42] Caloroso EE, Rouse MW. Occlusion therapy in clinical management of strabismus. Boston: Butterworth-Heinemann; 1993. p. 113–26.
[43] Tassinari JD. Binasal occlusion. J Beh Optom 1991;1:16–21.
[44] Rutstein RP, Daum KM. Amblyopia in anomalies of binocular vision: diagnosis and management. St. Louis: Mosby; 1998. p. 7–60.
[45] Greenwald I. Effective strabismus therapy. Santa Ana,CA: Opt Extension Prog; 1979.
[46] Yin X, Yang H, Chen Y, et al. Effect of Binasal Occlusion in Children with Concomitant Esotropia. Chin J Optom Ophthalmol Vis Sci 2020;22:764–8.

[47] Choe HR, Yang HE, Hwang J-M. Long-term outcomes of prismatic correction in partially accommodative esotropia. PLoS One 2019;14(12):e0225654.
[48] Chang F, Wang T, Yu J, et al. Prism treatment of acute acquired concomitant esotropia precipitated by visual confusion. Strabismus 2020;28:7–12.
[49] Veronneau-Troutman S. Fresnel prism and their effects on visual acuity and binocularity. Trans Am Ophthalmol Soc 1978;76:610–53.
[50] Caloroso EE, Rouse MW. Prism correction in clinical management of strabismus. Boston: Butterworth-Heinemann; 1993. p. 94–112.
[51] Birnbaum MH. Adverse response of prism therapy in strabismus. J Am Optom Assoc 1976;47:1195–9.
[52] Christenson GN, Rouse MW. Management of a young esotrope using vision therapy and prismatic prescription. J Am Optom Assoc 1987;58:592–6.
[53] Krumholtz I, FitzGerald DE. Outcome indicators in a strabismic sample treated by vision therapy. J Beh Optom 1999;10:143–6.
[54] Ziegler D, Huff D, Rouse MW. Success in strabismus therapy: a literature review. J Am Optom Assoc 1982;53:979–83.
[55] Griffin JR. 2nd edition.. Binocular anomalies: procedures for vision therapy, 168 Chicago: Professional Pres; 1982. p. 172–313.
[56] FitzGerald DE. Congenital esotropia: case report. J Beh Optom 1992;3:59–64.
[57] Hellerstein LF, Dowis RT, Maples WC. Optometric management of strabismus patients. J Am Optom Assoc 1994;65:621–5.
[58] Ludlam WM. Orthopic treatment of strabismus. Am J Optom Arch Am Acad Optom 1961;61:369–88.
[59] FitzGerald DE, Gruning CF. Vision therapy for a preschool child with acquired accommodative esotropia. J Beh Optom 1997;8:59–63.
[60] Wick B. Accommodative esotropia: efficacy of therapy. J Am Optom Assoc 1987;58: 562–6.
[61] Wick B. Visual therapy for small angle esotropia. Am J Optom Physiol Opt 1974;51: 490–6.
[62] Duane A. A new classification of the motor anomalies of the eyes based upon physiological principles. Ann Ophthalmol 1897;6:247–60.
[63] Rutstein RP, Daum KM. Strabismus in anomalies of binocular vision: diagnosis and management. St. Louis: Mosby; 1998. p. 189–204.
[64] Coffee B, Wick B, Cotter S, et al. Treatment options in intermittent exotropia: a critical appraisal. Optom Vis Sci 1992;69:386–404.
[65] Rutstein RP, Corliss DA. The clinical course of intermittent exotropia. Optom Vis Sci 2003;80:644–9.
[66] Nusz KJ, Monhney BG, Diehl NN. The course of intermittent exotropia in a population-based cohort. Ophthalmology 2006;113:1154–8.
[67] Buck D, Powell CJ, Rahi J, et al. The improving outcomes in intermittent exotropia study: outcomes at 2 years after diagnosis in an observational cohort. BMC Ophthalmol 2012;1; https://doi.org/10.1186/1471-2415-12-1.
[68] Haggerty H, Richardson S, Hrisos S, et al. The Newcastle Control Score: a new method of grading the severity of intermittent distance exotropia. Br J Ophthalmol 2004;88:233–5.
[69] Holmes JM, Hatt SR, Leske DA. Is intermittent exotropia a curable condition? Eye 2015;29: 171–6.
[70] Mohney BG, Cotter SA, Chandler DL, et al. Three-year observation of children 3 to 10 years of age with untreated intermittent exotropia. Ophthalmology 2019;126:1249–60.
[71] Figueira EC, Hing S. Intermittent exotropia comparison of treatments. Clin Exp Ophthalmol 2006;34:245–51.
[72] Caltrider N, Jampolsky A. Overcorrecting minus lens therapy for treatment of intermittent exotropia. Ophthalmology 1983;90:1160–5.

[73] Bayramlar H, Gurturk AY, Sari U, et al. Overcorrecting minus lens therapy in patients with intermittent exotropia: Should it be the first therapeutic choice? Int Ophthalmol 2017;37: 385–90.
[74] Kennedy JR. The correction of divergent strabismus with concave lenses. Am J Optom Arch Am Acad Optom 1954;31:605–14.
[75] Goodacre H. Minus overcorrection: conservative treatment of intermittent exotropia in the young child: a comparative study. Aust Orthopt J 1985;22:9–17.
76 Watts P, Tippings E, Al-Madfai H. Intermittent exotropia, overcorrecting minus lenses and the Newcastle scoring system. JAAPOS 2005;9:460–4.
[77] Kushner BJ. Does overcorrecting minus lens therapy for intermittent exotropia cause myopia? Arch Ophthalmol 1999;117:638–42.
[78] Chen AM, Erzurum AM, Chandler CL, et al. Overminus lens therapy for children 3 to 10 years of age with intermittent exotropia. JAMA Ophthalmol 2021;139:464–76.
[79] Mohney B, Holmes JM. An Office-based scale for assessing control in intermittent exotropia. Strabismus 2006;14:147–50.
[80] Freeman RS, Isenberg SJ. The use of part-time occlusion for early onset unilateral exotropia. J Pediatr Ophthalmol Strabismus 1989;26:94–6.
[81] Akberi MR, Mirzajani A, Moeinitabar MR, et al. The effect of alternate occlusion on control of intermittent exotropia in children. Eur J Ophthalmol 2020;30:275–9.
[82] Spoor DK, Hiles DA. Occlusion therapy of exodeviations occurring in infants and young children. Ophthalmology 1979;86:2152–7.
[83] Cotter SA, Mohney BG, Chandler DL, et al. A randomized trial comparing part-time patching with observation for children 3 to 10 years of age with intermittent exotropia. Ophthalmology 2014;121:2299–310.
[84] Cotter SA, Mohney BG, Chandler DL, et al. A randomized trial comparing part-time patching with observation for intermittent exotropia in children 12 to 35 months of age. Ophthalmology 2015;122:1718–25.
[85] Spoor DK, Hiles DA. Occlusion therapy of exodeviations occurring in infants and young children- a three year follow up. Am Orthopt J 1983;33:116–20.
[86] Choi H, Kim S, Jung J, et al. Factors associated with the effectiveness of part-time patching for intermittent exotropia in children. Eur J Ophthalmol 2021 Aug 10; https://doi.org/10.1177/1120672121110378 1120672121110378.
[87] Worrell BE, Hirsch MJ, Morgan MW. An evaluation of prism prescribed by Sheard's criterion. Optom Vis Sci 1971;48:373–6.
[88] El Gendy NMS, Nabi EA. Is inverse prism therapy comparable to conventional prism therapy for improving Newcastle scores in patients with basic intermittent exotropia? Semin Ophthalmol 2019;34:497–503.
[89] Jamplosky A. Characteristics of suppression in strabismus. Arch Ophthalmol 1955;54: 683–96.
[90] Hardesty HH. The use of prisms in the management of non paretic strabismus. Prisms in the management of intermittent exotropia. Am Orthopt J 1972;22:22–30.
[91] Feng Y, Jiang J, Bai X, et al. A randomized trial evaluating efficacy of overminus lenses combined with prism in the treatment of children with intermittent exotropia. BMC Ophthalmol 2021;21:73.
[92] Peddle A, Han E, Steiner A. Vision therapy for basic exotropia in adults: 2 case studies. Optometry 2011;82:467–74.
[93] Wick B. Visual therapy for constant exotropia with anomalous retinal correspondence – a case report. Am J Optom Physiol Opt 1974;51:1005–8.
[94] Wick B. "Forced elimination" of anomalous retinal correspondence in constant exotropia – a case report. Am J Optom Physiol Opt 1975;52:58–62.
[95] Gallaway M, Vaxmonsky T, Scheiman M. Management of intermittent exotropia using a combination of visual therapy and surgery. J Am Optom Assoc 1989;60:428–34.

[96] Frantz KA. The importance of multiple treatment modalities in a case of divergence excess. J Am Optom Assoc 1990;61:457–62.
[97] Flax N. Management of divergence excess intermittent exotropia. J Beh Optom 1996;7(66):72–3.
[98] Cooper J. A Viewpoint: intermittent exotropia of the divergence excess type. J Beh Optom 1996;7:67–72.
[99] Ma MM-L, Kang Y, Chen C, et al. Vision therapy for intermittent exotropia : a case series. J Optom 2021;14:247–53.
[100] Asadi R, Ghasemi-Falavarjani K, Sadighi N. Orthoptic treatment in the management of intermittent exotropia. Iranian J Ophthalmol 2009;21:35–40.
[101] Singh V, Roy S, Sinha S. Role of orthoptic treatment in the management of intermittent exotropia. Indian J Ophthalmol 1992;40:83–5.
[102] Ma MM-L, Ying K, Scheiman M, et al. Office-based vergence and accommodative therapy for the treatment of intermittent exotropia: a pilot study. Optom Vis Sci 2019;96:925–33.

# Pediatric

Advances in Ophthalmology and Optometry 7 (2022) 71–87

ADVANCES IN OPHTHALMOLOGY AND OPTOMETRY

# Update on Pediatric Optic Neuritis

Sravanthi Vegunta, MD*

Moran Eye Center, 65 Mario Capecchi Dive, Salt Lake City, UT 84132, USA

**Keywords**

• Pediatric neurology • Neuro-ophthalmology • Optic neuritis
• Acute demyelinating syndromes • Myelin oligodendrocyte glycoprotein
• Neuromyelitis optica • Multiple sclerosis

**Key points**

- Pediatric optic neuritis has a wide differential including clinically isolated syndrome, multiple sclerosis, myelin oligodendrocyte glycoprotein, neuro-myelitis optica spectrum disorder, infectious causes, and parainfectious causes.
- Acute and chronic treatment of these conditions varies, thus understanding the differences between these diseases and making the correct diagnosis is essential to preserve vision.
- Prospective studies are lacking in this field and are needed to better elucidate the need for long-term immunomodulatory therapies, monitoring antibody titers, and imaging surveillance.

## Abbreviations

| | |
|---|---|
| ON | Optic neuritis |
| MS | multiple sclerosis |
| MOGAD | myelin oligodendrocyte glycoprotein-associated disease |
| NMOSD | neuro myelitis optica spectrum disorder |
| CIS | clinically isolated syndrome |
| ADS | acute demyelinating syndromes |

## INTRODUCTION

The diagnosis of optic neuritis (ON) during the past 30 years has changed from indicating a possible risk factor for multiple sclerosis (MS) , infectious cause, or

The author has no commercial or financial conflicts or funding sources.

*Corresponding Author. *E-mail address:* srav.vegunta@hsc.utah.edu

https://doi.org/10.1016/j.yaoo.2022.03.001
2452-1760/22/

parainfectious cause to a consideration of a wide differential of neurologic autoimmune diseases. We now have a deeper understanding of the epidemiology and varied presentations of neuromyelitis optica spectrum disorders (NMOSD) and myelin oligodendrocyte glycoprotein-associated diseases (MOGAD) among children and adults. Typical ON includes clinically isolated syndrome (CIS) and MS, whereas atypical ON includes NMOSD, MOGAD, and rare infectious or parainfectious causes. Properly recognizing patterns of disease presentation and making the correct diagnosis is time-sensitive and paramount given that acute and chronic treatments to restore and preserve vision depend on the diagnosis.

The purpose of this article is to discuss pediatric ON. The diseases that will be discussed in detail are ON related to MS, CIS, NMOSD, and MOGAD. Given the recent ability to perform antibody (Ab) testing for the latter 2 diseases, a shifting paradigm has occurrred in the literature regarding clinical versus laboratory classification of these diseases to better study presentations and prognoses.

## SIGNIFICANCE

### Overview of pediatric optic neuritis

#### *Epidemiology*

ON is a unilateral or bilateral inflammation of the optic nerve(s). The disease can be a CIS and not associated with any disease. Alternatively, it can be associated with an infectious process, parainfectious process, or a central nervous system (CNS) demyelinating condition. The incidence of ON in the United States was found to be 1.66/100,000 person years, based on a multiethnic cohort in Southern California of 81 incident cases of acute demyelinating syndromes (ADS) over 4.87 million person years of observation [1]. In incidence of ON in Canada was lower at 0.2/100,000 person years, based on a national survey of pediatricians between 2004 and 2007 and 219 children with ADS [2]. The mean age of presentation among children is 9 to 11 years [3–7]. Younger children tend to present with bilateral disease. Older children, similar to adults, tend to present unilaterally. In Waldman and colleagues' meta-analysis of pediatric ON, bilateral ON was present in 72% of children aged 10 years or younger, whereas unilateral ON was present in 70% of children aged 10 years or older ($P < 0.001$) [8]. Among postpubertal children, the girl to boy ratio is 2:1, similar to that among adults [7,9,10]. However, among prepubertal children, the frequency is equal among girls and boys [9]. No prospective study of ON exists in children, so most of our knowledge of the disease is based on the results of the optic neuritis treatment trial (ONTT) [11].

#### *Signs and symptoms*

Patients may present with retrobulbar pain, headaches, or pain with eye movements. Children have more difficulty describing the above symptoms, so they may initially present with only decrease in central vision during the course of hours to days. Visual acuity (VA) and color vision loss can range at presentation. Twenty percent of children with ON have VA of ≥20/40, 20% have VA between 20/50 and 20/190, and 60% have VA of ≤20/200 [12,13]. Per the ONTT, only about 35% of adult cases of ON presented with papillitis, whereas the remaining cases presented with retrobulbar ON [11]. However, pediatric ON presents with papillitis in up to 73% of cases (Fig. 1) [10,14]. Unilateral ON can present with a moderate relative afferent pupillary defect. The most common visual field defect in children who can complete formal visual field testing is a central or cecocentral scotoma [4,15].

*Testing*

Because most pediatric patients present with papillitis and bilateral ON, findings concerning for possible papilledema, they should undergo magnetic resonance imaging (MRI) of the orbits and brain with and without contrast to evaluate for hydrocephalus, space occupying lesions, meningitis, and other demyelinating lesions. The minority of patients who have vision loss and relative afferent pupillary defect without papillitis should also have the above imaging to evaluate the cause of vision loss. Additionally, patients who have findings concerning for MOGAD and NMOSD should have spinal imaging (discussed below). The typical optic nerve findings on imaging consist of thickening of the nerves on T1 sequence and postgadolinium enhancement and hyperintense T2 signal along the optic nerve or chiasm [16].

Imaging of the optic nerve with optical coherence tomography retinal nerve fiber layer thickness (OCT RNFL) can be a quick and easy way to follow subtle changes in the optic nerves over time in the ophthalmology or neurology clinic. In typical ON (CIS, MS-ON, or nonantibody-mediated ON), OCT RNFL thinning occurs as a stepwise decrease with each episode (Figs. 2 and 3). The retinal nerve fiber layer (RNFL) is more severely thinned in Ab-mediated ON. Additionally, pediatric patients with MOGAD-ON can have

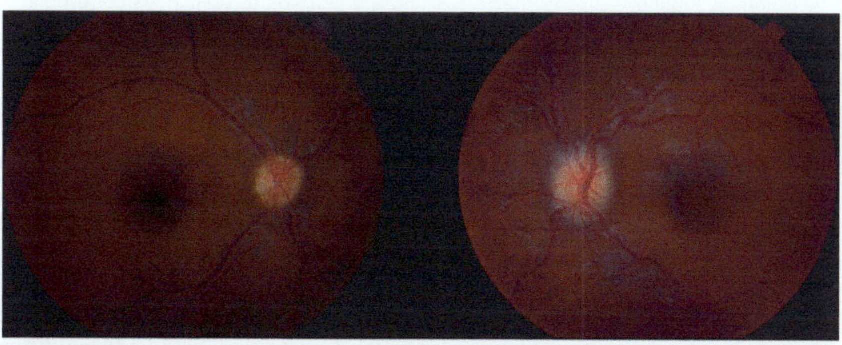

**Fig. 1.** Case 1: A 15-year-old girl presented with left eye pain. She had inferior visual field loss followed by superior field loss and eventually no light perception vision in the left eye. Fundus photos showing normal right optic nerve and left optic nerve swelling. She had positive serum aquaporin-4 antibody titer of 1:640.

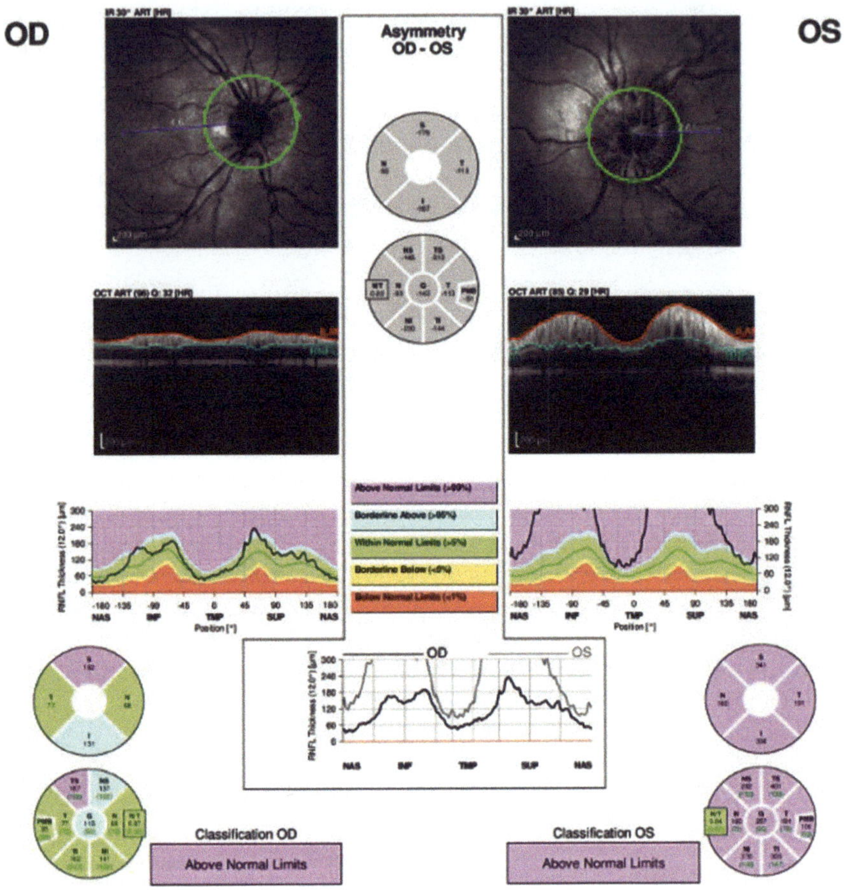


**Fig. 2.** Case 1: OCT RNFL scan of the left eye showing diffuse swelling. The right eye optic nerve is normal. Right eye superior nerve swelling is artifactual, as seen in the corresponding line scan.

progressive reduction in RNFL even without apparent clinical episodes and with preservation of VA [17,18].

Lumbar puncture with opening pressure is indicated because the differential includes elevated intracranial pressure, infection, and MS, among others. Cerebrospinal fluid (CSF) studies should include protein and glucose levels, cell count and differential, oligoclonal bands (OCB), and IgG index. If infection is suspected, additional CSF studies should include microbiology evaluation with viral polymerase chain reaction panel(s), Gram stain, and bacterial/fungal cultures [9,19].

Cell-based assays are the gold standard for the detection of MOG-IgG and aquaporin 4 (AQP4)-IgG. Serum testing is more sensitive than CSF testing [20]. The 2018 international recommendations on the diagnosis of MOGAD

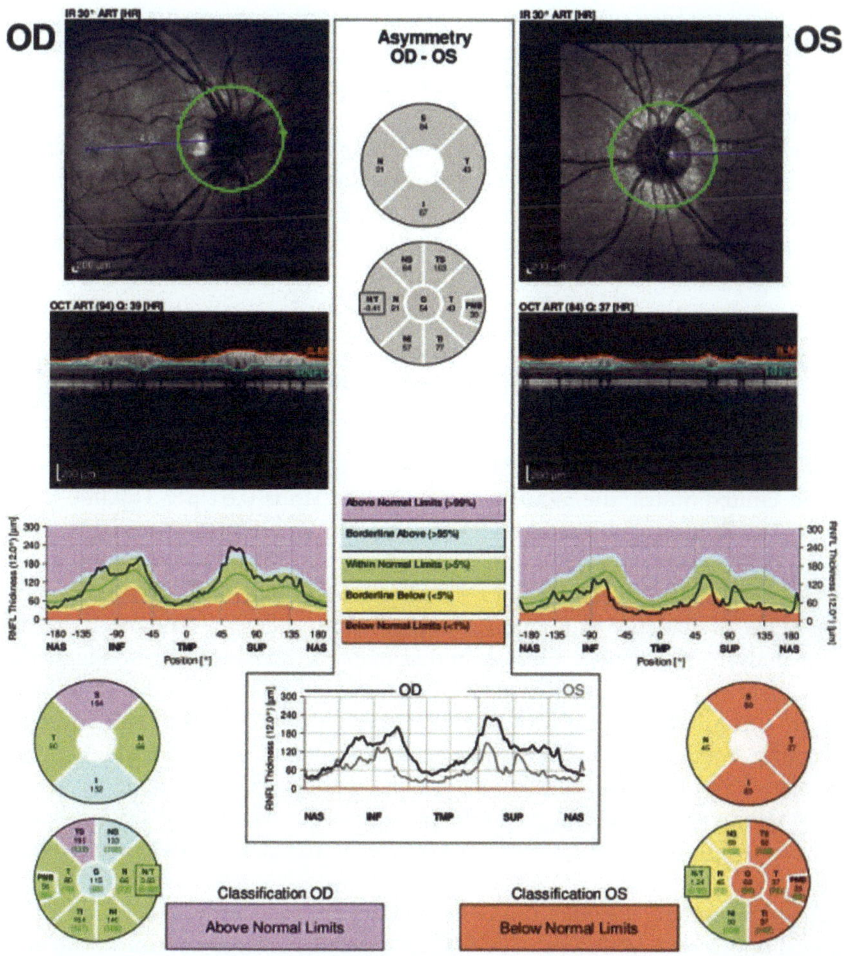


**Fig. 3.** Case 1: OCT RNFL scan one year after optic neuritis episode showing diffuse thinning of the left optic nerve and a stable right eye scan.

suggest selectively screening adults and adolescents for MOG-IgG because unscrupulously testing a rare biomarker can reduce its positive predictive value. However, MOG-IgG positivity is more common in children than adults, so children should more freely be tested for this antibody. Because simultaneously positive AQP4-IgG and MOG-IgG virtually does not exist, patients should be screened for the most likely biomarker with reflex testing to the other Ab [21,22]. Children with NMOSD can have negative AQP4-IgG Ab testing for up to 4 years after disease onset. Patients should have serial testing, if there is high clinical suspicion of NMOSD [23]. Positive antibodies have prognostic implications, as patients have a higher rate of relapses and worse visual outcomes compared with seronegative patients [24]. Pediatric NMOSD patients are less likely to have positive AQP4-IgG compared with adults. In a UK study, 50% of children with NMOSD had positive MOG-IgG and only 8% had positive AQP4-IgG [23].

Children with ON should have additional basic laboratory work up including serum and/or angiotensin-converting enzyme and chest X-ray for sarcoidosis, quantiferon gold, fluorescent treponemal Ab absorption and rapid plasma reagin, *Borrelia burgdorferi* antibodies, *Bartonella henselae* antibodies, and antinuclear Ab for lupus [25].

*Visual outcomes*

Full high-contrast visual acuity (HCVA) recovery ≥20/30 or 20/40 occurs in the majority (58%–97%) of children [26]. Patients experience this visual recovery by 3 months after the episode [27].

### Multiple sclerosis-associated optic neuritis

In the United States, the incidence of pediatric MS is 0.51 per 100,000 person years [1]. Children are less likely to convert to MS (22%–29% variable follow-up periods) compared with adults (50% more than 15 years, in setting of other CNS white matter lesions) [21]. ON is the presenting feature of pediatric MS in 10%–22% of patients [1,6,25]. Heussinger and colleagues reported in their meta-analysis of pediatric ON cases that every 1-year increase in age at diagnosis of ON was associated with a 32% increased risk of MS [8]. Risk factors for MS include MRI brain with white matter lesions on T2 and fluid-attenuated inversion recovery (FLAIR) sequences, sequential or recurrent ON, and elevated CSF OCB [25]. In the pediatric population where acute demyelinating encephalomyelitis (ADEM) is more common, the McDonald criteria can be applied to children aged 12 years or younger in the absence of encephalopathy [28].

Acute treatment includes intravenous (IV) or oral steroids. If no significant clinical improvement occurs with the first dose of steroids, a second dose of steroids, IV immunoglobulin (IVIG), or plasma exchange (PLEX) can be considered [29]. Children are 2 to 3 times more likely to experience relapse episodes of MS compared with adults; therefore, disease-modifying drugs (DMD) should be initiated early. First-line medications in children include interferon-β (INF-β) and glatiramer acetate. Second-line medications include natalizumab or rituximab and fingolimod [25].

### Myelin oligodendrocyte glycoprotein-associated disease optic neuritis

*Epidemiology*

According to Dutch studies, the incidence of pediatric MOGAD is between 0.14 and 0.31/100,000 person years [30,31]. The incidence among adults is 0.13/100,000 person years [32].

*Signs and symptoms*

Although the differences between typical and atypical ON are clear, the differences between MOGAD-ON and NMOSD-ON are less clear. The diagnosis of

NMOSD does not require AQP4-IgG positivity or MOG-IgG negativity [33]. Thus, patients can be diagnosed with MOG-IgG-positive NMOSD-phenotype. Other phenotypes of MOGAD in the literature include ADEM-phenotype, transverse myelitis (TM)-phenotype, longitudinally extensive transverse myelitis (LETM)-phenotype, ADEM + ON-phenotype, (LE)TM + ON-phenotype, and ADEM + (LE)TM + ON-phenotype. The latter 2 phenotypes are the same or similar to the NMOSD-phenotype. However, MOG-IgG positivity suggests a less severe disease course than AQP4-IgG positivity, as discussed below. The current dilemma is whether to consider MOG-IgG and AQP4-IgG-associated disorders separate diseases or the same disease under the general umbrella of NMOSD [23].

The clinical phenotype of MOGAD has a bimodal distribution. MOG is expressed in different regions of the brain in different age groups. Patients aged 9 years or younger tend to present with ADEM, and patients aged 9 years or older, including adults, tend to present with ON, TM, brainstem lesions, and/or NMOSD-phenotype [34]. ON is the most common presenting symptom in MOGAD. In an observational case series of 87 patients, pain with eye movements was present in 86%, and papillitis was present in 86% [35]. Among pediatric patients presenting with bilateral ON 73% had MOG-IgG, which is not typical of seronegative ON. Other studies have shown that bilateral simultaneous ON was present in 29% to 50% of pediatric patients with MOGAD [34]. Similar to seronegative and AQP4-IgG ON, patients with MOG-ON have severe visual loss ≤20/200 at nadir. However, patients with MOGAD usually have a better visual recovery than patients with AQP4-IgG and similar to patients with MS-ON at 6-month follow-up. Patients with MOGAD have visual recovery with VA of ≥20/25 in 89% of patients [36].

*Imaging*

Patients with MOGAD should have MRI brain, orbits, and whole spine imaging with contrast at the time of diagnosis.

MOGAD and AQP4-IgG patients have longitudinally extensive lesions of the optic nerve(s), involving the anterior optic nerve, more than half the length of the prechiasmatic nerve, and sometimes the chiasm. Specific to patients with MOGAD is perineural enhancement (Fig. 4) and orbital soft tissue inflammation [34]. Brain MRI typically shows T2-hyperintense, poorly demarcated subcortical, deep white matter, and deep gray matter supratentorial lesions. The lesions are usually greater than 2 cm in size. Brain and spinal lesions may not enhance or may enhance more diffusely than MS or AQP4-IgG NMOSD lesions. In ADEM, patients may have areas of restricted diffusion due to cytotoxic edema. However, this is not common in pediatric MOGAD. Brain and spinal lesions resolve on follow-up imaging, and new lesions develop during new neurologic episodes. Occasionally, new lesions can develop in asymptomatic patients [37].

OCT RNFL thinning of the optic nerves is similar in patients with MOGAD and AQP4-IgG ON and greater than in patients with seronegative ON (Figs. 5

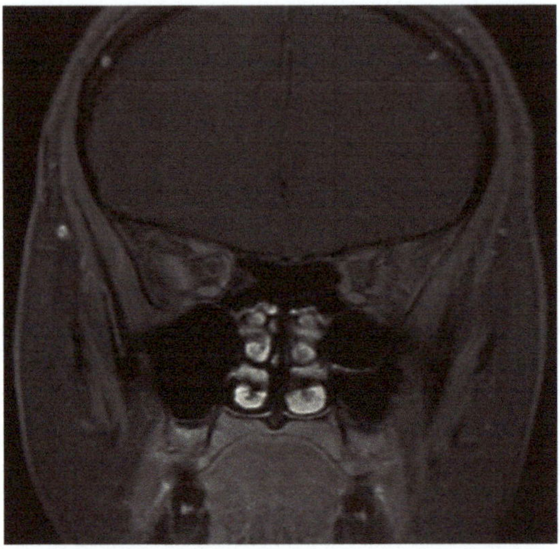

**Fig. 4.** Case 2: A 17-year-old girl admitted to the hospital with viral meningitis. Shortly after discharge from the hospital, she developed bilateral blurry vision. MRI orbital T1 postgadolinium fat-saturated coronal scan showing bilateral perineural enhancement. She tested positive for myelin oligodendrocyte glycoprotein antibodies.

and 6) [29]. However, patients with MOGAD have better visual outcomes than AQP4-IgG-positive patients. Theoretically, this may be due to the pathophysiology of MOGAD–demyelination with sparing of the ganglion cell axons. AQP4-IgG disease, an astrocytopathy, results in direct axon apoptosis [21].

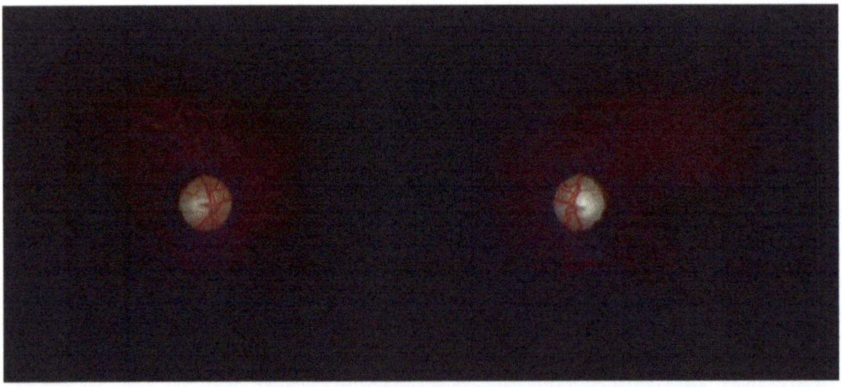

**Fig. 5.** Case 2: Fundus photos at presentation show diffuse bilateral optic nerve pallor, indicating that she may have had subclinical episodes of optic nerve demyelination prior to presentation.

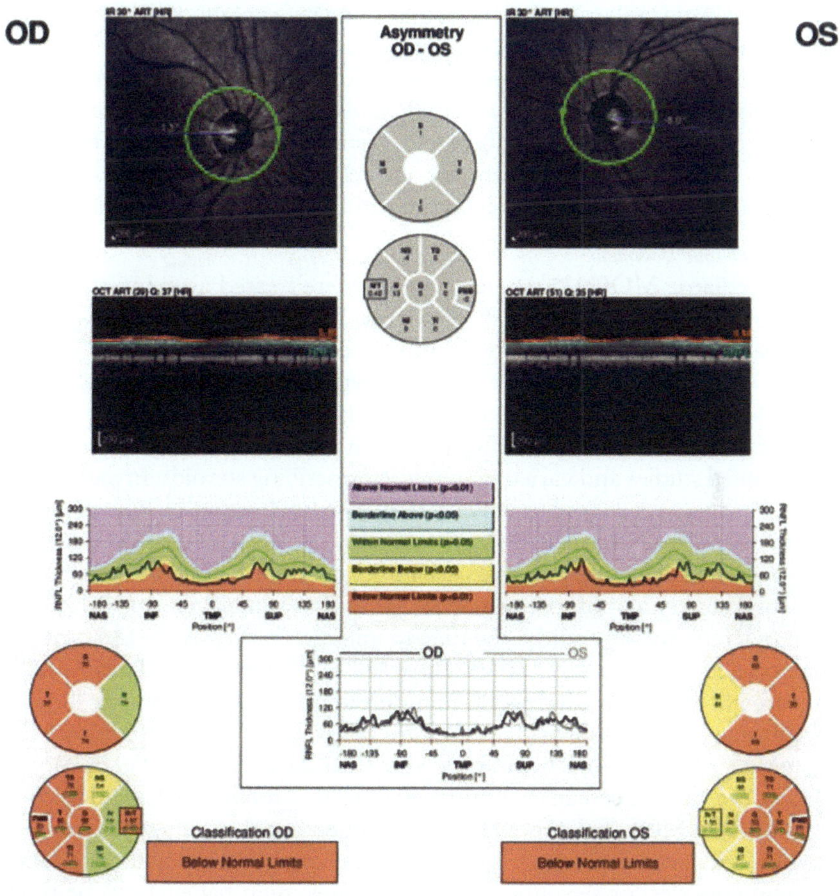


**Fig. 6.** Case 2: OCT RNFL scan showing diffuse optic nerve thinning bilaterally at time of presentation.

*Prognosis*

Two-thirds of MOGAD children have a monophasic disease course, and one-third of patients have relapsing disease. In children aged 9 years or older and adults, recurrent ON is the most frequent course. Adults more commonly have an isolated recurrent ON. Children aged less than 9 years can have relapses with recurrent ON, ADEM-ON, or NMOSD-phenotype [21,34]. Seropositivity on repeat serum MOG-IgG testing places patients at higher risk of relapse [34].

Additionally, the NMOSD-phenotype patients are more likely to have disease relapse with ON and/or (LE)TM. Among patients with NMOSD-phenotype, those with AQP4-IgG are more likely to relapse than patients with MOG-IgG [34].

Pediatric MOG-ON patients have relapses that are highly steroid-responsive, or even steroid-dependent. Therefore, relapsing MOG-IgG patients often meet criteria for chronic relapsing inflammatory optic neuropathy (CRION). Petzold and colleagues reported in a systematic review of 122 CRION cases with an age range of patients 14 to 69 years old [38]. The diagnostic criteria includes 2 ON episodes or more with decreased visual function, optic nerve enhancement on MRI, and negative laboratory testing for AQP4-IgG. The disease must also respond to steroid treatment and relapse on its withdrawal. Most patients present with ON, but patients also can have TM or encephalitis [29,34].

*Management and treatment*

In most pediatric MOGAD studies, patients were treated acutely with intravenous methylprednisolone (IVMP). Similar to seronegative or MS-ON, patients were treated with 20 to 30 mg/kg/d during 3 to 5 days up to 1 g/d. [41] Patients with MOGAD have a higher risk of relapse with fast taper. A slow taper during the course of 6 months reduced the risk of relapse [39]. However, the duration and dose of steroid taper and its effectiveness in preventing relapses is still unclear due to limited studies and varied practices in prescribing steroids. In patients who do not improve with steroid treatment, IVIG can be effective. IVIG is prescribed at 20 to 30 mg/kg/d up to 1 g/kg for 1 to 5 days. PLEX also can be added as an acute treatment; however, it is less well tolerated than IVIG. PLEX results in excellent recovery in most patients who do not show improvement with steroids alone. In a retrospective study, the time to initiation of PLEX (3–186 days) was not associated with the effect of the therapy [40,41]. Generally, patients with MOGAD are not placed on a long-term immunosuppressive therapy after the initial ON episode, because patients tend to have better visual recovery and less long-term visual loss compared to patients with NMOSD, seronegative, or MS ON. Relapses are rare in pediatric cohorts. Risk factors for relapses include consistently elevated MOG-IgG Ab markers, ON phenotype, older age, and short interval before next relapse [34]. If patients have severe neurologic compromise, recurrent episodes, or steroid-dependent relapses, then patients can be treated with the first-line agents, mycophenolate mofetil or azathioprine. Second-line agents include monthly IVIG and rituximab. If patients have a relapse while being treated with these medications, then they can switch to a different maintenance therapy, combination therapy, or low-dose steroid maintenance. Per European Union (E.U.) recommendations, if a patient does not have a relapse for 2 years, then they can consider deescalating maintenance therapy [41].

Patients with MOG-IgG ON should be tested and diagnosed separate from MS patients because patients with MOGAD will not have a reduction in relapses when treated with MS DMD such as INF-β, glatiramer acetate, or natalizumab. Importantly, alemtuzumab can worse MOGAD disease processes [21].

### Neuromyelitis optica spectrum disorder optic neuritis

*Epidemiology*

NMOSD diagnostic criteria published in 2015 by Wingerchuk and colleagues indicate that patients must meet a combination of clinical and imaging criteria but do not necessarily need to be seropositive for AQP4-IgG [33]. In fact, patients with MOG-IgG can be diagnosed with NMOSD, that is, MOG-IgG-positive NMOSD-phenotype. Wingerchuk's criteria apply to children with the exception that LETM is not specific to NMOSD. Children with ADEM and MS can also have LETM. NMOSD is generally an adult-onset disease with average age of onset in the fourth or fifth decades of life. Children only make up 3% to 5% of patients, and age of onset is 10 to 12 years. Rarely, NMOSD can present in children aged 16 months or younger [24]. This disease is more prevalent among Asian ethnicities. The incidence of NMOSD in children is 0.06/100,000 person years in Japan [42]. Among studies from Europe, Asia, and South America, the incidence of pediatric and adult-onset NMOSD is 0.05 to 4/100,000 per person years [23].

*Signs and symptoms*

NMOSD presents with ON in 50% to 75% of children, but recurrent attacks commonly present with TM [29]. Children have a 1% to 7% risk of developing NMO after an ON episode. A classic presentation of NMOSD in children and adults is intractable vomiting and hiccups due to area postrema syndrome. This presentation is more common in NMOSD and ADEM than in MS. Brainstem and cerebellar symptoms as seen in acute brainstem syndromes occur in 33% to 39% of adult and pediatric patients. Symptoms can include trigeminal neuralgia, diplopia, facial palsy, dysarthria, hypogeusia, pruritis, hearing loss, and vestibular ataxia [23].

Patients with NMOSD can have a more devastating neurologic course possibly due to direct astrocytopathy and neuronal necrosis caused by AQP4-Ab, whereas MS and MOGAD result in demyelination [21].

*Imaging*

A significant overlap exists between imaging findings in NMOSD and MOGAD. Adults and children with AQP4-IgG NMOSD have lesions in AQP4-rich areas in the brain such as the periaqueductal gray matter, dorsal brainstem, and periventricular region of the third ventricle. NMOSD patients can have white matter lesions in tumefactive and spindle-like patterns [24,29]. Patients can also have T1-hypointense lesions [37]. As in MOGAD, patients should have MRI brain, orbits, and full spine with contrast (Figs. 7 and 8).

*Treatment and management*

NMOSD ON is typically treated acutely with IVMP as it is in MS ON. However, adult patients are treated with IVIG or PLEX for episodes of NMOSD because it is more effective than steroids alone. Pediatric patients have low threshold to escalate therapy to PLEX or IVIG because vision loss can be severe. Subsequently, patients have a slow steroid taper during 2 to 6 months. During this time, children are started on immunotherapy with rituximab, mycophenolate mofetil, azathioprine, or monthly IVIG. Unlike in MOGAD, where patients may not be started on immunotherapy, patients with NMOSD must be started on immunotherapy as each attack can be significantly neurologically devastating with poor recovery. Patients are likely to be continued to this therapy even after years without relapses [21].

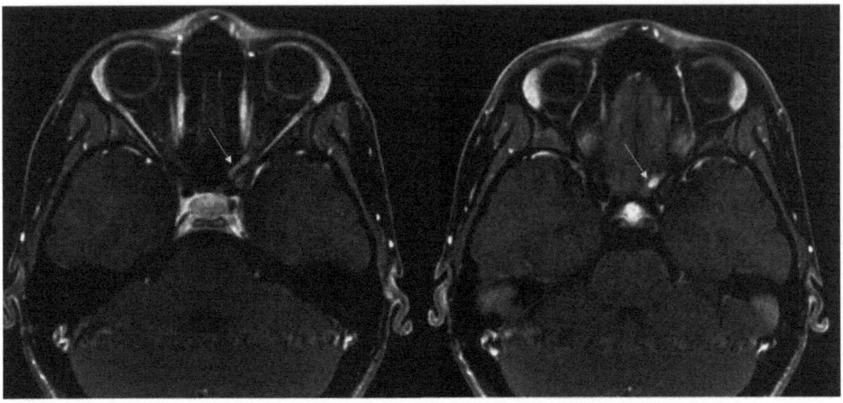

**Fig. 7.** Case 1: MRI orbits T1 postgadolinium fat-saturated axial scans showing enhancement of the left intracanalicular optic nerve .

Chronic immunotherapies under investigation currently include monoclonal antibodies such as tocilizumab, eculizumab, satralizumab, inebilizumab, and ofatumumab [23,24].

Similar to MOGAD, MS DMD may not prevent relapses in NMOSD and can even initiate recurrences. Dimethyl fumarate, INF-β, fingolimod, and natalizumab may be associated with relapses [21,24].

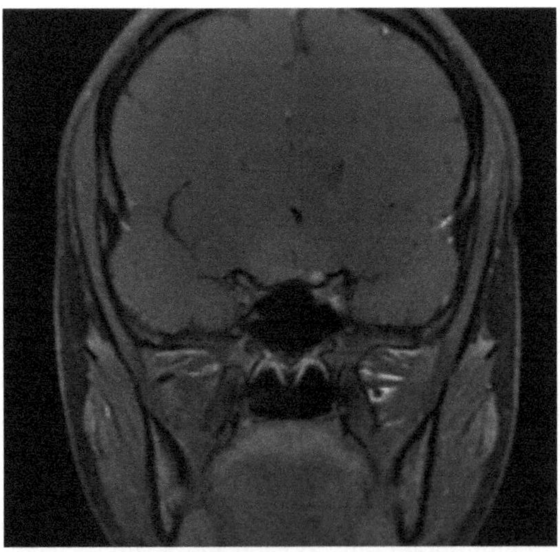

**Fig. 8.** Case 1: MRI orbits T1 postgadolinium fat-saturated coronal scans showing enhancement of the left optic nerve posteriorly to the chiasm.

*Visual outcomes and prognosis*

Pediatric NMOSD-ON results in severe and permanent visual loss. Median time to vision loss of <20/200 is 1.3 years [43]. Pediatric patients are more likely to have severe visual loss and brain lesions compared with adult patients [25]. AQP4-IgG seropositive children have greater than 50% risk of another episode of NMO in the year after their first episode and 90% risk of relapse overall [23,24].

Per Tenenbaum and colleagues, long-term follow-up for patients should include a complete neurologic assessment at baseline and at follow-up 3 to 6 months after presentation with routine follow-up every 6 to 12 months if asymptomatic. Patients may need interval laboratory testing based on their immunosuppressive therapy. Repeat imaging with MRI brain, orbits, and spine should be performed at 3 months after presentation, 6 months, 12 months, then yearly thereafter, or at time of acute attacks. To help with rehabilitation, patients may need multiple specialists including physiatry, physical therapy, occupational therapy, speech and language therapy, and cognitive testing [23].

## OTHER CAUSES OF OPTIC NEURITIS

Although autoimmune conditions are the most common causes of ON in children, other causes should be considered in the differential. Parainfectious or postvaccination ON, likely a systemic demyelinating process, is more common in children than adults. Measles, mumps, rubella, and pertussis vaccines and infections have been reported to be associated with ON in children. Other vaccines such as hepatitis B, diphtheria, tetanus, influenza, rabies, smallpox, and Bacillus Calmette-Guerin have also been associated with postvaccination ON. Infections associated with ON include varicella zoster virus, herpes simplex virus with acute retinal necrosis, progressive outer retinal necrosis, cytomegalovirus, syphilis, human immunodeficiency virus, tuberculosis, toxoplasma, toxocara, adenovirus, mononucleosis, Lyme disease, brucellosis, and mycoplasma pneumonia. These organisms have a variety of pathophysiologies including inflammatory, degenerative, or vascular processes. For example, herpes zoster can result in the inflammation of the optic nerve directly or ischemia leading to inflammatory thrombosis [25,44]. Parainfectious pediatric ON, which often presents with bilateral papillitis, can also be associated with ADEM and encephalomyelitis. Although no consensus exists on how to treat patients with parainfectious ON, they may need both antibiotics/antivirals and steroids [45].

Neuroretinitis presents with optic nerve swelling and a macular exudative star. Rather than optic nerve inflammation or a demyelinating process, neuroretinitis is an inflammation of the optic disc vasculature. It can be due to cat scratch disease or a monophasic or recurrent idiopathic neuroretinitis. It carries no increased risk of MS [46].

Children can have unilateral or bilateral optic disc swelling from a multitude of other causes such as the following. Papilledema due to idiopathic intracranial hypertension, meningitis, intracranial mass lesion, hydrocephalus, venous thrombosis; or compression due to optic nerve or optic nerve sheath tumor glioma, meningioma; adjacent infection, sinusitis, orbital cellulitis; or infiltration due to leukemia, lymphoma, sarcoidosis; or inflammation due to vasculitis, systemic lupus erythematosus, Leber hereditary optic neuropathy, or diabetic papillopathy; nonaccidental trauma; or pseudopapilledema [25].

### Relevance and future avenues to consider

Recent publications on pediatric ON have advocated for a prospective pediatric study akin to the ONTT. The Pediatric Eye Disease Investigator Group and Neuro-Ophthalmology Research Disease Investigator Consortium published the results of a multicenter prospective pilot study of the 6-month clinical outcomes of children aged 3 to 15 years with unilateral or bilateral ON. The goal was to recruit 100 patients within 2 weeks of symptom onset. Only 44 patients across 23 sites were able to be recruited during the 22-month period of the trial. The clinical data including Ab positivity, nadir of VA, and recovery of VA were within the ranges of previously reported retrospective studies. As previously reported, HCVA improved significantly in most patients, but low-contrast VA (LCVA) remained poor in patients even at the 6-month follow-up. The study was limited by the high percentage of patients who did not have Ab testing; 66% of patients did not have AQP4-IgG testing, and 70% did not have MOG-IgG testing. As the recruitment goal was not met in this study, the feasibility of a prospective study on the scale of the ONTT may be difficult to coordinate even across multiple sites. The difficulty in recruiting patients within the 2-week period after symptom onset has led to the study group to possibly reevaluate the admission criteria for a more involved prospective study.

A prospective study would be beneficial in helping to develop evidence-based follow-up protocols for pediatric patients with NMOSD and MOGAD. It is unclear if children should have frequent MOG-IgG levels or AQP4-IgG levels checked to better tailor long-term immunosuppression. Additionally, the frequency of imaging surveillance in asymptomatic children is unclear. The lifetime risk of relapses and other associated autoimmune diseases also are unknown.

Patients with MOGAD have been shown to have progressive OCT RNFL thinning without overt episodes of ON. It is unclear if these patients should be placed on chronic immunosuppressive therapy, and whether it would help to prevent progressive thinning of the optic nerve or atrophy of other areas of the brain.

## SUMMARY

Pediatric ON is a disease with a broad differential, most importantly CIS, MS, MOGAD, NMOSD, and infectious and parainfectious causes. Each of these conditions has been retrospectively studied and has different prognoses and associated neurologic conditions. The importance of properly recognizing these patterns disease and making the correct diagnosis is time-sensitive and paramount given that acute and long-term treatments vary.

In CIS ON, patients have an increased risk of MS with greater age at diagnosis. These patients should have MRI orbits and brain at the time of presentation. If features of MS, MOGAD, or NMOSD exist, patients should have further imaging of the spine and laboratory testing with cell-based assays of serum MOG-IgG and AQP4-IgG, CSF OCB, CSF studies, and other basic laboratories. Treatment with steroids for all of the above conditions is the mainstay of therapy. AQP4-Ab-positive patients should have a low threshold for escalated therapy with PLEX or IVIG and should be initiated on immunosuppressive therapy. Infectious and parainfectious ON may need additional treatment with antibiotics or antivirals. Most children with ON are likely to recover HCVA to baseline. LCVA continues to remain poor in about half of patients. CIS and MOGAD ON have the highest potential for visual recovery. AQP4-IgG ON is rare and often results in VA<20/200 at about 1 year after onset.

More prospective studies on the long-term prognosis, surveillance, and indications for chronic immunomodulatory therapy are needed.

## Acknowledgments

I have no funding sources. I would like to acknowledge my colleague Dr Meagan Seay, DO, Assistant Professor, Department of Ophthalmology and Visual Sciences and Department of Neurology, University of Utah School of Medicine for providing the patient cases and figures in this paper.

## References

[1] Langer-Gould A, Zhang JL, Chung J, et al. Incidence of acquired CNS demyelinating syndromes in a multiethnic cohort of children. Neurology 2011;77(12):1143–8.
[2] Banwell B, Kennedy J, Sadovnick D, et al. Incidence of acquired demyelination of the CNS in Canadian children. Neurology 2009;72(3):232–9.
[3] Lucchinetti CF, Kiers L, O'Duffy A, et al. Risk factors for developing multiple sclerosis after childhood optic neuritis. Neurology 1997;49(5):1413–8.
[4] Lana-Peixoto MA, de Andrade GC. The clinical profile of childhood optic neuritis. Arq Neuropsiquiatr 2001;59(2-B):311–7.
[5] Brady KM, Brar AS, Lee AG, et al. Optic neuritis in children: clinical features and visual outcome. J AAPOS 1999;3(2):98–103.
[6] Çakmakli G, Kurne A, Güven A, et al. Childhood optic neuritis: the pediatric neurologist's perspective. Eur J Paediatr Neurol 2009;13(5):452–7.
[7] Absoud M, Cummins C, Desai N, et al. Childhood optic neuritis clinical features and outcome. Arch Dis Child 2011;96(9):860–2.
[8] Waldman AT, Stull LB, Galetta SL, et al. Pediatric optic neuritis and risk of multiple sclerosis: Meta-analysis of observational studies. J AAPOS 2011;15(5):441–6.
[9] Boomer JA, Siatkowski RM. Optic neuritis in adults and children. Semin Ophthalmol 2003;18(4):174–80.
[10] Morales DS, Siatkowski RM, Howard CW, et al. Optic neuritis in children. J Pediatr Ophthalmol Strabismus 2000;37(5):254–9. Available at: https://pubmed-ncbi-nlm-nih-gov.proxy.ulib.uits.iu.edu/11020105/. Accessed December 23, 2021.
[11] Beck RW, Cleary PA, Anderson MM, et al. A randomized, controlled trial of corticosteroids in the treatment of acute optic neuritis. The Optic Neuritis Study Group. N Engl J Med 1992;326(9):581–8.

[12] Wilejto M, Shroff M, Buncic JR, et al. The clinical features, MRI findings, and outcome of optic neuritis in children. Neurology 2006;67(2):258–62.
[13] Bonhomme GR, Waldman AT, Balcer LJ, et al. Pediatric optic neuritis: brain MRI abnormalities and risk of multiple sclerosis. Neurology 2009;72(10):881–5.
[14] Jayakody H, Bonthius DJ, Longmuir R, et al. Pediatric optic neuritis: does a prolonged course of steroids reduce relapses? A preliminary study. Pediatr Neurol 2014;51(5):721–5.
[15] Kennedy C, Carroll FD. Optic neuritis in children. Arch Ophthalmol (Chicago) 1960;63(5): 747–55.
[16] Ramanathan S, Prelog K, Barnes EH, et al. Radiological differentiation of optic neuritis with myelin oligodendrocyte glycoprotein antibodies, aquaporin-4 antibodies, and multiple sclerosis. Mult Scler (Houndmills, Basingstoke, England) 2016;22(4):470–82.
[17] Narayan RN, McCreary M, Conger D, et al. Unique characteristics of optical coherence tomography (OCT) results and visual acuity testing in myelin oligodendrocyte glycoprotein (MOG) antibody positive pediatric patients. Mult Scler Relat Disord 2019;28:86–90.
[18] Peng A, Kinoshita M, Lai W, et al. Retinal nerve fiber layer thickness in optic neuritis with MOG antibodies: A systematic review and meta-analysis. J neuroimmunology 2018;325:69–73.
[19] El-Dairi MA, Ghasia F, Bhatti MT. Pediatric optic neuritis. Int Ophthalmol Clin 2012;52(3): 29–49.
[20] Armangue T, Capobianco M, de Chalus A, et al. E.U. paediatric MOG consortium consensus: Part 3 - Biomarkers of paediatric myelin oligodendrocyte glycoprotein antibody-associated disorders. Eur J Paediatr Neurol 2020;29:22–31.
[21] Lock JH, Newman NJ, Biousse V, et al. Update on pediatric optic neuritis. Curr Opin Ophthalmol 2019;30(6):418–25.
[22] Jarius S, Paul F, Aktas O, et al. MOG encephalomyelitis: international recommendations on diagnosis and antibody testing. J neuroinflammation 2018;15(1); https://doi.org/10.1186/S12974-018-1144-2.
[23] Tenembaum S, Chitnis T, Nakashima I, et al. Neuromyelitis optica spectrum disorders in children and adolescents. Neurology 2016;87(9 Suppl 2):S59–66.
[24] Gombolay GY, Chitnis T. Pediatric Neuromyelitis Optica Spectrum Disorders. Curr Treat Options Neurol 2018;20(6); https://doi.org/10.1007/S11940-018-0502-9.
[25] Chang MY, Pineles SL. Pediatric Optic Neuritis. Semin Pediatr Neurol 2017;24(2):122–8.
[26] Yeh EA, Graves JS, Benson LA, et al. Pediatric optic neuritis. Neurology 2016;87(9): S53–8.
[27] Wan MJ, Adebona O, Benson LA, et al. Visual outcomes in pediatric optic neuritis. Am J Ophthalmol 2014;158(3); https://doi.org/10.1016/J.AJO.2014.05.036.
[28] Wong YYM, de Mol CL, van der Vuurst De Vries RM, et al. Real-world validation of the 2017 McDonald criteria for pediatric MS. Neurol Neuroimmunol Neuroinflamm 2018;6(2); https://doi.org/10.1212/NXI.0000000000000528.
[29] Gise RA, Heidary G. Update on Pediatric Optic Neuritis. Curr Neurol Neurosci Rep 2020;20(3); https://doi.org/10.1007/s11910-020-1024-x.
[30] de Mol CL, Wong YYM, van Pelt ED, et al. The clinical spectrum and incidence of anti-MOG-associated acquired demyelinating syndromes in children and adults. Mult Scler 2020;26(7):806–14.
[31] de Mol CL, Wong YYM, van Pelt ED, et al. Incidence and outcome of acquired demyelinating syndromes in Dutch children: update of a nationwide and prospective study. J Neurol 2018;265(6):1310–9.
[32] Höftberger R, Sepulveda M, Armangue T, et al. Antibodies to MOG and AQP4 in adults with neuromyelitis optica and suspected limited forms of the disease. Mult Scler (Houndmills, Basingstoke, England) 2015;21(7):866–74.
[33] Wingerchuk DM, Banwell B, Bennett JL, et al. International consensus diagnostic criteria for neuromyelitis optica spectrum disorders. Neurology 2015;85(2):177–89.

[34] Bruijstens AL, Breu M, Wendel EM, et al. E.U. paediatric MOG consortium consensus: Part 4 - Outcome of paediatric myelin oligodendrocyte glycoprotein antibody-associated disorders. Eur J Paediatr Neurol 2020;29:32–40.
[35] Chen JJ, Flanagan EP, Jitprapaikulsan J, et al. Myelin Oligodendrocyte Glycoprotein Antibody–Positive Optic Neuritis: Clinical Characteristics, Radiologic Clues, and Outcome. Am J Ophthalmol 2018;195:8.
[36] Bruijstens AL, Lechner C, Flet-Berliac L, et al. E.U. paediatric MOG consortium consensus: Part 1 - Classification of clinical phenotypes of paediatric myelin oligodendrocyte glycoprotein antibody-associated disorders. Eur J Paediatr Neurol 2020;29:2–13.
[37] Baumann M, Bartels F, Finke C, et al. E.U. paediatric MOG consortium consensus: Part 2 - Neuroimaging features of paediatric myelin oligodendrocyte glycoprotein antibody-associated disorders. Eur J Paediatr Neurol 2020;29:14–21.
[38] Petzold A, Plant GT. Chronic relapsing inflammatory optic neuropathy: a systematic review of 122 cases reported. J Neurol 2014;261(1):17–26.
[39] Pandit L, Mustafa S, Nakashima I, et al. MOG-IgG-associated disease has a stereotypical clinical course, asymptomatic visual impairment and good treatment response. Mult Scler J 2018;4(3); https://doi.org/10.1177/2055217318787829.
[40] Savransky A, Rubstein A, Rios MH, et al. Prognostic indicators of improvement with therapeutic plasma exchange in pediatric demyelination. Neurology 2019;93(22):E2065–73.
[41] Bruijstens AL, Wendel EM, Lechner C, et al. E.U. paediatric MOG consortium consensus: Part 5 - Treatment of paediatric myelin oligodendrocyte glycoprotein antibody-associated disorders. Eur J Paediatr Neurol 2020;29:41–53; https://doi.org/10.1016/j.ejpn.2020.10.005, Epub 2020 Nov 4. PMID: 33176999.
[42] Yamaguchi Y, Torisu H, Kira R, et al. A nationwide survey of pediatric acquired demyelinating syndromes in Japan. Neurology 2016;87(19):2006–15.
[43] Collongues N, Marignier R, Zéphir H, et al. Long-term follow-up of neuromyelitis optica with a pediatric onset. Neurology 2010;75(12):1084–8.
[44] Sarkar P, Mehtani A, Gandhi HC, et al. Atypical optic neuritis: An overview. Indian J Ophthalmol 2021;69(1):27–35.
[45] Rappoport D, Goldenberg-Cohen N, Luckman J, et al. Parainfectious optic neuritis: manifestations in children vs adults. J neuro-ophthalmology 2014;34(2):122–9.
[46] Purvin V, Sundaram S, Kawasaki A. Neuroretinitis: review of the literature and new observations. J neuro-ophthalmology 2011;31(1):58–68.

Advances in Ophthalmology and Optometry 7 (2022) 89–118

ADVANCES IN OPHTHALMOLOGY AND OPTOMETRY

# Genetics of Congenital Cataract

Reddin Ahmad, BMBS, iBSc[a],
Suzannah Bell, MBChB, DTMH, MSc[b],
Mariya Moosajee, MBBS, BSc, PhD, FRCOphth[c,d,e,*]

[a]Bradford Teaching Hospitals NHS Foundation Trust, Bradford, West Yorkshire, United Kingdom; [b]Queen Alexandra Hospital, Portsmouth PO6 3LY, United Kingdom; [c]Moorfields Eye Hospital NHS Foundation Trust, London, United Kingdom; [d]University College London Institute of Ophthalmology, London, United Kingdom; [e]The Francis Crick Institute, London, United Kingdom

**Keywords**

• Cataract • Congenital cataract • Genetics • Inherited cataract
• Pediatric ophthalmology

**Key points**

- 20,000 to 40,000 children worldwide are born with cataract each year.
- Inherited cataract is a common cause of bilateral congenital cataract and can present as nonsyndromic, with other ocular abnormalities (complex) or with systemic features (syndromic).
- Next-generation sequencing has been shown to accelerate diagnosis, streamline care pathways, and facilitate tailored genetic counseling.
- Early surgery and frequent follow-up are vital to avoid amblyopia and optimize visual potential.
- A multidisciplinary team approach involving ophthalmic, pediatric, and genetic teams is vital and should also include school and local pediatric visual support services.

## INTRODUCTION

Up to 40,000 children are born with cataracts every year worldwide, with approximately 200,000 children blind from bilateral cataracts [1]. Incidence of childhood cataracts is estimated at 3 per 10,000 in the United Kingdom, with most of these occurring within the first year of life [2]. The most common

*Corresponding author. Moorfields Eye Hospital, 162 City Road, London EC1V 2PD, United Kingdom *E-mail address:* m.moosajee@ucl.ac.uk

https://doi.org/10.1016/j.yaoo.2022.03.004
2452-1760/22/

cause of bilateral cataracts is genetic mutations (in 61% of UK families), mainly inherited in an autosomal dominant mode [3,4].

Other causes include the following:

- Congenital infections, such as:
  - Toxoplasma
  - Rubella
  - Cytomegalovirus (CMV)
  - Herpes simplex virus I and II (HSV I + II)
- Iatrogenic causes, such as:
  - Medication
  - Radiation exposure
- Trauma

Inherited cataracts may be isolated (70%), occur with other ocular disease (complex, 15%), or as part of a syndrome (15%) [5]. As a variety of conditions are linked with congenital cataracts, a large number of investigations frequently are performed to establish the diagnosis. Currently, the investigative pathways for childhood cataract are unstandardized, with some patients not receiving any investigation despite a positive family history. Wasteful and inappropriate use of screening tests, such as for TORCH infections, is an issue, whereby incomplete tests are sent or results are interpreted incorrectly [6]. Screening of cataract-causing genes using next-generation sequencing has been shown to streamline this process and alter clinical outcomes for patients and their families [4,6,7].

Early interdisciplinary input, good parental engagement, and regular frequent follow-up are required for patients receiving cataract surgery to facilitate good long-term visual outcomes. Pediatrician involvement is important to help identify any syndromic features and arrange any further investigations. They also help support families through any developmental challenges that may arise throughout childhood. Parents have a key role in their child's management both preoperatively and postoperatively, including administering drops and patching.

## CAUSE AND CLASSIFICATION

During fetal development, the human lens arises from surface ectoderm. The cells enlarge to form the lens placode, then invaginate and pinch off to make the lens vesicle by day 33 of gestation [8]. The posterior epithelial cells lengthen anteriorly to obstruct the lumen of the lens vesicle, thereby forming the primary lens fibers. Secondary lens fibers are formed when the anterior epithelial cells at the equatorial area of the lens divide. This process continues throughout life [9].

Cataract arises when the normal lens structure or function is disrupted, thereby resulting in opacity. This could be due to stressors applied to lens proteins during in utero or childhood. However, the majority are due to genetic mutations encoding lens proteins, which directly affect their function [8]. Numerous congenital cataract morphologies have been described, such as posterior/anterior polar, posterior subcapsular, pulverulent lamella, nuclear, or cerulean (blue dot) cataract.

A cataract can be classified by age of presentation; cataracts presenting at or shortly after birth are typically described as congenital, and those presenting later can be described as developmental, infantile, or juvenile cataract with different criteria for these classifications [10]. Classification can be challenging, as a less visually significant cataract may be present since birth but not identified until later during eye screening or when the cataract has progressed.

## SIGNIFICANCE

Current genetic testing makes it possible to identify a genetic mutation in approximately 60% to 90% of bilateral cataract cases [3,4]. This will increase as genetic testing is more widely available to patients, and more cataract-causing genes/variants are discovered. Inherited cataracts display great genetic and phenotypic heterogeneity with significant variation seen both between and within families who possess the same mutation. Pleiotropic effects can be observed in some lens protein mutations, for example, the *NHS* gene has an intricate pattern of regulated gene expression affecting the development of neural, ocular, and craniofacial structures causing Nance-Horan syndrome [11]. Similar phenotypic variation can be observed in other cataract-causing genes, such as LSS (encoding lanosterol synthase), depending on the location of the nucleotide change where mutations occurring at the C-terminus of this gene are linked with lens defects, but those occurring toward the N terminus are linked with hair loss [12].

## NONSYNDROMIC CONGENITAL CATARACT

The main lens proteins linked with congenital cataracts are as follows:

- Crystallins
- Membrane proteins
- Cytoskeletal structural proteins
- Transcription factors

Some of these genes also are associated with the development of other ocular structures; hence, ~15% of cases has associated eye abnormalities, such as glaucoma, myopia, microphthalmia, microcornea, coloboma, anterior segment dysgenesis (ASD), corneal dystrophy, vitreoretinal degeneration, retinal abnormalities, and optic atrophy [10].

### Crystallins

α, β, and γ-crystallins are the main structural proteins involved in maintaining lens transparency and refraction. They have a highly organized molecular structure, and some have specific interactions with other proteins. For example, α-crystallins also act like molecular chaperones, promoting folding/unfolding of other denatured or damaged proteins and inhibiting apoptosis [13]. More than 100 mutations (mostly missense) exist encoding 12 different human α, β, and

**Table 1**
Genetic mutations associated with isolated cataract

| Gene name/locus | Gene/locus MIM number | Inheritance | Disease MIM number | Disease name | Phenotype |
|---|---|---|---|---|---|
| *AGK* | 610,345 | AR | 614,691 | Cataract 38, congenital cataract | Congenital cataract. |
| *BFSP1* | 603,307 | AD/AR | 611,391 | Cataract 33, multiple types | Cortical, nuclear, punctate lamellar cataracts |
| *BFSP2* | 603,212 | AD | 611,597 | Cataract 12, multiple types | Lamellar, cortical, nuclear embryonic, "scattered lens opacities" |
| *CHMP4B* | 610,897 | AD | 605,387 | Cataract 31, multiple types | Posterior subcapsular cataract, progressing to affect nucleus and anterior subcapsular regions. Posterior polar cataracts |
| *CRYAA* | 123,580 | AD/AR | 604,219 | Congenital cataract; cataract 9, multiple types | Nuclear, zonular, central nuclear, laminar, lamellar, anterior polar, posterior polar, cortical, embryonal, anterior subcapsular, fan-shaped, total cataracts |
| *CRYAB* | 123,590 | AD/AR | 613,763 | Cataract 16, multiple types | Nuclear, posterior polar, nuclear, lamellar cataracts |
| *CRYBA1* | 123,610 | AD | 600,881 | Cataract 10, multiple types; cataract congenital zonular with sutural opacities | Cataract 10, cataract congenital zonular with sutural opacities, nuclear, lamellar cataract |
| *CRYBA2* | 600,836 | AD | 115,900 | Cataract 42 | Multifocal cataract, congenital, juvenile, posterior polar, early cataract |
| *CRYBA4* | 123,631 | AD | 610,425 | Cataract 23 | Lamellar and nuclear cataracts |
| *CRYBB1* | 600,929 | AD/AR | 611,544 | Congenital nuclear cataract; cataract 17, multiple types | Congenital nuclear cataract, pulverulent cataracts |
| *CRYBB2* | 123,620 | AD | 601,547 | Cataract 3, multiple types | Coppock-like cataract, cerulean cataracts |
| *CRYBB3* | 123,630 | AD/AR | 609,741 | Congenital nuclear cataract; cataract 22 | Congenital, cortical, nuclear cataract |
| *CRYGB* | | | | | |
| *CRYGC* | 123,680 | AD | 604,307 | Cataract 2, multiple types; AD cataract Coppock-like | Cataract, variable zonular pulverulent, Coppock-like cataract |

| | | | | | |
|---|---|---|---|---|---|
| *CRYGD* | 123,690 | AD | 115,700 | Cataracts; cataract 4, multiple types, congenital cerulean cataract | Aculeiform, progressive, congenital cerulean cataract |
| *CRYGS* | 123,730 | AD | 116,100 | Cataract 20, multiple types | Progressive polymorphic cortical cataract, progressive "opalescent" cataract |
| *CYP51A1* | 601,637 | AR | N/A | Autosomal recessive cataract due to abnormal sterol metabolism | Not otherwise specified, congenital cataract total white cataracts |
| *DNMBP* | 611,282 | AR | 618,415 | Cataract 48 | Infantile onset cataracts |
| *EPHA2* | 176,946 | AD | 116,600 | Age-related cortical cataract; cataract 6, multiple types | Age-related cortical cataract. Persistent fetal vasculature, posterior polar, posterior subcapsular cataracts |
| *FOXE3* | 601,094 | AD/AR | 612,968 | Autosomal dominant cataracts, cataract 34 multiple types | Membranous, posterior subcapsular cataracts |
| *FYCO1* | 607,182 | AR | 610,019 | Congenital cataract; cataract 18 | Nuclear cataract, congenital cataracts |
| *GJA3* | 121,015 | AD | 601,885 | Zonular pulverulent cataract; cataract 14, multiple types | Nuclear pulverulent, zonular pulverulent cataract posterior polar, nuclear coralliform, embryonal nuclear, Coppock-like cataracts |
| *GJA8* | 600,897 | AD | 116,200 | Cataract 1, multiple types | Zonular pulverulent, nuclear progressive |
| *HSF4* | 602,438 | AD/AR | 116,800 | Cataracts; cataract 5, multiple types | Lamellar, zonular stellate, anterior polar cataracts |
| *LEMD2* | 616,312 | AR | 212,500 | Cataract 46, juvenile-onset | Juvenile-onset "Hutterite-type cataract" |
| *LIM2* | 154,045 | AR | 615,277 | Cortical pulverulent cataract; cataract 19 | Cortical pulverulent cataract, congenital total cataract, nuclear cataract |
| *LSS* | 600,909 | AR | 616,509 | Cataract 44 | Total cataract |
| *MAF* | 177,075 | AD | 610,202 | Cataract, pulverulent or cerulean, without microcornea, cataract 21, multiple types | Cataract, pulverulent, or cerulean, without microcornea, cataract 21, cortical pulverulent, nuclear pulverulent with progression to posterior subcapsular cataract. Lamellar, anterior polar, nuclear, anterior subcapsular cataracts |

(*continued on next page*)

**Table 1**
**(*continued*)**

| Gene name/locus | Gene/locus MIM number | Inheritance | Disease MIM number | Disease name | Phenotype |
|---|---|---|---|---|---|
| *MIP* | 154,050 | AD | 615,274 | Cataracts; cataract 15, multiple types | Cataract 15, anterior and posterior polar, cortical cataract, progressive punctate lamellar, nonprogressive congenital lamellar and sutural cataracts, embryonal nuclear cataracts |
| *NHS* | 300,457 | XL | 302,200 | Cataract 40, X-linked | Total nuclear, sutural, lamellar, zonular, perinuclear, posterior stellate cataracts |
| *PITX3* | 602,669 | AD, AR | 610,623 | Cataract 11, multiple types | Cataract 11, posterior polar, total and cortical cataracts |
| *TDRD7* | 611,258 | AR | 613,887 | Cataract 36 | Congenital cataracts |
| *UNC45 B* | 611,220 | AD | 616,279 | ?Cataract 43 | Posterior subcapsular and central cataracts |
| *VIM* | 193,060 | AD | 116,300 | Cataract 30, pulverulent | Pulverulent cataracts |
| *WFS1* | 606,201 | AD/AR | 116,400 | ?Cataract 41 | Congenital nuclear cataract |

Detailed phenotype data from Genomics England PanelApp and OMIM cataract databases and associated relevant publications.

*Abbreviations:* AD, autosomal dominant; AR, autosomal recessive; N/A, not applicable; XL, x-linked.

*From* Bell SJ, Oluonye N, Harding P, Moosajee M. Congenital cataract: a guide to genetic and clinical management. Therapeutic Advances in Rare Disease. January 2020.

$\gamma$-crystallin genes (Table 1), which are responsible for around half of nonsyndromic hereditary cataract [14].

### Cytoskeletal structural proteins

Beaded filament structural proteins (BFSPs) are intermediate filament proteins that are expressed in various cells of the body (eg, glial, epithelial, and muscle cells). Two BFSPs are solely expressed in the lens, BFSP1 (Filensin) and BFSP2 (Phakinin), both of which combine with crystallins to maintain lens structure integrity. Homozygous *BFSP2* mutations cause childhood cataract, but heterozygous mutations also are linked to age-related cataract and myopia (Table 2) [15].

### Membrane proteins

Lens membrane proteins have a key role in the integrity and metabolic homeostasis of the avascular lens. Genetic mutations in these membrane proteins cause disruption in transport of solutes and ions between cells resulting in clouding of the lens (see Table 1). A list of membrane proteins and associated mutations leading to cataracts are mentioned in later discussion.

*Gap junctions*

- Comprise 6 connexin protein subunits [16]
  - Play a major part in lens microcirculation
    - Supply metabolites and nutrients to the lens center
    - Transport unwanted ions and by-products to the periphery [17]
- Three mutations *GJA3* and *GJA8* result in amplified hemichannel activity, and 2 mutations reduce hemichannel activity (usually missense).
  - Often associated with nuclear and zonular pulverulent cataracts with varying progression [18]
- Associated with microcornea and the development of cataract [18]

Mutations in membrane proteins, such as major intrinsic proteins, account for approximately 5% of inherited cataract [19].

*Aquaporin-0/Major intrinsic protein (MIP)*

- Most expressed membrane protein in the human lens
- Autosomal dominant Aquaporin-0/Major intrinsic protein (MIP) is expressed in lens fiber cells
- Leads to several different cataract phenotypes, such as anterior and posterior polar, cortical, progressive punctate lamellar, nonprogressive congenital lamellar, sutural, embryonal, and nuclear cataracts (see Table 1) [20]

*Lens intrinsic membrane protein-2*

- Encodes MP19; a membrane protein with 4 transmembrane domains
- Contributes to lens transparency [21]
- Three *LIM2* missense mutations have been documented to cause autosomal recessive cataract:
  - c.313 T > G, p.(Phe105Val) associated with cortical cataract
  - c.587 G > A, p.(Gly154Glu) mutation in a family causing autosomal recessive cataract

**Table 2**
Genetic mutations associated with isolated cataract

| Gene symbol | Gene/locus MIM number | Inheritance | Disease MIM number | Disease name | Ocular comorbidities (besides cataract) |
|---|---|---|---|---|---|
| *CRYBA1* | 123,610 | AD | 600,881 | Cataract 10, multiple types | Nystagmus, esotropia |
| *CRYBA2* | 600,836 | AD | 115,900 | Cataract 42 | Eccentric pupil, glaucoma, myopia |
| *CRYBA4* | 123,631 | AD/AR | 610,425 | Cataract 23 | Microcornea, microphthalmia |
| *CRYBB1* | 600,929 | AD/AR | 611,544 | — | Microcornea, nystagmus, iris and choroid coloboma |
| *CRYBB2* | 123,620 | AD | 601,547 | Cataract 3, multiple types | Microphthalmia, microcornea, coloboma (posterior segment), glaucoma |
| *CRYGC* | 123,680 | AD | 604,307 | Cataract 2, multiple types; AD cataract Coppock-like | Microcornea |
| *CRYGD* | 123,690 | AD | 115,700 | Cataract 4, multiple types | Microcornea |
| *DNMBP* | 611,282 | AR | 618,415 | Cataract 48 | Nystagmus, amblyopia, exotropia |
| *EPHA2* | 176,946 | AD | 116,600 | Cataract 6, multiple types | Microcornea, microphthalmia |
| *FOXE3* | 601,094 | AD/AR | 610,256 | Peters anomaly | ASD, ocular dysgenesis, corneal opacity, Peters anomaly, microphthalmia, microcornea, nystagmus |
| *GJA3* | 121,015 | AD | 601,885 | Cataract 14, multiple types | Microphthalmia, microcornea |
| *GJA8* | 600,897 | AD | 116,200 | Cataract-microcornea syndrome | Microcornea, microphthalmia, glaucoma, ASD, coloboma, sclerocornea, total corneal opacification |
| *MAF* | 177,075 | AD | 610,202 | - | Microcornea, iris coloboma, microcornea, glaucoma, microphthalmia, myopia, nystagmus, Peters anomaly |

| | | | | | |
|---|---|---|---|---|---|
| *NHS* | 300,457 | XL | 302,200 | Cataract 40, X-linked | Microcornea, microphthalmia |
| *OPA3* | 258,501 | AD | 258,501 | Autosomal dominant optic atrophy with cataract (ADOAC) | Optic atrophy |
| *P3H2* | 610,341 | AR | 614,292 | — | High myopia, lens dislocation, retinal detachment, vitreoretinal degeneration |
| *PAX6* | 607,108 | AD | 106,210 | — | Cataract with late-onset corneal dystrophy |
| *PITX3* | 602,669 | AD | 610,623 | — | Anterior segment dysgenesis |
| *PXDN* | 605,158 | AR | 269,400 | — | Corneal opacity, developmental glaucoma; corneal opacification associated with other ocular anomalies (COPA) |
| *VSX2* | 142,993 | AR | 610,092 | — | Microphthalmia and iris abnormalities<br>Microphthalmia with coloboma type 3, microphthalmia isolated type 2 |

Detailed phenotype data from Genomics England PanelApp and OMIM cataract databases and associated relevant publications XL, X-linked.

*From* Bell SJ, Oluonye N, Harding P, Moosajee M. Congenital cataract: a guide to genetic and clinical management. Therapeutic Advances in Rare Disease. January 2020.

  - c.233 G > A, p.(Gly78Asp) mutation in a consanguineous Pakistani family with nuclear cataracts [22]

EPHA2 and Dynamin binding protein (DNMBP) are membrane proteins that are associated with inherited cataracts.

*Ephrin receptor A2 (*EPHA2*)*
- Encodes a membrane-bound protein tyrosine kinase [23]
- Mutations in EPHA2 frequently linked with autosomal dominant posterior polar cataracts and newly associated with microphthalmia [24,25]
- Mutations arising in the sterile-a-motif area of the molecule alter its structure
  - Hinders cell migration in human and mouse fibroblast lens epithelial cells [26]

*Dynamin binding protein (*DNMBP*)*
- DNMBP encodes a protein that modulates the structure of cell junctions by binding to tight junction protein 1
- Biallele loss-of-function variants cause a complex cataract phenotype, including nystagmus, strabismus, and pupil abnormalities [24]

### Transcription factors

Mutations in transcription factor genes can lead to inherited cataracts. Some examples are listed as follows:

Heat shock transcription factor 4 (HSF4)

- Helps regulate the differentiation of lens fiber cells
- Shields the lens protein from cell stressors
- Autosomal dominant or recessive mutations commonly cause lamellar cataract
  - May be present at birth or arise during infancy
  - Inheritance can be either dominant or recessive
  - Sixteen mutations have been identified with *HSF4*
    - Thirteen are missense
    - Eleven occurred in the protein's DNA binding domain
- Signifies this area is vital for normal protein function [27]

*MAF* affect the basic-leucine zipper (bZIP) domain of a transcription faction.

- Most (7/18) of the known mutations are linked with several ocular abnormalities [27]
  - Indicating the bZIP domain has an essential role in eye development
- *MAF* mutations in the N-terminus upstream of a transactivation domain encoding area also cause Ayme-Gripp syndrome and Asperger syndrome (Table 3) [27].

*FOXE3*
- Encodes transcription factors with a "forkhead" DNA binding area
- Involved in lens embryology
- Twenty-four mutations found to impact various ocular structures, such as the cornea, iris, lens, and retina (see Table 2) [27]
  - Most of these mutations are missense
  - Ten occur in the forkhead DNA binding domain

**Table 3**
Genetic mutations associated with syndromic cataract

| Gene symbol | Gene/locus MIM number | Inheritance | Disease MIM number | Disease name | Frequent associated systemic features |
|---|---|---|---|---|---|
| *ADAMTS10* | 608,990 | AR | 277,600 | Weill-Marchesani syndrome | Short stature, brachycephaly, joint stiffness |
| *AGK* | 610,345 | AR | 212,350 | Sengers syndrome | Hypertrophic cardiomyopathy, skeletal myopathy, exercise intolerance |
| *AGPS* | 603,051 | AR | 600,121 | Rhizomelic chondrodysplasia punctata type 3 | Short stature, broad nasal bridge, epicanthus, high-arched palate, dysplastic external ears, micrognathia, congenital contractures, dwarfism, severe mental disability with spasticity |
| *ALDH18A1* | 138,250 | AD/AR | 616,603 | Autosomal dominant/recessive cutis laxa-3 (ADCL3/ARCL3) | Mental disability, joint hypermobility, skin hyperelasticity, metabolic abnormalities: hyperammonemia/prolinemia/ornithinemia |
| *B3GLCT* | 610,308 | AR | 261,540 | Peters-plus syndrome | Peters anomaly, growth retardation, short stature, brachydactyly, developmental delay |
| *BCOR* | 300,166 | X-linked (dominant) | 300,485 | Oculofaciocardiodental syndrome | Eye anomalies (microphthalmia, glaucoma), facial abnormalities (long narrow face, high nasal bridge, pointed nose, cleft palate), cardiac anomalies (atrial/ventricular septal defect, floppy mitral valve), dental abnormalities (canine radiculomegaly, delayed dentition, oligodontia) |

(*continued on next page*)

**Table 3 (*continued*)**

| Gene symbol | Gene/locus MIM number | Inheritance | Disease MIM number | Disease name | Frequent associated systemic features |
|---|---|---|---|---|---|
| *COL2A1* | 120,140 | AD | 609,508 | Stickler syndrome type I nonsyndromic ocular | Congenital vitreous abnormality (vestigial gel in retrolental space) with midline clefting, flat midface, hearing loss, mild spondyloepiphyseal dysplasia, early-onset arthritis |
| *COL4A1* | 120,130 | AD | 175,780 | — | Brain small-vessel disease with or without ocular anomalies; microphthalmia |
| *COL4A5* | 303,630 | X-linked | 301,050 | Alport syndrome | Progressive renal failure, hearing loss and lenticonus, corneal erosions, retinal flecks |
| *COL11A1* | 120,280 | AD | 154,780 | Marshall syndrome; Stickler syndrome | Hearing loss, retinal detachment, midfacial hypoplasia, palatal hypoplasia |
| *COL18A1* | 120,328 | AR | 267,750 | Knobloch syndrome | High myopia, vitreoretinal degeneration, retinal detachment |
| *CRYAB* | 123,590 | AD/AR | 613,763 | — | Myofibrillar myopathy, adult-onset cardiomyopathy, dilated cardiomyopathy |
| *CYP27A1* | 606,530 | AR | 213,700 | Cerebrotendinous xanthomatosis | Childhood cholestasis, tendon xanthomas. Neurologic complications in adulthood, including neuropsychiatric disturbance, increased muscle tone, ataxia, dystonia, seizures |
| *CYP51A1* | 601,637 | AR | — | — | Developmental delay, spastic diplegia, and cryptogenic neonatal liver cirrhosis, neonatal cholestatic jaundice |

| | | | | | |
|---|---|---|---|---|---|
| *DCR* | — | IC | 190,685 | Down syndrome | Mental disability, characteristic facies, cardiac anomalies, GI tract disorders, leukemia, hearing loss, early Alzheimer disease |
| *DHCR7* | 602,858 | AR | 270,400 | Smith-Lemli-Opitz syndrome | Hypotonia, microcephaly, micrognathia, craniofacial abnormalities, postaxial polydactyly, syndactyly, hypospadias, developmental delay |
| *DMPK* | 605,377 | AD | 160,900 | Myotonic dystrophy 1 | Myotonia muscular dystrophy, cataracts, hypogonadism, frontal balding, ECG changes |
| *EED* | 605,984 | AD | 617,561 | Cohen-Gibson syndrome | Dysmorphic facial features, advanced bone age, skeletal anomalies, large hands, long fingers and camptodactyly, scoliosis, and cervical spinal abnormalities |
| *EIF2B2* | 606,454 | AR | 603,896 | Leukoencephalopathy with vanishing white matter | Variable neurologic features, including progressive cerebellar ataxia, spasticity, cognitive impairment associated with white matter lesions on brain imaging |
| *EPHA2* | 176,946 | AD | 116,600 | — | Microcornea, phacodonesis, neurodevelopmental delay, mild dysmorphic features |

(*continued on next page*)

**Table 3**
**(*continued*)**

| Gene symbol | Gene/locus MIM number | Inheritance | Disease MIM number | Disease name | Frequent associated systemic features |
|---|---|---|---|---|---|
| *ERCC2* | 126,340 | AR | 610,756 | Cerebrooculofacioskeletal syndrome (COFS2); trichothiodystrophy 1 (TTD1) | COFS2: Microcephaly, prominent nose, microphthalmia, blepharophimosis, large ears, overlapping upper lip, long philtrum, micrognathia<br>TTD1: Brittle sulphur-deficient hair, cutaneous, neurologic and growth abnormalities |
| *ERCC3* | 133,510 | AR | 616,390 | Trichothiodystrophy 2 (TTD2) | Brittle sulphur-deficient hair, cutaneous, neurologic and growth abnormalities |
| *ERCC6* | 609,413 | AR | 133,540 | Cockayne syndrome type B (CSB) Cerebrooculofacioskeletal syndrome 1 (COFS1) | CSB: Progeroid appearance, cachectic dwarfism, failure to thrive, mental disability, loss of adipose tissue, joint contractures, sensorineural hearing loss<br>COFS1: Microcephaly, mental disability, facial dysmorphism, arthrogryposis |
| *ERCC8* | 609,412 | AR | 216,400 | Cockayne syndrome type A MIMID | Progeroid appearance, cachectic dwarfism, mental disability, loss of adipose tissue, sensorineural hearing loss |
| *FAM126A* | 610,531 | AR | 610,532 | Leukodystrophy hypomyelinating 5 | Hypomyelination resulting in psychomotor regression, mental disability, sensorimotor peripheral neuropathy |

| | | | | | |
|---|---|---|---|---|---|
| *FBN1* | | AD | | Marfan syndrome | Skeletal, ocular, and cardiovascular abnormalities. Long limbs and fingers, high arched palate, aortic dilatation/regurgitation, myopia, subluxation of lens |
| *FOXE3* | 601,094 | AD | 612,968 | Cataract 34, multiple types | Vitreoretinal dysplasia, neurodevelopmental delay, joint laxity |
| *FTL* | 134,790 | AD | 600,886 | Hyperferritinemia-cataract syndrome | Hyperferritinemia, microcytic anemia |
| *GALK1* | 604,313 | AR | 230,200 | Galactokinase deficiency with cataracts | Elevated plasma galactose with milder features of galactosemia |
| *GALT* | 606,999 | AR | 230,400 | Galactosemia | Elevated plasma galactose with poor feeding with poor weight gain, vomiting and diarrhea, liver cell damage, and lethargy |
| *GCNT2* | 600,429 | AR | 116,700 | Adult I blood group with congenital cataract | Adult I blood group |
| *GEMIN4* | 606,969 | AR | 617,913 | — | Neurodevelopmental disorder with microcephaly, renal abnormalities |
| *GNPAT* | 602,744 | AR | 222,765 | Rhizomelic chondrodysplasia punctata type 2 | Rhizomelic skeletal dysplasia, mental disability |
| *GTF2H5* | 608,780 | AR | 616,395 | Trichothiodystrophy 3, photosensitive | Brittle sulphur-deficient hair, cutaneous, neurologic, and growth abnormalities |
| *HMX1* | 142,992 | AR | 612,109 | Oculoauricular syndrome | Microphthalmia, microcornea, corneal opacity, coloboma, external ear abnormalities |
| *HTRA2* | 606,441 | AR | 617,248 | 3-methylglutaconic aciduria, type VIII | Death in infancy. Hypotonia, abnormal movements, respiratory insufficiency, lack of development with seizures |

(*continued on next page*)

**Table 3**
**(*continued*)**

| Gene symbol | Gene/locus MIM number | Inheritance | Disease MIM number | Disease name | Frequent associated systemic features |
|---|---|---|---|---|---|
| *INPP5K* | 607,875 | AR | 617,404 | Congenital muscular dystrophy with cataracts and mild cognitive impairment (MDCCAID) | Muscular dystrophy with progressive muscle weakness in childhood and mild cognitive impairment |
| *JAM3* | 606,871 | AR | 613,730 | — | Hemorrhagic destruction of the brain, subependymal calcification |
| *LONP1* | 605,490 | AR | 600,373 | CODAS syndrome (cerebral, ocular, dental, auricular, skeletal) | Developmental delay, craniofacial abnormalities, ptosis, median nasal groove, delayed tooth eruption, anomalous cusp morphology, malformed helices, hearing loss, short stature, delayed epiphyseal ossification, metaphyseal hip dysplasia, vertebral coronal clefts |
| *LSS* | 616,509 | AR | 600,909 | - | Congenital cataract, hypotrichosis |
| *MAF* | 177,075 | AD | 610,202 | Ayme-Gripp syndrome | Sensorineural hearing loss, intellectual disability, seizures, brachycephaly, a distinctive flat facial appearance, and reduced growth |
| *MAN2B1* | 609,458 | AR | 248,500 | Mannosidosis alpha types I and II | Progressive mental disability, immune deficiency, impaired hearing, and Hurler-like skeletal changes |

| | | | | | |
|---|---|---|---|---|---|
| *MSMO1* | 607,545 | AR | 616,834 | — | Microcephaly, psoriasiform dermatitis |
| *MYH9* | 160,775 | AD | 155,100 | Epstein syndrome; Fechtner syndrome | Nephritis, mild hearing loss, thrombocytopenia |
| *NDP* | 300,658 | X-linked (recessive) | 310,600 | Norrie disease | Very early childhood blindness due to degenerative and proliferative changes of the neuroretina with or without progressive mental disability and psychosis and deafness |
| *NF2* | 607,379 | AD | 101,000 | Neurofibromatosis type 2 | Multiple neoplasia syndrome. Tumors of either cranial nerve (usually bilateral), meningiomas, and schwannomas |
| *NHS* | 300,457 | X-linked (dominant) | 302,200 | Nance-Horan syndrome | Microcornea, dental anomalies, for example, Hutchinsonian incisors, mesiodens, dysmorphic features, for example, large anteverted pinna, mental disability |
| *OCRL* | 300,535 | X-linked (recessive) | 309,000 | Lowe syndrome | Hydrophthalmia, mental disability, vitamin D-resistant rickets, amino aciduria, reduced ammonia produced by kidney |
| *PEX1* | 602,136 | AR | 214,100 | Peroxisome biogenesis disorder 1A (Zellweger) (ZS) | Neurologic abnormalities, characteristic dysmorphism and hepatomegaly, death in infancy |
| | | | | Refsum disease infantile; adrenoleukodystrophy neonatal | Symptoms similar to ZS with survival to early childhood |
| | | | | | Symptoms similar to ZS with longest survival 3–11 y of age |

(*continued on next page*)

**Table 3**
**(*continued*)**

| Gene symbol | Gene/locus MIM number | Inheritance | Disease MIM number | Disease name | Frequent associated systemic features |
|---|---|---|---|---|---|
| *PEX2* | 170,993 | AR | 614,866 | Peroxisome biogenesis disorder 5A (Zellweger) | Neurologic abnormalities, characteristic dysmorphism and hepatomegaly, death in infancy |
| *PEX3* | 603,164 | AR | 614,882 | Peroxisome biogenesis disorder 10A (Zellweger) | Neurologic abnormalities, characteristic dysmorphism and hepatomegaly, death in infancy |
| *PEX5* | 600,414 | AR | 214,110/202,370/616,716 | Peroxisome biogenesis disorder 2A (Zellweger)<br>Peroxisome biogenesis disorder 2B<br>Rhizomelic chondrodysplasia punctata, type 5 | Neurologic abnormalities, characteristic dysmorphism and hepatomegaly, death in infancy<br>Rhizomelic skeletal dysplasia, mental disability |
| *PEX6* | 601,498 | AR | 614,862 | Peroxisome biogenesis disorder 4A (Zellweger) | Neurologic abnormalities, characteristic dysmorphism and hepatomegaly, death in infancy |
| *PEX7* | 601,757 | AR | 215,100 | Rhizomelic chondrodysplasia punctata type 1<br>Refsum disease<br>Peroxisome biogenesis disorder | Rhizomelic skeletal dysplasia, mental disability<br>Symptoms similar to ZS with survival to early childhood<br>Neurologic abnormalities, characteristic dysmorphism and hepatomegaly, death in infancy |
| *PEX10* | 602,859 | AR | 614,870 | Peroxisome biogenesis disorder 6A (Zellweger)<br>Adrenoleukodystrophy neonatal | Neurologic abnormalities, characteristic dysmorphism and hepatomegaly, death in infancy<br>Symptoms similar to ZS with longest survival 3–11 y of age |

| | | | | | |
|---|---|---|---|---|---|
| *PEX11 B* | 603,867 | AR | 614,920 | Peroxisome biogenesis disorder | Neurologic abnormalities, characteristic dysmorphism and hepatomegaly, death in infancy |
| *PEX12* | 614,859 | AR | 614,859 | Peroxisome biogenesis disorder 3A (Zellweger); peroxisome biogenesis disorder complementation group 3 | Neurologic abnormalities, characteristic dysmorphism and hepatomegaly, death in infancy |
| *PEX13* | 601,789 | AR | 614,883 | Peroxisome biogenesis disorder 11A (Zellweger); adrenoleukodystrophy neonatal | Neurologic abnormalities, characteristic dysmorphism and hepatomegaly, death in infancy<br>Symptoms similar to ZS with longest survival 3–11 y of age |
| *PEX14* | 601,791 | AR | 614,887 | Peroxisome biogenesis disorder 13A | Neurologic abnormalities, characteristic dysmorphism and hepatomegaly, death in infancy |
| *PEX16* | 603,360 | AR | 614,876 | Peroxisome biogenesis disorder 8A (Zellweger) | Neurologic abnormalities, characteristic dysmorphism and hepatomegaly, death in infancy |
| *PEX19* | 600,279 | AR | 614,886 | Peroxisome biogenesis disorder 12A (Zellweger) | Neurologic abnormalities, characteristic dysmorphism and hepatomegaly, death in infancy |
| *PEX26* | 608,666 | AR | 614,872 | Peroxisome biogenesis disorder 7A (Zellweger) (ZS)<br>Refsum disease infantile; adrenoleukodystrophy neonatal | Neurologic abnormalities, characteristic dysmorphism and hepatomegaly, death in infancy<br>Symptoms similar to ZS with survival to early childhood<br>Symptoms similar to ZS with longest survival 3–11 y of age |
| *PITX3* | 602,669 | AD, AR | 610,623 | — | Mental disability, choreiform movements, increased muscle tone, deep tendon reflexes of lower extremities |

(*continued on next page*)

**Table 3 (*continued*)**

| Gene symbol | Gene/locus MIM number | Inheritance | Disease MIM number | Disease name | Frequent associated systemic features |
|---|---|---|---|---|---|
| *POMT1* | 607,423 | AR | 236,670 | Walker-Warburg syndrome | Cobblestone (type II) lissencephaly, cerebellar malformations, retinal malformations |
| *RAB18* | 602,207 | AR | 614,222 | Warburg microsyndrome 3 | Congenital microcephaly, cortical dysplasia, microcornea, optic atrophy, severe mental disability, hypotonic diplegia, hypogenitalism |
| *RAB3GAP1* | 602,536 | AR | 600,118 | Warburg microsyndrome 1 | Congenital microcephaly, cortical dysplasia, microcornea, optic atrophy, severe mental disability, hypotonic diplegia, hypogenitalism |
| *RAB3GAP2* | 609,275 | AR | 212,720 | Warburg microsyndrome 2 (WMS2)<br>Martsolf syndrome | Congenital microcephaly, cortical dysplasia, microcornea, optic atrophy, severe mental disability, hypotonic diplegia, hypogenitalism<br>Milder phenotype of WMS2. Microphthalmia, postnatal microcephaly, developmental delay |
| *RECQL4* | 603,780 | AR | 268,400 | Rothmund-Thompson syndrome, type 2 | Poikiloderma, congenital bone defects, increased risk of osteosarcoma in childhood, skin cancer in adulthood |

| | | | | | |
|---|---|---|---|---|---|
| *SC5D* | 602,286 | AR | 607,330 | Lathosterolosis | Facial dysmorphisms, severe microcephaly, micrognathia, neonatal jaundice, mental disability, hexadactyly, syndactyly, liver disease |
| *SEC23 A* | 610,511 | AR | 607,812 | Craniolenticulosutural dysplasia | Facial dysmorphism, late closing fontanelle, skeletal defects |
| *SIL1* | 608,005 | AR | 248,800 | Marinesco-Sjogren syndrome | Cerebellar ataxia, progressive myopathy |
| *SLC2A1* | 138,140 | AD | 608,885 | Stomatin-deficient cryohydrocytosis with neurologic defects | Delayed psychomotor development, seizures, pseudohyperkalemia |
| *SLC33A1* | 603,690 | AR | 614,482 | — | Congenital cataracts, hearing loss, and neurodegeneration |
| *SRD5A3* | 611,715 | AR | 612,713 | Kahrizi syndrome | Mental disability, coloboma, kyphosis |
| *TFAP2A* | 107,580 | AD | 113,620 | Branchiooculofacial syndrome | High arched palate, prominent philtrum, narrow ear canals, abnormal pinnae, periorbital and scalp cysts |
| *WRN* | 604,611 | AR | 277,700 | Werner syndrome | Accelerated aging appearance and disorders associated with aging, including diabetes mellitus, osteoporosis, premature atherosclerosis, benign and malignant neoplasms |
| *XYLT2* | 608,125 | AR | 605,822 | Spondyloocular syndrome | Bone fragility, hearing defects, retinal detachment, facial dysmorphism, immobile spine, platyspondyly |

Detailed phenotype data from Genomics England PanelApp and OMIM cataract databases and associated relevant publications.

*From* Bell SJ, Oluonye N, Harding P, Moosajee M. Congenital cataract: a guide to genetic and clinical management. Therapeutic Advances in Rare Disease. January 2020.

*Pituitary homeobox 3 proteins*

- Transcription factors
- Known to play a vital role in regulating lens epithelial cell maintenance and fiber cell differentiation in mice [28]
- Contain the homeobox and the otp, aristaless, rax domains
  - No mutations causing cataracts have been recorded in either domain
- Pituitary homeobox 3 (*PITX3*) mutations usually result in posterior polar cataract ± ASD
- Can also lead to other ocular abnormalities, such as corneal opacity, glaucoma, microcornea, microphthalmia, and nystagmus [27]

## SYNDROMIC CONGENITAL CATARACT

Syndromic congenital cataract can present owing to several different types of genetic mutations, including chromosomal rearrangements, mitochondrial mutations, and triplet repeat disorders [22]. Cataracts present with phenotypic variation and are linked with numerous systemic dysmorphic features [29].

Chromosomal abnormalities involving cataracts include the following:

### Down syndrome (Trisomy 21)

- Born with characteristic features
- Prone to numerous health issues (see Table 3)
- Cataract found in 15% of children
- Ocular abnormalities include amblyopia, astigmatism, blepharitis, hypermetropia, iris abnormalities, lacrimal system obstruction, myopia, nystagmus, retinal abnormalities, strabismus, and up-slanting palpebral fissures [30]

### Patau syndrome (trisomy 13)

- Commonly present with cataract, microphthalmia, and ocular coloboma
- Rarely live more than a few weeks owing to numerous significant congenital abnormalities of other organs and structures

### Lowe syndrome

- X-linked recessive
- Caused by mutations in the *ORCL* gene
  - Encodes inositol polyphosphate 5-phosphatase ORCL-1
  - Involved in multiple intracellular processes that impact actin stress fibers, polymerization, and distribution
  - Triad of congenital cataracts, intellectual disability, and proximal tubular dysfunction. Hypotonia and cataract may be seen in the neonatal period. May not be identified until later in childhood when renal issues become more obvious

### Norrie disease

- X-linked
- Caused by mutation in the *NDP* gene
  - Encodes norrin
  - Genotype-phenotype correlations with missense mutations in exon 3 leading to a less severe phenotype than nonsense mutations [31]
- Blindness commonly present in the first few weeks of life

- Bilateral retrolental vascularized masses seen with normal sized eyes
- Cataracts, corneal opacity, shallow anterior chamber, iris atrophy all are common features
- Eyes become phthisical over time [31]

### Nance-horan syndrome

- X-linked involving the *NHS* gene with loss-of-function mutations causing systemic features but translocations like duplications resulting in isolated nonsyndromic cataract [32]
  - It is theorized this protein may be involved in the controlling of actin remodeling, tight junction proteins, and preserving cell morphology
  - The exact function is unknown [33]
- Typical facial dysmorphic features
  - Long face, large ears, prominent nose
- Ocular and dental issues, including cataract and developmental delay
- Female carrier children may show a milder phenotype with Y-sutural lens opacities with cortical "riders"
  - May also have milder dental and facial features [34].

### Myotonic dystrophy 1

- Autosomal dominant
- Occurs owing to cytosine-thymine-guanine repeat disorder in Myotonic dystrophy protein kinase (DMPK)
- Linked with numerous ocular features: cataract, corneal lesions, epiphora, reduced intraocular pressure, eyelid ptosis, retinal degeneration, extraocular myotonia and weakness, abnormal central control of eye movement [35]
- Cataracts are commonly nonspecific and present as punctate opacities [36]

### Neurofibromatosis type 2

- Autosomal dominant
- *NF2* gene mutation
- Presents in adulthood with bilateral vestibular schwannoma
- In children, most commonly seen with small posterior capsular or cortical edge cataracts as well as nonvestibular schwannoma neurologic features and subtle skin tumors [37]

Metabolic conditions are an essential differential to consider in congenital cataracts. They are frequently autosomal recessive. In these conditions, cataracts may be the initial feature, whereas systemic signs are mild. Several rare autosomal recessive diseases are linked with cataract development.

### Zellweger spectrum disorder

- Autosomal recessive
- Mutation in PEX genes that encode proteins needed for peroxisome biogenesis [38]
- Metabolic peroxisome biogenesis disorder
- Usually presents with severe abnormalities leading to early death (see Table 3)
- Milder phenotypic presentation includes neonatal adrenoleukodystrophy and infantile Refsum disease [39]

### Rothmund-thompson syndrome

- Only 300 recorded cases
- Two-third of cases owing to mutations in the *RECOL4* gene
  - Involved in DNA replication and repair
- Widespread changes in skin, connective tissue, and bone
- Higher incidence of childhood and adolescence cancers
  - Specifically, bone malignancies (osteosarcomas) and skin cancers (basal or squamous cell carcinomas)

### Cockayne syndrome

- Rare autosomal recessive condition with variable severity
- *ERCC6* or *ERCC8* mutations
  - Impact repair of mitochondria and DNA damage (such as from environmental stressors like sunlight leading to photosensitivity) [40].

### Cerebrotendinous xanthomatosis

- *CYP27A1* mutations
  - Build-up of cholesterol and cholestenol in tissues leading to CTX [41]
- Developmental cataract commonly an early ocular feature of this disease
- Systemic signs include infantile diarrhea and tendon xanthomas
- Diagnosis frequently not made until adulthood when patient develops progressive neurologic signs
- Early diagnosis and management with daily chenodeoxycholic acid can stop or even reverse severe neurologic complications and significantly improve prognosis [42]

### Galactosemia

- Rare inherited disorder of galactose metabolism
- Part of screening process at birth in the United Kingdom
- Galactokinase (GALK1) and galactose-1-phosphate (GALT) gene mutations lead to GALK1 and classic galactosemia, respectively (see Table 3)
- Almost 200 mutations in the GALT gene have been identified
- Presentation is commonly severe in first few weeks of life owing to infants being exposed to breast/formula milk [43]
- Build-up of galactitol in the lens results in characteristic "oil droplet" cataract
- Anterior and posterior cataract can arise [44]
- Early diagnosis and commencement of galactose-free diet can reverse lens opacification and avert severe systemic complications [45]
- GALK1 deficiency is viewed as a mild form of galactosemia, and pediatric cataract is commonly the main clinical sign [46]

## ACQUIRED CAUSES

### Congenital infections

Worldwide, rubella is the leading cause of congenital cataract and is a public health problem particularly in countries lacking in national immunization programs [47]. During pregnancy, infection of the mother with rubella would place the fetus in danger of developing clinical rubella syndrome (cardiac disease, cataract, and deafness). Further infections that cause cataract include but are not limited to toxoplasmosis, CMV, and HSV I + II. A TORCH screen is often part of the investigation for congenital cataract. However, these tests are often used and interpreted incorrectly. Many factors can influence the positivity of the investigation, such as maternal antibodies in neonates [48]. More recently, evidence suggests specific investigations for individual cases depending on the vaccination status, child comorbidities, and maternal antenatal history are more effective [49].

### Trauma

Trauma is another important cause of childhood cataract, and its presentation and management have specific considerations. Traumatic cataract usually is unilateral and may present with damage to other ocular structures, for example, angle recession, which may lead to secondary glaucoma. Surgery may be more challenging, but patients often suffer less dense amblyopia and a better visual outcome [50]. Objects causing trauma differ globally, with bow and arrows being the most likely cause of ocular trauma in India, whereas sticks, stones, and thorns are more frequent in East Africa [50].

## OTHER COMMON CAUSES OF CATARACT IN CHILDREN

### Uveitic cataract and steroid-related cataract

Anterior uveitis is an inflammation of the iris and ciliary body. Juvenile idiopathic arthritis (JIA) is the most common systemic association in children with uveitis and is linked with HLAB27 positivity. JIA is a group of arthritides seen in childhood, and an extra-articular sign is uveitis, seen in 11% to 13% of patients. It is more common in women and in patients with oligoarthritis and positive antinuclear antibodies. Inflammation in the anterior chamber or the use of steroids can lead to the formation of cataracts [51]. The exact mechanism by which steroids cause cataract (typically posterior subcapsular cataract) is unknown, but it is theorized glucocorticoids play an essential role in gene transcription in lens epithelial cells [52].

### Radiation cataract

Radiation exposure, particularly at higher doses, can lead to cataracts. Therefore, children receiving radiotherapy for pediatric cancers (commonly in leukemia, lymphoma, tumors of the central nervous system, kidney, soft tissue, and bone) are at risk. Doses greater than 3 Gy can lead to cataract developing more quickly, although, more recently, it has been found that cataract can occur at even lower doses of radiation (0.5 Gy), with increasing risk following a linear pattern [1]. Measures can be taken to reduce the chance of cataract in high-risk patients by shielding the eye and using accurate radiation dose estimates [1].

## RELEVANCE

### Management of childhood cataract

Pediatric cataract management has more considerations than cataract in adults. Decisions are made to facilitate optimal visual development during an amblyogenic phase and balanced with the risks of early surgery. Pediatric cataract surgery can be done with or without anterior capsulotomy, posterior capsulotomy, and anterior vitrectomy [53].

There is debate regarding insertion of intraocular lens (IOL) during cataract surgery. A 5-year follow-up study indicated that for patients less than 2 years old, inserting an IOL leads to comparable postoperative vision when compared with contact lens only. IOL insertion did not favorably protect against postoperative glaucoma and meant a further step during surgery. The study recommended patients be left aphakic, especially those younger than 6 months of age, until further research is completed [54]. In the pediatric population, choosing an IOL is complex, as the eye continues to grow throughout childhood; power calculations are more difficult, as attaining precise measurements are more challenging in a young child. The study advised cataract should be performed at 6 to 8 weeks of age for bilateral cataract and at 6 weeks for unilateral cataract [55].

Stringent postoperative care and frequent follow-up are vital for good long-term visual outcomes. Lensectomy at an earlier age leads to improved visual outcomes and lower risk of strabismus; however, the risk of developing glaucoma is greater [55]. Medical management can be considered with dilating drops to increase light entering the eye in less visually significant cataracts. In some cases, nonsurgical management can be used, such as dietary changes and enzyme replacement in galactosemia that can halt or reverse the formation of cataract [56].

*Genetic testing*

Genetic panel testing of known cataract-causing genes is a vital investigation in congenital cataract, with recent studies showing between 60% and 90% molecular diagnostic rates in bilateral cases [3,4]. The latest next-generation sequencing technology allows more than 90% coverage, and whole-genome sequencing has been estimated to increase rate of diagnosis by another 40% [57]. Recent studies have shown that initial panel testing of patients with cataract improves diagnosis rates and allows for personalized care with tailored genetic counseling to support future family planning decisions [6].

*Multidisciplinary care*

A multidisciplinary approach is essential for children with cataracts. General pediatrician assessment is required to identify causes, systemic features that may be life-threatening, particularly while waiting for genetic testing results. Regular ophthalmology follow-up is needed with input from ophthalmologists, optometrists, and orthoptists to monitor the visual development and general eye health and to minimize development of amblyopia. Pediatric patients with moderate reduction in vision in the United Kingdom are referred to specialist advisory services to support the family with advice and access to educational services.

## SUMMARY

Congenital cataract is a heterogenous disease with genetic, infectious, and other causes that need to be considered. Establishing a diagnosis is challenging, and many families remain without a diagnosis. Advances in genomic technology have sped up the continuing discovery of new cataract-causing mutations and strengthened genotype-phenotype correlations. CAT-MAP is a database that contains a list of more than 350 human and mouse genes and loci including at least 16 human loci where the primary causal gene remains unknown [22]. It also contains a list of genes known to cause cataract phenotype in mice. Although there may be genotype-phenotype discrepancies between humans and mice, this list indicates more genes are yet to be discovered. Research now aims to deliver high-quality evidence of the clinical application of genomic testing to support its successful integration and use in clinical practice [58]. Accurate and early diagnosis of congenital cataracts is vital for families, as it allows individualized genetic counseling. Newer online resources, such as gene.vision, provide families with information about their condition and keep them informed of new developments [59]. It facilitates a multidisciplinary approach to support the best possible development of the child during the critical early period, educate families, and allow them to plan for the future.

## CLINICS CARE POINTS

- When presented with a child with cataracts, take a careful birth, medical, and family history (examine family members where possible) to elucidate cause of cataracts.
- Refer children with a new diagnosis of cataracts to specialist genetics services for genetic testing and counseling.
- Children with cataracts require specialized multidisciplinary care. Ensure patients are referred to a general pediatrician for assessment and have a regular review by the ophthalmologist, optometrist, and orthoptist to minimize the risk of amblyopia.

## Disclosure

The authors have nothing to disclose.

## References

[1] Chodick G, Sigurdson AJ, Kleinerman RA, et al. The risk of cataract among survivors of childhood and adolescent cancer: a report from the Childhood Cancer Survivor Study. Radiat Res 2016;185(4):366–74.
[2] Rahi JS, Dezateux C, British Congenital Cataract Interest Group. Measuring and interpreting the incidence of congenital ocular anomalies: lessons from a national study of congenital cataract in the UK. Invest Ophthalmol Vis Sci 2001;42(7):1444–8.
[3] Patel A, Hayward JD, Tailor V, et al. The Oculome panel test: next-generation sequencing to diagnose a diverse range of genetic developmental eye disorders. Ophthalmology 2019;126(6):888–907.
[4] Bell S, Malka S, Lloyd IC, et al. Clinical spectrum and genetic diagnosis of 54 consecutive patients aged 0-25 with bilateral cataracts. Genes 2021;12(2):1–11.

[5] Yi J, Yun J, Li ZK, et al. Epidemiology and molecular genetics of congenital cataracts. Int J Ophthalmol 2011;4(4):422–32.
[6] Musleh M, Hall G, Lloyd IC, et al. Diagnosing the cause of bilateral paediatric cataracts: comparison of standard testing with a next-generation sequencing approach. Eye (Lond) 2016;30(9):1175–81.
[7] Gillespie RL, Urquhart J, Anderson B, et al. Next-generation sequencing in the diagnosis of metabolic disease marked by pediatric cataract. Ophthalmology 2016;123(1):217–20.
[8] Pichi F, Lembo A, Serafino M, et al. Genetics of congenital cataract. Dev Ophthalmol 2016;57:1–14.
[9] Bassnett S, Shi Y, Vrensen GFJM. Biological glass: structural determinants of eye lens transparency. Philos Trans R Soc Lond B Biol Sci 2011;366(1568):1250–64.
[10] Hejtmancik JF. Congenital cataracts and their molecular genetics. Semin Cell Dev Biol 2008;19(2):134–49.
[11] Ling C, Sui R, Yao F, et al. Whole exome sequencing identified a novel truncation mutation in the NHS gene associated with Nance-Horan syndrome. BMC Med Genet 2019;20(1):14.
[12] Romano MT, Tafazzoli A, Mattern M, et al. Bi-allelic mutations in LSS, encoding lanosterol synthase, cause autosomal-recessive hypotrichosis simplex. Am J Hum Genet 2018;103(5): 777–85.
[13] Augusteyn RC. Alpha-crystallin: a review of its structure and function. Clin Exp Optom 2004;87(6):356–66.
[14] Shiels A, Hejtmancik JF. Molecular genetics of cataract. Prog Mol Biol Translational Sci 2015;134:203–18.
[15] Perng MD, Zhang Q, Quinlan RA. Insights into the beaded filament of the eye lens. Exp Cell Res 2007;313(10):2180–8.
[16] Nielsen PA, Baruch A, Shestopalov VI, et al. Lens connexins alpha3Cx46 and alpha8Cx50 interact with zonula occludens protein-1 (ZO-1). Mol Biol Cell 2003;14(6):2470–81.
[17] Beyer EC, Ebihara L, Berthoud VM. Connexin mutants and cataracts. Front Pharmacol 2013;4:43.
[18] Berthoud VM, Ngezahayo A. Focus on lens connexins. BMC Cel Biol 2017;18(Suppl 1):6.
[19] Shiels A, Hejtmancik JF. Mutations and mechanisms in congenital and age-related cataracts. Exp Eye Res 2017;156:95–102.
[20] Agre P, Brown D, Nielsen S. Aquaporin water channels: unanswered questions and unresolved controversies. Curr Opin Cell Biol 1995;7(4):472–83.
[21] Shiels A, King JM, Mackay DS, et al. Refractive defects and cataracts in mice lacking lens intrinsic membrane protein-2. Invest Ophthalmol Vis Sci 2007;48(2):500–8.
[22] Shiels A, Bennett TM, Hejtmancik JF. Cat-Map: putting cataract on the map. Mol Vis 2010;16:2007–15.
[23] Dave A, Martin S, Kumar R, et al. EPHA2 mutations contribute to congenital cataract through diverse mechanisms. Mol Vis 2016;22:18–30.
[24] Ansar M, Chung HL, Taylor RL, et al. Bi-allelic loss-of-function variants in DNMBP cause infantile cataracts. Am J Hum Genet 2018;103(4):568–78.
[25] Harding P, Toms M, Schiff E, et al. EPHA2 Segregates with microphthalmia and congenital cataracts in two unrelated families. Int J Mol Sci 2021;22(4):1–14.
[26] Park JE, Son AI, Hua R, et al. Human cataract mutations in EPHA2 SAM domain alter receptor stability and function. PLoS ONE 2012;7(5):e36564.
[27] Anand D, Agrawal SA, Slavotinek A, et al. Mutation update of transcription factor genes FOXE3, HSF4, MAF, and PITX3 causing cataracts and other developmental ocular defects. Hum Mutat 2018;39(4):471–94.
[28] Ho HY, Chang KH, Nichols J, et al. Homeodomain protein Pitx3 maintains the mitotic activity of lens epithelial cells. Mech Dev 2009;126(1–2):18–29.
[29] Cassidy L, Taylor D. Congenital cataract and multisystem disorders. Eye 1999;13(3): 464–73.

[30] Bull MJ. Health supervision for children with Down syndrome. Pediatrics 2011;128(2): 393–406.
[31] Walker JL, Dixon J, Fenton CR, et al. Two new mutations in exon 3 of theNDP gene: S73X and S101F associated with severe and less severe ocular phenotype, respectively. Hum Mutat 1997;9(1):53–6.
[32] Coccia M, Brooks SP, Webb TR, et al. X-linked cataract and Nance-Horan syndrome are allelic disorders. Hum Mol Genet 2009;18(14):2643–55.
[33] Brooks SP, Coccia M, Tang HR, et al. The Nance–Horan syndrome protein encodes a functional WAVE homology domain (WHD) and is important for co-ordinating actin remodelling and maintaining cell morphology. Hum Mol Genet 2010;19(12):2421–32.
[34] Bixler D, Higgins M, Hartsfield J. The Nance-Horan syndrome: a rare X-linked ocular-dental trait with expression in heterozygous females. Clin Genet 2008;26(1):30–5.
[35] Ikeda KS, Iwabe-Marchese C, França MC Jr, et al. Myotonic dystrophy type 1: frequency of ophthalmologic findings. Arquivos de Neuro-Psiquiatria. 2016;74(3):183–8.
[36] Thornton CA. Myotonic dystrophy. Neurol Clin 2014;32(3):705–19.
[37] Ruggieri M, Praticò AD, Serra A, et al. Childhood neurofibromatosis type 2 (NF2) and related disorders: from bench to bedside and biologically targeted therapies. Acta Otorhinolaryngol Ital 2016;36(5):345–67.
[38] Distel B, Erdmann R, Gould SJ, et al. A unified nomenclature for peroxisome biogenesis factors. J Cell Biol 1996;135(1):1–3.
[39] Klouwer FCC, Berendse K, Ferdinandusse S, et al. Zellweger spectrum disorders: clinical overview and management approach. Orphanet J Rare Dis 2015;10(1):151.
[40] Khobta A, Epe B. Repair of oxidatively generated DNA damage in Cockayne syndrome. Mech Ageing Dev 2013;134(5–6):253–60.
[41] Cali JJ, Hsieh CL, Francke U, et al. Mutations in the bile acid biosynthetic enzyme sterol 27-hydroxylase underlie cerebrotendinous xanthomatosis. J Biol Chem 1991;266(12): 7779–83.
[42] Nie S, Chen G, Cao X, et al. Cerebrotendinous xanthomatosis: a comprehensive review of pathogenesis, clinical manifestations, diagnosis, and management. Orphanet J Rare Dis 2014;9:179.
[43] Coelho AI, Rubio-Gozalbo ME, Vicente JB, et al. Sweet and sour: an update on classic galactosemia. J Inherit Metab Dis 2017;40(3):325–42.
[44] Khokhar S, Pillay G, Dhull C, et al. Pediatric cataract. Indian J Ophthalmol 2017;65(12): 1340.
[45] Stambolian D. Galactose and cataract. Surv Ophthalmol 1988;32(5):333–49.
[46] Demirbas D, Coelho AI, Rubio-Gozalbo ME, et al. Hereditary galactosemia. Metabolism 2018;83:188–96.
[47] Singh MP, Ram J, Kumar A, et al. Infectious agents in congenital cataract in a tertiary care referral center in North India. Diagn Microbiol Infect Dis 2016;85(4):477–81.
[48] de Jong EP, Vossen ACTM, Walther FJ, et al. How to use... neonatal TORCH testing. Arch Dis Child Educ Pract Ed 2013;98(3):93–8.
[49] Mc Loone E, Joyce N, Coyle P. TORCH testing in non-familial paediatric cataract. Eye 2016;30(9):1275–6.
[50] Khokhar S, Gupta S, Yogi R, et al. Epidemiology and intermediate-term outcomes of open- and closed-globe injuries in traumatic childhood cataract. Eur J Ophthalmol 2014;24(1): 124–30.
[51] Durrani OM. Degree, duration, and causes of visual loss in uveitis. Br J Ophthalmol 2004;88(9):1159–62.
[52] Jobling AI, Augusteyn RC. What causes steroid cataracts? A review of steroid-induced posterior subcapsular cataracts. Clin Exp Optom 2002;85(2):61–75.
[53] Lim ME, Buckley EG, Prakalapakorn SG. Update on congenital cataract surgery management. Curr Opin Ophthalmol 2017;28(1):87–92.

[54] Lambert SR, Aakalu VK, Hutchinson AK, et al. Intraocular lens implantation during early childhood. Ophthalmology 2019;126(10):1454–61.
[55] Russell B, DuBois L, Lynn M, et al. The infant aphakia treatment study contact lens experience to age 5 years. Eye Contact Lens 2017;43(6):352–7.
[56] Scientific Department TRC of O. Cataract Surgery Guidelines.; 2010.
[57] Clark MM, Stark Z, Farnaes L, et al. Meta-analysis of the diagnostic and clinical utility of genome and exome sequencing and chromosomal microarray in children with suspected genetic diseases. NPJ Genomic Med 2018;3(1):16.
[58] Lenassi E, Clayton-Smith J, Douzgou S, et al. Clinical utility of genetic testing in 201 preschool children with inherited eye disorders. Genet Med 2020;22(4):745–51.
[59] Yeong JL, Thomas P, Buller J, et al. A newly developed web-based resource on genetic eye disorders for users with visual impairment (Gene.Vision): usability study. J Med Internet Res 2021;23(1):e19151.

Advances in Ophthalmology and Optometry 7 (2022) 119–137

ADVANCES IN OPHTHALMOLOGY AND OPTOMETRY

# Pediatric Graft-Versus-Host Disease

Kerri McInnis-Smith, BA[a,1], Holly K. Miller, DO[b,c], Aparna Ramasubramanian, MD[b,*]

[a]Mayo Clinic Alix School of Medicine, 13400 E. Shea Boulevard, Scottsdale, AZ 85259, USA; [b]Phoenix Children's Hospital, 1919 E Thomas Road, Phoenix, AZ 85016, USA; [c]Mayo Clinic Arizona, 13400 E. Shea Boulevard, Scottsdale, AZ 85259, USA

**Keywords**

• Dry eye • Graft-vs-host • Keratoconjunctivitis sicca • Stem cell • Transplant

**Key points**

- The risk of chronic graft-versus-host disease (GVHD) in the pediatric population is around 25%.
- Early detection of ocular GVHD is important as it causes poor quality of life due to discomfort and vision loss and is also an indicator of systemic GVHD, which leads to increased morbidity and mortality.
- Sequential systemic treatment of ocular manifestation of GVHD is important, and a multidisciplinary approach enables systemic and ocular treatments to be synergistic.

## BACKGROUND

Hematopoietic stem cell transplant (HSCT) is the process of infusing stem cells following a conditioning regimen and is used with curative intent in the pediatric population for conditions such as malignancy, bone marrow failure, hemoglobinopathies, immunodeficiencies, and certain metabolic syndromes [1–4]. Although HSCT is a potentially life-saving measure, severe complications are common. For malignancy, a desired effect of HSCT is achieved through graft-versus-leukemia (GvL), caused by the recognition of host antigens by donor T-cells. However, that same principle also underlies one of the treatment's most prevalent

[1]19635 N. Cave Creek Road. Apt. 206. Phoenix. AZ 85024.

*Corresponding author. 1920 E Cambridge Avenue, Phoenix, AZ 85006-1464. *E-mail address:* aramasubramanian@phoenixchildrens.com

https://doi.org/10.1016/j.yaoo.2022.03.002
2452-1760/22/

toxicities and a major cause of nonrelapse mortality–graft-versus-host disease (GVHD).

What would eventually become known as GVHD was initially recognized in 1956 by Dick van Bekkum and colleagues in their study of mice receiving intravenous autologous or allogeneic bone marrow (BM) cells following total body irradiation; it was termed "secondary disease." Barnes and colleagues were the first group to rename secondary disease as GVHD in 1962. Although the disease had already been described in mice, the first successful nonsyngeneic (i.e., nonidentical twin) allogeneic bone marrow transplant in humans did not occur until 1968 [5]. The ocular manifestations that accompanied GVHD were initially recognized as a Sjögren-type syndrome affecting normal tear function and, in 1983, Franklin and colleagues better captured the extent of these ophthalmologic complications secondary to GVHD [6].

Unfortunately, there remain many serious complications following HSCT, the most prominent of which is GVHD. Acute GVHD (aGVHD) and chronic GVHD (cGVHD) were historically differentiated by their time to onset, with 100 days after HSCT serving as the cutoff. More recently, the distinction between the two syndromes relies on clinical symptoms and was officially reclassified by the National Institutes of Health (NIH) in 2005 [7]. Acute GVHD most commonly affects the skin, liver, and gastrointestinal (GI) tract whereas chronic disease can be limited to one organ system but often has much more diffuse involvement. Less than 10% of patients with aGVHD ever develop ocular involvement, so this article will focus mainly on cGVHD, given its greater predilection for the eyes [8]. The degree of human leukocyte antigen (HLA) matching and stem cell source carry different risks of GVHD, but the overall risk of cGVHD in the pediatric population receiving HSCT has been estimated to be around 22% to 29% [9].

Not only does GVHD have prominent clinical signs and symptoms, but the disease is associated with a high mortality rate. In fact, cGVHD is one of the leading contributors to morbidity and causes of nonrelapse mortality in patients who survive for more than 2 years after allogeneic HSCT [10]. The ability to identify symptoms of GVHD and effectively manage patients is a critical skill of all ophthalmologists, especially as ocular symptoms occasionally are the presenting sign of underlying widespread GVHD and can extensively undermine the patient's quality of life.

## Hematopoietic stem cell transplant

The process of HSCT has been markedly refined since the first successful human transplant over 50 years ago and now is a commonly performed medical practice. According to the Center for International Blood and Marrow Transplant Research, over 23,000 HSCT were performed nationwide in 2019, with 10% in children under 18 years of age [11]. There are numerous pediatric conditions for which HSCT is the only potentially curative option, including [1–4]:

- Malignancy
- Bone marrow failure

- Hemoglobinopathies
- Immunodeficiencies
- Various metabolic syndromes

According to studies by Hoehn and colleagues, the most common indications for HSCT in children under 7 years of age are acute lymphocytic leukemia (ALL) and acute myelogenous leukemia (AML); for children 7 to 18 years old, the top indications are ALL, chronic myelogenous leukemia (CML), and aplastic anemia [3,4].

Certain distinctions must be made as to the source of stem cell harvesting. Firstly, cells can be harvested from the patient's own body (autologous), from the patient's identical twin (syngeneic), or from another healthy human donor (allogeneic). Secondly, there are multiple tissue sites from which stem cells can be transplanted, including bone marrow (BM), peripheral blood (PB), and cord blood (CB). From 2015 to 2019, the predominant cell sources for transplant in adults were PB (88%), followed by BM (9%) and CB (3%) [11]. These donor sources have varying degrees of risk for the development of GVHD.

## Pathophysiology of systemic GVHD

GVHD occurs when donor T-cells are stimulated by host antigens, which is the same principle that underlies the advantageous graft-versus-leukemia (GvL) phenomenon. The goal, therefore, is to maximize GvL benefit while minimizing the risk of GVHD.

There are three phases in the pathogenesis of GVHD [8].

1. Conditioning: HSCT preconditioning regimen causes local destruction of host tissue, resulting in increased levels of proinflammatory cytokines (TNF-alpha, IL-1, IL-6, etc.), which activate host antigen-presenting cells (APCs).
2. Donor T-cell activation: APCs present antigens to donor T-cells, which results in T-cell stimulation and rapid proliferation of cellular and inflammatory mediators.
3. Effector phase: It is a cascade of soluble and cellular mediators that further promote inflammation and host tissue destruction or apoptosis.

Although this explanation of the pathophysiology of GVHD mainly centers around T-cells, more recent evidence has suggested that B-cells play a supporting role in its development [2,12,13].

## Incidence of Chronic GVHD

Approximately 23,000 HSCT are performed annually in the United States, and one group estimated that cGVHD occurs in 40% to 70% of the adult allogeneic HSCT. Of note, this study was completed before the definition of acute versus chronic disease transitioned from one based on time to that on symptoms and also focused on the adult population [12]. It has been shown that the risk of cGVHD is significantly lower in the pediatric population (22%–29%) than in adults, and any occurrence of aGVHD increases the risk of subsequently developing cGVHD [9]. However, the various stem cell sources are associated with different risks for GVHD, and the recent increased use of alternative sources [such as peripheral blood stem cells (PBSCs)] has resulted in a slightly higher risk of disease in the pediatric population than previously [1]. The following stem cell sources are listed in order from the highest to lowest risk of cGVHD: PBSC, BM, and CB [2,9]. One study estimated that the rate of cGVHD in children is as low as 6% in matched sibling cord blood transplants and as high as 25% in matched unrelated donor PBSC transplants [2].

The incidence of ophthalmologic manifestations of disease is very high and reported to occur in 60% to 90% of patients with diagnosed cGVHD [6].

## Diagnosis and Classification of Systemic GVHD

The NIH consensus criteria, developed in 2005, served to both standardize diagnostic criteria for cGVHD and propose clinical scoring systems for disease severity. It also recommended that the distinction of acute versus chronic disease be based on clinical signs rather than the time to onset. In addition to classic aGVHD and classic cGVHD, two other subcategories were proposed: (1) late-onset aGVHD, with acute-like symptoms developing past 100 days and (2) overlap syndrome, involving features of both acute and chronic disease (Fig. 1) [7,14].

Per the NIH recommendations, the diagnosis of systemic cGVHD requires [7,14]

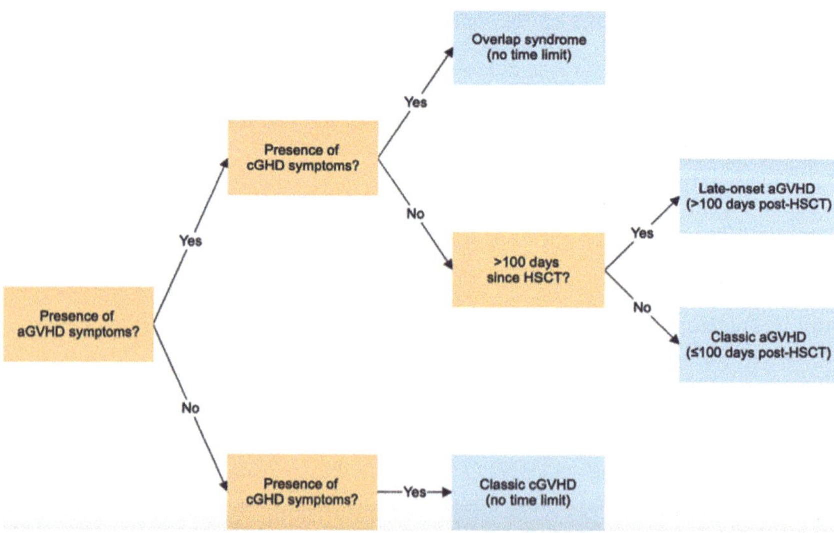


**Fig. 1.** Classifications of graft-versus-host disease, per the NIH consensus criteria. (*Data from* Filipovich AH, Weisdorf D, Pavletic S, et al. National Institutes of Health consensus development project on criteria for clinical trials in chronic graft-versus-host disease: I. diagnosis and staging working group report. Biology of Blood and Marrow Transplantation. 2005;11(12):945–956.)

- at least 1 diagnostic clinical sign of cGVHD or
- at least 1 distinctive manifestation along with a confirmed biopsy or other relevant tests in the same or another organ.

Although biopsy and additional testing are always encouraged and provide further diagnostic value, they are not necessarily required if other diagnostic criteria are met. The specific diagnostic and distinctive symptoms of cGVHD are listed in Table 1, along with typical symptoms of acute GVHD (adapted from Jagasia) [7,14]. It is evident that acute disease often affects three organ systems (skin, liver, and gastrointestinal tract) whereas chronic disease can have much more extensive involvement, frequently involving the eyes.

**Table 1**
Diagnostic and distinctive signs/symptoms of chronic GVHD and acute GVHD

| Organ or site | Acute GVHD | Chronic GVHD |
|---|---|---|
| Skin | Erythema, maculopapular rash, pruritus | Diagnostic: poikiloderma, lichen planus-like features, sclerotic features, morphea-like features, lichen sclerosis-like features<br>Distinctive: depigmentation, papulosquamous lesions |
| Nails | | Diagnostic: none<br>Distinctive: dystrophy; longitudinal ridging, splitting, or brittle nails; onycholysis; pterygium unguis; nail loss |
| Scalp and hair | | Diagnostic: none<br>Distinctive: alopecia (after recovery from induction chemoradiotherapy), loss of body hair, scaling |
| Oral | Erythema, pain following resolution of mucositis | Diagnostic: lichen planus-like changes<br>Distinctive: xerostomia, mucoceles, mucosal atrophy, ulcers, pseudomembranes |
| Eyes | | Diagnostic: none<br>Distinctive: new onset dry, gritty, or painful eyes; cicatricial conjunctivitis; keratoconjunctivitis sicca; confluent areas of punctate keratopathy; photophobia; periorbital hyperpigmentation; blepharitis |
| Gastro-intestinal | Anorexia, nausea, vomiting, diarrhea, weight loss, failure to thrive | Diagnostic: esophageal web; strictures or stenosis in the upper to mid-third of the esophagus<br>Distinctive: none |

(*continued on next page*)

**Table 1**
**(*continued*)**

| Organ or site | Acute GVHD | Chronic GVHD |
|---|---|---|
| Genitals | | Diagnostic: lichen planus-like features, lichen sclerosus-like features, vaginal scarring or clitoral/labial agglutination, phimosis or uretheral/meatus scarring or stenosis<br>Distinctive: erosions, fissures, ulcers |
| Liver | Elevation of total bilirubin, ALP, ALT, or AST to >2x ULN with no other cause | Same features as acute (no diagnostic or distinctive features) |
| Lung | | Diagnostic: bronchiolitis obliterans diagnosed with biopsy, bronchiolitis obliterans syndrome<br>Distinctive: air trapping and bronchiectasis on chest CT |
| Muscles, joints | | Diagnostic: fasciitis, joint stiffness, or contractures secondary to fasciitis or sclerosis<br>Distinctive: myositis or polymyositis |

*Adapted from* Jagasia MH, Greinix HT, Arora M, et al. National Institutes of Health consensus development project on criteria for clinical trials in chronic graft-versus-host disease: I. The 2014 diagnosis and staging working group report. Biol Biology of Blood and Marrow Transplantation. 2015;21(3):389-401.e1.

The median onset of cGVHD is 6 months post-transplant although no specific time limitation exists for classic cGVHD [2]. Three different patterns of onset of cGVHD occur as follows, which have been associated with differing prognosis (see Prognosis section) [15].

1. Progressive: active aGVHD merges into cGVHD
2. Quiescent: aGVHD resolves completely but is followed later by cGVHD
3. De novo: cGVHD develops without prior aGVHD

## Grading of Systemic Disease Severity

The most accepted grading system of cGVHD severity, known as the NIH Global Scoring System, uses the extent of organ involvement and functional impairment to group cases into mild, moderate, or severe disease [7].

- Mild: Two or lesser sites of involvement with no clinically significant functional impairment and without lung symptoms
- Moderate: one or more sites with clinically significant but no major disability, less than 2 organs with no clinically significant functional impairment, or mild lung symptoms
- Severe: major disability caused by cGVHD or moderate/severe lung symptoms

## Risk Factors for Systemic GVHD

In recent decades, significant research efforts have been aimed at identifying the risk factors for the development of cGVHD. The following factors are shown to increase the probability of acquiring cGVHD [1,2,9,12,13,16]. Those denoted with an asterisk were found to be risk factors for disease in the pediatric population specifically [17].

- Severe aGVHD*
- Histocompatibility—antigen disparity between the donor and recipient
- Older donor or recipient age*
- Malignant indication for transplant, especially CML*
- Use of total body irradiation (TBI) in the preparative regimen
- Female donor to male recipient*
- Immunosuppression other than ciclosporin/methotrexate
- Latent viral infection
- Stem cell source (PBSC > BM > CB)
- Genetic susceptibility (see Identification of genetic associations section)
- Receiving subsequent donor leukocyte infusions

## Prognosis

The probability of achieving cGVHD remission depends on the severity of disease, with a cumulative remission incidence of 44.6%. Most patients with mild and moderate disease achieve remission, whereas only one-third of those with severe cGVHD achieve remission after 8 years [14]. It remains controversial whether the ability of the NIH severity score to predict mortality holds true in the pediatric population [10,18]. Of note, children typically have improved outcomes compared with the adult population, with a 68% disease-free survival rate at 6 years in the pediatric population with cGVHD [1]. It is important to remember is that ophthalmologic manifestations often persist after remission of other systemic disease (see Ocular GVHD section). In a study of 55 patients with aqueous tear deficiency secondary to cGVHD, none of the patients had resumption of normal tear function 4 years after remission [19]. This phenomenon is probably compounded by factors other than GVHD, including the underlying disease, medical therapy, and radiation therapy.

## Ocular GVHD

Ocular signs and symptoms are extremely common in cGVHD, occurring in 60% to 90% of patients with diagnosed chronic GVHD [6]. Chronic GVHD can affect nearly all parts of the eye and result in varying effects on a patient's vision and quality of life. Although ocular symptoms often develop within 2 years of cGVHD diagnosis, patients who do not have eye involvement at disease onset still remain at high risk of developing such symptoms later on [20].

### *Clinical Presentation of Ocular GVHD*

The most common manifestation of ocular GVHD (oGVHD) is keratoconjunctivitis sicca, or dry eye, which occurs in 40% to 75% of all patients with ocular signs and typically develops within 6 to 9 months post-HSCT [12,21].

It often is accompanied by other inflammatory signs of the conjunctiva, such as conjunctival edema, chemosis, or pseudomembrane formation. This process can subsequently cause "secondary epithelial changes," such as punctate keratopathy, filament formation, corneal infections, and even corneal erosions and ulcerations [8]. Four stages of conjunctival GVHD have been described [22].

1. Conjunctival hyperemia without other changes (Fig. 2)
2. Chemotic response, serosanguinous exudates, or both
3. Formation of conjunctival pseudomembrane
4. Sloughing of corneal epithelium

Involvement of the conjunctiva in GVHD has been associated with worse outcomes, including higher mortality and decreased quality of life [20].

Other possible ophthalmologic signs of GVHD include the following [2,6,8,12,23]:

- Lacrimal gland: fibrosis leading to irreversible dry eye
- Eyelid: ectropion or entropion development, meibomian gland dysfunction (Fig. 3), lagophthalmos, symblepharon, and trichiasis
- Cornea: superior limbic keratoconjunctivitis, limbal stem cell deficiency, filamentary keratitis, corneal neovascularization, and corneal ulceration or perforation
- Lens: cataract formation (often confounded by corticosteroids and TBI)
- Posterior segment: microvascular retinopathy, central serous retinopathy, posterior scleritis, optic disc edema, and infections
- Cutaneous: dermatitis, poliosis, madarosis, and vitiligo

The symptoms experienced by patients depend on the structures most affected and often begin with irritation and dry eye sensation although it can alternatively present with excessive tearing [1,8,21]. The difficulty in evaluating ocular symptoms in the pediatric population is that young children rarely report dry eye symptoms and require more specific history-taking and examination. Children with chronic oGVHD often present with photophobia as the chief complaint [24]. Other symptoms include burning, painful eyes, redness, and blurry vision. Although permanent vision loss is exceedingly rare even in ocular GVHD, it potentially can occur in cases of conjunctival infection, blepharitis, keratitis, or endophthalmitis [8].

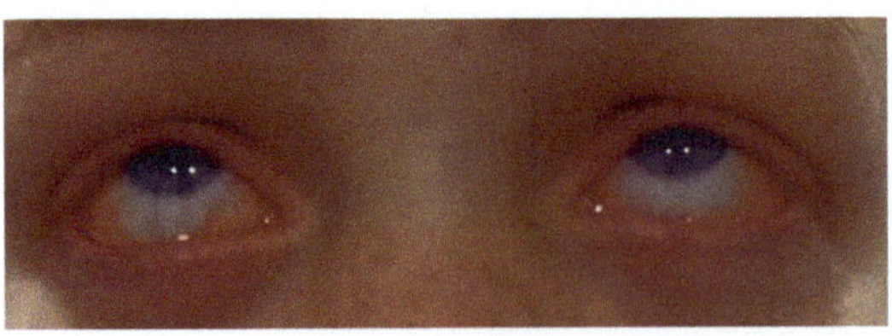

**Fig. 2.** Conjunctival hyperemia and corneal epithelial changes in a child with chronic GVHD.

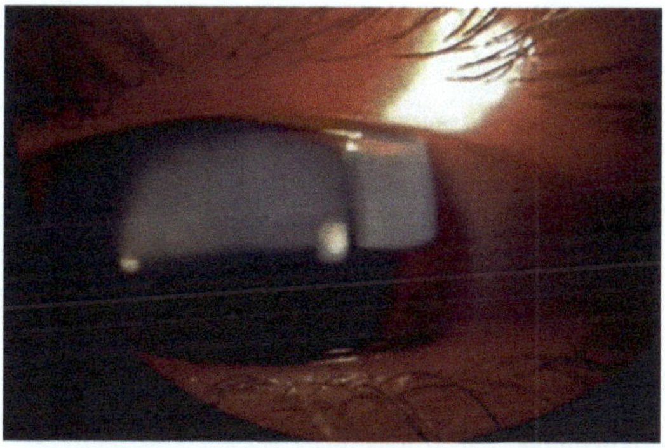

**Fig. 3.** Meibomian gland disease in GVHD.

*Diagnosis of Ocular GVHD*

The lack of pathognomic symptoms or clinical signs for chronic oGVHD contributes to the difficulty in diagnosis. There are three main diagnostic criteria published by the NIH, International Consensus Criteria on Ocular GVHD (ICCGVHD) and TFOS Dry Eye Workshop (DEWS) II.

Multiple diagnostic tools and tests are variably implemented in the three guidelines described below. The sensitivity and specificity of each of these tests when used alone is listed in Table 2 [25].

Per the NIH consensus criteria, the eye manifestations of cGVHD are distinctive rather than diagnostic and therefore require a biopsy or other

**Table 2**
Sensitivity and specificity of diagnostic tools when used alone for diagnosis of oGVHD per NIH criteria

| Diagnostic tool | Description | Sensitivity (%) | Specificity (%) |
|---|---|---|---|
| Schirmer's test, $\leq 5$ mm | Measures moisture content on a piece of filter paper after 5 min inside the lower eyelid | 81 | 100 |
| Ocular surface disease index (OSDI), $\geq 13$ | 12 patient-reported questions related to dry eyes | 31 | 82 |
| Corneal staining, $\geq$ grade 1 | Use of fluorescein to evaluate corneal epitheliopathy | 62 | 90 |
| Tear film breakup time (TBUT), $\leq 5$ s | Interval of time between complete blink and appearance of first break in tear film | 64 | 71 |
| Tear film osmolarity, $\geq 308$ mOsm/L | | 67 | 41 |

*Adapted from* Pathak M, Diep PP, Lai X, Brinch L, Ruud E, Drolsum L. Ocular findings and ocular graft-versus-host disease after allogeneic stem cell transplantation without total body irradiation. Bone Marrow Transplant. 2018;53(7):863–872.

relevant test to confirm the diagnosis of cGVHD (see Table 1). The updated NIH diagnostic criteria are [14]

1. Schirmer test smaller than 5 mm at 5 min or
2. Schirmer test 6 to 10 mm at 5 min with KCS diagnosed by slit-lamp examination

The ICCGVHD guidelines use the ocular surface disease index (OSDI), Schirmer's test, corneal fluorescein staining, conjunctival injection, and the presence of systemic GVHD to determine the likelihood of oGVHD [26]. Finally, the TFOS DEWS II criteria published in 2013 state that the OSDI be larger than 13, along with one of the following [27,28]:

- Tear film breakup time (TBUT) less than 10 s
- Tear osmolarity greater than 308 mOsm/L in either eye or interocular difference greater than 8 mOsm/L
- Ocular surface staining: more than 5 corneal spots, more than 9 conjunctival spots or lid margin

*Grading of Ocular Disease Severity*

Multiple grading systems for chronic oGVHD severity have been proposed, including one from the NIH consensus criteria (Table 3) and another based solely on conjunctival findings (Table 4).

*Pathophysiology and Histology of Ocular GVHD*

The actual etiology of ocular symptoms in a patient diagnosed with GVHD can be difficult to determine as many potential confounding factors may be present, including underlying disease, concomitant medical therapy, or prior radiation therapy. Akin to the pathogenesis of systemic GVHD, chronic oGVHD consists of a T-cell-mediated inflammatory process followed by an immune cascade.

Certain histopathologic changes occur mostly in the tissue of the conjunctiva and lacrimal glands and coincide with the experienced symptoms. These include fibrosis and atrophy of the tubuloalveolar glands and ducts in the

**Table 3**
Grading of chronic oGVHD, per NIH consensus criteria

| Severity grade | Dry eye symptoms | Effects on ADLs | Lubricant eye drops |
|---|---|---|---|
| Grade 0 | Asymptomatic patient with KCS confirmed by ophthalmologist | | |
| Grade 1 | Mild | Not affected | $\leq 3\times$ daily |
| Grade 2 | Moderate | Partially affected | $>3\times$ daily or punctal plug |
| Grade 3 | Severe | Significantly affected, unable to work, or loss of vision due to KCS | Special eyewear required |

*Adapted from* Jagasia MH, Greinix HT, Arora M, et al. National Institutes of Health consensus development project on criteria for clinical trials in chronic graft-versus-host disease: I. The 2014 diagnosis and staging working group report. Biology of Blood and Marrow Transplantation. 2015;21(3):389-401.e1.

**Table 4**
Grading of chronic oGVHD based on conjunctival findings

| Severity grade | Conjunctival findings |
|---|---|
| Grade 1 | Conjunctival hyperemia occurring on the bulbar or palpebral conjunctiva in at least one eyelid |
| Grade 2 | Palpebral conjunctival fibrovascular changes occurring along the superior border of the upper eyelid, or the lower border of the tarsal plate of the lower eyelid, with or without conjunctival epithelial sloughing, involving <25% of the total surface area in at least one eyelid |
| Grade 3 | Palpebral conjunctival fibrovascular changes occurring along the superior border of the upper eyelid, or the lower border of the tarsal plate of the lower eyelid, involving 25%–75% of the total surface area in at least one eyelid |
| Grade 4 | >75% of the total surface area with or without a cicatricial entropion in at least one eyelid |

*Data from* Robinson MR, Lee SS, Rubin BI, et al. Topical corticosteroid therapy for cicatricial conjunctivitis associated with chronic graft-versus-host disease. Bone Marrow Transplant. 2004;33(10):1031–1035.

lacrimal gland, accumulation of PAS-positive material within the lumina of acina and ductules, lymphocytic infiltration, and an increased number of CD34+ fibroblasts [8,12,21].

*Risk Factors for Ocular GVHD*

Separate risk factors other than those discussed earlier have been shown to increase the risk of developing ocular manifestations of cGVHD, including [8,20,29]

- History of acute GVHD
- Multiorgan GVHD involvement, especially oral, pulmonary, and cutaneous
- Use of PBSCs
- Female donor to male recipient
- Absence of anti-T-cell globulin (ATG) in conditioning regimen
- Ebstein Barr Virus-seropositive donor

It remains controversial whether the underlying disease predisposes a child to chronic oGVHD development.

*Prevention and Screening of GVHD*

The most effective way to prevent chronic oGVHD is to prevent cGVHD via improved cross-matching techniques and T-cell depletion. Substantial improvements in high-fidelity molecular typing of HLA loci combined with the vast increase in the number of donors available worldwide in recent decades have made HSCT a much more feasible and potentially curative option than previously. The modern technique of HLA matching further increases reliability and thoroughness. Although a perfect match is not always available, particularly in minority cultures, we now have the ability to estimate HSCT efficacy and risk of complications such as GVHD based on the degree of allele/antigen mismatch [2].

Cyclosporine A (CsA) or tacrolimus combined with mycophenolate mofetil or methotrexate is administered to patients following HSCT to deactivate donor T lymphocytes [8]. CsA and tacrolimus are both calcineurin inhibitors that block T-cell proliferation and IL-2 production to halt T lymphocytes. Methotrexate is a folate antagonist that blocks T-cell activation, and mycophenolate mofetil inhibits IMP dehydrogenase, a key enzyme in nucleotide synthesis [30]. Antithymocyte globulin is also added for patients with higher degrees of HLA mismatching.

It is fundamental that all patients, including children, undergo a comprehensive eye examination before HSCT to assess their baseline ophthalmologic health and allow the clinician to better differentiate preexisting eye symptoms from active ocular manifestations of cGVHD. Additionally, Hebert and colleagues found that almost 50% of children who were diagnosed with oGVHD were asymptomatic at the time of diagnosis, highlighting the importance of systematic eye screening following HSCT [29]. This screening should start no later than 6 months post-transplant and occur every 3 to 12 months thereafter. It is important to always recommend comprehensive eye examination at the time of initial diagnosis of cGVHD in other sites [23].

## Mainstays and recent developments in therapy

### *Systemic Treatment*

The management of ocular signs of cGVHD begins with systemic treatment tailored to the individual, often including corticosteroids and calcineurin inhibitors such as cyclosporine A [8,15,16,23]. As initially suggested by the NIH consensus criteria and supported by multiple subsequent studies, systemic therapy is recommended for patients with moderate or severe cGVHD whereas topical therapy is used for those with mild cGVHD (see Grading of Disease Severity section) [14]. Clinicians should start with high-dose steroids (1–2 mg/kg/d), with the aim to wean until the lowest allowable dose of steroids without a cGHVD symptom flare is achieved [2].

It has been shown that the vast majority (90%) of patients who would respond to therapy will do so within 3 months of beginning treatment [2]. Unfortunately, up to 50% of patients continue to require immunosuppression past 5 years after their initial diagnosis, with the average duration of therapy being 1 to 3 years [2]. It is important to consider the added toxicities that both long-term steroid use and immunosuppression can cause, including infections, splenic dysfunction, diabetes mellitus, muscle weakness, osteoporosis, avascular necrosis, and cushingoid features. One study showed that the major cause of death in cGVHD is opportunistic infection, secondary to the long-term immunosuppression [10]. Further, calcineurin inhibitors such as cyclosporine A can cause renal impairment, hypertension, and neurologic paresthesias [15].

*Local Treatment*

In addition to systemic therapy, various local treatments are available that are focused on four main goals: (1) lubrication; (2) decrease in inflammation; (3) drainage control; and (4) evaporation control. The management of patients with ocular manifestations of cGVHD is outlined in Fig. 4 (used with permission from Blackburn and colleagues)

*Lubrication*

The first goal of improving symptoms of chronic oGVHD is increasing ocular surface moisture. Preservative-free artificial tears should be offered to all patients with ophthalmologic signs. Other options for improving lubrication include viscous ointment at night, hyaluronic acid and dexpanthenol-containing eye drops, mucin-secretagogue eye drops, and hydroxypropyl methylcellulose pellets. The utility of oral omega-3-fatty acids in improving dry eye symptoms remains controversial. Two drugs that have been shown to improve KCS in Sjögren syndrome, oral cevimeline and pilocarpine, are occasionally used for oGVHD. Another option includes autologous serum eye drops, which have both lubricating and anti-inflammatory benefits and were shown to improve symptoms in 91% of patients and objective findings in 32% of patients with oGVHD [21,23].

*Inflammation Control*

The second goal of ocular GVHD symptom control is to reduce ocular surface inflammation.

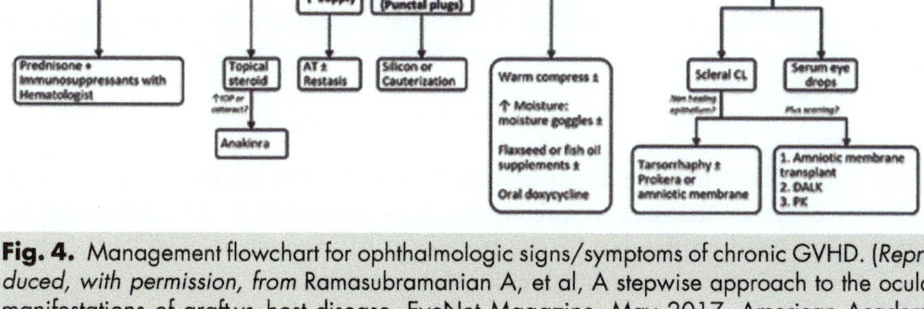


**Fig. 4.** Management flowchart for ophthalmologic signs/symptoms of chronic GVHD. (*Reproduced, with permission, from* Ramasubramanian A, et al, A stepwise approach to the ocular manifestations of graft-vs.-host disease. EyeNet Magazine, May 2017, American Academy of Ophthalmology.)

Cyclosporine eye drops should be given to all patients with inflammatory signs of GVHD, given their ability to improve Schirmer test results and TBUT, increase conjunctival goblet cells and decrease punctate keratopathy. The recommended long-term dose of topical cyclosporine is 0.05% or 0.1% twice daily [21].

Acute exacerbations of ocular GVHD require intensive treatment often consisting of topical corticosteroids. Although effective, this approach should only be considered short term and always be closely monitored as long-term steroids are associated with complications such as glaucoma, cataract formation, corneal thinning, and severe infections. A safe and feasible alternative to steroids is topical tacrolimus (0.05% or 0.02%), which does not have the ocular hypertensive consequences of topical corticosteroids [21,23].

Other drugs shown to help with inflammation control in chronic oGVHD include [21,23]

- topical tranilast: inhibits TGF-beta
- topical anakinra 2.5%: IL-1 receptor antagonist
- topical lifitegrast: inhibits LFA-1/ICAM-1 interaction
- topical inhibitors of Janus and spleen tyrosine kinases (JAK and SYK)

*Evaporation Control*

The third goal of local treatment for ocular GVHD consists of evaporation control, aiming to minimize meibomian gland blockage. It is important to emphasize proper eyelid hygiene to patients, including removing all makeup before bed and applying frequent warm compresses. Some topical antibiotics and dietary supplementation of fish and flaxseed oil have been shown to improve meibomian gland function [23].

*Drainage Control*

The fourth and final goal of symptomatic treatment for chronic oGVHD is drainage control. This is often achieved via punctal occlusion with collagen or silicone plugs but can occasionally require permanent surgical occlusion or thermal cauterization.

*Control of Epithelial Disease*

The cornea develops changes from chronic keratoconjunctivitis that can hamper long term vision by causing scarring. The options to conserve the corneal epithelium include scleral contact lens, moisture chamber goggles, or amniotic membrane devices such as the *Prokera* corneal bandage device or *Ambiodisk* [21,23].

*Refractory Cases*

Very rarely, there may be patients with symptoms that are refractory to all the above treatment measures, requiring surgical intervention. The following surgeries have been performed in the treatment of chronic oGVHD symptoms: partial tarsorrhaphy, superficial epithelial debridement, amniotic membrane transplantation, corneal transplantation, lysis of membranes and symblepharon, and deep anterior lamellar or penetrating keratoplasty [21,23].

*Future trends*

*Standardization of Guidelines.* As mentioned previously, numerous different diagnostic and staging criteria have been proposed. The NIH report on cGVHD diagnosis and staging, first published in 2005 and then updated in 2014, was the first concerted effort to standardize the diagnostic criteria for chronic oGVHD. Then, the more detailed and arguably less subjective ICCGVHD guidelines were proposed in 2013, followed by the DEWS II set in 2017. Each of these three grading systems incorporate different clinical parameters to gauge the probability and severity of ocular involvement. Multiple studies have been published analyzing the homogeneity between the different guidelines and their diagnostic and grading outcomes. One group found that the diagnosis of ocular GVHD varied significantly depending on which diagnostic criteria was applied. The most disagreement occurred with the DEWS II criteria, and "moderate" agreement was found between the NIH and ICCGVHD criteria [25].

Additional studies aimed at comparing the multiple diagnostic and grading approaches are needed to determine which is the most sensitive and specific for chronic oGVHD. The standardization of these criteria will not only allow for early detection and better patient care but also for more accurate population-wide estimations of disease incidence and contributing risk factors.

*Identification of Genetic Associations*

Recent analysis has suggested that there are multiple genetic factors that may play a role in the development of GVHD. For example, Ansari and colleagues identified 4 novel loci that contribute to aGVHD [13].

- ERC1: participates in the DNA damage response signaling pathway
- PLEK: protein kinase C substrate, inducibly expressed by macrophages
- SPRED1: tumor suppressor, negative regulator of the Ras/mitogen activated protein kinase (MAPK) pathway
- NOP9: participates in RNA recognition and processing

Although this study focused on acute GVHD and its genetic underpinnings, there are most likely similar genetic factors associated with chronic GVHD and its ocular manifestations.

*Discovery of cGVHD Biomarkers*

Several biomarkers for the presence of organ-specific aGVHD have been discovered and proved since the early 2000's, with algorithms in place based on the presence and levels of these biomarkers providing the risk of mortality. Several researchers are collaborating to identify specific biomarkers for cGVHD as the detection of sensitive biomarkers for cGVHD could be a game-changing breakthrough. Not only would it reveal potential targets for pharmacologic therapies but allow for better selection of a therapeutic regimen individualized to the specific patient. Some currently promising candidates as disease biomarkers include [16]

- suppressor of tumorigenicity 2 (ST2)
- B-cell activating factor (BAFF)
- CXCL9, CXCL10, CXCL11

- matrix metalloproteinase 3
- osteopontin
- gene polymorphisms in CTLA4, HPSE, IL1R1, CCR6

*Novel Therapeutic Approaches*

The mainstays of therapy and recommended approach to management for patients with ocular manifestations of cGVHD were discussed above. However, as new drugs for systemic GVHD and dry eye disease are approved, it is important to assess the potential for these drugs in the treatment of the more nuanced setting of chronic oGVHD.

Until recently, little advancement occurred in the field of systemic GVHD treatment, with no novel therapies approved by the FDA for patients with steroid-dependent or steroid-refractory disease over the last few decades [16]. As mentioned previously, recent evidence highlights a greater role for B-cells in the development of GVHD than previously thought, bringing more interest to medications that affect B-cells, their differentiation and downstream signaling. One such mechanism of B-cell receptor downstream signaling occurs via Bruton's tyrosine kinase (BTK). Ibrutinib, a BTK inhibitor, was the first FDA-approved drug for steroid-resistant cGVHD [16]. Other potential cGVHD drugs currently in clinical trial have the following biochemical targets [16]:

- spleen tyrosine kinase (SYK), active in B-cell receptor downstream signaling
- ROCK2, involved in T-cell activation
- JAK1 and JAK2, required for cytokine production and APC function
- IL-6 receptor, involved in the activation of macrophages and fibroblasts
- TGF-beta receptor, involved in Th1 and Th17 activity
- CD30, expressed by many inflammatory cells
- CTLA-4, involved in T-cell activation
- platelet-derived growth factor receptor (PDGFR), activated in fibrosis

Likewise, novel therapies for the treatment of non-GVHD-related dry eye disease have been proposed in recent years. For example, anakinra and lifitegrast were both initially proposed for the treatment of primary dry eye disease before they were found to be safe and effective for chronic oGVHD [21]. Other recently published studies propose the following approaches to dry eye disease [31]:

- Medication: lacritin, lubricin, Thymosin beta-4, amniotic membrane extract eye drops (AMEED), varenicline nasal spray
- Devices: intranasal tear neurostimulation
- Procedures: intense pulsed light (IPL), vectored thermal pulsation (*LipiFlow*), meibomian gland probing, Mibo Thermoflo, BlephEx, TearCare system

Additional studies will be required to determine the efficacy of these new cGVHD and dry eye disease treatments in improving the specific ophthalmologic symptoms of oGVHD.

## SUMMARY

The importance of clinician familiarity with the varied possibility of clinical signs and symptoms of cGVHD cannot be overstated, especially given its high prevalence, and mortality. The involvement of a multidisciplinary care team is of paramount importance in caring for patients with suspect GVHD. This team should include providers from a multitude of specialties, including ophthalmology, dermatology, pulmonology, urology/gynecology, endocrinology, dentistry, physical therapy, and so on. Some institutions have special multidisciplinary care centers, solely focused on this idea of bringing together a team of specialists to better care for patients with cGVHD.

As discussed earlier, the field of transplant medicine is constantly evolving, with ongoing research efforts focused on disease prevention, biomarker identification, and novel therapeutic options. Each of these study areas is interconnected, for example, with biomarker identification affording new insights into potential drug targets and prevention techniques. Additionally, as the pathophysiology of GVHD development is better understood, these findings will allow us to identify drug targets more efficiently and perhaps decrease the rate of cGVHD prevention by improving transplant practices and donor/recipient matching.

## CLINICS CARE POINTS

- In the clinical management of patients with GVHD, it is useful to use the NIH criteria during every patient visit and routinely use OSDI for older children.
- The two main goals in treatment are to improve lubrication and to decrease inflammation.
- The treatment of GVHD needs both systemic and local control and hence close collaboration with the oncologist is important.

## DISCLOSURE

No disclosures. No funding support.

### References

[1] Jacobsohn DA. Optimal management of chronic graft-versus-host disease in children: Review. Br J Haematol 2010;150(3):278–92.

[2] Baird K, Cooke K, Schultz KR. Chronic graft-versus-host disease (GVHD) in children. Pediatr Clin North Am 2010;57(1):297–322.

[3] Hoehn ME, Vestal R, Calderwood J, et al. Ocular complications in school-age children and adolescents after allogeneic bone marrow transplantation. Am J Ophthalmol 2020;213:153–60.

[4] Hoehn ME, Calderwood J, Gannon E, et al. Ocular complications in a young pediatric population following bone marrow transplantation. J Am Assoc Pediatr Ophthalmol Strabismus 2018;22(2):102–6.e1.

[5] Vriesendorp HM, Heidt PJ. History of graft-versus-host disease. Exp Hematol 2016;44(8):674–88.

[6] Fung SS, Elbaz U, Mireskandari K, et al. Graft versus host disease: a pediatric perspective. Expert Rev Ophthalmol 2019;14(2):89–99.
[7] Filipovich AH, Weisdorf D, Pavletic S, et al. National Institutes of Health Consensus Development Project on Criteria for Clinical Trials in Chronic Graft-versus-Host Disease: I. Diagnosis and Staging Working Group Report. Biol Blood Marrow Transplant 2005;11(12): 945–56.
[8] Riemens A, te Boome L, Imhof S, et al. Current insights into ocular graft-versus-host disease. Curr Opin Ophthalmol 2010;21(6):485–94.
[9] Zecca M. Chronic graft-versus-host disease in children: incidence, risk factors, and impact on outcome. Blood 2002;100(4):1192–200.
[10] Inagaki J, Moritake H, Nishikawa T, et al. Long-term morbidity and mortality in children with chronic graft-versus-host disease classified by national institutes of health consensus criteria after allogeneic hematopoietic stem cell transplantation. Biol Blood Marrow Transplant 2015;21(11):1973–80.
[11] Transplant Activity Report. Center for International Blood and Marrow Transplant, a contractor for the C.W. Bill Young Cell Transplantation Program operated through the U. S. Department of Health and Human Services, Health Resources and Services Administration. Healthcare Systems Bureau; 2021.
[12] Nicholas GA, Carl R. Ocular manifestations of graft versus host disease. Current Opinion in Ophthalmology 2004, 15(6):503-7.
[13] Ansari M, Petrykey K, Rezgui MA, et al. Genetic susceptibility to acute graft versus host disease in pediatric patients undergoing HSCT. Bone Marrow Transplant 2021;56(11): 2697–704.
[14] Jagasia MH, Greinix HT, Arora M, et al. National Institutes of Health Consensus Development Project on Criteria for Clinical Trials in Chronic Graft-versus-Host Disease: I. The 2014 Diagnosis and Staging Working Group Report. Biol Blood Marrow Transplant 2015;21(3):389–401.e1.
[15] Liu YM, Hockenberry M. Review of chronic graft-versus-host disease in children after allogeneic stem cell transplantation: nursing perspective. J Pediatr Oncol Nurs 2011;28(1):6–15.
[16] Zeiser R, Blazar BR. Pathophysiology of chronic graft-versus-host disease and therapeutic targets. Longo DL, ed. N Engl J Med. 2017;377(26):2565-2579.
[17] Kondo M, Kojima S, Horibe K, et al. Risk factors for chronic graft-versus-host disease after allogeneic stem cell transplantation in children. Bone Marrow Transpl 2001;27(7): 727–30.
[18] Lee JW, Lee DH, Jang PS, et al. Prognostic Implications of the NIH Consensus Criteria in Children with Chronic Graft-versus-Host Disease. Yonsei Med J 2011;52(5):779.
[19] Hirst L, Jabs D, Tutschka P, et al. The Eye in Bone Marrow Transplantation: I. Clinical Study. Arch Ophthalmol 1983;101(4):580–4.
[20] Sun YC, Chai X, Inamoto Y, et al. Impact of ocular chronic graft-versus-host disease on quality of life. Biol Blood Marrow Transplant 2015;21(9):1687–91.
[21] Inamoto Y, Valdés-Sanz N, Ogawa Y, et al. Ocular graft-versus-host disease after hematopoietic cell transplantation: expert review from the Late Effects and Quality of Life Working Committee of the CIBMTR and Transplant Complications Working Party of the EBMT. Bone Marrow Transpl 2019;54(5):662–73.
[22] Jabs D, Wingard J, Green W. The eye in bone marrow transplantation. III. Conjunctival graft-vs-host disease. Arch Ophthalmol 1989;107:1343–8.
[23] Blackburn R, Mueller B, Ramasubramanian A. A stepwise approach to the ocular manifestations of graft-vs.-host disease. EyeNet Magazine; 2017.
[24] Lawitschka A, Ball L, Peters C. Nonpharmacologic treatment of chronic graft-versus-host disease in children and adolescents. Biol Blood Marrow Transplant 2012;18(1):S74–81.
[25] Pathak M, Diep PP, Lai X, et al. Ocular findings and ocular graft-versus-host disease after allogeneic stem cell transplantation without total body irradiation. Bone Marrow Transpl 2018;53(7):863–72.

[26] Ogawa Y, Kim SK, Dana R, et al. International Chronic Ocular Graft-vs-Host-Disease (GVHD) Consensus Group: Proposed Diagnostic Criteria for Chronic GVHD (Part I). Sci Rep 2013;3(1):3419.
[27] Wolffsohn JS, Arita R, Chalmers R, et al. TFOS DEWS II Diagnostic Methodology report. Ocul Surf 2017;15(3):539–74.
[28] Robinson MR, Lee SS, Rubin BI, et al. Topical corticosteroid therapy for cicatricial conjunctivitis associated with chronic graft-versus-host disease. Bone Marrow Transpl 2004;33(10):1031–5.
[29] Hébert M, Archambault C, Doyon C, et al. Risk factors for ocular involvement in pediatric graft-versus-host disease. Cornea 2021;40(9):1158–64.
[30] Hamilton BK. Current approaches to prevent and treat GVHD after allogeneic stem cell transplantation. Hematology 2018;2018(1):228–35.
[31] O'Neil EC, Henderson M, Massaro-Giordano M, et al. Advances in dry eye disease treatment. Curr Opin Ophthalmol 2019;30(3):166–78.

# Ophthalmic Pathology & Ocular Oncology

Advances in Ophthalmology and Optometry 7 (2022) 139–149

ADVANCES IN OPHTHALMOLOGY AND OPTOMETRY

# Fluorescence In Situ Hybridization in Ocular Oncology

Seema Sen, MD[a,*], Shahzan Anjum, MSc[a], Mehar Chand Sharma, MD[b]

[a]Ocular Pathology Services, Dr. Rajendra Prasad Centre for Ophthalmic Sciences, All India Institute of Medical Sciences, New Delhi, Delhi, India; [b]Department of Pathology, All India Institute of Medical Sciences, New Delhi, Delhi, India

**Keywords**

• Fluorescence In situ hybridization (FISH) • Lymphoma • Uveal melanoma • Adenoid cystic carcinoma • Ocular tumors

**Key points**

- Ocular tumors including lymphoma, uveal melanoma and adenoid cystic carcinoma of lacrimal gland are aggressive and metastatic tumors.
- Immunoexpression combined with study of genetic rearrangement studies are considered an ideal approach for better patient management.
- Study of chromosomal abnormalities are useful for diagnosis, prognosis and for targeted therapy in ocular malignancies.

## INTRODUCTION

Fluorescence in situ hybridization (FISH) is a gold standard in cytogenetics for the detection of chromosomal rearrangements or aberrations in diseased or malignant cells. In diagnostics, FISH involves the binding of the probe to the target of interest, which enables its detection and visualization. FISH can be performed on suspended cells, cultured cells, and frozen or formalin-fixed paraffin-embedded (FFPE) tissue sections. However, during the fixation of any of the samples for FISH, it is important to preserve nucleic acid and cellular integrity [1]. The advantage of FISH over karyotyping is that it does not

*Corresponding author. Ocular Pathology Services, Dr. Rajendra Prasad Centre for Ophthalmic Sciences, All India Institute of Medical Sciences, New Delhi 110029, India. *E-mail address:* drseemasen@gmail.com

https://doi.org/10.1016/j.yaoo.2022.03.003

require fresh tissues, and FFPE sections as old as 25 years can be used [2]. With improvements in labeling of probes and high-resolution imaging systems, FISH has been renovated for analysis of nuclear structures and gene function [3].

Although its use has diminished in the era of array comparative genomic hybridization (CGH) and next-generation sequencing (NGS), FISH continues to be an extremely powerful tool because absolute copy number quantification is obtained at the single-cell level within the tumor-section architecture. In the era of precision cancer medicine, efficient genotyping is critical [4]. Use of panels of gene-specific probes for somatic losses, gains, and translocations are routinely used for hematologic and solid tumors and are one of the fastest-growing areas in cancer diagnosis [3]. The most important advantage of FISH lies in its high specificity and sensitivity in recognizing DNA and RNA sequences, it can be used for both metaphase and interphase nuclei and visualization at the level of a single cell. By FISH technology, conventional cytogenetics has been upgraded to molecular cytogenetics [3].

Joseph Gall and Mary Lou Pardue demonstrated that molecular hybridization could be used to identify the position of DNA sequences *in situ* (ie, within their natural chromosome positions). In 1969, these 2 scientists showed that in the nucleus of a frog's eggs, radioactive copies of a ribosomal DNA sequence could be used to detect complementary DNA sequences. Following this key observation, there have been many refinements in the procedure to the extent that in situ hybridization is now considered an essential tool in cytogenetics [4].

Fluorescent labels replaced radioactive labels in hybridization probes because of their safety, stability, and ease of detection. Most in situ hybridization tests presently are performed using FISH procedures. Synthetic FISH probes can easily be designed and synthesized and have become popular. Chromosomal regions from oligonucleotide libraries can detect targets in the range of tens of kilobases to megabases.

Selected DNA strands incorporated with fluorophore-coupled nucleotides can be used as probes to hybridize onto the complementary sequences in tested cells and tissues and then visualized through a fluorescence microscope or an imaging system. This hybridization-based macromolecule recognition tool is very effective in mapping genes and polymorphic loci onto metaphase chromosomes for constructing a physical map of the human genome. This technology was initially developed as a physical mapping tool to delineate genes within chromosomes. Its high analytical resolution to a single gene level and high sensitivity and specificity has enabled its immediate application for genetic diagnosis of constitutional common aneuploidies, microdeletion/microduplication syndromes, and subtelomeric rearrangements. Cas9-mediated FISH (CASFISH) allows in situ labeling of repetitive sequence and single-copy sequences without the disruption of nuclear genomic organization in fixed or living cells [4].

## SIGNIFICANCE OF FLUORESCENCE IN SITU HYBRIDIZATION

FISH is a useful tool both in research and diagnostic applications as it provides quantitative information about nucleic acid distribution including spatial information within cells. In ophthalmic pathology, it can be useful in the management of lymphomas, uveal melanomas (UMs), and orbital tumors including adenoid cystic carcinomas (ACCs) and other malignant tumors.

## General Principle of Fluorescence In Situ Hybridization (Fig. 1)

- Make fluorescent copy of probe sequence
- Denature both probe and target sequences by heat or chemicals so that new hydrogen bonds form between target and probe during hybridization
- Mix the probe and target to allow hybridization to complementary sequences on chromosome
- Visualize hybrids using a fluorescent microscope.

## Detailed Fluorescence In Situ Hybridization Protocol for Tissue Sections

- Unstained 3-4 μm sections are deparaffinized and rehydrated
- The deparaffinized tissue sections are air dried and placed in prewarmed (98°C) 1X pretreatment solution for 50 minutes in a water bath. The slides are immersed in 2X standard saline citrate I (SSC I) solution for 5 minutes followed

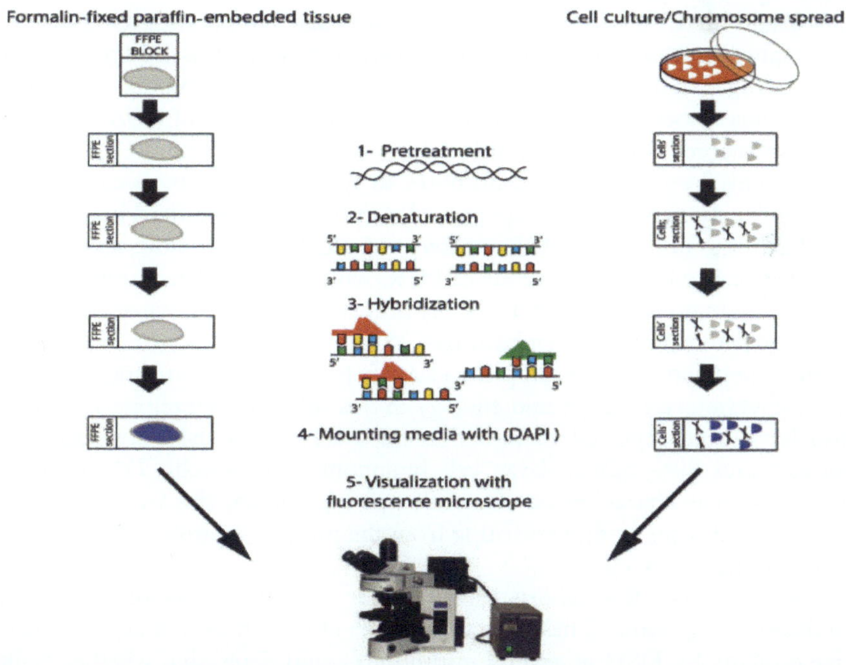


**Fig. 1.** Protocol of FISH: The target DNA and fluorochrome-labeled DNA probe are denatured and allowed to hybridize. The slide is then washed, counterstained, and viewed by a fluorescence microscope. (*From* Alamri A, Nam JY, Blancato JK. Fluorescence In Situ Hybridization of Cells, Chromosomes, and Formalin-Fixed Paraffin-Embedded Tissues. Methods Mol Biol. 2017;1606:265-279.)

by digestion in 0.1% pepsin solution by putting slides at 37°C for 17 minutes in Thermo Brite (Abbott Park, IL, USA).

- Immediately after digestion, the slides are immersed in 2X standard saline citrate II (SSC II) solution for 3 minutes and dehydrated using ethanol at room temperature. The slides are air dried and the section is marked by selecting the area on a light microscope.
- Now add 5 μL of probe on the marked section in the dark and cover with coverslip. The slides are kept in Thermo Brite (Abbott Park, IL, USA) and the program is set as denature at 85°C for 5 minutes and hybridized at 37°C for overnight.
- Next day, following hybridization, slides are removed from Thermo Brite and placed in prewarmed wash buffer I at 72°C for 5 minutes. Then the slides are placed in wash buffer II for 1 minute at room temperature.
- Now rinse the slides with distilled water and air dry at room temperature in the dark. The slides are then stained with 4′,6-diamidino-2-phenylindole (DAPI; CytoTest, USA), and coverslip is placed for microscopic review. Visualization of the FISH signals is accomplished by using a fluorescence microscope and pictures captured by using a FISH imaging system. Thirty to hundred nuclei are scored for each case [5]. The slides are stored in a dark box at −20°C.

## Ocular lymphomas

Low-grade MALTomas are the commonest ocular lymphomas. Classification of lymphomas based on somatic mutations is important as this may reduce the etiologic heterogeneity of lymphomas for epidemiologic research. Lymphoma-associated translocations include juxtaposition of (*IGH*) promoter on chromosome 14(14;18) translocation with an oncogene BCL2 gene at 18q21. This overexpression contributes to lymphomagenesis because of the constitutive expression of antiapoptotic bcl2 protein. By standard karyotyping, it is difficult to distinguish. As compared with PCR, FISH is more sensitive and specific because of the limitations of PCR, which cannot detect translocations outside the regions bound by the PCR primer region and because of the possibility to detect rare non-neoplastic t(14;18) positive lymphocytes. FISH is very useful in population-based samples to classify lymphomas according to t(14;18) for discovering risk factors and etiology in this subset of lymphomas. FISH assays have been reported to have identified t(14;18) in 84% follicular lymphomas and 39% diffuse large cell lymphomas [2]. Cyclin D1 (CCND1) translocation is characteristic of mantle cell lymphoma, this can be detected by FISH and helps in differentiating from the morphologically similar chronic lymphoid leukemia [3].

There are very few reports on molecular or cytogenetics of ocular non-Hodgkin's lymphoma. These account for 8% of total lymphomas, and molecular profiling by FISH at several institutions could determine whether ocular MALTomas are homogenous entities. Tanimoto and colleagues have reported various karyotypic abnormalities seen in MALT lymphomas including the commonest t(11;18)(q21;q21), which results from the fusion of the apoptosis inhibitor-2 (API2) gene and the MALT1 gene at the 11q21 and 18q21 breakpoints. The other commonly reported abnormality includes (14;18)(q32;q21) in 24% cases. However, Tanimoto and colleagues have reported trisomy 18 in 10% to 50% cases (Fig. 2). They attribute FISH in interphase as being more sensitive. Further they have reported morphologic differences based on primary site of involvement, presence of large lymphoid cells, lymphoepithelial lesions, and degree of nodularity in this subset of cases. The authors believe that trisomy 18 may represent a unique subgroup of primary ocular adnexal MALT lymphomas. Trisomy 18 was strongly related to the recurrence-free survival rate [6].

## Uveal Melanomas

UM is the commonest primary intraocular tumor, and 50% of patients die of late-appearing metastasis. Genetic factors can reliably predict high risk of metastasis and poor prognosis. The loss of 1 copy of chromosome 3 (monosomy 3 [M3]) or class 2 in choroidal melanoma patients is most strongly associated with metastatic death. Patients with disomy 3 or class I by molecular profiling have a better prognosis. Reduction of survival is 50% to 100%. Molecular testing for UM cases has become a standard in patient management 7]. FISH testing for the centromere region of chromosome 3 is a reliable option among many others (Fig. 3). Initially karyotyping was used and subsequently other technologies, including FISH, CGH, spectral karyotyping, microsatellite analysis, multiplex ligation-dependent probe amplification, and single nucleotide polymorphisms. Similarly, chromosome 8q gains and loss of chromosome 1 significantly correlates with reduced survival [8]. Most common chromosomal aberrations encountered in UM chromosome include 1p loss 28% to

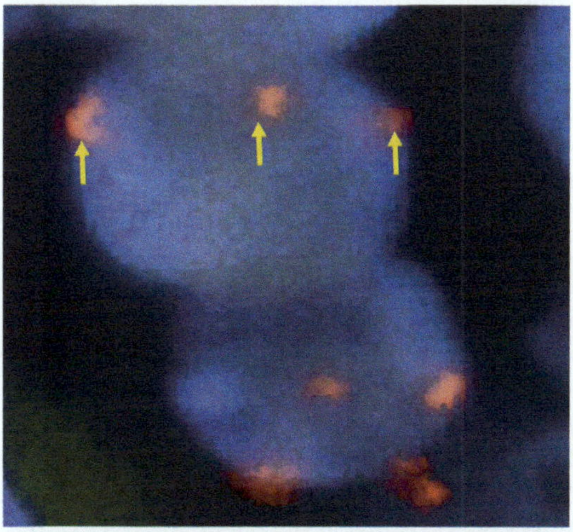

**Fig. 2.** Trisomy 18 as seen by 3 orange signals by chromosomal enumeration probes (CEP) in ocular MALTomas (*arrows*). (*Adapted from* Tanimoto K, Sekiguchi N, Yokota Y, Kaneko A, Watanabe T, Maeshima AM, Matsuno Y, Harada M, Tobinai K, Kobayashi Y. Fluorescence in situ hybridization (FISH) analysis of primary ocular adnexal MALT lymphoma. BMC Cancer. 2006 Oct 20;6:249.)

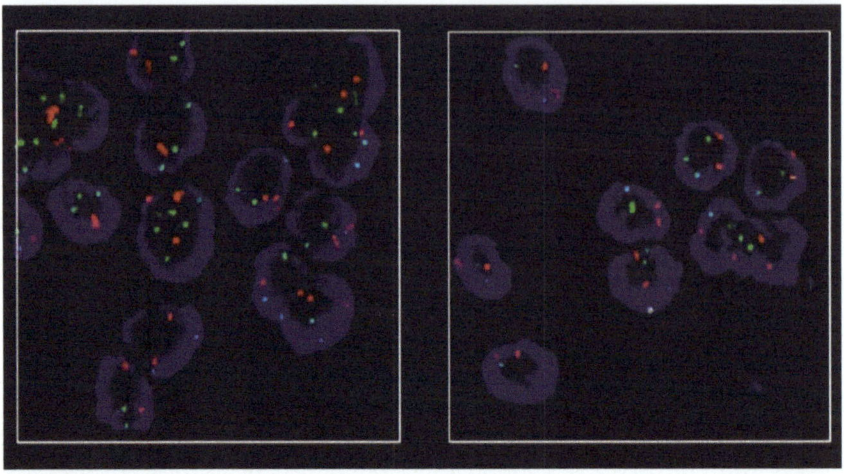

**Fig. 3.** Representative image of FISH analysis in human uveal melanoma. Nuclei were stained with blue fluorescent DAPI. Specific signals for chromosome 3 are indicated in red; chromosome 4-specific signals are indicated in green. (*From* Sipos E, Hegyi K, Treszl A, et al. Concurrence of chromosome 3 and 4 aberrations in human uveal melanoma. Oncol Rep. 2017;37(4):1927-1934.)

34%, 1q gain 24%, 3 loss 50% to 61%, 6p gain 28% to 54%, 6q loss 35% to 37%, 8p loss 17% to 28%, and 8q gain 36% to 63%. The percentage of cells showing monosomy correlates with prognosis. Patients with poor prognostic molecular abnormalities detected by FISH are candidates for adjuvant therapy that may prevent the development of metastasis [9].

## Adenoid Cystic Carcinoma

ACC is the commonest malignant lacrimal gland epithelial tumor. Myb, a nuclear transcription factor, is overexpressed in 60% to 80% of ACCs and correlates with a genetic translocation of the MYB gene to the transcription factor gene NFIB, resulting in the MYB-NFIB fusion, an important oncogene (t[6, 9]) (Fig. 4). This key oncogenic event was first discovered in 2009 by Persson and colleagues in Goran Stenman's laboratory [10]. Autocrine stimulation controls the expression of the MYB-NFIB fusion in ACC cells, increasing proliferation and generating changes in the cell cycle and RNA processing [10–12]. This fusion has been postulated as the main driver of tumor proliferation in ACC [13]. This translocation results in overexpression of MYB through deletion of target sites, which repress MYB expression. This, in turn, activates MYB targets [14–16]. Persson and coworkers demonstrated that the translocation results in an MYB–NFIB fusion oncogene in ACC of the breast and head and neck [16]. Subsequent studies have shown that MYB–NFIB is expressed in more than 85% of ACCs and that the major consequence of the fusion is activation of the MYB oncogene [17–19].

Recurrent translocations often result in the formation of tumor type-specific fusion oncogenes that may be used as diagnostic biomarkers. The products of

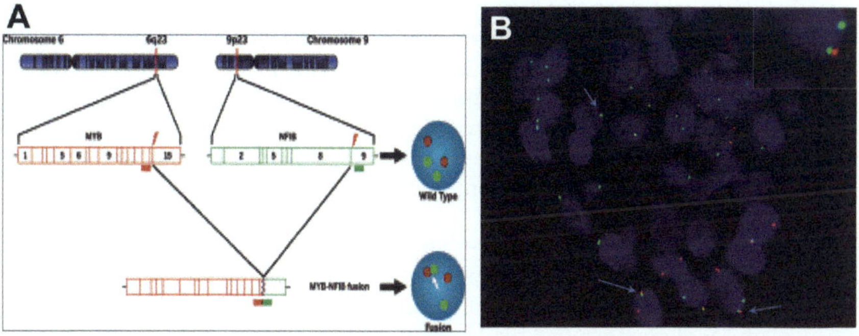


**Fig. 4.** MYB-NFIB fusion gene in lacrimal gland adenoid cystic carcinoma. (*A*) Schematic illustration represents the MYB and NFIB gene as well as the MYB-NFIB fusion gene and the resulting protein. (*B*) FISH analysis using 5′MYB (orange) and 3′NFIB (green) probe in fusion-positive ACC case. Note the overlap of the MYB and NFIB probe in fusion-positive ACC (inset).

these gene fusions can cause the abnormal expression of transcription factors or the unregulated activation of tyrosine kinases (TKs), both of which lead to uncontrolled cell growth, ultimately causing cancer. Some fusion genes have been developed as therapeutic targets. Fusion genes involving proto-oncogenes such as TKs are some of the most popular molecular targets. TKs can be overexpressed through fusion with another stronger promoter, resulting in the misregulation of cellular proliferation, survival, differentiation, and motility. The first fusion-targeted drug, imatinib, a TK inhibitor, was approved in 2001 for the treatment of Philadelphia chromosome (BCR-ABL)-positive CML. EWS-FLI1 is another oncogenic fusion gene expressed in Ewing sarcoma. siRNA targeting the junction sequence of EWS-FLI1 was tested in NIH/3T3 EWS-FLI1 cells and mice xenografted with an EWS-FLI1-expressing tumor. In both in vitro and in vivo experiments, such siRNAs were found to have a high efficiency of tumor growth inhibition [20].

## PRESENT RELEVANCE AND FUTURE OF FLUORESCENCE IN SITU HYBRIDIZATION

As FISH provides both genomic and transcriptome information in the spatial context, it has applications both in clinical diagnosis and genomic research. The binding of the complementary probes helps in the detection of several medical conditions including different chromosomal aberrations as translocations, insertions, or deletions. This includes diseases such as cystic fibrosis, trisomies, and leukemias, among others.

- FISH has a wide spectrum of diagnostic and research applications. Orbital alveolar rhabdomyosarcomas with 1;13 translocation has prognostic value as well. Sarcomas may have distinctive, recurrent diagnostic translocations as seen in prognostic implications [21].

- FISH is an important ancillary diagnostic test and represents an alternative to RT-PCR as in the case of clear cell sarcoma and its mimic malignant melanoma when fresh tissue is unavailable. Commercially available dual-color break-apart for FISH probes EWS (22q12) gene [22].
- Guide in cancer treatment-Herceptin-targeted therapy is effective in HER2 overexpressed breast cancer. Gene amplifications like human epidermal growth factor2 (HER2) gene copy number changes as prognostic markers for breast and ovarian cancer.
- FISH assays could guide effective targeted therapy as translocations involving the TFE3 gene at XP11.2 in papillary renal cell carcinoma.
- With advances in fluorescence microscopy and digital imaging, as well as the availability of genomic and bioinformatic resources, there has been a diversification of the original FISH protocol. This visually appealing technique has the advantage of its combined cytologic and molecular approach and its unique ability to provide resolution, which is in between DNA analysis and chromosomal techniques, while retaining the information generated at the single-cell level.
- Quantification of gene copy numbers is critical for understanding tumor biology and management of patients with cancer. DNA FISH is the gold standard for detecting copy number alterations, FISH is limited by the number of genes one can quantify simultaneously. Single-cell NGS is another powerful tool but very expensive. To overcome this, the authors have devised a multiplex approach for metaphase spreads of tumor cell lines and cultured cell lines [23].
- The study of genetic heterogeneity of cancer cells is greatly helped by multiplex FISH. Work on glioblastoma has shown intermingled tumor populations having amplifications of EGFR, MET, or PDGFRA. Mosaicism can be detected only by FISH as CGH and NGS are not sensitive to detect minor amplified subpopulations. A multiplex FISH will have clinical implications for simultaneously assaying actionable copy number changes in tumor samples when the tumor cells are limited as in circulating tumor cells [23].
- Disadvantages of FISH assays in FFPE sections include presence of overlapping cells, which hinder scoring. Also, commercial FISH probes are costly and require training to perform and score. Despite the high specificity and possibility of quantitative imaging, another disadvantage of FISH includes the assay time and probe consumption, which needs to be addressed to promote its extensive usage.
- Microfluidic techniques hold great promise in improving these drawbacks. These can resolve the limitations in probe consumption and hybridization time [4].

## CLINICS CARE POINTS

- FISH has the advantage of being useful in metaphase and interphase nuclei.
- Microarrays can be made from FFPE tissues for FISH. Tissue microarrays allow large numbers of cases that require less probe and reagents and are less time consuming, conserve tissues, and are reproducible [22].

- Both karyotyping and FISH are useful for screening and follow-up of clonal abnormalities. FISH panels provide rapid evaluation of targeted abnormal patterns and their percentage. The chromosomal analysis then provides clonal abnormalities [3].
- Rapid prenatal testing of common aneuploidy and genomic disorders. Useful in diagnostic assays of uncultured interphase cells from amniotic fluid or chorionic villus samples.
- Interphase FISH is particularly fruitful for cancer cytogenetics for classifying tumors, selecting treatment protocols, as well as monitoring response to treatment.
- It is both cost and time-efficient method in which formalin-fixed paraffin-embedded tissues can be used. However, it is still not widely used in many diagnostic laboratories because of the high cost of the probes, fluorescent microscope, high sensitivity cooled camera with high-resolution images, and imaging software (platform) needed for capturing the images.
- FISH will continue to be an integral part of genetic diagnosis despite availability of newer technologies such as microarray and exome sequencing.
- The multiplex FISH assay serves as a complementary test performed side by side with NGS mutational panels in genotyping laboratories.
- For leukemias such as acute promyelocytic leukemia, which require early therapy, rapid FISH results are mandatory for targeted therapy for the administration of all-trans retinoic acid. Targeted treatment against ABL1/BCR fusion protein by tyrosine inhibitors, which have increased survival from 20% to 80% to 90%.
- There are 20 to 30 genes associated with amplification and deletion events in various malignancies. Development of a robust multiplex reproducible FISH assay holds the key to providing a simple and accurate methodology to simultaneously assay multiple genes [3].
- Its wider use in ocular oncology will be useful to identify oncogenes and expression of their downstream target genes in various ocular malignancies. Creation of commercial platforms for FISH would encourage its usage and would provide useful information regarding the pathogenic mechanism as well as to elucidate their aggressive biological behavior and more importantly to identify novel therapeutic targets.
- Advances in microfluidic devices for miniaturized and automatic FISH are under development and once validated, will pave the way for more disease-specific probes and widen the spectrum for diagnostic FISH applications.
- Further novel FISH techniques, including imaging systems with improved resolution for intranuclear genomic organization-CASFISH and oligopaint FISH, are mainly for genetic research applications [4].
- These single-molecule, single-cell–based FISH techniques will become translated into cell-based genetic diagnosis resulting in an improvement from chromosomal, genomic, and epigenetic alterations [3].

## DISCLOSURE

Shahzan Anjum is grateful to ICMR, New Delhi for providing her Senior Research Fellowship (No.3/2/2/30/2018/Onlne Pathology Fship/NCD-III).

## References

[1] Fluorescence In Situ Hybridization (FISH). Clare O'Connor, Nature Education Citation: O'Connor, C. Fluorescence in situ hybridization (FISH). Nat Educ 2008;1(1):171.
[2] Chang CM, Schroeder JC, Huang WY, et al. Non-Hodgkin's lymphoma (NHL) subtypes defined by common translocations: utility of fluorescence in situ hybridization (FISH) in a case-control study. Leuk Res 2010;34(2):190–5.
[3] Cui C, Shu W, Li P. Fluorescence in situ hybridization: cell-based genetic diagnostic and research applications. Front Cell Dev Biol 2016;(4):89.
[4] Huber D, Voith von Voithenberg L, Kaigala GV. Fluorescence in situ hybridization (FISH): History, limitations and what to expect from micro-scale FISH? Micro Nano Eng 2018;(1):15–24.
[5] Von Holstein SL, Fehr A, Heegaard S, et al. CRTC1-MAML2 gene fusion in mucoepidermoid carcinoma of the lacrimal gland. Oncol Rep 2012;27:1413–6.
[6] Tanimoto K, Sekiguchi N, Yokota Y, et al. Fluorescence in situ hybridization (FISH) analysis of primary ocular adnexal MALT lymphoma. BMC Cancer 2006;(6):249.
[7] Klufas MA, Richter E, Itty S, et al. Comparison of Gene Expression Profiling and Chromosome 3 Analysis by Fluorescent in situ Hybridization and Multiplex Ligation Probe Amplification in Fine-Needle Aspiration Biopsy Specimens of Uveal Melanoma. Ocul Oncol Pathol 2017;4(1):16–20.
[8] Coupland SE, Lake SL, Zeschnigk M, et al. Molecular pathology of uveal melanoma. Eye (Lond) 2013;27(2):230–42.
[9] Thomas van den B, van Beek Jackelien GM, Vaarwater J, et al. Higher Percentage of FISH-Determined Monosomy 3 and 8q Amplification in Uveal Melanoma Cells relate to Poor Patient Prognosis. Invest Ophthalmol Vis Sci 2012;53(6):2668–74.
[10] Andersson MK, Åman P, Stenman G. IGF2/IGF1R signaling as a therapeutic target in MYB-positive adenoid cystic carcinomas and other fusion gene-driven tumors. Cells 2019;8: 913.
[11] Wang Y, Zhang CY, Xia RH, et al. The MYB/miR-130a/NDRG2 axis modulates tumor proliferation and metastatic potential in salivary adenoid cystic carcinoma. Cell Death Dis 2018;9:917.
[12] Almeida-Pinto YD, Costa SFDS, de Andrade BAB, et al. t(6;9) (MYB-NFIB) in head and neck adenoid cystic carcinoma: a systematic review with meta-analysis. Oral Dis 2019;25: 1277–82.
[13] Xu L, Zhao F, Yang W, et al. MYB promotes the growth and metastasis of salivary adenoid cystic carcinoma. Int J Oncol 2019;54:1579–90.
[14] Andersson MK, Afshari MK, Andren Y, et al. Targeting the oncogenic transcriptional regulator MYB in adenoid cystic carcinoma by inhibition of IGF1R/AKT signaling. J Natl Cancer Inst 2017;109; https://doi.org/10.1093/jnci/djx017.
[15] Ho AS, Kannan K, Roy DM, et al. The mutational landscape of adenoid cystic carcinoma. Nat Genet 2013;45:791–8.
[16] Persson M, Andren Y, Mark J, et al. Recurrent fusion of MYB and NFIB transcription factor genes in carcinomas of the breast and head and neck. Proc Natl Acad Sci U S A 2009;106:18740–4.
[17] Brill LB, Kanner WA, Fehr A, et al. Analysis of MYB expression and MYB-NFIB gene fusions in adenoid cystic carcinoma and other salivary neoplasms. Mod Pathol 2011;24: 1169–76.
[18] Mitani Y, Rao PH, Futreal PA, et al. Novel chromosomal rearrangements and break points at the t(6;9) in salivary adenoid cystic carcinoma: association with MYB NFIB chimeric fusion, MYB expression, and clinical outcome. Clin Cancer Res 2011;17:7003–14.

[19] West RB, Kong C, Clarke N, et al. MYB expression and translocation in adenoid cystic carcinomas and other salivary gland tumors with clinicopathologic correlation. Am J Surg Pathol 2011;35:92–9.
[20] Rowley JD. Chromosome translocations: dangerous liaisons revisited. Nat Rev Cancer 2001;1:245–50.
[21] Mudhar HS. Ocular Pathology. In: Chaugule S, Honavar S, Finger P, editors. Surgical ophthalmic oncology. Cham (Switzerland): Springer; 2019. p. 175–80.
[22] Patel RM, Downs-Kelly E, Weiss SW, et al. Dual-color, break-apart fluorescence in situ hybridization for EWS gene rearrangement distinguishes clear cell sarcoma of soft tissue from malignant melanoma. Mod Pathol 2005;18(12):1585–90.
[23] Onozato ML, Yapp C, Richardson D, et al. Highly Multiplexed Fluorescence in Situ Hybridization for in Situ Genomics. J Mol Diagn 2019;21(Issue 3):390–407.

Advances in Ophthalmology and Optometry 7 (2022) 151–160

ADVANCES IN OPHTHALMOLOGY AND OPTOMETRY

# Intra-arterial Chemotherapy for Retinoblastoma: An Update

Bhavna Chawla, MD[a,*], Navneet Sidhu, MD[a], Shailesh Gaikwad, MD[b]

[a]Ocular Oncology Service, RP Centre for Ophthalmic Sciences, All India Institute of Medical Sciences, New Delhi, Delhi 110029 India; [b]Department of Neuroimaging and Interventional Neuroradiology, All India Institute of Medical Sciences, New Delhi, Delhi 110029, India

**Keywords**

• Retinoblastoma • Intra-arterial chemotherapy (IAC) • Ophthalmic artery • Melphalan • Topotecan

**Key points**

- Retinoblastoma is the most common primary intraocular tumor in children.
- Intra-arterial chemotherapy is a form of targeted drug therapy that involves direct administration of chemotherapy drugs via the ophthalmic artery.
- IAC has improved globe salvage rates for refractory retinoblastoma.
- In selected cases, it is also used as a first-line treatment.
- Its administration requires a skilled and experienced multidisciplinary team.

## INTRODUCTION

Retinoblastoma is the most common primary intraocular tumor in children. It also is one of the most successfully treated malignancies. Intra-arterial Chemotherapy (IAC), also known as superselective ophthalmic artery chemotherapy or chemosurgery, is one of the upcoming treatment modalities for retinoblastoma. Since its introduction, IAC has been found to be an effective treatment modality in salvaging globes that would otherwise have been enucleated. As a result, the procedure has gained popularity worldwide and is currently available in many countries and centers treating retinoblastoma.

In this procedure, the chemotherapy drug is injected directly into the ophthalmic artery of the affected eye. The primary aim is to deliver a

*Corresponding author. *E-mail address:* bhavna2424@hotmail.com

https://doi.org/10.1016/j.yaoo.2022.03.005

high concentration of chemotherapy drug into the eye, thus minimizing the side effects of systemic toxicity, which would occur with intravenous chemotherapy. IAC administration is technically challenging and requires a skilled and experienced multidisciplinary team comprising of ocular oncologist, interventional neuroradiologist, and a pediatric oncologist.

## HISTORY

The first report of chemotherapy delivered to the eye via the intra-arterial route was by Reese and colleagues in 1954 using triethylene melamine (TEM) [1]. In this procedure, TEM, which is a nitrogen mustard analog, was directly injected into the ipsilateral internal carotid artery by placing a suture ligation to provide traction and hemostasis [2]. However, because of associated systemic toxicities, this procedure was discontinued. In 1968, a retrograde infusion of anticancer drugs into the ophthalmic artery through the external carotid artery was described [3]. This procedure showed significant tumor regression.

In 2004, Mohri et al described the Japanese technique of "selective ophthalmic arterial infusion" (SOAI) therapy by using a micro-balloon catheter positioned into the internal carotid artery by a transfemoral artery approach [3,4]. In the Japanese technique, a 4F vascular catheter was introduced from the femoral artery using the Seldinger technique and advanced into the internal carotid artery of the affected side after which a micro-balloon catheter was passed through the vascular catheter to a position beyond the orifice of the ophthalmic artery [4]. After that, temporal occlusion was achieved by inflating the balloon, and the anticancer drug was then injected into the ophthalmic artery.

The Japanese technique of SOAI was further developed into "direct intra-arterial ophthalmic artery infusion" by Abramson and Gobin with their respective team in New York [5,6]. In a study that began in 2006, it was reported that direct catheterization of the ophthalmic artery was quick, efficient, reliable, and safe when used in children [6].

Indications for Intra-arterial Chemotherapy: [7]

1. Refractory retinoblastoma (group D or E)
2. Recurrent tumor (group C or D), with or without subretinal seeds
3. Primary retinoblastoma (unilateral group C or D)
4. Bilateral group D or E, along with focal therapy

Contraindications of IAC include [7]

1. Eyes with vitreous hemorrhage, preseptal or orbital cellulitis, prephthisical or phthisical eyes, neovascular glaucoma
2. Extraocular retinoblastoma (ie, optic nerve or scleral extension)
3. Trilateral retinoblastoma (involvement of pineal gland)
4. Systemic metastasis (hematogenous or central nervous system)
5. Tortuous ophthalmic artery or failure to catheterize the artery).

**Table 1**
Various terminologies used in IAC

| | |
|---|---|
| Primary IAC | IAC is used as the first line of treatment |
| Secondary IAC | Administered after a failed previous treatment (eg, intravitreal chemotherapy, plaque brachytherapy, external beam radiotherapy, or systemic chemotherapy). |
| Tandem IAC | When bilaterally administered simultaneously |
| Bridge IAC | Treatment of retinoblastoma is initiated with intravitreal chemotherapy, followed later by IAC |
| Rescue IAC | Repeat IAC after an initial IAC for recurrent tumor or subretinal/vitreous seeds |

*Data from* Refs. [8–10]

## INTRA-ARTERIAL CHEMOTHERAPY TERMINOLOGY

The various terminologies used in IAC are summarized in Table 1.

## PROCEDURE

The main aim of treatment with IAC is to achieve tumor regression with minimal side effects. Hence, the number of sessions required should be decided on a case-to-case basis. History of previous treatments and subsequent follow-ups are essential to determine the exact treatment protocol. In a review by Yousef and colleagues, IAC was administered every 4 weeks for 3 sittings, and complete resolution of the tumor was observed [11]. Shields and colleagues, Suzuki and colleagues, and Gobin and colleagues, in different studies, reported the number of median sessions as 3 [2,4,5].

The procedure is performed under general anesthesia. Before the procedure, intravenous heparin (50–100 IU/kg body weight) is given. The femoral artery on the side of the tumor is catheterized, and the catheter is advanced under fluoroscopy guidance into the ophthalmic artery (Fig. 1). In most cases, the microcatheter is positioned at the ostium of the ophthalmic artery.

In a few patients, it may be difficult to catheterize the ophthalmic artery because of various factors. These factors include small size of the ophthalmic artery as seen in young patients, alternative vascular supply to the eye by the middle meningeal artery as seen in 1% to 5% of patients, ophthalmic artery vasospasm intraoperatively, and difficulty catheterizing the ophthalmic artery because of its steep rise from the internal carotid artery [12–14]. In such a case where the ophthalmic artery cannot be accessed, alternative routes may be tried. The external carotid artery circulation is accessed to catheterize the orbital branch of the middle meningeal artery, and a selective angiogram is performed to determine if this branch is well developed, which may then be used to administer chemotherapy. If the middle meningeal artery route cannot be accessed, a temporary balloon occlusion of the internal carotid artery just distal to the origin of the ophthalmic artery may be tried.

Once the catheter is in place, chemotherapy drugs are injected directly into the involved eye. The drugs are diluted in 30 cc of normal saline before

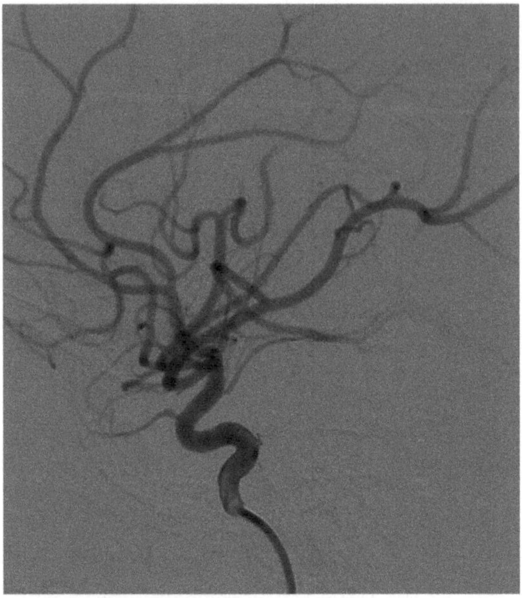

**Fig. 1.** IAC procedure to cannulate the ophthalmic artery.

infusion and manually injected in a pulsatile manner for over 30 minutes. The pulsatile manner of injection allows the disruption of laminar flow and an even distribution of the drugs to the vascular territory. If a balloon occlusion technique is used, alternate infusion (4 minutes of balloon inflation) and reperfusion (2 minutes of balloon deflation) is followed to ensure adequate cerebral perfusion. After the procedure is complete, it is essential to rule out a thromboembolic event by performing another fluoroscopy, after which the microcatheter and guide wire are removed. The femoral artery is compressed manually for 10 to 15 minutes to achieve hemostasis. The patient is to be observed for 4 to 6 hours after the procedure. IAC usually is avoided in neonates and infants younger than 6 months because of difficult femoral artery cannulation. A complete blood count with platelets is recommended for all patients 7 to 10 days after IAC to monitor for myelosuppression. Ophthalmic examinations should be performed every 3 to 4 weeks after the treatment. Visual acuity, pupillary reaction, fundus examination with RetCam digital photography, and ocular ultrasonography (B by A scan) are used to monitor the treatment response and to determine the need for further therapies.

## INTRA-ARTERIAL CHEMOTHERAPY DRUGS

The 3 principal chemotherapeutic drugs used in IAC are melphalan, topotecan, and carboplatin. Recent treatment regimens include single-drug, 2-drug, or 3-drug regimen based on the group and previous treatments received. The drugs used are summarized in Table 2.

**Table 2**
Drugs used for intra-arterial chemotherapy

| Drug | Type of drug | Dose | Indications |
|---|---|---|---|
| Melphalan | Alkylating agent | 3–7.5 mg | Group B and C retinoblastoma |
| Topotecan | Topoisomerase 1 inhibitor | 1–2 mg | Advanced retinoblastoma with vitreous seeds |
| Carboplatin | Platinum-based derivative | 15–30 mg | Recurrence, suboptimal response to previous IAC |

*Adapted from* Manjandavida FP, Stathopoulos C, Zhang J, et al. Intra-arterial chemotherapy in retinoblastoma - A paradigm change. Indian J Ophthalmol. 2019;67(6):740-754.

The alkylating agent melphalan, which is a nitrogen mustard derivative, is the most commonly used intra-arterial chemotherapy agent in the treatment of advanced retinoblastoma. A few in vitro studies on melphalan with human cultured retinoblastoma cells using clonogenic assays showed that melphalan was the most effective drug compared with other chemotherapeutic drugs [15]. Systemic intravenous use of melphalan is associated with severe myelosuppression, hence limiting its use. Because melphalan is commercially available in a powder form, which is reconstituted before administration, it is essential to filter melphalan injection as the particles can embolize the intraocular vessels. Topotecan, which is a topoisomerase inhibitor, has been increasingly used intra-arterially now for aggressive cases that are nonresponsive to melphalan. Topotecan successfully halts tumor progression. It also has less intraocular toxicity. Carboplatin, which is a platinum-based derivative, usually is added as a multiagent triple therapy (melphalan + topotecan + carboplatin) in eyes with failed single- or double-agent IAC or systemic intravenous chemotherapy. Carboplatin is preferred in the triple-regimen drug protocol for bilateral retinoblastoma with a reduced dose of melphalan to avoid the cumulative toxicity of melphalan. The drug dosage is determined on a case-to-case basis depending on the age and body weight of the child. The number and dose of the chemotherapeutic agents are determined based on the extent of the disease, vitreous and subretinal seedings, and the clinical response to previous treatments.

## SIGNIFICANCE OF INTRA-ARTERIAL CHEMOTHERAPY

Accurate diagnosis and staging of the disease are important for management of retinoblastoma. Before the advent of IAC, the most common treatment for advanced or refractory retinoblastoma was enucleation. Enucleation is a cosmetically disfiguring surgery. With the evolution of IAC, the requirement for enucleation has reduced significantly. IAC has been shown to be effective in treating tumors that have failed to respond to intravenous chemotherapy (Fig. 2). Although initially used in eyes with previously failed treatment, it now is being increasingly used as a primary therapy in the treatment of naïve eyes (ie, eyes that have not received any treatment before).

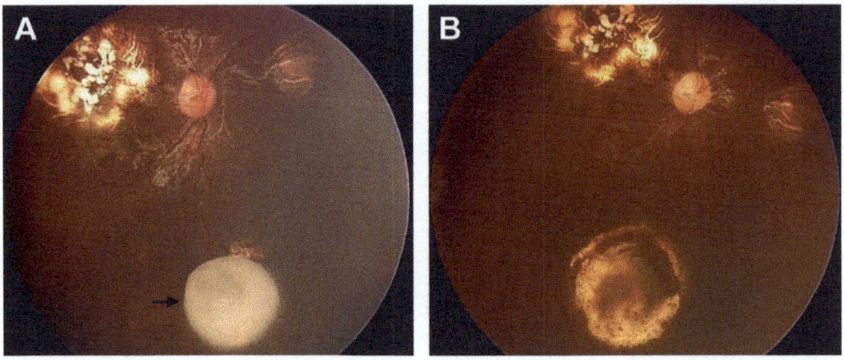


**Fig. 2.** Fundus image of the right eye in a 3-year-old child. (*A*) Active tumor (*arrow*) that failed to regress after 6 cycles of intravenous chemotherapy. (*B*) Regressed tumor following IAC with melphalan.

Vitreous or subretinal seeding, although associated with poor prognosis, has been found to be effectively managed by intra-arterial chemotherapy. Also, studies indicate that IAC can resolve a partial retinal detachment in almost 100% of cases and total retinal detachment in 43%–75% of cases [16,17]. IAC administered after an initial IAC for primary or secondary retinoblastoma was termed as rescue IAC by Shields and colleagues [10]. They have reported tumor control in 75% of cases and globe salvage in 67% of cases [10]. They concluded that rescue IAC can be considered in patients with failed initial IAC, especially in one-eyed or unilateral retinoblastoma. In another study, Shields and colleagues reported that IAC alone provided a good tumor regression with complete control in 88%, control of subretinal seeds in 82% ,and vitreous seeds in 67% following 3 sessions [2,18]. Francis and colleagues reported the recurrence-free survival after IAC at 1 and 2 years as 76.3% and 70%, respectively [19].

It should be emphasized that IAC is indicated for the treatment of intraocular disease only and should be strictly avoided in tumors with extraocular involvement.

## COMPLICATIONS OF INTRA-ARTERIAL CHEMOTHERAPY

### Local

IAC can lead to local and systemic complications [20–22]. The most common side effects are periocular erythema, blepharoptosis, and temporary madarosis. It can lead to vascular toxicities such as ophthalmic artery thrombosis, choroidal nonperfusion, subretinal hemorrhages, and vitreous hemorrhage. It also may lead to ischemic optic atrophy resulting in compromised visual acuity.

### Systemic

It can lead to transient femoral artery occlusion characterized by localized swelling and pain at the catheter insertion site on the leg. This can be treated using aspirin. If not resolved, it can lead to gangrene and loss of the limb. Nausea, vomiting, and fever rarely may be seen.

## WHAT'S NEW IN INTRA-ARTERIAL CHEMOTHERAPY?

### Treatment Approaches

At present, research on retinoblastoma is focused on newer targeted treatment approaches that maximize the efficacy with minimal side effects. Currently, the newer treatment options include the combination of IAC with intravitreal chemotherapy, which has led to further improvement in tumor regression [23]. Dalvin and colleagues have reported a regression of tumor and subretinal seeds when IAC was administered along with intravitreal chemotherapy [24]. In the study, the need for enucleation or radiation therapy was eliminated in 75% of patients with IAC alone and in 65% of patients when IAC was combined with intravitreal chemotherapy.

In recent studies by Sweid and colleagues and Al Saiegh and colleagues, a transradial approach for IAC was described, which is an improvement in the technique [25,26]. They found that the transradial approach was much easier, and no thromboembolic events or access site complications were noted. It was noted that the transradial approach was easier in younger children.

### Drugs

A study published by Area and colleagues described the continuous infusion of verapamil [27]. In the study, they concluded that infusion decreased fluoroscopy time, dose area product, and radiation doses during the procedure.

It has been seen that the addition of topotecan to melphalan has led to an effective reduction in the requirement for intravitreal or periocular injections or focal therapy like cryotherapy or transpupillary thermotherapy [28]. The use of topotecan reduces the cumulative toxicity associated with melphalan.

A few studies have demonstrated the antitumor activity of cardenolide glycosides like digoxin against retinoblastoma, both in vitro and in vivo. A case report in which digoxin was administered orally showed insufficient intraocular levels to have therapeutic effect, but a modest response was seen with intra-arterial delivery of digoxin [29].

Methotrexate has been tried intra-arterially in a few studies, but a higher dose of 6 to 12 mg is required, which can lead to more intraocular toxicity [5]. Hence, methotrexate in IAC is not yet approved.

### Patient profile

IAC has been tried in infants younger than than 3 months or less than 10 kg in a few studies with successful regression of tumor [30,31]. These studies suggest that IAC can be tried safely and successfully even in infants younger than 3 months with promising results and minimal intraocular side effects.

## SUMMARY

IAC has been found to successfully salvage globes in eyes that otherwise would have been enucleated, as in advanced retinoblastoma. It now is a widely used treatment modality. It usually is indicated for group C, D, or E retinoblastoma (International Classification of Retinoblastoma) refractory to standard treatment modalities. It also can be used as a primary treatment. IAC is efficient for subretinal seeds as well. Because the procedure is associated with certain risks, careful case selection is very important. It is to be avoided in patients with extraocular extension or with optic nerve involvement.

It can be given as a single-, double-, or triple-drug regimen involving melphalan, topotecan, and carboplatin. These drugs are highly effective for tumor regression as well as for regression of the vitreous seeds. IAC, however, may be associated with a few complications as well such as periocular erythema, blepharoptosis, and temporary madarosis. It also may lead to ophthalmic artery thrombosis, nonperfusion of the retina, or vitreous hemorrhage. Local site thrombosis may be seen in rare cases.

Proper delivery of IAC requires an integrated management between an ocular oncologist, neurointerventional radiologist, anesthesiologist, pediatric oncologist, nursing, and other ancillary staff. A proper protocol with detailed planning should be set up before proceeding for the therapy. Because it is comparable to a complex surgical procedure, IAC is rightly labeled as "chemosurgery." A major concern in the low- and middle-income countries is the financial constraint due to high treatment cost and the infrastructure involved.

With newer techniques and drugs being used in IAC, it has become a better and safer treatment modality for management of retinoblastoma. The combination of IAC with intravitreal chemotherapy has led to further improvement in tumor regression. Newer advances in IAC delivery techniques and drugs hold promise for the future.

## CLINICS CARE POINTS

- IAC is a form of targeted drug therapy that involves direct administration of chemotherapy drugs into the eye via the ophthalmic artery.
- This route allows for achieving a higher concentration of anticancer drugs in the eye than systemic chemotherapy as well as minimizing the systemic side effects.
- IAC is most commonly indicated for refractory group C or D retinoblastoma.
- It may also be used as primary therapy in advanced group D or E retinoblastoma.
- Careful case selection is very important.
- The conventional method of drug administration is via the transfemoral route.
- The most commonly used drugs are melphalan, topotecan, and carboplatin.
- IAC can also be used in combination with intravitreal chemotherapy to achieve significant tumor regression.

## Disclosure

The authors have nothing to disclose. They have no commercial or financial conflicts of interest. They do not have any funding sources.

## References

[1] Reese AB, Hyman GA, Tapley ND, et al. The treatment of retinoblastoma by x-ray and triethylene melamine. AMA Arch Ophthalmol 1958;60(5):897–906.
[2] Shields CL, Bianciotto CG, Jabbour P, et al. Intra-arterial chemotherapy for retinoblastoma: report No. 1, control of retinal tumors, subretinal seeds, and vitreous seeds. Arch Ophthalmol 2011;129(11):1399–406.
[3] Jabbour P, Chalouhi N, Tjoumakaris S, et al. Pearls and pitfalls of intraarterial chemotherapy for retinoblastoma. J Neurosurg Pediatr 2012;10(3):175–81.
[4] Suzuki S, Yamane T, Mohri M, et al. Selective ophthalmic arterial injection therapy for intraocular retinoblastoma: the long-term prognosis. Ophthalmology 2011;118(10):2081–7.
[5] Gobin YP, Dunkel IJ, Marr BP, et al. Intra-arterial chemotherapy for the management of retinoblastoma: four-year experience. Arch Ophthalmol Chic Ill 1960 2011;129(6):732–7.
[6] Abramson DH, Dunkel IJ, Brodie SE, et al. A phase I/II study of direct intraarterial (ophthalmic artery) chemotherapy with melphalan for intraocular retinoblastoma initial results. Ophthalmology 2008;115(8):1398–404.
[7] Zanaty M, Barros G, Chalouhi N, et al. Update on intra-arterial chemotherapy for retinoblastoma. ScientificWorldJournal 2014;2014:869604.
[8] Abramson DH, Dunkel IJ, Brodie SE, et al. Bilateral Superselective Ophthalmic Artery Chemotherapy for Bilateral Retinoblastoma: Tandem Therapy. Arch Ophthalmol 2010;128(3):370–2.
[9] Gobin YP, Dunkel IJ, Marr BP, et al. Combined, sequential intravenous and intra-arterial chemotherapy (bridge chemotherapy) for young infants with retinoblastoma. PLoS One 2012;7(9):e44322.
[10] Shields CL, Say EA, Pointdujour-Lim R, et al. Rescue intra-arterial chemotherapy following retinoblastoma recurrence after initial intra-arterial chemotherapy. J Fr Ophtalmol 2015;38(6):542–9.
[11] Yousef YA, Soliman SE, Astudillo PPP, et al. Intra-arterial Chemotherapy for Retinoblastoma: A Systematic Review. JAMA Ophthalmol 2016;134(5):584–91.
[12] Hayreh SS. Orbital vascular anatomy. Eye (Lond) 2006;20(10):1130–44.
[13] Hayreh SS, Dass R. The Ophthalmic Artery: I. Origin and Intra-Cranial and Intra-Canalicular Course. Br J Ophthalmol 1962;46(2):65–98.
[14] Manjandavida FP, Stathopoulos C, Zhang J, et al. Intra-arterial chemotherapy in retinoblastoma - A paradigm change. Indian J Ophthalmol 2019;67(6):740–54.
[15] Inomata M, Kaneko A. Chemosensitivity profiles of primary and cultured human retinoblastoma cells in a human tumor clonogenic assay. Jpn J Cancer Res 1987;78(8):858–68.
[16] Abramson, DH. Lessons Learned After 5 Years (and 500 infusions) of Chemosurgery: Predictors of Success and Failure. in ISOO 2011 Biannual Meeting. 2011. Buenos Aires, Argentina.
[17] Shields, CL. Intra-arterial Chemotherapy for Retinoblastoma: Exposures, Tumor Control, Complications - New Observations. in ISOO 2011 Biannual Meeting. 2011. Buenos Aires, Argentina.
[18] Shields CL, Kaliki S, Rojanaporn D, et al. Intravenous and intra-arterial chemotherapy for retinoblastoma: what have we learned? Curr Opin Ophthalmol 2012;23(3):202–9.
[19] Francis JH, Levin AM, Zabor EC, et al. Ten-year experience with ophthalmic artery chemosurgery: Ocular and recurrence-free survival. PLoS One 2018;13(5):e0197081.
[20] Munier FL, Beck-Popovic M, Balmer A, et al. Occurrence of sectoral choroidal occlusive vasculopathy and retinal arteriolar embolization after superselective ophthalmic artery chemotherapy for advanced intraocular retinoblastoma. Retina Phila Pa 2011;31(3):566–73.

[21] Monroy JE, Orbach DB, VanderVeen D. Complications of intra-arterial chemotherapy for retinoblastoma. Semin Ophthalmol 2014;29(5–6):429–33.
[22] Marr B, Gobin PY, Dunkel IJ, et al. Spontaneously Resolving Periocular Erythema and Ciliary Madarosis Following Intra-arterial Chemotherapy for Retinoblastoma. Middle East Afr J Ophthalmol 2010;17(3):207–9.
[23] Tuncer S, Sencer S, Kebudi R, et al. Superselective intra-arterial chemotherapy in the primary management of advanced intra-ocular retinoblastoma: first 4-year experience from a single institution in Turkey. Acta Ophthalmol (Copenh) 2016;94(7):e644–51.
[24] Dalvin LA, Lim L-AS, Chang M, et al. Circumscribed choroidal hemangioma: Clinical features and outcomes by age category in 458 cases. Saudi J Ophthalmol 2019;33(3): 219–28.
[25] Sweid A, Jabbour P. Intra-arterial chemotherapy for retinoblastoma: transradial and transfemoral approach. J Neurointerventional Surg 2020;12(8):828.
[26] Al Saiegh F, Chalouhi N, Sweid A, et al. Intra-arterial chemotherapy for retinoblastoma via the transradial route: Technique, feasibility, and case series. Clin Neurol Neurosurg 2020;194:105824.
[27] Area C, Yen CJ, Chevez-Barrios P, et al. Technical and anatomical factors affecting intra-arterial chemotherapy fluoroscopy time and radiation dose for intraocular retinoblastoma. J Neurointerventional Surg 2019;11(12):1273–6.
[28] Stacey AW, De Francesco S, Borri M, et al. The Addition of Topotecan to Melphalan in the Treatment of Retinoblastoma with Intra-arterial Chemotherapy. Ophthalmol Retina 2021;5(8):824–30.
[29] Patel M, Paulus YM, Gobin YP, et al. Intra-arterial and oral digoxin therapy for retinoblastoma. Ophthalmic Genet 2011;32(3):147–50.
[30] Chen M, Zhao J, Xia J, et al. Intra-Arterial Chemotherapy as Primary Therapy for Retinoblastoma in Infants Less than 3 Months of Age: A Series of 10 Case-Studies. PLoS One 2016;11(8):e0160873.
[31] Sweid A, Hammoud B, Weinberg JH, et al. Intra-Arterial Chemotherapy for Retinoblastoma in Infants ≤10 kg: 74 Treated Eyes with 222 IAC Sessions. AJNR Am J Neuroradiol 2020;41(7):1286–92.

Advances in Ophthalmology and Optometry 7 (2022) 161–176

ADVANCES IN OPHTHALMOLOGY AND OPTOMETRY

# Advances in Pediatric Periocular Vascular Neoplasms

Kasturi Bhattacharjee, MS, FRCSEd*, Aditi Mehta, MD, Vatsalya Venkatraman, MD

Department of Ophthalmic Plastic and Reconstructive Surgery and Oculofacial Aesthetics, Sri Sankaradeva Nethralaya, Guwahati, Assam 781028, India

**Keywords**

• Infantile hemangioma • Pediatric vascular lesions • Propranolol • ISSVA • Bleomycin

**Key points**

- Pediatric vascular lesions include congenital malformations from mesenchymal stem cells as well as neoplastic tumors arising from transformed endothelial cells.
- The International Society for the Study of Vascular Anomalies (ISSVA) Classification is helpful in characterizing the lesions and provides standardized nomenclature.
- With involvement of the periocular area, the presentation may be dramatic and potentially disfiguring, in addition to carrying a risk of stimulus deprivation amblyopia.
- Clinical diagnosis usually is sufficient for infantile hemangiomas. Imaging helps assess extensive involvement, characterize intralesional vasculature, and diagnose rare infiltrative/malignant tumors.
- Management has to be optimized and often is multidisciplinary, with some patients having systemic involvement and/or syndromic associations.

## INTRODUCTION

Pediatric periocular vascular lesions broadly include 2 categories: malformations and neoplasms [1]. Vascular neoplasms usually are benign and originate from transformed endothelial and other vascular cells, which exhibit an increased proliferation. Commonest of these is the infantile hemangioma

*Corresponding author. Department of Ophthalmic Plastic and Reconstructive Surgery and Oculofacial Aesthetics, Sri Sankaradeva Nethralaya, Beltola, Guwahati, Assam 781028, India. *E-mail address:* kasturibhattacharjee44@hotmail.com

https://doi.org/10.1016/j.yaoo.2022.03.006

(IH), which usually presents within the first year of life. Other lesions include congenital hemangioma (rapidly involuting, partially involuting, and noninvoluting types), pyogenic granuloma, spindle-cell hemangioma, and epitheloid hemangiomas. Locally infiltrative lesions are rare and even rarer in the periocular region. These include tufted angioma, reticular/composite/polymorphous/epitheloid/Kaposiform hemangioendotheliomas, papillary intralymphatic angioendothelioma, and Kaposi sarcoma. Large hemangioendotheliomas may sequester platelets and exhibit the Kasabach-Merritt phenomenon (KMP), commonly seen with Kaposiform hemangioendotheliomas. Malignant tumors like angiosarcomas and epitheloid hemangioendothelioma are extremely rare. When they occur, they exhibit a high metastatic potential.

Vascular neoplasms need to be differentiated from congenital vascular malformations that are noninvoluting, exhibit growth commensurately with age, do not demonstrate endothelial proliferation, and have the ability to expand hemodynamically [2]. These lesions consist of small and/or large vascular channels lined by a flat endothelium with a unilamellar basement membrane. The International Society for the Study of Vascular Anomalies (ISSVA) (2018) serves as a useful guide to categorize these lesions based on the demographics, clinical features, imaging findings, and/or histopathology [3]. Using the ISSVA system for classification is considered the clinical gold standard, as misdiagnosis and wrong nomenclature are common [4].

## SIGNIFICANCE

In this section, we shall discuss the associated red flags and syndromes that may be heralded by the periorbital vascular lesions. We also will discuss the decision-making process for watchful observation and indications for instituting therapy.

### Vascular tumors

Depending on the nature of the tumor, watchful observation may be useful especially in cases of small IHs, which usually present within 6 months of life, and after a period of rapid growth, it may exhibit spontaneous regression [5]. When a diagnostic dilemma arises, imaging followed by biopsy for histopathological confirmation may be required. IHs are positive for GLUT-1 (GLUcose Transporter 1) on immunohistochemistry. Intervention for IH is indicated when the lesion leads to complications like visual axis obstruction, amblyopia secondary to induced astigmatism, optic nerve compression, exposure keratopathy, severe cosmetic blemish, necrosis, or infection [6–8]. In cases of associated facial IH, it is important to rule out complications including compromised airways arising as a mass effect of extensive perioral/nasal/subglottic lesions.

Congenital hemangiomas differ in their epidemiology from IHs as they are fully developed at birth and do not proliferate thereafter. They are immunohistochemically negative for GLUT-1 in comparison to IHs [4].

Systemic involvement including visceral hemangiomas should be suspected in the presence of large lesions or a high number of cutaneous lesions ($\geq 5$).

Cardiac function assessment is important as these high-flow tumors may produce high-output cardiac failure due to large shunt flow [9]. In addition, cardiac evaluation for ruling out heart block and rhythm abnormalities is important before instituting beta blocker therapy in case of IH. Rarely, there may be consumption coagulopathy due to platelet entrapment in the highly vascular tumors–the KMP. Microangiopathic hemolytic anemia may develop in association with large hemangiomas of the periocular region, digestive tract, and the liver because of destruction of erythrocytes resulting from coagulation or sheer stress while passing through the anastomosing channels of the hemangiomas. The "PHACES" syndrome includes posterior fossa malformation, segmental hemangiomas of the face/neck, arterial stenosis/aneurysm/occlusion, cardiovascular anomalies, eye abnormalities, sternal cleft, and supraumbilical raphe and is characterized by a flat, telangiectatic facial hemangioma.

Multidisciplinary approach is important for optimizing treatment outcomes. Oral propranolol has gained FDA approval in 2017 as the first-line therapy for IH for children older than 5 weeks. The recommended dose is 1.7 mg/kg/d in 2 to 3 divided doses for about 6 months. Institution as well as discontinuation should be gradual in a step-up dosing over a period of 1 to 2 weeks while watching for symptoms like bradycardia, lethargy, and poor feeding [10]. Guidelines for initiating propranolol in syndromic cases including PHACES syndrome are established. For localized skin surface lesions, topical beta blockers like timolol maleate gel have shown promising results while minimizing systemic complications. A third alternate route is intralesional beta blocker (propranolol/labetalol), which can be injected under topical anesthesia plus sedation with high efficacy in small localized hemangiomas (Fig. 1) [11]. Other drugs used previously include systemic as well as local glucocorticoids. Biological immune response modifiers including imiquimod and becaplermin have been experimentally tried for ulcerated hemangiomas [12,13]. Pulsed-dyed laser is useful for treating superficial lesions. For partially involuted lesions, the use of nonablative fractional photothermolysis for anetodermic fibrofatty residua has been advocated [14].

Lesions like pyogenic granuloma may have a prior history of minor trauma preceding their onset, which occurs after the first 4 to 6 months of life. They consist of intravenous lobular capillary hemangioma and have a tendency to bleed, and surgical curettage/excision is definitive (Fig. 2) [15].

Tufted angioma and Kaposiform hemangioendothelioma are considered to be part of a spectrum of the same disease and exhibit lymphatic antigens, while being negative for GLUT-1 [16]. These lesions involve extremities, and their presence in head and neck region is rare. Magnetic resonance imaging (MRI) features include poorly demarcated, vascularized lesions with feeder vessels and frequent flow voids. Arteriovenous shunting disappears. Associated lymphedema may be observed along with dilated draining veins. Treatment involves embolization followed by chemotherapy with vincristine and prednisolone. Surgery may help in debulking the lesion but carries high morbidity especially if coagulopathy (KMP) has developed. Newer advances include

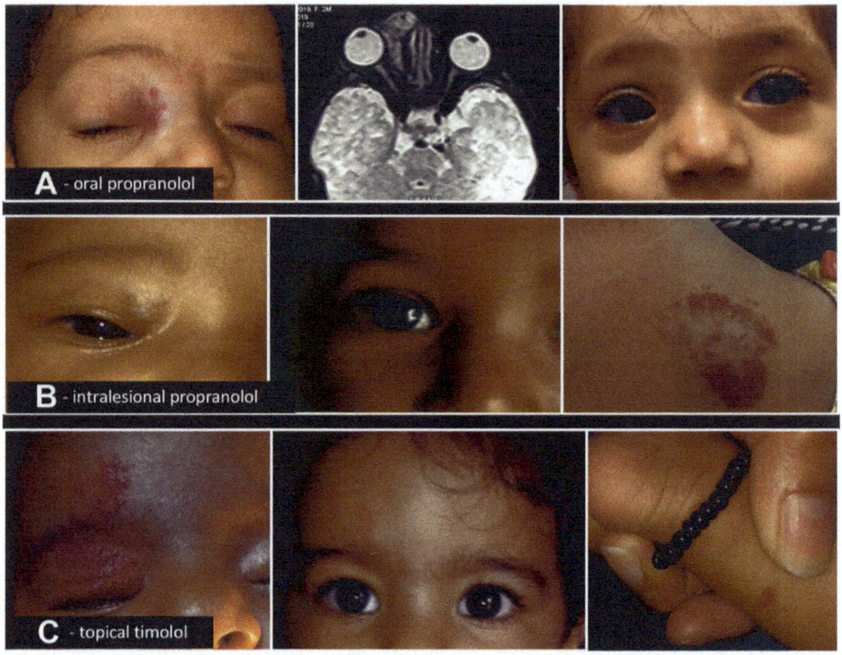


**Fig. 1.** Infantile hemangioma (IH): (*A*) This panel shows pretreatment and posttreatment images of a 3-month-old child with right anterior orbital and cutaneous IH. Contrast-enhanced MRI confirms the vascular nature and extent of the lesion. (*B*) The response of a right side superonasal anteriorly located lesion to 3 doses of intralesional propranolol. The child also has a cutaneous lesion on the neck, which is under observation. (*C*) Response to topical timolol applied for an extensive cutaneous lesion involving the right upper eyelid and forehead in a 6-month-old girl. Note the residual reddish hue on forehead after 5 months. Another cutaneous lesion along right foot also responded well to topical timolol.

the use of mammalian target of rapamycin (mTOR) inhibitors like sirolimus in conjunction with antiplatelet therapy with acetylsalicylate acid [4].

Kaposi sarcoma is extremely rare in the pediatric age group, exhibits a low-grade malignant potential, and is associated with HHV-8 virus infecting the endothelial cells and leading to a lymphatic reprogramming [17]. When the eyelid is involved, metastatic workup followed by debulking and cryotherapy or intralesional bleomycin is recommended. Angiosarcoma of the eyelid is extremely rare and may mimic a chalazion. Although the peak incidence is in the sixth-seventh decade, rarely they present in childhood. Risk factors include chronic lymphedema in the Stewart Treves syndrome, postradiation therapy, exposure to arsenic or vinyl chloride, and genetic predisposition in neurofibromatosis type 1, BReast CAncer Gene 1/2 mutations, Maffucci syndrome, and Klippel-Trenaunay syndrome [4]. Cutaneous angiosarcomas may present as a bruise or papule with ill-defined borders and may be multifocal and mimic benign vascular lesions. Clinical examination for fine vessels may

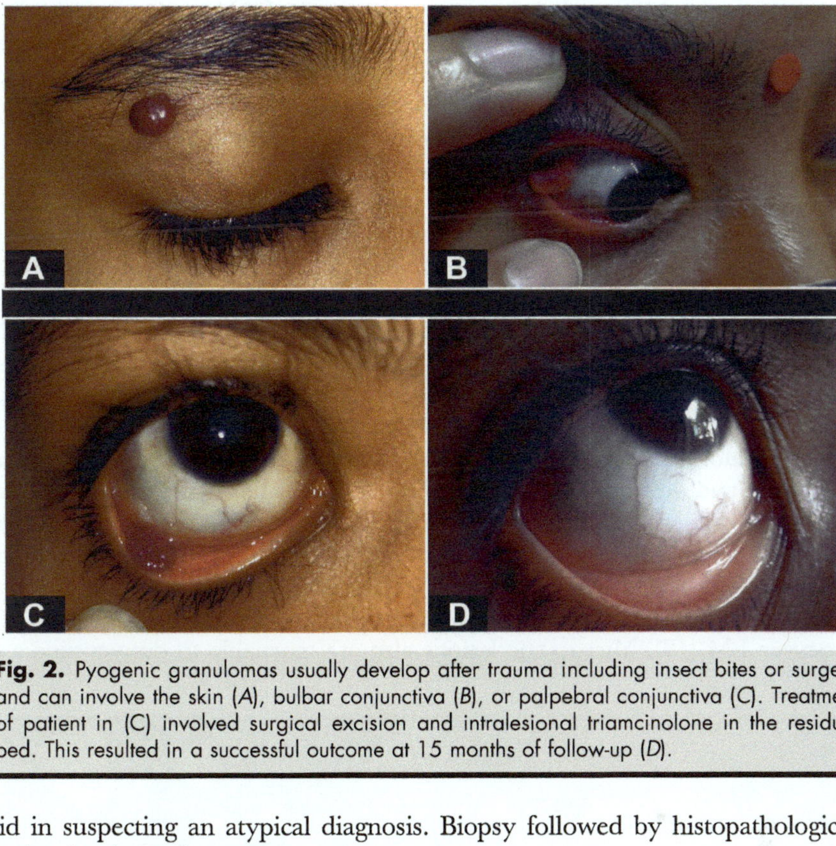


**Fig. 2.** Pyogenic granulomas usually develop after trauma including insect bites or surgery and can involve the skin (*A*), bulbar conjunctiva (*B*), or palpebral conjunctiva (*C*). Treatment of patient in (C) involved surgical excision and intralesional triamcinolone in the residual bed. This resulted in a successful outcome at 15 months of follow-up (*D*).

aid in suspecting an atypical diagnosis. Biopsy followed by histopathological evaluation is confirmatory.

Hemangiopericytoma arises from vascular pericytes and is a part of the spectrum of solitary fibrous tumors, characterized by staghorn-shaped vessels and spindle cells [18]. In children, these manifest as self-limiting lesions with low malignant potential in contrast to adults where likelihood of metastasis is high. Treatment involves surgery followed by radiotherapy in combination with systemic therapy. Because they are highly vascular, presurgical embolization can reduce risk of bleeding.

## Vascular malformations

In contrast to tumors, the vascular malformations do not exhibit spontaneous regression and hence pose a management challenge. Some malformations, including lymphangiomas, have a waxing and waning course with periods of growth and hemorrhage, coinciding with respiratory tract infections. Others may be present at birth but exhibit rapid growth during puberty, possibly due to hormonal influences.

Lymphatic (lymphangiomas) and venous malformations (VMs; including cavernous VM) are considered to be no-flow and slow-flow lesions angiographically. An overlap exists and previously was termed solitary encapsulated venolymphatic malformation. Now according to the ISSVA update, the malformations are classified as follows: simple, combined, named as per major vessels, and those associated with other anomalies [3]. By angiographic characteristics, they are divided into no/minimal flow-lymphatic malformation (LM), which can be microcystic or macrocystic and capillary malformations; slow-flow distensible varices; slow-flow nondistensible cavernous VM; and high-flow arterio-VM.

Lymphangiomas commonly involving the facial region usually present at birth (60%) or by 2 years of age (>90%) [1]. Lesions may be confined to the skin/ocular surface or involve deeper tissues (Fig. 3). When a periocular lymphangioma is suspected, careful evaluation of buccal mucosa for associated lesions is required. Clinical presentation is diverse, and large lesions may produce facial asymmetry, neurovascular dysfunction, or even airway obstruction. Enlargement and painful proptosis may be associated with periods of upper respiratory tract infections leading to intralesional hemorrhage. Urgent aspiration and debulking may be required if the lesions cause a compartment syndrome and vision decline. Treatment is largely symptomatic rather than curative. Percutaneous drainage and ablation are the first-line management. Oral sirolimus inhibits the mTOR, a regulator of cell growth and vascular endothelial growth factor (VEGF) expression. It has shown good results in microcystic LM [19]. Microcystic lesions also are amenable to doxycycline and

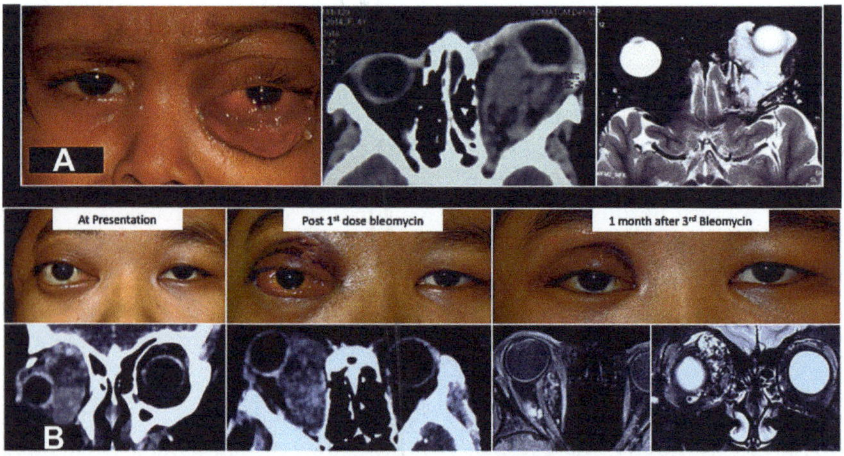


**Fig. 3.** Lymphatic malformations (LM): (*A*) This panel depicts a 2-year-old boy with left-sided proptosis, chemosis, and extensive orbital LM, confirmed on axial CT and MRI scans. (*B*) Serial follow0up of a 12-year-old girl who had previously undergone orbitotomy and debulking 4 years prior. She presented with recurring proptosis due to a large right orbital LM, seen on CT scans. She was undertaken for incision biopsy to confirm the diagnosis followed by 3 sessions of intralesional bleomycin. After the first dose, she developed a compartment-like syndrome, and oral steroids were added. There was significant resolution of proptosis and improvement in cosmesis after the third bleomycin, which was also confirmed on the follow-up MRI.

surgery. Intralesional bleomycin has shown promising results in macrocystic lesions although repeat injections are required. Macrocystic lesions also respond well to sodium tetradecyl sulfate and various sclerosant agents including bleomycin, picibanil (OK-432), or alcohol [20].

Primary lymphedema including the hereditary lymphedema, Nonne-Milroy disease, lymphedema-distichiasis syndrome, microcephaly-chorioretinopathy-lymphedema, the Hennekam lymphangiectasia-lymphedema syndrome, and lymphedema with myelodysplasia may have pediatric onset and require multidisciplinary management [3].

Capillary malformations are sporadic, as are congenital venule malformations. They usually are asymptomatic, and laser can be offered to reduce the cosmetic blemish. A classic port-wine stain is encountered in a capillary malformation associated with the Sturge-Weber syndrome, and evaluation for ipsilateral glaucoma as well as intracranial pial angioma is necessary (Fig. 4). This association is seen in up to 25% with a unilateral ophthalmic dermatomal distribution of the port wine stain and in up to 33% when the lesion affects bilaterally [1].

VMs of the distensible type include varices and may affect the conjunctiva, eyelid, and orbit. The deeper orbital lesions may cause proptosis and visible swelling, which usually appears as a bluish hue on the overlying skin. Enophthalmos may be noted in long-standing lesions because of repeated distension and collapse causing orbital fat atrophy. Evaluation for compressibility, postural variation, and enlargement on Valsalva maneuver is diagnostic [21]. Small asymptomatic lesions may be observed serially. The conjunctival lesions consist of dilated venous channels and have a bunch of grapes appearance (Fig. 5). These may bleed on trivial trauma, presenting with subconjunctival hemorrhage, and may have deeper orbital extensions. Surgery of the infiltrative ill-defined lesions may not be curative and carries a risk of bleeding.

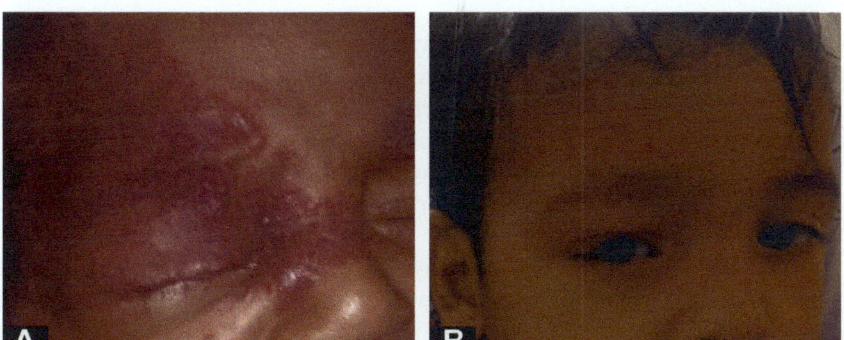


**Fig. 4.** Extensive capillary malformation involving right orbit in a case of Sturge-Weber Syndrome (A). The lesion responded well to topical timolol application (B). The child was also diagnosed with ipsilateral glaucoma, which responded partially to medical management with timolol maleate eyedrops.

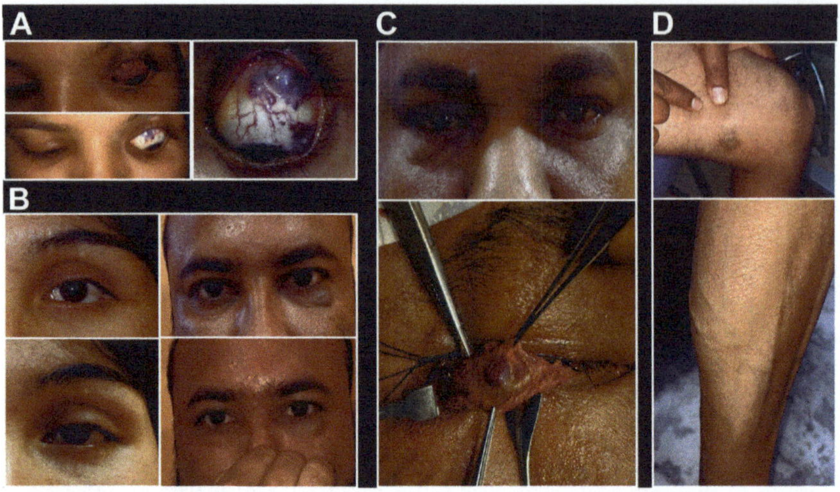


**Fig. 5.** Distensible venous malformation (VM) or varices: (*A*) Clinical presentations: Quiescent conjunctival lesions may develop extensive subconjunctival hemorrhage after trivial trauma and have a dramatic appearance as seen in this 14-year-old girl. Once the hemorrhage resolves, the lesion lies in the superonasal fornix and extends into the anterior orbit. Another typical presentation is a bunch of grapes pattern, seen in a 12-year-old boy. (*B*) Long-standing lesions due to repeated distension and collapse cause orbital fat atrophy leading to enophthalmos as seen in this 22-year-old lady with a left-sided congenital orbital varix (*left*). Varices enlarge on maneuvers causing increased venous pressure including crying or Valsalva maneuver (*right*, 22-year-old man). (*C*) Clinical and intraoperative photograph of a 30-year-old man who had a blue hued right lower eyelid lesion since childhood and was causing a cosmetic concern. Preoperative imaging ruled out postseptal extension, and surgical excision was performed. Intraoperatively, the bleeders were carefully cauterized to prevent excessive hemorrhage. (*D*) Syndromic associations of VM include the Klippel-Trenaunay syndrome with peripheral limb varices, usually developing in the popliteal fossa.

Intralesional sclerotherapy with bleomycin has shown effective results. Some syndromic associations of these VMs include Klippel-Trenaunay, Parkes Weber, Servelle-Martorell syndromes characterized by limb hypertrophy, Maffucci syndrome with VM and enchondromas, Proteus syndrome with VM/LM, and asymmetric somatic overgrowth and congenital lipomatous overgrowth, vascular malformation, epidermal nevi, scoliosis/skeletal, and spinal syndrome (CLOVES) [3].

Nondistensible cavernous VM may be present since birth and remain asymptomatic. They usually present in middle-aged population with a female preponderance. Sometimes, they may present early at puberty or during pregnancy, due to growth under hormonal influences (Fig. 6). These lesions usually are intraconal in location, and radiology is diagnostic. Surgical excision with cryo-assisted extraction is the treatment of choice. Recently, surgical excision with intraluminal cyanoacrylate glue application aids in solidifying the lesion and reducing intraoperative bleeding [22].

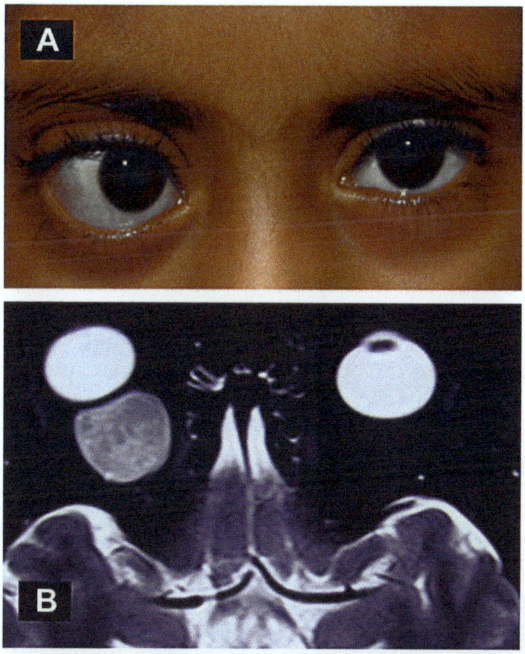


**Fig. 6.** (*A*) Eleven-year-old girl presented with gradual onset right-sided proptosis and blurring of vision. She had her menarche 1 year prior. Imaging (*B*) revealed an intraconal well-defined venous malformation (cavernous hemangioma).

Arterio-VMs (AVMs) can cause functional morbidity, cosmetic disfigurement, and high-output cardiac failure [1]. When an AVM is suspected, retinal evaluation is essential for associated Wyburn-Mason syndrome. Widespread cutaneous telangiectasia may be found in hereditary hemorrhagic telangiectasia (HHT) or Osler-Weber-Rendu syndrome with multiple AVMs affecting the brain, liver, lungs, and orbit. Treatment involves obliteration of the nidus percutaneously, endovascularly, or surgically [3].

Once the diagnosis is established, proper counseling regarding the chronicity of the disease in case of malformations especially those with syndromic associations is important. The ophthalmologist must keep in mind the psychological impact, especially when the parents/caregivers are anxious about the associated cosmesis and long-term prognosis [1].

## Secondary orbital involvement

Rarely, an intracranial vascular lesion may initially present with periocular symptoms like proptosis, exposure keratopathy, and conjunctival chemosis, developing due to congestive orbitopathy. Timely neuroimaging is paramount in such cases.

Vein of Galen malformation is a rare congenital cerebral vascular malformation resulting from maldevelopment of the embryonic median prosencephalic vein of Markowski and is diagnosed in the fetal or early neonatal period. It may present with high-output cardiac failure, macrocephaly, audible bruits, developmental delay, hydrocephalus, seizures, subarachnoid hemorrhage, and failure to thrive. Orbital involvement is in the form of proptosis with dilated orbital veins due to multiple high-flow fistulas (Fig. 7) [23].

Acquired (traumatic) carotid cavernous fistulas after blunt head trauma may be encountered in the pediatric population. Presentation involves proptosis, orbital congestion, chemosis, dilated corkscrew scleral vessels, persistent headaches, and diplopia. Owing to extensive communication of the cavernous sinuses, presentation may be variable and can involve both orbits (Fig. 8) [24]. Although not usually life-threatening, there is a risk of vision loss. Imaging of orbit reveals a dilated tortuous superior ophthalmic vein, increased bulk of extraocular muscles, and dilated cavernous venous sinus. Surgical and endovascular treatment is aimed at ligation of the external and/or internal carotid arteries and fistula embolization with glue, balloons, micro-coils, and stents [25].

## PRESENT RELEVANCE AND FUTURE AVENUES TO CONSIDER

Vascular lesions commonly affect the periocular and head and neck regions in the pediatric age group. It is important for the clinician to keep in mind that

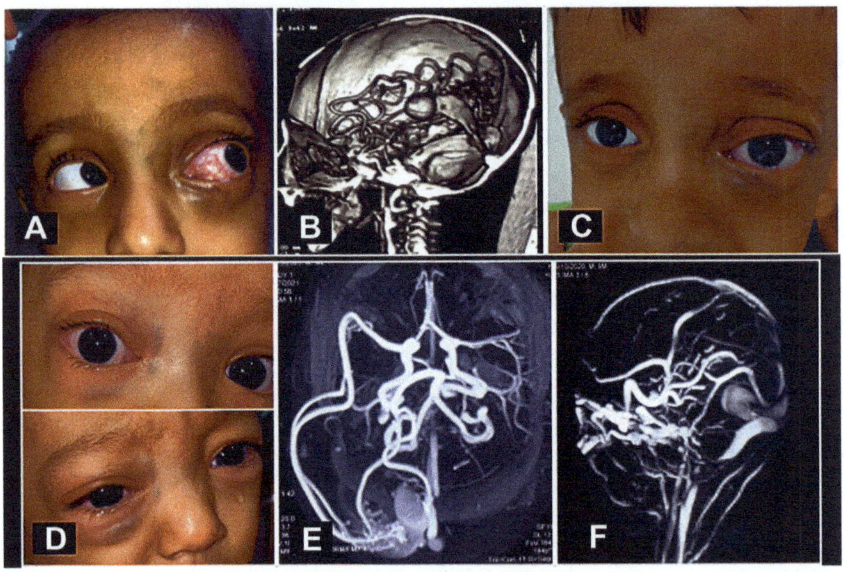


**Fig. 7.** (*A*) A 13-month-old child with left-sided proptosis, dilated corkscrew episcleral vessels, and congestive orbitopathy presented to the ophthalmic emergency. Systemic history was significant for failure to thrive and seizures. (*B*) Digital subtraction angiography (DSA) revealed an intracranial vein of Galen malformation, draining into the straight sinus. Embolization was performed with partial resolution of proptosis at the 6-month follow-up visit (*C*). (*D*) A 2-year-old boy with distensible cerebral venous malformation extending into the left orbit. The lesions distend on crying. DSA reveals aneurysm in left occipital lobe (*E*) and anteriorly in the left orbit (*F*).

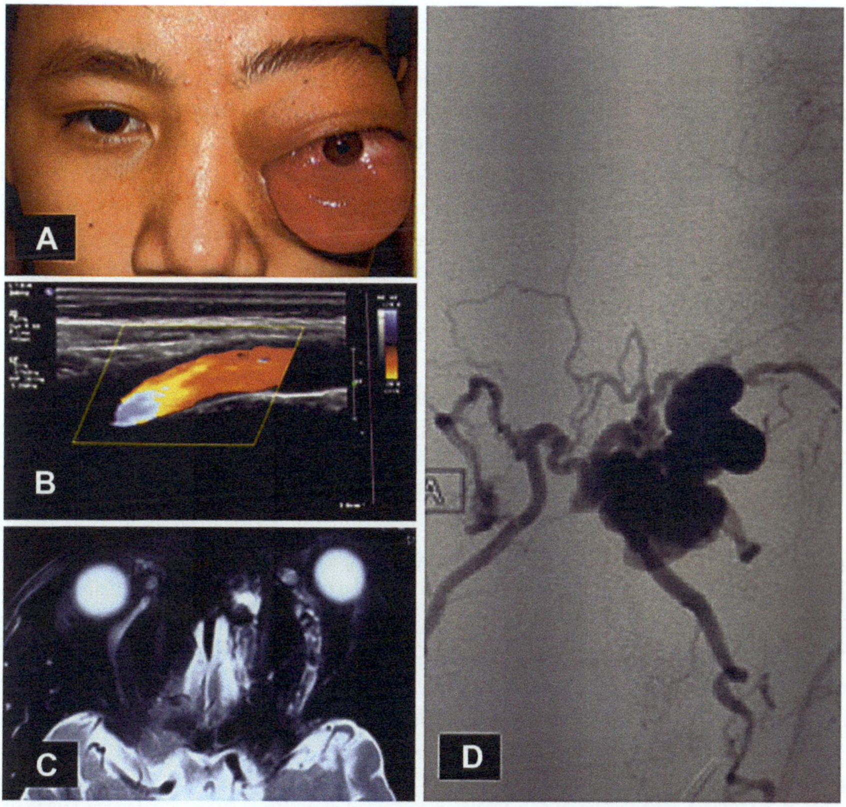


**Fig. 8.** (*A*): A 12-year-old boy presented with persistent chemosis of left eye following blunt trauma with bricks, 4 months prior. Episcleral vessels were dilated and tortuous, and there was left-sided proptosis. Doppler ultrasonography (*B*) of left internal carotid artery was performed. MRI (*C*) revealed a dilated tortuous thrombosed "S-shaped" left superior ophthalmic vein. (*D*) DSA confirmed a left direct type carotid-cavernous fistula.

although it is very common, not all pediatric periocular vascular lesions are IHs. The development of an improved classification and nomenclature system (ISSVA) along with insights into pathogenesis of tumor pathways have resulted in a clear understanding of these lesions [3]. Improvement in radiological imaging along with interventional techniques has allowed for multidisciplinary management of complex lesions, especially in situations where there is systemic involvement or syndromic association. Targeted therapy and personalized medicine have provided safer treatment options, and ongoing research in this field will help in better management of these complex lesions [26].

Research into the origin of IH has led to the discovery of an origin from hemangioma stem cells differentiating into 3 cell types. These include the endothelial cells, pericytes, and adipocytes, which proliferate under the influence of

VEGF-1. Excessive VEGF expression is noted in the proliferative phase of IH, and it decreases rapidly during the involutional phase [27]. This hypothesis may pave the way for therapy with anti-VEGF drugs, which have a good safety profile and have been used extensively for retinal disorders including retinopathy of prematurity and retinal and choroidal hemangiomas. Experimental studies have shown comparable efficacy of bevacizumab (monoclonal antibody against VEGF) and intralesional triamcinolone in early proliferative IH [28]. Malignant transformation of IH to angiosarcoma (seen very rarely) has been successfully managed with systemic chemotherapy along with bevacizumab [29]. Anti-VEGF agents suppress proangiogenic signaling pathways and also have shown promising results in treating angiosarcoma and Kaposi sarcoma [30,31].

Other signal pathways in IH include Notch, β-adrenergic signaling, HIF-α (hypoxia induced factor - alpha) mediated pathway, PI3K/Akt/mTOR, and Platelet Derived Growth Factor B (PDGF-B)/ Platelet Derived Growth Factor Receptor (PDGFR) [32]. IH endothelial cells also express GLUT-1, which also is noted in placental endothelial cells, postulating a possible placental origin. IHs also express neural crest and mesenchymal stem cell–derived proteins that may give rise to the fibrofatty residua of IH and affect its common occurrence in the head and neck region. Tissue hypoxia upregulates GLUT-1, induces vasculogenesis and angiogenesis, and is associated with prematurity. In accordance, a history of prematurity, low birth weight, placental anomalies, and multiple pregnancies is shown to have a higher incidence of IHs [26].

After a serendipitous discovery by Léauté-Labrèze, wherein propranolol being administered for cardiac disorders led to rapid clearance of IH, oral propranolol now has become the FDA-approved first-line therapy for IH [10,33]. It acts on hemangioma stem cells, suppresses proliferation, and promotes apoptosis in a dose-dependent fashion. The recommended duration of therapy is 6 months to achieve a 90% to 95% resolution.

VEGF-receptor expression has been variably demonstrated in orbital cavernous venous, lymphatic, and lymphaticovenous malformations, potentially paving way for alternative therapy with anti-VEGF drugs in these lesions [34].

The use of intraoperative cyanoacrylate glue to solidify VMs to facilitate surgical resection recently has been described. It is preferred to perform the embolization under image guidance as a hybrid procedure with direct intraoperative mapping as well as visualization of the lesion in the endovascular operating room [22].

An increased expression of the programmed cell death 1 receptor (PD-1) has been displayed in both IHs and VMs. This may potentially pave a path for immunotherapy with PD-1 ligands including pembrolizumab, nivolumab, and avelumab [35].

Increased understanding of the genetic basis of vascular malformations has led to discovery of somatic and mosaic mutations involving activation of 2 major intracellular signal pathways: the proliferation pathway via RAS/MAPK/

ERK (Ras/mitogen-activated protein kinase/extracellular signal-regulated kinase) and the antiapoptosis pathway via PI3K/protein kinase B (AKT)/mTOR (phosphatidylinositol 3 kinase/protein kinase B/mammalian target of rapamycin). Mutations in various genes of the PI3K/AKT/mTOR pathway are involved in congenital hemangiomas, including Rapidly Involuting Congenital Hemangioma (RICH) and Non Involuting Congenital Hemangioma (NICH), Kaposiform hemangioendotheliomas, tufted angiomas, and pyogenic granulomas. Somatic mutations in GNAQ gene affecting the RAS/MAPK/ERK are seen in Sturge-Weber Syndrome as well as in isolated capillary malformations. High-flow AVMs are driven by mutations involving the RAS/MAPK/ERK pathway [36]. This insight has paved avenues for molecular targeted therapy directed at the downstream signal pathways.

Sirolimus, discussed previously, is a direct inhibitor of mTOR. It obstructs downstream signaling and protein synthesis, leading to antitumoral and antiangiogenic effects. The VASE trial is a phase III clinical trial evaluating the efficacy and safety of sirolimus in vascular anomalies that are refractory to standard care in both adult and pediatric populations [37]. Everolimus, another mTOR inhibitor, has been used off-label in Kaposiform hemangioendothelioma; diffuse lymphatic, venous, and arteriovenous malformations; and congenital segmental lymphedema.

PIK3CA inhibitors under development include BYL719 (alpelisib). These have been tried successfully in the CLOVES syndrome. PI3K/AKT pathway inhibitors, such as ARQ 092 (miransertib), have been tried in the Proteus syndrome (the MOSAIC trial). MEK inhibitors, which inhibit the MAPK pathway, include trametinib. A prospective phase II trial, TRAMAV studying the use of trametinib in high-flow AVMs, is underway [36].

Mutations in endoglin or activin receptor-like kinase gene have been observed in HHT/Osler-Weber-Rendu syndrome. These genes affect the transforming growth factor-β signaling pathway, which acts in parallel to the VEGF pathway, paving way for the use of bevacizumab in these lesions. Thalidomide, lenalidomide, and pomalidomide also cause direct VEGF inhibition and have been tried for sporadic AVMs. Pazopanib, which inhibits tyrosine kinase receptors including the VEGF receptor-2, has shown promising results in HHT with uncontrolled bleeding [36,38].

Thus, the era of theranostics (therapeutics + diagnostics) for personalized medicine and targeted therapy is going to provide innovative treatment options for vascular anomalies with the establishment of genetic and molecular basis of disease origin.

## SUMMARY

Vascular anomalies of the head and neck are no longer blanketly termed as hemangiomas. Early clinical assessment including presenting age, growth, and proliferation can help classify the lesions into vascular tumors and vascular malformations. Radiological imaging with MRI can help aid in classification of the lesions. The ISSVA 2018 nomenclature system helps in systematic characterization of these lesions to understand their nature and decide the management. While histologic diagnosis is confirmatory, it may not always be possible. In such situations, radiology, including digital angiography and study of flow characteristics of the lesions, will help establish provisional diagnosis.

Both types of vascular anomalies of the head and neck region cause significant disfigurement and disability. Presence of large lesions obscuring the eyes can in fact have a severe psychological impact on patients as well as on their families. Syndromic associations must be suspected, and the patient needs to be evaluated by a multidisciplinary team. The understanding of genetic basis and molecular pathways of these lesions has provided novel insights into newer therapies.

While most lesions can be managed conservatively, with some, such as IH showing spontaneous resolution, treatment is imperative to prevent complications such as visual loss, amblyopia, optic nerve compression, exposure keratopathy, and in rare cases, emergent situations like airway obstruction. Patients with high-flow lesions must undergo cardiac evaluation. The same is also required before initiating oral propranolol therapy in IH.

Medical therapy is useful in most cases. When surgical intervention is planned, case selection is critical. The goals of surgery must be realistic, and the extent may vary from excision to debulking or just obtaining a specimen for histopathological confirmation, without causing significant morbidity.

Molecular targeted therapy is under evolutionary research and will soon pave the way for better management of these complex lesions.

## CLINICS CARE POINTS

- When a child presents with a periorbital vascular lesion, clinical examination should include history of progression/spontaneous regression of lesion, postural variation, change in size on crying, as well as detailed systemic evaluation for associated syndromes and cutaneous and visceral lesions.
- Visual assessment is important as visual axis obstruction or induced astigmatism may lead to amblyopia, warranting timely intervention.
- Radiology (ultrasonography, computed tomography, and/or magnetic resonance imaging) is useful for studying the flow characteristics.
- The gold standard 2018 updated International Society for the Study of Vascular Anomalies (ISSVA) classification and nomenclature system should be followed to appropriately classify the lesion as tumor or malformation and hence avoid misdiagnosis.
- Multidisciplinary management involving ophthalmologists, pediatricians, and radiologists is recommended.

## Disclosure

The authors have nothing to disclose.

## References

[1] Mahady K, Thust S, Berkeley R, et al. Vascular anomalies of the head and neck in children. Quant Imaging Med Surg 2015;5(6):886–97.
[2] Adams DM, Brandão LR, Peterman CM, et al. Vascular anomaly cases for the pediatric hematologist oncologists-An interdisciplinary review. Pediatr Blood Cancer 2018;65(1); https://doi.org/10.1002/pbc.26716.
[3] Available at: http://www.issva.org/UserFiles/file/ISSVA-Classification-2018.pdf accessed January 2, 2022.
[4] Wildgruber M, Sadick M, Müller-Wille R, et al. Vascular tumors in infants and adolescents. Insights Imaging 2019;10(1):30.
[5] Kanski JJ, Bowling B, Nischal KK, et al. 7th ed.. Clinical ophthalmology : a systematic approach, ix Edinburgh ; New York: Elsevier/Saunders; 2014. p. 909.
[6] Tambe K, Munshi V, Dewsbery C, et al. Relationship of infantile periocular hemangioma depth to growth and regression pattern. J AAPOS 2009;13(6):567–70.
[7] Stigmar G, Crawford JS, Ward CM, et al. Ophthalmic sequelae of infantile hemangiomas of the eyelids and orbit. Am J Ophthalmol 1978;85(6):806–13.
[8] Cuttone JM, Durso F, Miller M, et al. The relationship between soft tissue anomalies around the orbit and globe and astigmatic refractive errors: a preliminary report. J Pediatr Ophthalmol Strabismus 1980;17(1):29–36.
[9] Bang GM, Setabutr P. Periocular capillary hemangiomas: indications and options for treatment. Middle East Afr J Ophthalmol 2010;17(2):121–8; https://doi.org/10.4103/0974-9233.63071.
[10] Pierre Fabre Pharmaceuticals I. HIGHLIGHTS OF PRESCRIBING INFORMATION for Hemangeol. 2014. Available at: https://www.accessdata.fda.gov/drugsatfda_docs/label/2014/205410s000lbl.pdf. Accessed November 22, 2021.
[11] Mehta A, Bajaj MS, Pushker N, et al. To compare intralesional and oral propranolol for treating periorbital and eyelid capillary hemangiomas. Indian J Ophthalmol 2019;67(12): 1974–80.
[12] Mascarenhas R, Guiote V, Agro J, et al. Ulcerated infantile hemangioma treated with imiquimod. Dermatol Online J 2011;17(9):13.
[13] Metz BJ, Rubenstein MC, Levy ML, et al. Response of ulcerated perineal hemangiomas of infancy to becaplermin gel, a recombinant human platelet-derived growth factor. Arch Dermatol 2004;140(7):867–70.
[14] Laubach HJ, Anderson RR, Luger T, et al. Fractional photothermolysis for involuted infantile hemangioma. Arch Dermatol 2009;145(7):748–50.
[15] Patrice SJ, Wiss K, Mulliken JB. Pyogenic granuloma (lobular capillary hemangioma): a clinicopathologic study of 178 cases. Pediatr Dermatol 1991;8(4):267–76.
[16] van Vugt LJ, van der Vleuten CJM, Flucke U, et al. The utility of GLUT1 as a diagnostic marker in cutaneous vascular anomalies: a review of literature and recommendations for daily practice. Pathol Res Pract 2017;213(6):591–7.
[17] Abalo-Lojo JM, Abdulkader-Nallib I, Pérez LM, et al. Eyelid Kaposi Sarcoma in an HIV-negative Patient. Indian J Ophthalmol 2018;66(6):854–5.
[18] Gengler C, Guillou L. Solitary fibrous tumour and haemangiopericytoma: evolution of a concept. Histopathology 2006;48(1):63–74.
[19] Adams DM, Trenor CC 3rd, Hammill AM, et al. Efficacy and safety of sirolimus in the treatment of complicated vascular anomalies. Pediatrics 2016;137(2):e20153257.
[20] Balakrishnan K, Edwards TC, Perkins JA. Functional and symptom impacts of pediatric head and neck lymphatic malformations: developing a patient-derived instrument. Otolaryngol Head Neck Surg 2012;147:925–31.
[21] Smoker WR, Gentry LR, Yee NK, et al. Vascular lesions of the orbit: more than meets the eye. Radiographics 2008;28(1):185–325.
[22] Cheng AC, Li EY, Chan TC, et al. Hybrid procedure for orbital venous malformation in the endovascular operation room. Eye (Lond) 2015;29(8):1069–75.

[23] Puvabanditsin S, Mehta R, Palomares K, et al. Vein of Galen malformation in a neonate: A case report and review of endovascular management. World J Clin Pediatr 2017;6(1): 103–9.
[24] Jain C, Mehta A, Bhatia V, et al. Isolated contralateral abducens palsy in direct carotid-cavernous fistula. BMJ Case Rep 2020;13(12):e238746.
[25] Sundar G. Vascular lesions of the orbit: conceptual approach and recent advances. Indian J Ophthalmol 2018;66(1):3–6.
[26] Sullivan TJ. Vascular anomalies of the orbit–a reappraisal. Asia Pac J Ophthalmol (Phila) 2018;7(5):356–63.
[27] Boscolo E, Mulllikan JB, Bischoff J. VEGFR-1 mediates endothelial differentiation and formation of blood vessels in a murine model of infantile hemangioma. Am J Pathol 2011;179: 2266–77.
[28] Jin E, Luo L, Bai Y, et al. Comparative effectiveness of intravitreal bevacizumab with or without triamcinolone acetonide for treatment of diabetic macular edema. Ann Pharmacother 2015;49(4):387–97.
[29] Jeng MR, Fuh B, Blatt J, et al. Malignant transformation of infantile hemangioma to angiosarcoma: response to chemotherapy with bevacizumab. Pediatr Blood Cancer 2014;61(11):2115–7.
[30] Pourazizi M, Kabiri S, Abtahi-Naeini B. Intralesional bevacizumab (avastin®) as a novel addition to infantile hemangioma management: a medical hypothesis. J Res Pharm Pract 2017;6(3):190–1.
[31] Sabry HH, Sorour NE, Akl EM. Intralesional injection of bevacizumab versus triamcinolone acetonide in infantile hemangioma. J Dermatolog Treat 2020;31(3):279–84.
[32] Ji Y, Chen S, Li K, et al. Signaling pathways in the development of infantile hemangioma. J Hematol Oncol 2014;7:13.
[33] Leaute-Labreze C, Dumas de la Roque E, Hubiche T, et al. Propranolol for severe hemangiomas of infancy. N Engl J Med 2008;358(24):2649–51.
[34] Tran AQ, Shoji MK, Levitt A, et al. Vascular endothelial growth factor receptor expression in orbital cavernous malformations and lymphatic malformations. Ophthalmol Vis Care 2021;1(1):1003.
[35] Amaya CN, Wians FH Jr, Bryan BA, et al. Enhanced expression of Programmed cell death 1 (PD-1) protein in benign vascular anomalies. Pathology 2017;49(3):292–6.
[36] Van Damme A, Seront E, Dekeuleneer V, et al. New and emerging targeted therapies for vascular malformations. Am J Clin Dermatol 2020;21(5):657–68.
[37] Dong J, Han D, Wang D, et al. Efficacy and safety of sirolimus in the treatment of vascular malformations: a protocol for systematic review and meta-analysis. Medicine (Baltimore) 2020;99(40):e22596.
[38] Robert F, Desroches-Castan A, Bailly S, et al. Future treatments for hereditary hemorrhagic telangiectasia. Orphanet J Rare Dis 2020;15(1):4.

# Cataract & Refractive Surgery

Advances in Ophthalmology and Optometry 7 (2022) 177–186

ADVANCES IN OPHTHALMOLOGY AND OPTOMETRY

# Femtosecond Laser-Assisted Cataract Surgery

Emily Chang, MD, Amy Zhang, MD*

Kellogg Eye Center, University of Michigan, Ann Arbor, MI, USA

**Keywords**

• Femtosecond • Cataract surgery • Arcuate keratotomy • Nuclear fragmentation • Anterior capsulectomy • Clear corneal incision

**Key points**

- Femtosecond laser has been adapted in cataract surgery to assist with lens fragmentation, and the creation of incisions, capsulectomies, and astigmatism-correcting arcuate keratotomies.
- Femtosecond laser is a useful surgical tool in complex cataract surgery, specifically in zonulopathy and dense lenses.
- Despite its precision, in its current state, femtosecond laser-assisted cataract surgery (FLACS) surgical outcomes remain nonsuperior to the conventional phacoemulsification surgery in routine cases, making the financial cost of FLACS hard to justify.

## INTRODUCTION

The current gold standard for cataract surgery involves phacoemulsification, which utilizes ultrasound energy, to break up the cataractous lens so that it can be removed by suction. When femtosecond laser technology was initially introduced in ophthalmology in the early 2000s, it was used to create lamellar flaps in laser in situ keratomileusis. Approximately 10 years later, it was adapted to assist with multiple steps during cataract surgery [1]. Since femtosecond laser-assisted cataract surgery (FLACS) first became commercially available approximately a decade ago, it has continued to provoke much interest as well as controversy. When patients present to clinic interested in "laser cataract surgery," they are often under the impression that cataract surgery will be performed

*Corresponding author. Kellogg Eye Center, University of Michigan, 1000 Wall Street, Ann Arbor, MI 48105. *E-mail address:* amydz@med.umich.edu

https://doi.org/10.1016/j.yaoo.2022.04.002

solely with a laser. However, only certain steps of cataract surgery can be performed by the laser. This article will highlight the different FLACS options.

## FEMTOSECOND LASER TECHNOLOGY

The optically clear layers of the eye–the cornea and the lens–do not typically absorb electromagnetic radiation in the visible or near infrared spectrum [2]. Therefore, when light is shone on these structures, it simply passes through without altering tissue. However, if the light is highly concentrated with a short-pulsed duration, it will be absorbed by the tissue, causing focal disruption [2]. The femtosecond laser uses neodymium:glass at the near-infrared wavelength of 1053 nm. When tissue absorbs the photon energy from the highly focused laser, it turns into a plasma of free electrons and ionized molecules, which subsequently rapidly expands, creating cavitation bubbles that separate the targeted tissue. This process of converting light energy to mechanical energy is called photodisruption [3]. The femtosecond laser fires at the ultrashort duration of $10^{-15}$ seconds (femtosecond), which allows it to create microcavitation bubbles with minimal adjacent tissue damage [4]. In contrast, the Neodymium: yttrium aluminum garnet laser (Nd:YAG) laser fires with a longer, nanosecond duration that results in more collateral tissue damage. The femtosecond laser also is focused at a specific depth within the cornea or lens and causes no damage along its path because near-infrared light is not absorbed by the surrounding tissue. This allows the femtosecond laser to cut tissue at specified depths with virtually no heat development.

Currently 4 steps of cataract surgery occur where the femtosecond laser can be used. At the level of the cornea, the laser can be used to make the tunneled main clear corneal incision (CCI) or the side port incision. Additionally, the femtosecond laser can be used to create corneal stromal incisions for astigmatic correction. In terms of the lens, the femtosecond laser can be used to create a precise anterior capsular opening as well as assist in the fragmentation and softening of the lens.

The femtosecond laser is used in conjunction with optical coherence tomography (OCT) or 3-dimentional (3D) ray-tracing reconstruction to map the treatment plan [3]. This mapping ensures appropriate orientation of the cornea before creating CCIs or arcuate incisions. Imaging of the anterior segment (AS) is important when creating the anterior capsulectomy because poor identification of the AS structures can lead to a decentered capsulorhexis. The surgeon also defines a safety zone–the distance of nuclear fragmentation from the posterior capsule–to prevent hitting the posterior capsule. OCT or 3D ray-tracing detect cataractous lens tilt, preventing nicking the anterior or posterior capsule [5].

## CLEAR CORNEAL INCISION

The careful construction of a CCI in cataract surgery is an important aspect in maintaining a stable anterior chamber and a sutureless surgery. The main wound is used to gain access to the anterior chamber as instruments repeatedly enter and exit the main wound. A leaky wound is a risk factor for endophthalmitis [6]. Studies examining the sealability of manual CCIs have shown that square-shaped multiplanar wounds provide the most structurally sound wounds [7].

With manual CCI, it can be difficult to precisely control the length and architecture of the incision. In a comparative case series, as low as 19% of manually created CCI were truly triplanar because of inadequate depth of the first stage of the incision [8]. Femtosecond laser can automate the creation of a main wound, ensuring precision of CCI creation. In rabbit and cadaveric human eyes, femtosecond laser penetrating incisions had more predictable outcomes with less postoperative scarring than manual incisions [9]. Using AS-OCT of in vivo CCIs, femtosecond CCIs resulted in a lower incidence of localized Descemet membrane detachment, a lower incidence of endothelial gape, and a more reliable triplanar rather than biplanar wound architecture [8].

Despite the multitude of studies demonstrating the superior precision and predictability of femtosecond CCIs, a discrepancy exists in real-world practice. Most surgeons still do not use the femtosecond laser for creation of CCIs when they are using the femtosecond laser for other steps in their cataract surgery. It is also still up for debate whether the increased predictability of CCI created by femtosecond laser in fact leads to superior sealability of the wound. The wound deformation rate from an I/A probe in cadaveric eyes was significantly higher in femtosecond-created wounds than in manually created wounds, resulting in poorer self-sealing properties in femtosecond-created wounds [10]. In a large retrospective study of more than 1000 eyes in vivo, femtosecond CCIs were found to leak twice as frequently as manual CCIs (17.6% vs 8.7%) [11]. However, when the parameters of femtosecond CCIs were optimized in this single surgeon study, risk of leakage became equivalent to manual CCIs [11].

A well-constructed CCI also induces minimal astigmatism. Both preexisting corneal astigmatism as well as surgically induced astigmatism contribute to postoperative corneal astigmatism. Femtosecond CCIs are an attractive option to reverse preexisting corneal astigmatism by creating reproducible on-axis incisions to correct moderate levels of astigmatism [12]. However, when comparing surgically induced astigmatism in manual versus femtosecond CCI, Mastropasqua and colleagues and Diakonis and colleagues found no statistically significant superiority in reducing surgically induced astigmatism (SIA) with femtosecond CCI [13,14]. Zhu and colleagues actually found that femtosecond CCIs induced more astigmatism and produced thicker CCI than manual incisions [15]. This was because femtosecond CCIs distance from the limbus was more unpredictable and on average further than the manual CCI group. Although theoretically femtosecond CCIs should create less SIA, until the laser incision location system becomes more predictable, manual CCIs remain superior.

## ANTERIOR CAPSULECTOMY

The continuous curvilinear capsulorhexis (CCC) in the phacoemulsification cataract surgery may be the most important yet most difficult step to master in cataract surgery. A well-constructed capsulorhexis improves the safety of hydrodissection, nuclear emulsification, and cortical cleanup [16]. Ideally, it captures the optic and both haptics, allowing for centration of theintraocuar lens (IOL) in the visual axis. An overlapping capsulorhexis also lowers the rate of posterior capsule opacification by allowing the capsular bag to envelop the optic, causing the posterior optic edge to create an indentation in the posterior capsule, creating a mechanical barrier for posteriorly migrating epithelial cells [17]. Ideally, the overlap around the optic edge is 0.5 mm 360°, allowing the capsule to contain the IOL close to the effective lens position.

In an era where premium IOLs (toric, multifocal, and accommodating IOLs) are increasingly popular, a well-centered and appropriately sized anterior capsulectomy is even more critical. Capsulectomy architecture directly affects effective lens position, a major source of postcataract surgery refractive error [18]. A capsulectomy that is too small is prone to contraction, effectively pushing the IOL posteriorly. A capsulectomy that is too large does not create enough overlap with the IOL, allowing the IOL to bow forward or tilt. Laser-created capsulectomies are significantly more precise in size, with a much smaller deviation from intended diameter than when manual technique is used (29 μm ± 26 vs 337 ± 258 μm) [16].

A femtosecond laser-created anterior capsulectomy can create a perfectly circular opening. This theoretically increases the tensile strength of the resulting capsule opening because tags in the capsulorhexis end up creating focal areas of weakness. A noncircular capsulorhexis is at higher risk of a radial tear that can wrap around to the posterior capsule leading to vitreous loss. Femtosecond lasers more consistently produce circular capsulectomies, with a deviation from circularity of 6% compared with 20% for manual capsulectomies [16].

However, the perfectly circular capsulectomy created by the femtosecond laser can make removal of cortical material by irrigation and aspiration more difficult. This is because when the capsulectomy is created by the laser, it also cuts a circular disc of cortex immediately below it. This underlying circular disc can make it more difficult to visualize the residual cortex, making final cortical extraction a new challenge [3].

Reports exist of increased anterior capsular tears occurring in femtosecond capsulectomies when compared with manual CCC despite creation of a complete capsulectomy in 100% of cases. In a prospective cohort study of more than 1000 patients, anterior capsule tears occurred in 1.87% of femtosecond cases and 0.12% of manual cases [19]. Subsequent scanning electron microscopy of laser-cut capsules revealed tags and skip lesions on the capsulectomy edges. These postage-stamp perforations increase the risk for anterior capsule tears. Aberrant misfired pits also were noted at locations other than the edge of the capsule. These irregularities are thought to be due to minute irregularities in laser pulse energy introduced by folds in Descemet when docking, corneal or anterior capsule opacities, patient movement, or inaccurate OCT tracking [20]. Arbisser and colleagues have proposed a dimple-down maneuver involving applying gentle central posterior pressure on the capsulectomy to not only identify the location of tags but also to break the tag without causing a radial tear [20].

Conflicting evidence has been presented by Day and colleagues, suggesting that femtosecond capsulectomies are noninferior to manual CCC in creating anterior capsular tears. In a study of 1000 cases, the rate of anterior capsule tear was 0.1% (1 in 1000), comparable to manual cases [21]. This discrepancy in rates may be reconciled by an upgrade in software for the femtosecond laser wherein the time to create a capsulectomy decreased by 66% (from 4.5 seconds to 1.5 seconds). A decrease in capsulectomy creation time limits the potential impact of eye movement. This study suggests that as femtosecond laser technology continues to improve, prior limitations may no longer be relevant.

Today, the femtosecond laser is not the only device used to create automated capsulectomies. Because the femtosecond laser can be both cost-prohibitive and space-prohibitive, the precision pulse capsulectomy (PPC) is a feasible alternative [22]. It also can be used in eyes with corneal opacities, where laser use is contraindicated. Commercially available as the Zepto PPC device, this disposable capsulectomy device consists of a soft foldable silicone suction cup that can be delivered through a CCI (>2.2 mm). After suction is achieved and the nitinol capsulectomy ring is apposed to the capsule, a 4 millisecond electrical waveform is delivered [22]. It is important to note that the Zepto is still prone to skip areas within the capsulectomy and capsulectomy tags, with a reported 4.9% rate of capsulorhexis runoff in a study of 123 eyes [23]. However, the Zepto remains a good option for poorly dilated pupils, zonular dialysis, or intumescent cataracts.

## NUCLEAR FRAGMENTATION

Techniques that reduce the effective phacoemulsification time (EPT) diminish the total number of joules delivered to the eye, limiting the damage to ocular structures. In vitro studies have shown that phacoemulsification energy induces creation of free radicals leading to oxidative tissue damage of corneal endothelial cells [24,25]. In vivo, endothelial cell loss is directly correlated with total emitted ultrasound energy during cataract surgery [26]. Minimizing injury to endothelial cells is especially important in patients with preexisting endothelial cell dysfunction, such as in Fuchs dystrophy.

The femtosecond laser has been used to pretreat the lens through either segmentation or fragmentation. Linear segmentation divides the lens into more manageable pieces. Fragmentation uses cube-shaped patterns of laser pulses to break up the nucleus into small cubes, so that these cubes can be aspirated from the eye instead of requiring phacoemulsification energy [2]. Different grid patterns can be used in fragmentation according to surgeon preference. In a study of 400 eyes (200 femtosecond, 200 conventional), nuclear fragmentation by femtosecond laser reduced EPT by 70% [27]. The reduction in EPT with femtosecond nuclear fragmentation was noted to be greatest in lenses with denser crystalline lens opacification [28]. Palanker and colleagues demonstrated that 30% of femtosecond cases can reach 0 EPT, whereas 0% of conventional cases reached 0 EPT [29].

A reduction in EPT may be particularly helpful in hypermature or dense cataracts. However, there are theoretic issues that may arise with the femtosecond laser. A release of liquefied lens material during capsulectomy may lead to poor laser penetration or posterior capsule rupture due to changes in lens position when liquefied material is released [3]. When nuclear fragmentation occurs, it also introduces air bubbles that can be trapped between the lens and posterior lens capsule. Therefore, before hydrodissection, the surgeon should carefully tap on the lens to release the air bubbles and prevent blowing out the posterior capsule [3].

The advantages of reduction in EPT concerning visual outcomes seem to be limited to the immediate postoperative period. At both 3 weeks and 6 months, postoperatively, despite the reduction of EPT, femtosecond laser pretreatment has not led to long-term improved visual outcomes [29,30]. Similarly, at both 1 month and 6 months, postoperatively, it is controversial whether the difference in endothelial cell loss is preserved because certain studies have shown there is no statistically significant difference in endothelial cells between femtosecond and conventional groups, despite significant differences in EPT [30,31].

Despite the reduction of EPT in laser-assisted surgery, concern exists that the laser energy delivered during laser-assisted surgery may contribute to an increased risk of postoperative cystoid macular edema (CME). Increased prostaglandin levels have been identified in the aqueous humor of patients after laser-assisted cataract surgery compared with those with conventional surgery [32]. Prostaglandins are thought to be an inflammatory mediator that causes the breakdown of the blood–aqueous and blood–retina barrier, contributing to accumulation of transudate. Intraoperative miosis following femtosecond laser also has been observed and is thought to be due to the release of prostaglandins [33]. Constricted pupils subsequently may require increased surgical manipulation during phacoemulsification, further contributing to the release of inflammatory mediators.

In a study of 1390 eyes, at 2 months, postoperatively, no statistically significant difference occurred in the reported incidence of clinical CME between cohorts having laser-assisted versus conventional cataract surgery [34]. Most patients with CME after cataract surgery in both cohorts had preexisting risk factors for postoperative CME, suggesting that the risk for these patients remains elevated regardless of the surgical technique used [34]. However, in another study of 1291 patients, 0.8% of eyes in the femtosecond group developed postoperative CME, whereas 0.2% of the conventional group developed postoperative CME [35]. Although not statistically significant, on subgroup analysis of the laser surgery cases that developed CME, interestingly a correlation occurred with a software speed upgrade to the laser. This finding suggests that faster laser treatment speeds might be a potential risk factor for subthreshold (nonvisible) retinal damage [35]. The femtosecond platforms in these studies used high energy (microjoule) delivered at low-frequency (kHz) pulses. Van Nuffel and colleagues propose a low-energy femtosecond laser alternative that uses low energy (nanojoule) and high pulse rate (>1 MHz) [36]. They found that this low-energy alternative led to a lower rate of postoperative CME compared with the conventional phacoemulsification group [36].

## ASTIGMATISM MANAGEMENT

In modern day cataract surgery, an important goal is decreasing a patient's spectacle dependence. Approximately one-third of patients have greater than 0.75 diopters of preoperative corneal astigmatism [37]. Therefore, it becomes important not only to minimize surgically induced astigmatism but also find methods to reduce preexisting astigmatism. Options to address corneal astigmatism during cataract surgery include placing main incisions "on-axis" (with or without opposite CCIs), performing limbal relaxing incisions (LRIs), creating femtosecond laser arcuate keratotomies (FS-AK), inserting toric intraocular lenses, and performing postcataract surgery excimer laser refractive surgery [4]. LRIs to correct mild-moderate amounts of astigmatism (<2.5–3.0 D) are popular due to ease of performance and low cost [38]. However, LRIs are subject to inaccuracies due to the lack of reproducible depth and length of the incision.

In a study directly comparing LRIs with femtosecond arcuate keratotomies, FS-AK had a greater correction index (SIA was 73% of the targeted induced astigmatism [TIA]) compared with LRI (SIA was 43% of the TIA) [39]. Forty-four percentage of the patients in the FS-AK group achieved a postoperative cylinder less than 0.5 D compared with only 20% in the LRI group [39]. This study was limited in its length of follow-up of 1 month, postoperatively. However, other studies have shown stability of femtosecond arcuate keratotomy at both 1 and 5 years, postoperatively [40,41].

Another advantage of FS-AK over LRIs is that the corneal incisions placed by FS-AK can be either penetrating or intrastromal. Nonpenetrating FS-AK theoretically minimizes postoperative pain and eliminates the risk of postoperative infection [42]. Intrastromal AK is an effective method of correcting astigmatism as demonstrated by Day and colleagues where the mean astigmatism correction was 63% when using a nomogram that aimed to provide 70% astigmatic magnitude correction [42].

Despite the advantages of FS-AK, for higher levels of astigmatism, toric IOL are oftentimes a better option for correcting astigmatism due to the inherent limitations of astigmatic keratotomy. Exact positioning of the toric IOL is critical to its function. Rotation of a toric IOL by 10° away from its intended axis results in a 30% decrease in effectiveness. The current method of marking toric axis involves preoperative ink marking of the conjunctiva. However, this is subject to dissolution of the ink, smudging, and eye rotation. The femtosecond laser can be used to create 2 intrastromal incisions to mark the steep axis of the cornea to ensure exact toric IOL placement [43].

## SUMMARY

FLACS is able to improve the precision and accuracy of certain steps of cataract surgery. Nevertheless, in its current state, the clinical outcomes of FLACS are nonsuperior to the conventional phacoemulsification surgery, making the financial cost hard to justify. FLACS currently is a useful surgical tool in complex scenarios of zonular loss or hypermature cataracts but is not indicated for routine cases. In some health-care settings, enthusiasm for FLACS has been driven by revenue opportunities, reputation, and marketing opportunities. However, its substantial cost has limited its broader adoption. In addition, FLACS requires patient transfer from the laser to the surgical suite, reducing surgical productivity. This loss of efficiency, in terms of number of cases able to be performed in a day, has important monetary ramifications in all surgical settings. As femtosecond laser technology continues to evolve, its adoption may continue to increase as we come closer to fully automated robotic cataract surgery. Regardless, FLACS has demonstrated that it is here to stay.

## CLINICS CARE POINTS

- Currently, the femtosecond laser can be used during 4 steps of cataract surgery to improve accuracy and precision—clear corneal incision (CCI) creation, anterior capsulotomy, nuclear fragmentation, and astigmatism correction.
- Despite the precision of femtosecond-created CCIs, most surgeons will still opt for manual CCI because it is still up for debate whether the femtosecond laser indeed leads to a superiorly constructed wound.
- When dealing with complex scenarios, femtosecond anterior capsulotomy as well as femtosecond nuclear fragmentation can help ease the removal of hypermature cataracts or cataracts in the setting of zonular loss.
- In an era where cataract surgery is also a refractive procedure, femtosecond laser arcuate keratotomies offer a precise and reproducible method to correct mild-moderate amounts of astigmatism.

## DISCLOSURE

The authors have nothing to disclose.

### References

[1] Nagy Z, Takacs A, Filkorn T, et al. Initial clinical evaluation of an intraocular femtosecond laser in cataract surgery. J Refract Surg Thorofare NJ 1995 2009;25(12):1053–60.
[2] Kullman G, Pineda R. Alternative applications of the femtosecond laser in ophthalmology. Semin Ophthalmol 2010;25(5–6):256–64.
[3] Donaldson KE, Braga-Mele R, Cabot F, et al. Femtosecond laser–assisted cataract surgery. J Cataract Refract Surg 2013;39(11):1753–63.
[4] Roberts HW, Day AC, O'Brart DP. Femtosecond laser–assisted cataract surgery: a review. Eur J Ophthalmol 2020;30(3):417–29.
[5] Krueger RR, Talamo JH, Lindstrom RL. Textbook of refractive laser assisted cataract surgery (ReLACS). Springer Science & Business Media; 2012.
[6] Wallin T, Parker J, Jin Y, et al. Cohort study of 27 cases of endophthalmitis at a single institution. J Cataract Refract Surg 2005;31(4):735–41.
[7] Masket S, Belani S. Proper wound construction to prevent short-term ocular hypotony after clear corneal incision cataract surgery. J Cataract Refract Surg 2007;33(3):383–6.

[8] Grewal DS, Basti S. Comparison of morphologic features of clear corneal incisions created with a femtosecond laser or a keratome. J Cataract Refract Surg 2014;40(4):521–30.
[9] Gray B, Binder PS, Huang LC, et al. Penetrating and intrastromal corneal arcuate incisions in rabbit and human cadaver eyes: manual diamond blade and femtosecond laser-created incisions. Eye Contact Lens 2016;42(4):267–73.
[10] Kojima T, Takagi M, Ichikawa K, et al. Clinical and ex vivo laboratory comparison of the self-sealing properties and dimensional stability between the femtosecond laser and manual clear corneal incisions. Acta Ophthalmol (Copenh) 2018;96(4):e510–4.
[11] Benard-Seguin É, Bostan C, Fadous R, et al. Optimization of femtosecond laser-constructed clear corneal wound sealability for cataract surgery. J Cataract Refract Surg 2020;46(12): 1611–7.
[12] Chen W, Ji M, Wu J, et al. Effect of femtosecond laser-assisted steepest-meridian clear corneal incisions on preexisting corneal regular astigmatism at the time of cataract surgery. Int J Ophthalmol 2020;13(12):1895–900.
[13] Mastropasqua L, Toto L, Mastropasqua A, et al. Femtosecond laser versus manual clear corneal incision in cataract surgery. J Refract Surg Thorofare NJ 1995 2014;30(1):27–33.
[14] Ferreira TB, Ribeiro FJ, Pinheiro J, et al. Comparison of surgically induced astigmatism and morphologic features resulting from femtosecond laser and manual clear corneal incisions for cataract surgery. J Refract Surg Thorofare NJ 1995 2018;34(5):322–9.
[15] Zhu S, Qu N, Wang W, et al. Morphologic features and surgically induced astigmatism of femtosecond laser versus manual clear corneal incisions. J Cataract Refract Surg 2017;43(11):1430–5.
[16] Friedman NJ, Palanker DV, Schuele G, et al. Femtosecond laser capsulotomy. J Cataract Refract Surg 2011;37(7):1189–98.
[17] Ram J, Pandey SK, Apple DJ, et al. Effect of in-the-bag intraocular lens fixation on the prevention of posterior capsule opacification. J Cataract Refract Surg 2001;27(7):1039–46.
[18] Ho JD, Liou SW, Tsai RJF, et al. Estimation of the effective lens position using a rotating Scheimpflug camera. J Cataract Refract Surg 2008;34(12):2119–27.
[19] Abell RG, Davies PEJ, Phelan D, et al. Anterior capsulotomy integrity after femtosecond laser-assisted cataract surgery. Ophthalmology 2014;121(1):17–24.
[20] Arbisser LB, Schultz T, Dick HB. Central dimple-down maneuver for consistent continuous femtosecond laser capsulotomy. J Cataract Refract Surg 2013;39(12):1796–7.
[21] Day AC, Gartry DS, Maurino V, et al. Efficacy of anterior capsulotomy creation in femtosecond laser–assisted cataract surgery. J Cataract Refract Surg 2014;40(12):2031–4.
[22] Waltz K, Thompson VM, Quesada G. Precision pulse capsulotomy: Initial clinical experience in simple and challenging cataract surgery cases. J Cataract Refract Surg 2017;43(5):606–14.
[23] Kelkar JA, Mehta HM, Kelkar AS, et al. Precision pulse capsulotomy in phacoemulsification: Clinical experience in Indian eyes. Indian J Ophthalmol 2018;66(9):1272–7.
[24] Shin YJ, Nishi Y, Engler C, et al. The effect of phacoemulsification energy on the redox state of cultured human corneal endothelial cells. Arch Ophthalmol Chic Ill 1960 2009;127(4): 435–41.
[25] Murano N, Ishizaki M, Sato S, et al. Corneal endothelial cell damage by free radicals associated with ultrasound oscillation. Arch Ophthalmol Chic Ill 1960 2008;126(6):816–21.
[26] Hayashi K, Hayashi H, Nakao F, et al. Risk factors for corneal endothelial injury during phacoemulsification. J Cataract Refract Surg 1996;22(8):1079–84.
[27] Abell RG, Kerr NM, Vote BJ. Femtosecond laser-assisted cataract surgery compared with conventional cataract surgery. Clin Experiment Ophthalmol 2013;41(5):455–62.
[28] Mayer WJ, Klaproth OK, Hengerer FH, et al. Impact of crystalline lens opacification on effective phacoemulsification time in femtosecond laser-assisted cataract surgery. Am J Ophthalmol 2014;157(2):426–32.e1.
[29] Abell RG, Kerr NM, Vote BJ. Toward zero effective phacoemulsification time using femtosecond laser pretreatment. Ophthalmology 2013;120(5):942–8.

[30] Krarup T, Ejstrup R, Mortensen A, et al. Comparison of refractive predictability and endothelial cell loss in femtosecond laser-assisted cataract surgery and conventional phaco surgery: prospective randomised trial with 6 months of follow-up. BMJ Open Ophthalmol 2019;4(1): e000233.
[31] Takács AI, Kovács I, Miháltz K, et al. Central corneal volume and endothelial cell count following femtosecond laser-assisted refractive cataract surgery compared to conventional phacoemulsification. J Refract Surg Thorofare NJ 1995 2012;28(6):387–91.
[32] Schultz T, Joachim SC, Kuehn M, et al. Changes in prostaglandin levels in patients undergoing femtosecond laser-assisted cataract surgery. J Refract Surg Thorofare NJ 1995 2013;29(11):742–7.
[33] Mirshahi A, A Ponto K. Changes in pupil area during low-energy femtosecond laser-assisted cataract surgery. J Ophthalmic Vis Res 2019;14(3):251–6.
[34] Levitz L, Reich J, Roberts TV, et al. Incidence of cystoid macular edema: Femtosecond laser–assisted cataract surgery versus manual cataract surgery. J Cataract Refract Surg 2015;41(3):683–6.
[35] Ewe SYP, Oakley CL, Abell RG, et al. Cystoid macular edema after femtosecond laser–assisted versus phacoemulsification cataract surgery. J Cataract Refract Surg 2015;41(11):2373–8.
[36] Van Nuffel S, Claeys MF, Claeys MH. Cystoid macular edema following cataract surgery with low-energy femtosecond laser versus conventional phacoemulsification. Clin Ophthalmol Auckl NZ 2020;14:2873–8.
[37] Hoffmann PC, Hütz WW. Analysis of biometry and prevalence data for corneal astigmatism in 23,239 eyes. J Cataract Refract Surg 2010;36(9):1479–85.
[38] Lim R, Borasio E, Ilari L. Long-term stability of keratometric astigmatism after limbal relaxing incisions. J Cataract Refract Surg 2014;40(10):1676–81.
[39] Roberts HW, Wagh VK, Sullivan DL, et al. Refractive outcomes after limbal relaxing incisions or femtosecond laser arcuate keratotomy to manage corneal astigmatism at the time of cataract surgery. J Cataract Refract Surg 2018;44(8):955–63.
[40] Schwarzenbacher L, Schartmüller D, Röggla V, et al. One-year results of arcuate keratotomy in patients with low to moderate corneal astigmatism using a low-pulse-energy femtosecond laser. Am J Ophthalmol 2021;224:53–65.
[41] Chan TCY, Ng ALK, Wang Z, et al. Five-year changes in corneal astigmatism after combined femtosecond-assisted phacoemulsification and arcuate keratotomy. Am J Ophthalmol 2020;217:232–9.
[42] Day AC, Lau NM, Stevens JD. Nonpenetrating femtosecond laser intrastromal astigmatic keratotomy in eyes having cataract surgery. J Cataract Refract Surg 2016;42(1):102–9.
[43] Dick HB, Schultz T. Laser-assisted marking for toric intraocular lens alignment. J Cataract Refract Surg 2016;42(1):7–10.

Advances in Ophthalmology and Optometry 7 (2022) 187–199

ADVANCES IN OPHTHALMOLOGY AND OPTOMETRY

# Advanced Technology Intraocular Lenses

Mariam S. Hamid, MD[a,*], Man Li Jin, MD[a], Kevin J. Everett, MD[a,b]

[a]Henry Ford Hospital Department of Ophthalmology, 2799 West Grand Boulevard, K10 Department of Ophthalmology, Detroit, MI 48202, USA; [b]Henry Ford OptimEyes Super Vision Center - Sterling Heights, 44987 Schoenherr Road, Sterling Heights, MI 48313, USA

**Keywords**

• Presbyopia correcting lenses • Multifocal intraocular lenses • Extended depth-of-focus lenses • Accommodative intraocular lenses • Phakic intraocular lenses • Light adjustable lenses

**Key points**

- Intraocular lenses (IOLs) have been in use since 1949 to correct for presbyopia and include accommodative, multifocal, and extended depth-of-focus lenses.
- Multifocal lenses typically are either diffractive, refractive, or use qualities of both in an attempt to achieve spectacle freedom; however, they also induce photic phenomena including glare, halos, and starbursts as a consequence of multiple images focused simultaneously on the retina.
- Extended depth-of-focus IOLs have been developed to correct presbyopia to a certain degree while reducing the risk of photic phenomena.
- Light adjustable IOLs allow the spherical and cylinder power of the implant to be adjusted after cataract surgery.
- Phakic IOLs may be considered in young patients with a clear crystalline lens who do not meet criteria for excimer laser eye surgery.

## INTRODUCTION

Cataract surgery has a surprisingly long history, dating back to as early as 600 BC. Intraocular lenses (IOLs) were not introduced until 1949, when the first IOLs were created out of polymethylmethacrylate. Although riddled with

Financial Disclosures: M.S. Hamid and M.L. Jin: None. K.J. Everett: Consultant & Speaker for Alcon.

*Corresponding author. *E-mail address:* mariamshamid@gmail.com

https://doi.org/10.1016/j.yaoo.2022.04.003

complications such as glaucoma, inflammation, and IOL dislocations, this technology paved the way for modern cataract surgery. Monofocal lenses have a fixed power and require the use of glasses to fully correct for refractive error including myopia, hyperopia, and astigmatism.

Multiple intraocular lens technologies have been developed to help patients functionally restore the ability to see at near as well as distance to achieve partial or complete spectacle independence and improve their quality of life. The first multifocal intraocular lens was Food and Drug Administration (FDA) approved in 1997 to help provide satisfactory vision at distance, intermediate distance, and near after cataract surgery or refractive lens exchange [1,2]. Some limitations exist to the use of multifocal IOLs, namely photic phenomena including glare, halos, and/or starbursts, which are a consequence of having images simultaneously focused on the retina.

One technology emerging in the realm of presbyopia-correcting IOLs is the extended depth-of-focus (EDOF) lens. These lenses create a single elongated focal point, contrasted to the multiple foci of multifocal IOLs, and aim to reduce photic side effects such as glare and halos. The elongated focus aims to improve intermediate vision while retaining distance vision, however, often at the expense of near visual performance when compared with multifocal lenses [3].

The development of the advanced technology intraocular implants for presbyopic correction has garnered intense interest for the potential of spectacle independence after cataract surgery. The cataract extraction procedure for implantation of a multifocal and EDOF lenses is the same as that for a monofocal lens and has similar safety profiles. In this article, recent developments in advanced technology IOLs will be discussed.

Phakic IOLs have emerged for use in patients with clear crystalline lenses, allowing young patients to preserve accommodation. They are used to correct refractive error for patients that may not meet the corneal thickness or curvature requirements to safely undergo excimer laser surgery. They also have the benefit of correcting a larger refractive error, beyond the limits of safe LASIK (*laser-assisted in situ keratomileusis*) or PRK correction.

## SIGNIFICANCE

### Accommodative Lenses

Accommodative IOLs are either single-optic or dual-optic systems. The only available accommodative intraocular lens in the United States is the Crysta-Lens that uses a single-optic system. In this system, a single optic has flexible haptic that allows anterior movement of the lens to change the focal length and increase the dioptric power of the eye [1,4]. Clinical trials have demonstrated up to 1 diopter of accommodation [1].

In contrast, in the dual-optic system, as the name suggests there are two separate optic; the anterior lens has a high power, and the posterior lens has a negative power. Their relationship to each other defines the dioptric power of the eye and changes based on the zonular tension. When the ciliary muscles contract with accommodation, the zonular fibers relax, causing the lenses in the dual-optic system to separate in the anterior–posterior direction, increasing the dioptric power of the eye [1,4]. The mean accommodative range in one such lens, the Synchrony, which is not available in the United States, is 3.22 ± 0.88 diopters [1]. One disadvantage of the Synchrony is that it requires a relatively large 3.7 mm incision, which can induce unplanned postoperative astigmatism [1].

## Multifocal Lenses

Multifocal lenses use light rays at distance, intermediate, and near points to be simultaneously focused on the retina. Diffractive, refractive, or hybrid physical principles are used to create multiple distinct focal points to achieve spectacle freedom [4,5]. Multifocal IOLs are additionally differentiated as either rotationally symmetric or rotationally asymmetric and apodized or non-apodized. Studies have shown multifocal IOLs to have 3 to 5 diopters between primary and secondary focal points, achieving a depth of field of 2-3x that of a monofocal IOL [6].

Diffractive IOLs are the most commonly implanted multifocal lenses [7]. These lenses have a series of concentric rings on the surface of the lens resulting in discontinuity in optical density, allowing light particles to change direction when they encounter the rings using the Huygens–Fresnel principle [6–9]. The distance between each sequential ring is called a step height [1]. Varying the size and pattern of step heights allows the relative distribution of light energy at each focal point. At the first step height, the smallest concentric ring in the center of the lens, all light rays are focused at near [1]. The step height gradually decreases toward the periphery of the lens, where a smaller proportion of the wavelength as the discontinuity in the rings causes a change in the direction and speed of the light [1,7], allowing multiple focal points rather than the one focal point seen in traditional monofocal IOLs [7].

Apodized lenses, such as the Restor (which has hybrid diffractive and refractive qualities), have a gradual decrease in diffractive step heights from the center to the periphery [7]. When looking at a near object, the pupil is miotic due to the near triad (miosis, accommodation, convergence) allowing only the central concentric rings to be exposed to light, making the focal point at near [1,7]. When looking at distance, the pupil is mydriatic allowing more of the concentric rings of smaller step heights to be exposed, allowing light to diffract at a focal point of distance [1,7]. Seeing distance targets in bright light settings is a challenge of apodized IOLs, as bright lights constrict the pupil allowing only the central rings for near targets to be exposed. In contrast, non-apodized lenses such as the Tecnis multifocal IOL, AT LISA 809, step heights are uniform from central to periphery [7]. Therefore, the light distribution is independent of pupil size, and an equal amount of light is distributed to both the near and distant focal points [1,7].

Rotationally symmetric lenses are more commonly inserted than rotationally asymmetric lenses, which have an embedded inferior add power, similar to that of a bifocal spectacle. They are available outside of the United States. Rotationally asymmetrical lenses, such as the Lentis Mplus LS-313 (a refractive IOL), were first developed in 2009; they have an embedded inferior segmental near add segment and aim to reduce the photic phenomena seen in the rotationally symmetric IOLs [2,7]. One such example is the LENTIS Mplus [1]. The IOL is independent of pupil size greater than 2 mm [1]. It is a single piece IOL with a +3.0D or +1.5D add. Despite attempts to minimize photic phenomena, asymmetrical IOLs still can have pupil-dependent photic phenomena as the center of the pupil moves slightly nasally while constricting, so the amount of light distributed between the near and distance portions of the IOL, and subsequently the vision, can be unpredictable [2] (Fig. 1).

Refractive IOLs have concentric zones of different dioptric powers [7]. This is achieved by varying the curvature of the anterior or posterior surface of the lens [6]. They are pupil dependent [7] (Fig. 2).

An example of a hybrid diffractive–refractive multifocal IOL is the Alcon Panoptix. It is a one-piece aspheric IOL [7]. It has a 4.5 mm diffractive area in the center with 15 diffractive zones and an outer refractive rim, resulting in +2.17D intermediate add power and +3.25 near add [7]. As a compromise

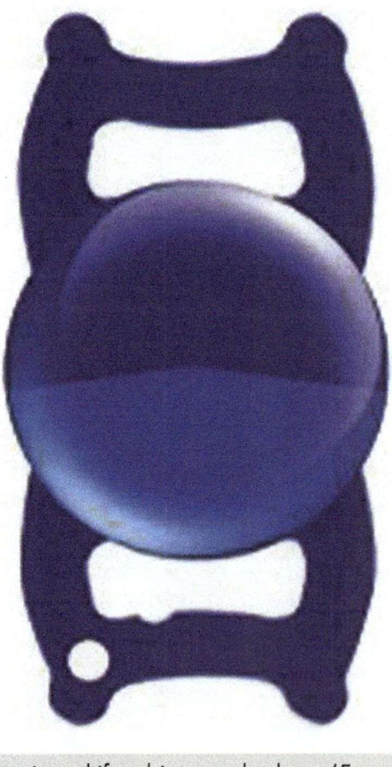

**Fig. 1.** Rotationally asymmetric multifocal intraocular lens. (*From* Pazo EE, McNeely RN, Richoz O, Nesbit MA, Moore TCB, Moore JE. Pupil influence on the quality of vision in rotationally asymmetric multifocal IOLs with surface-embedded near segment. J Cataract Refract Surg. 2017;43(11):1420-1429.)

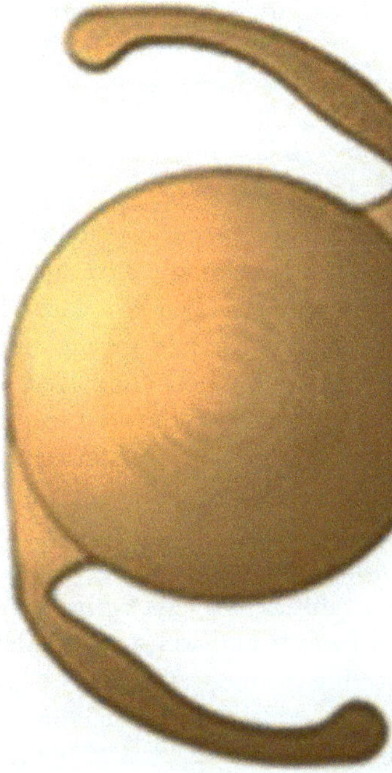

**Fig. 2.** AcrySof Restor SN6AD3, an example of an apodized diffractive lens. (Alió JL, Pikkel J. Multifocal Intraocular Lenses: The Art and the Practice. Springer Nature 2014.)

for multiple focal points, there is splitting of light, with a distribution of 25% at near (40 cm), 25% at intermediate (60 cm), and 50% at distance [7]. It also employs a fourth focal point at 1.20 m due to light from the first focal point diffracting further than the focal length that is not visible but allows intermediate vision to be at a more comfortable distance [7].

## Optical Side Effects in Multifocal Intraocular Lenses

Because light is distributed among multiple focal points, photic phenomena or undesired light images in the visual field occur in multifocal IOLs [7]. These include glare, halos, and/or starbursts [7]. In addition, the light in the out-of-focus image reduces the contrast of the in-focus image [1,7]. Multifocal IOLs are also associated with a reduction in contrast sensitivity as the light in the out-of-focus image reduces the contrast of the in-focus image. When comparing multifocal IOLs to monofocal IOLs, a higher incidence of reported glare and halos occurs in the multifocal groups, RR (relative risk) 1.41 (95% CI 1.03–1.93) and 3.58 (1.99–6.46), respectively [5]. Patients typically adapt to the unwanted optical phenomena in a 6-month period in a process called neuroadaptation in which the brain suppresses the unwanted image, but some patients have persistent symptoms [1,7]. Multifocal IOLs overall have a high satisfaction rate with more than 90% of postoperative patients indicating that they would choose the same intraocular lens again; however, up to 10% of patients are intolerant of the photic phenomena, and some require IOL explantation [1,9].

## Extended-Vision Intraocular Lens

EDOF lenses are a new technology emerging in the realm of presbyopia-correcting IOLs. These lenses create a single elongated focal point, contrasted to the multiple foci of multifocal IOLs The elongated focus aims to improve intermediate vision while retaining distance vision; however, this often is at the cost of near visual performance when compared with multifocal lenses. They aim to reduce photic phenomena compared to multifocal IOLs.

The first EDOF IOL was produced by Johnson and Johnson Vision (Symfony) in 2014, later FDA approved for use in the United States in 2016. Since then, several EDOF IOLs have been released to the market.

Vivity is a new EDOF intraocular lens using Alcon's proprietary X-wave technology. It is a novel, non-diffractive lens with a 6-mm biconvex, aspheric optic. The lens is produced from a high refractive index hydrophobic acrylic material with blue-light-filtering properties [10,11]. The anterior surface of the Vivity lens is designed with negative spherical aberration and created using the wavefront shaping technology, and its central optical element achieves the extended depth of field vision. The light rays passing through the central 2.2 mm of the wavefront-shaping zone of the optic are stretched and shifted compared with the peripheral light rays, extending the range of focus [10]. A toric version of the Vivity is also available, which achieves astigmatic correction with the biconic structure of the posture surface of the lens [10] (Fig. 3).

The Vivity DFT015 lens provided a greater negative range of binocular defocus when compared with the SN60WF monofocal lens, with no abrupt drop in visual acuity. Clinical studies show that the Vivity lens achieved the improvement of uncorrected binocular intermediate and near visual acuity of 1 line better versus the Alcon SN60WF monofocal lens 6 months postoperatively in patients aiming for emmetropia [12]. At 6 months, the percentage of patients in the Vivity group reporting no visual disturbance was comparable to patients in the SN60WF group. The same study reported lower average mesopic contrast sensitivity in the DFT015 when compared with the SN60WF group.

Since then, other studies published have supported the improvement of intermediate vision with the DFT015 lens [13,14]. Kohnen and colleagues found that 63% of patients with bilateral Vivity IOL implantation reported no optical phenomena at 3 months postoperatively [14]. In this study, 38% of patients reported needing reading spectacles, whereas 50% of the patients are entirely spectacle independent at all distances [14]. In another study, where patients were bilaterally implanted with the Vivity IOL, with a target of emmetropia in the dominant eye and a target of −0.75 in the non-dominant eye, 76% of all patients had binocular distance-corrected VA of 0.2 logMAR (Logarithm

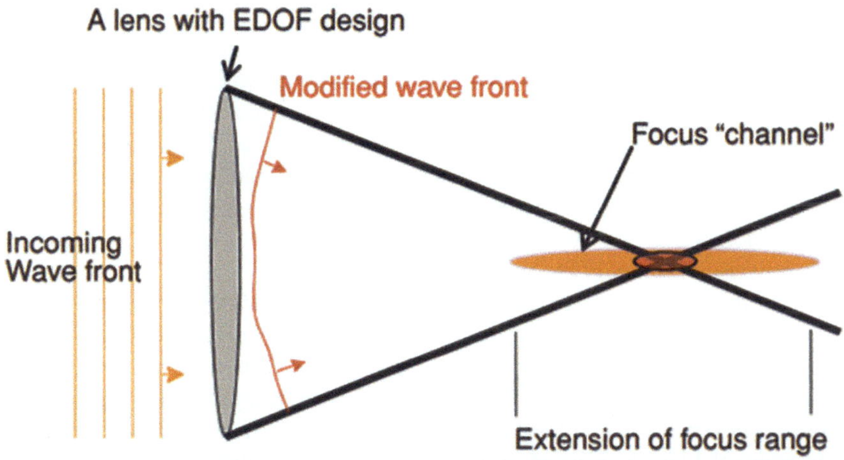


**Fig. 3.** Visual representation of the mechanism of an EDOF IOLan extended depth of focus IOL modifies the light wavefront and creates an elongated focal point (*From* Zeev Zalevsky "Extended depth of focus imaging: a review," SPIE Reviews 1(1), 018001 (1 January 2010).)

of the Minimum Angle of Resolution) or better at distance, intermediate, and near [15].

## Monofocal Intraocular Lenses with Increased Depth of Focus

The Tecnis Eyhance is a new, advanced monofocal IOL produced by Johnson & Johnson. It is a 1-piece, biconvex aspheric lens with a 6.0 mm optic, with a continuous 360-degree posterior square edge design [16]. The lens is similar to the Tecnis monofocal lens ZCB00; however, it is distinguished by a continuous change in power from the periphery to the center of the lens. In addition to this, the lens is built with negative spherical aberration to extend its depth of focus. A study on Eyhance lens found that the power profile at the center 2 mm of the lens grants a myopic defocus of −0.5D with a 2 mm pupil [17].

Several studies have found the Tecnis Eyhance lens to be superior to the Tecnis 1-piece monofocal lens for intermediate vision without compromising distance vision while retaining a photic side effect profile similar to a traditional monofocal lens [18–22]; however, it has not yet been proven to be superior in near vision. When comparing the Tecnis Eyhance to the Tecnis Symfony (an EDOF lens), the two lenses seem to have comparable distance and intermediate vision while the Symfony achieves superior near vision and higher rates of spectacle independence [23]. This, however, is at the expense of more photic phenomena [23–25].

## Light Adjustable Intraocular Lenses

Light adjustable IOLs are the only type of intraocular implants that allow adjustments of lens power after cataract surgery to improve refractive accuracy. This lens is based on the principles of diffusion. The light adjustable lens is composed of a silicone matrix embedded with photosensitive macromers. After lens implantation, ultraviolet (UV) light is directed at an area of the lens, which would turn the macromers into polymers. This creates a diffusion gradient, drawing macromers to diffuse into the light-exposed area until equilibrium is reached, resulting in a predictable shift in lens curvature and is capable of changing both the spherical and cylinder power of the lens. The adjustable range varies between −2D to +2D sphere and up to 3D cylinder. Up to four sessions of light treatment may be needed to achieve the desired lens power. After the target vision has been achieved, UV light is directed to the optic to secure the final power [26]. An FDA study of 600 participants found that those who received the light adjustable lens are twice as likely to achieve a uncorrected distance vision of 20/20 when compared with a standard monofocal lens [26].

This new technology of light adjustable lenses comes with a few caveats. Light adjustment procedures require full view of the IOL optic and require good pupillary dilation. Patients are also required to adhere strictly to full-time wear of UV-blocking glasses for several weeks after cataract surgery, as any unintended exposure may prevent future adjustments of the lens power. In addition, the implantation of this lens is contraindicated in patients with certain eye diseases such as macular disease and prior history of herpes eye infection [26].

### Phakic Intraocular Lenses

An additional advanced technology utilizing intraocular lens placement is the use of phakic IOLs in patients with clear crystalline lenses. In this technique, artificial lenses are placed in phakic eyes allowing preservation of the architectural integrity of the cornea in patients who do not meet eligibility criteria for excimer laser treatment in laser-assisted in situ keratomileusis or photorefractive keratectomy [27]. In addition, phakic IOLs can correct a refractive spherical error ranging from −20D to +22D, which is a significantly larger range compared to that which can be corrected with an excimer laser (approximately −12D to +6D) [27]. Early attempts at the use of phakic IOLs started in 1950 but resulted in untoward side effects including corneal decompensation due to endothelial cell loss, uveitis-glaucoma-hyphema syndrome due to iris chafing, accelerated cataract formation, and astigmatism induced by a large surgical wound required for lens insertion [27]. In 2004, the FDA approved the first phakic IOL for use in myopia. Present day, phakic IOLs are categorized by their placement: anterior chamber supported, iris-fixated in the anterior chamber, or sulcus-fixated like in the implantable collamer lens [27]. Newer phakic lens models may still result in corneal decompensation and glaucoma like in earlier models, but improved architecture have allowed them to be safer and have predictable refractive outcomes [27].

## DISCUSSION, FUTURE CONSIDERATIONS, AND SUMMARY

Over the years, new advancements in intraocular lens implant technology broadened the options for presbyopia correction in patients undergoing cataract surgery. The advent of the computer and internet age led to increasing demand for intermediate vision, as our daily lives became more intertwined with the digital screen. As the technology for modern cataract surgery has matured, new options for advanced technology IOLs have been developed.

The more commonly used presbyopia-correcting lens is the multifocal lens, which presents the earliest attempts to correct for presbyopia using IOLs. These lenses take advantage of optical properties including diffraction, refraction, or combination of the two to allow images from different distances to be simultaneously focused on the retina to try to make patients spectacle-free. As a consequence, out-of-focus images can contribute to reduced contrast sensitivity and photic phenomena, including glare, halos, and starbursts. The photic phenomena typically resolve within 6 months in a process called neuroadaptation; however, up to 10% of patients are intolerant of the side effects, and some result in lens explantation. Multifocal lenses create distinct peaks on the defocus curve correlating to improved visual acuity at determined distances, with comparatively blurrier vision in between. As a consequence, out-of-focus images can contribute to reduced contrast sensitivity. The Tecnis Synergy IOL, a hybrid diffractive multifocal and EDOF lens that was FDA approved in May 2021, has anecdotal evidence of improved contrast sensitivity compared with other multifocal IOLs, though this has not yet been formally published. In the future, it would be advantageous to create multifocal IOLs that are pupil-independent and lack the photic phenomena seen in current models.

Given the optical side effects of multifocal IOLs, eligible patients should be selected and consented carefully to ensure no preexisting ocular disease that could limit visual acuity. Lifestyle and occupational choices should be discussed with patients before implantation as patients that do activities in low light settings may be especially intolerant of the reduced contrast sensitivity [1]. A thorough slit-lamp examination and supplemental imaging should be ordered to explore pathology that could exacerbate the ability for multifocal IOLs to work most effectively. Macular pathology should be ruled out before the implantation of multifocal IOLs, such as with optical coherence tomography, as even small macular abnormalities can result in reduced contrast sensibility that can be worsened by implantation of a multifocal IOL [7]. Patients with corneal disease such as epithelial basement membrane disease, particularly in the central visual axis, should also avoid multifocal IOLs [1]. Glaucoma is a relative contraindication and may be acceptable if mild stage [7]. High hyperopes may also have a large angle kappa after implantation and centration of a multifocal IOL and may not tolerate them [1]. Lastly, as many of the multifocal IOLs are pupil dependent, pupil reactivity should be assessed before implantation [6].

Data on the CrystaLens, which is the only approved accommodating IOL in the United States, demonstrate a mean uncorrected near visual acuity of 0.19 logMAR (Snellen equivalent, 20/31), a mean uncorrected intermediate visual acuity of 0.07 logMAR (Snellen equivalent, 20/23), and a mean uncorrected distance visual acuity of 0.08 logMAR (Snellen equivalent, 20/24) [28]. Compared with monofocal IOLs, accommodative IOLs seem to allow patients to achieve better near visual acuity at 6 months postoperatively (on average, an improvement of 3.20 Jaeger units), and at 12 months postoperatively. Although accommodative lenses were found to have improved distance visual acuity at 6 months compared with monofocal lenses (0.04 standard deviations better), accommodative lenses comparatively had worse vision with time, with 12 months or more compared with monofocal lenses (0.12 log-MAR worse). The decreased vision is possibly attributed to a higher rate of posterior capsular opacification [4].

EDOF IOLs provide a wider range of uncorrected vision when compared with monofocal lenses. They provide some degree of spectacle independence by delivering improved intermediate vision without compromising distance visual acuity. As the increasing commodity of smartphone and computer use, many patients find the intermediate vision range to be increasingly important. In addition, as the Vivity EDOF uses a non-diffractive technology and does not split the light like a diffractive lens might, contrast sensitivity may be preserved [29]. All of these properties can make the EDOF IOLs an attractive option for patients who value spectacle independence at intermediate distances while reducing the chance of glare and halos.

Patients with preexisting ocular disease who might not otherwise qualify for a multifocal lens may benefit from an EDOF lens or a monofocal with EDOF properties due to its relatively preserved contrast sensitivity and reduced photic phenomenon. Additionally, depending on the specific needs of the patient, one may further extend the depth of focus by using a monovision approach with the EDOF IOLs by targeting one eye for emmetropia and the other eye for mild myopia [30,31], granting some degree of spectacle independence at near. In addition, one may take advantage of the myopic defocus curve of the EDOF to aim for true plano for distance vision, as any potential postoperative hyperopia may be tolerated thanks to the extended focus depth of the lens.

Compared with traditional monofocal IOLs, the Tecnis Eyhance provides approximately a −0.5D of myopic defocus, providing some uncorrected intermediate vision. Although its intermediate range is less than a traditional EDOF IOL, it comes with the advantage of being considered a monofocal IOL and incurs no extra out of pocket cost for the patient.

Compared with monofocal IOLs, no statistically significant difference occurs in unaided distance visual acuity in multifocal IOLs [5]. Multifocal IOLs showed the improved near vision compared with monofocal IOLs as well as a higher incidence of spectacle independence [5]. Comparing rotationally asymmetric refractive multifocal IOLs to apodized diffractive multifocal IOLs, the diffractive multifocal IOL group had better near visual acuity outcomes and a lower incidence of aberrations [28]. The rotationally asymmetric refractive multifocal IOL group had better intermediate visual acuity outcomes and contrast sensitivity [28].

Reviewing data comparing visual outcomes within the subcategory of multifocal and EDOF lenses has been challenging as the lenses have different near focal points [32]. Most studies show no statistically significant difference in best corrected distance visual acuity among the multifocal platforms [32]. For intermediate distances, all lenses have an average visual outcome in the 20/20 to 20/30 range from 50 to 80 cm [32]. Overall, studies comparing presbyopia-correcting lenses including multifocal and EDOF IOLs have demonstrated a higher prevalence of spectacle independence compared with monofocal IOLs [29,32]. Comparing the degree of visual quality at distance, near, and intermediate distances, the level of spectacle independence and side effect profile between multifocal and EDOF IOLs may be an interesting area of future research which can further delineate the differing visual profiles between the two types of IOLs.

Many new IOL technologies are on the horizon, including an intraocular capsular implant, which allows for exchange of IOLs and also may eliminate the variable of effective lens position by controlling the X, Y, and Z plane within the eye [33]. Ongoing clinical trials exist evaluating the efficacy of fluid-filled, shape-changing IOLs designed to mimic natural accommodation [34]. As developing technologies bring forth an abundance of new lens technologies to correct presbyopia, it is important to consider the patient's expectations and baseline ocular function to choose a lens which would ultimately best suit their lifestyle and visual needs.

## CLINICS CARE POINTS

- Explore the patient's expectations of spectacle independence and side effect profile before choosing a presbyopia correcting intraocular lense (IOL)
- When choosing a presbyopia correcting lens, take care to review the full ocular history.
- The ideal candidate for a multifocal lens is a healthy eye with no other ocular diseases
- For patients who are not a good candidate for multifocal lenses, extended depth-of-focus IOLs may be an option to provide some level of spectacle independence for distance and intermediate tasks.

## References

[1] Stein RM, Stein RL. The ophthalmic assistant. Elsevier; 2018 chap 32 Surgical correction of presbyopia.
[2] Pazo EE, McNeely RN, Richoz O, et al. Published October 31, 2017. Volume 43, Issue 11. Pages 1420-1429. © 2017.
[3] Rocha KM. Extended Depth of Focus IOLs: The Next Chapter in Refractive Technology? J Refract Surg 2017;33(3):146–9.
[4] Ong HS, Evans JR, Allan BD. Accommodative intraocular lens versus standard monofocal intraocular lens implantation in cataract surgery. Cochrane Database Syst Rev 2014;5: CD009667.

[5] de Silva SR, Evans JR, Kirthi V, et al. Multifocal versus monofocal intraocular lenses after cataract extraction. Cochrane Database Syst Rev 2016;(12):CD003169. Accessed February 28, 2022.
[6] Plaza-Puche AB, Alió JL. Refractive surgery. Elsevier; 2020 chap 39 Multifocal Intraocular Lenses.
[7] Fragoso VV, Alió JL. Ophthalmology. Elsevier; 2019 chap 3.10 Surgical Correction of Presbyopia.
[8] Alió J, Pikkel J. Multifocal intraocular lenses. The art and the practice. 1st edition.
[9] Salmon JF. Kanski's clinical ophthalmology. Elsevier; 2020 chap 8 Corneal and Refractive Surgery.
[10] AcrySoft IQ Vivity Extended Vision IOL Product information.
[11] Zeev Zalevsky "Extended depth of focus imaging: a review. SPIE Rev 2010;1(1):018001.
[12] McCabe C. Clinical outcomes of a novel non-diffractive extended vision IOL. Paper presented at: International Society of Presbyopia2019.
[13] Gundersen KG, Potvin R. Clinical Outcomes and Quality of Vision Associated with Bilateral Implantation of a Wavefront Shaping Presbyopia Correcting Intraocular Lens. Clin Ophthalmol 2021;15:4723–30.
[14] Kohnen T, Petermann K, Böhm M, et al. Nondiffractive wavefront-shaping extended depth-of-focus intraocular lens: visual performance and patient-reported outcomes. J Cataract Refract Surg 2022;48(2):144–50.
[15] Newsom TH, Potvin R. Evaluation of Quality of Vision and Visual Outcomes with Bilateral Implantation of a Non-Diffractive Extended Vision Intraocular Lens with a Target of Slight Myopia in the Non-Dominant Eye. Clin Ophthalmol 2022;16:183–90.
[16] Tecnis Eyhance Specifications Information Sheet. Available at: https://www.jnjvisionpro.-com/sites/us/files/public/surgical/IOLs/pp2020ct5377_tecnis_eyhance_spec_-sheet_v3_final.pdf. Accessed March 7, 2022.
[17] Vega F, Millán MS, Gil MA, et al. Optical Performance of a Monofocal Intraocular Lens Designed to Extend Depth of Focus. J Refract Surg 2020;36(9):625–32.
[18] Unsal U, Sabur H. Comparison of new monofocal innovative and standard monofocal intraocular lens after phacoemulsification. Int Ophthalmol 2021;41(1):273–82.
[19] de Luis Eguileor B, Martínez-Indart L, Martínez Alday N, et al. Differences in intermediate vision: monofocal intraocular lenses vs. monofocal extended depth of focus intraocular lenses. Arch Soc Esp Oftalmol (Engl Ed) 2020;95(11):523–7.
[20] Yangzes S, Kamble N, Grewal S, et al. Comparison of an aspheric monofocal intraocular lens with the new generation monofocal lens using defocus curve. Indian J Ophthalmol 2020;68(12):3025–9.
[21] Lopes D, Loureiro T, Carreira R, et al. Comparative evaluation of visual outcomes after bilateral implantation of an advanced or conventional monofocal intraocular lens. Eur J Ophthalmol 2022;32(1):229–34.
[22] Huh J, Eom Y, Yang SK, et al. A comparison of clinical outcomes and optical performance between monofocal and new monofocal with enhanced intermediate function intraocular lenses: a case-control study. BMC Ophthalmol 2021;21(1):365.
[23] Lee JH, Moon SY, Chung HS, et al. Clinical outcomes of a monofocal intraocular lens with enhanced intermediate function compared with an extended depth-of-focus intraocular lens. J Cataract Refract Surg 2022;48(1):61–6.
[24] Jeon YJ, Yoon Y, Kim TI, et al. Comparison Between an Intraocular Lens With Extended Depth of Focus (Tecnis Symfony ZXR00) and a New Monofocal Intraocular Lens With Enhanced Intermediate Vision (Tecnis Eyhance ICB00). Asia Pac J Ophthalmol (Phila) 2021;10(6):542–7.
[25] Corbelli E, Iuliano L, Bandello F, et al. Comparative analysis of visual outcome with 3 intraocular lenses: monofocal, enhanced monofocal, and extended depth of focus. J Cataract Refract Surg 2022;48(1):67–74.

[26] FDA.gov. LAL Summary of Safety and Effectiveness. Available at: https://www.accessdata.fda.gov/cdrh_docs/pdf16/P160055B.pdf. Accessed March 6 2022.
[27] Ghanem RC, Ghanem VC, Allemann N, et al. Ophthalmology. Elsevier; 2019 chap 3.7 Phakic Intraocular Lenses.
[28] Alió J, Plaza-Puche AB, Javaloy J, et al. Comparison of the visual and intraocular optical performance of a refractive multifocal IOL with rotational asymmetry and an apodized diffractive multifocal IOL. J Refract Surg 2012;28:100–5.
[29] Schallhorn JM. Multifocal and Extended Depth of Focus Intraocular Lenses: A Comparison of Data from the United States Food and Drug Administration Premarket Approval Trials. J Refract Surg 2021;37(2):98–104.
[30] van Amelsfort T, Webers VSC, Bauer NJC, et al. Visual outcomes of a new nondiffractive extended depth-of-focus intraocular lens targeted for minimonovision: 3-month results of a prospective cohort study. J Cataract Refract Surg 2022;48(2):151–6.
[31] Coassin M, Mori T, Di Zazzo A, et al. Effect of minimonovision in bilateral implantation of a novel non-diffractive extended depth-of-focus intraocular lens: defocus curves, visual outcomes, and quality of life. Eur J Ophthalmol 2021; https://doi.org/10.1177/11206721211064018.11206721211064018.
[32] Schallhorn JM, Pantanelli SM, Lin CC, et al. Multifocal and Accommodating Intraocular Lenses for the Treatment of Presbyopia: A Report by the American Academy of Ophthalmology. Ophthalmology 2021;128(10):1469–82.
[33] The Gemini Refractive Capsule. Omega Ophthalmics ®. (2018, August 7). Omega Ophthalmics ®. Available at: https://www.omegaophthalmics.com/. Accessed March 6, 2022.
[34] Juvene Intraocular Lens. (n.d.). LensGen. Available at: http://lensgen.com/services/. Accessed March 7, 2022.

# Vitreoretinal Disease

Advances in Ophthalmology and Optometry 7 (2022) 201–218

ADVANCES IN OPHTHALMOLOGY AND OPTOMETRY

# Diagnostic and Treatment Considerations for Macular Holes

Rupak Bhuyan, MD[a], Jeffrey Brown, MD[a], Robin Ginsburg, MD[a,b,*]

[a]Department of Ophthalmology, Icahn School of Medicine at Mount Sinai Hospital, One Gustave L. Levy Place, Box 1183, New York, NY 10029, USA; [b]Department of Ophthalmology, New York Eye and Ear Infirmary at Mount Sinai, New York, NY 10003, USA

**Keywords**

• Macular holes • Gass stage • ILM peel

**Key points**

- Macular holes can be classified into stages according to the depth of the defect and separation of vitreous from retina.
- Stage 1 holes may be observed given a high rate of spontaneous closure.
- Small stage 2 holes can be treated with either nonsurgical or surgical methods.
- Stage 3 and 4 holes should undergo surgery.

**Video content accompanies this article at http://www.advancesinophthalmology.com**

## INTRODUCTION

Macular holes (MHs) are foveal neurosensory disruptions that develop over weeks to months. Vitreomacular traction (VMT) is the most common cause [1]. Known risk factors include myopia, ocular inflammation, and age. Most MHs are idiopathic, although some are traumatic. Women are more commonly affected, with age of presentation usually greater than 55 years. Incidence is 8.69 eyes per 1,000,000 population per year. Prevalence ranges from 0.02% to 7%. About 15% to 20% of MHs are bilateral [2].

*Corresponding author. One Gustave L. Levy Place, Box 1183, New York, NY 10029. *E-mail address:* robin.ginsburg@mssm.edu

https://doi.org/10.1016/j.yaoo.2022.03.018

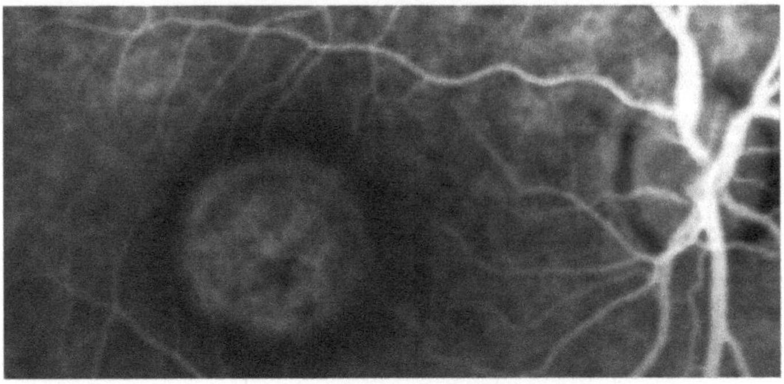

**Fig. 1.** Fluorescein angiogram (late phase) showing a hyperfluorescent transmission defect through a large macular hole. (*From* Freund KB, Sarraf D, Mieler WF, et al. Chapter 9: Vitreomacular traction, epiretinal membranes, and macular holes. In: Freund KB, Sarraf D, Mieler WF, et al, editors. The retinal atlas. 2nd edition. Elsevier; 2017. p. 913–35.)

Symptoms may include decreased visual acuity (VA), metamorphopsia, and a central scotoma. A Watzke-Allen test is useful for distinguishing full-thickness macular holes (FTMHs) from lamellar holes (inner foveal defect) and pseudoholes (defect in an epiretinal membrane [ERM]). A positive Watzke sign features an observed absolute discontinuity in a light beam projected vertically across the fovea. Other findings may include a grayish macular rim, a surrounding cuff of subretinal fluid, yellow deposits, and/or retinal pigment epithelim (RPE) changes at the hole's base and the adjacent ERM [2].

Additional findings may include a hyperfluorescent transmission defect through a macular defect on fluorescein angiography (Fig. 1), cystoid macular edema (CME) of the outer plexiform and inner nuclear layers as well as photoreceptor thinning on pathology (Fig. 2), and an anvil-shaped deformity of the edges of the hole on optical coherence tomography (OCT) [2].

Multiple staging systems for MHs have been described. The Gass system, described in the 1990s, is clinically focused and represents how the vitreomacular interface affects the fovea [3]. Four stages are described, with stage 1, an impending MH, subdivided into 1A and 1B. Stage 1A represents a foveolar detachment with a central yellow spot and loss of foveal depression. Stage 1B features an encircling yellow-colored ring. Stage 2 represents a smaller FTMH less than 400 μm in diameter with an inner retinal "roof" or pseudo-operculum. Stage 3 MHs are greater than 400 μm with a frank operculum; they may also possess a rim of RPE hyperpigmnetation/hypopigmentation, subretinal fluid cuff, and an ERM. Stage 4 holes are distinguished by a complete posterior vitreous detachment [4].

The International Vitreomacular Traction Study (IVTS) created a new classification system based on OCT findings, using size and presence or absence of VMT to further characterize pathology. IVTS features vitreomacular adhesion (VMA) without foveal distortion, analogous to stage 1. Stage 2 is described as VMT with foveal contour disruption but no hole, whereas stage 3 is

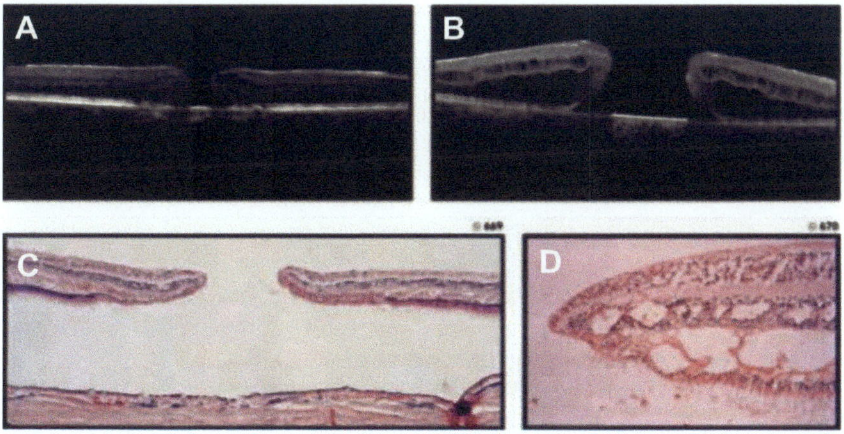


**Fig. 2.** OCT images showing a full-thickness macular hole with cystic intraretinal edema (*A, B*). Anvil-shaped deformity (*B*). Hematoxylin-eosin–stained section of human neurosensory retina with a full-thickness macular hole under low (*C*) and high magnification (*D*). Note the cystic spaces representative of edema and photoreceptor layer thinning. (*From* Freund KB, Sarraf D, Mieler WF, et al. Chapter 9: Vitreomacular traction, epiretinal membranes, and macular holes. In: Freund KB, Sarraf D, Mieler WF, et al, editors. The retinal atlas. 2nd edition. Elsevier; 2017. 913–35.)

represented by an FTMH seen as a defect from internal limiting membrane (ILM) to RPE with VMT [5]. A comparison of Gass and IVTS staging is shown in Fig. 3.

## SIGNIFICANCE

### Nonsurgical treatment

#### *Observation*

MHs exhibit a 4% to 11.5% rate of spontaneous closure. Stage 1 MH can be observed with almost half undergoing spontaneous closure after vitreomacular separation (Fig. 4) [4].

#### *Cystoid dehydration*

Topical off-label steroids, nonsteroidal anti-inflammatory agents, and carbonic anhydrase inhibitors can dehydrate retinas with small FTMHs. Trials looked at prednisolone acetate 1%, difluprednate 0.05%, ketorolac-tromethamine 0.5%, bromfenac 0.07%, brinzolamide 1%, and dorzolamide 2% with dosing varying from 1 to 4 times daily. Decreases in cystoid spaces were observed within 2 to 4 weeks of therapy initiation, with most successful hole closures occurring at 2 to 8 weeks. Treatment duration continued until hole closure, with mean duration of 5.6 weeks. There was an 86% closure rate and average VA change from 20/70 at diagnosis to 20/40 at the time of closure [6]. Fig. 5 shows successful closure after combination therapy with prednisolone and ketorolac 4 times daily and dorzolamide twice daily.

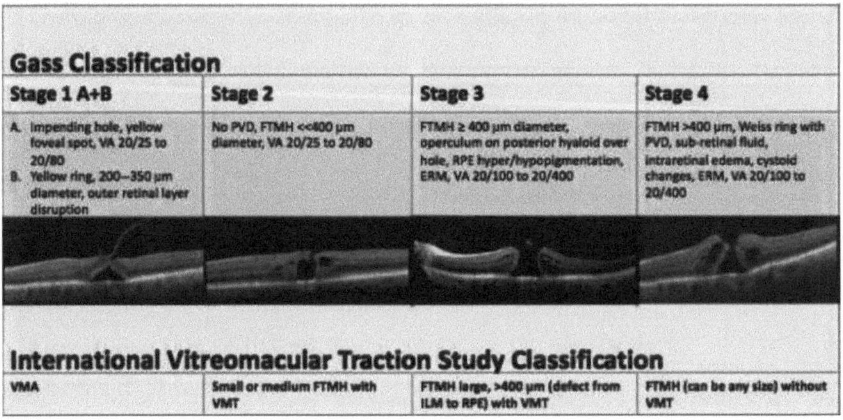


**Fig. 3.** Comparison of the Gass and International Vitreomacular Traction Study staging systems for macular holes. PVD, posterior vitreous detachment. *(Adapted from* Freund KB, Sarraf D, Mieler WF, et al. Chapter 9: Vitreomacular traction, epiretinal membranes, and macular holes. In: Freund KB, Sarraf D, Mieler WF, et al, editors. The retinal atlas. 2nd edition. Elsevier; 2017. p. 913–35.)

*Ocriplasmin*

Ocriplasmin (Jetrea) is a recombinant protease that cleaves proteins at the vitreoretinal interface. Ocriplasmin was approved by the US Food and Drug Administration in 2012 to treat symptomatic VMT. The Trial of Microplasmin Intravitreal Injection for Non-surgical Treatment of Focal Vitreomacular Adhesion (MIVI-TRUST) revealed a 41% MH closure rate with ocriplasmin versus 11% with placebo [7]. Fig. 6 demonstrates successful closure.

*Pneumatic vitreolysis*

Pneumatic vitreolysis (PVL) with perfluoropropane (C3F8) gas was introduced for symptomatic VMT and small stage 2 MHs with a closure rate of 57%. Additional studies revealed success rates of 50% to 80% for small MHs using either C3F8 or sulfur hexafluoride (SF6). A 7% adverse event rate occurred, including retinal flap tears, conversion of impending MHs into FTMHs, and rhegmatogenous retinal detachment (rRD). Nonetheless, all patients obtained final VA of 20/40 or better with laser and/or pars plana vitrectomy (PPV) [8].

## Surgery

*Internal limiting membrane peel*

The ILM forms the inner boundary of the retina and the basement membrane of Muller cells. The ILM can serve as a scaffold for contractile tissue (eg, myofibroblasts, fibrocytes, RPE cells) that has been implicated in VMT. Thus, surgery without ILM removal may lead to failure of primary MH closure or reopening of successfully closed holes [1].

Fig. 7 diagrams the steps of ILM removal. A variety of instruments including a bent microvitreoretinal blade, pick, ILM forceps, diamond-dusted membrane

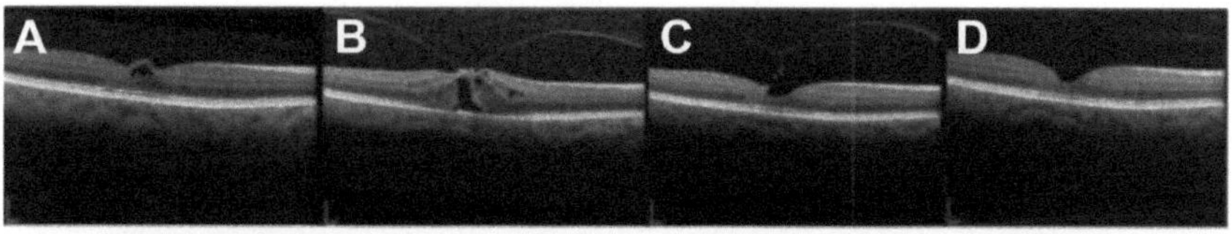


**Fig. 4.** Spontaneous closure of a macular hole on OCT. Stage 1A with VMT at diagnosis (*A*), Stage 1B at 7 months after diagnosis (*B*), resolving (*C*), and with successful closure (*D*).

scraper, or microserrated nitinol loop can be used to pinch and pull the membrane tangentially to create a flap. Although the optimal point of peel initiation is unknown, starting 1000 μm above or below the foveola seems advantageous because the ILM is thickest there and avoids the nasal papillomacular nerve fiber bundle and thinner temporal retina. The optimal extent of ILM peeling is not known, although at least 1 disc diameter circumferentially around the MH is most common [9].

A Cochrane review favored ILM removal over PPV alone, but the evidence was less compelling for small MHs [10]. There is also added benefit to ILM removal for MHs in myopic eyes, particularly with staphyloma or retinoschisis. The American Academy of Ophthalmology (AAO) reaffirmed the benefit of ILM peeling issuing a recommendation in its Preferred Practice Pattern (PPP) (Fig. 8) [1].

*Internal limiting membrane staining*

Dyes such as indocyanine green (ICG), brilliant blue (BB), and triamcinolone acetonide (TA) have been used to improve ILM visualization (Fig. 9). A meta-analysis revealed no difference in closure rates between ILM peeling with and without staining. Visual outcomes also did not differ 6 months after removal among patients receiving ICG, BB, or TA. Owing to lack of large randomized controlled trials (RCTs), no recommendations regarding dye use other than surgeon preference exist. If using ICG, however, it is imperative to use low concentrations (2.5 mg/mL) and short exposure times (5–10 seconds) to avoid retinal toxicity [1].

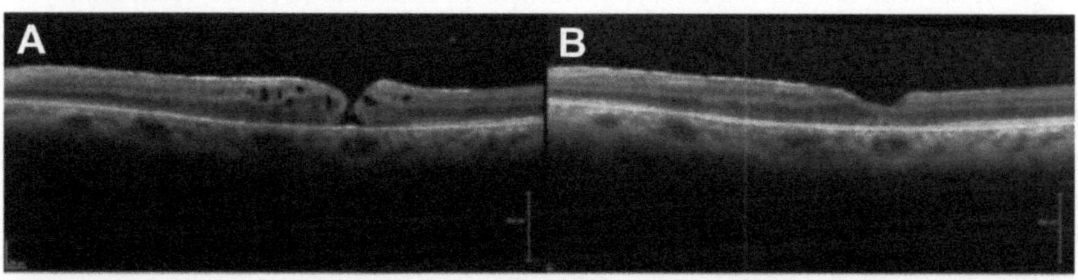


**Fig. 5.** OCT images of a macular hole before (*A*) and 1 month after (*B*) treatment with topical prednisolone acetate, ketorolac, and dorzolamide.

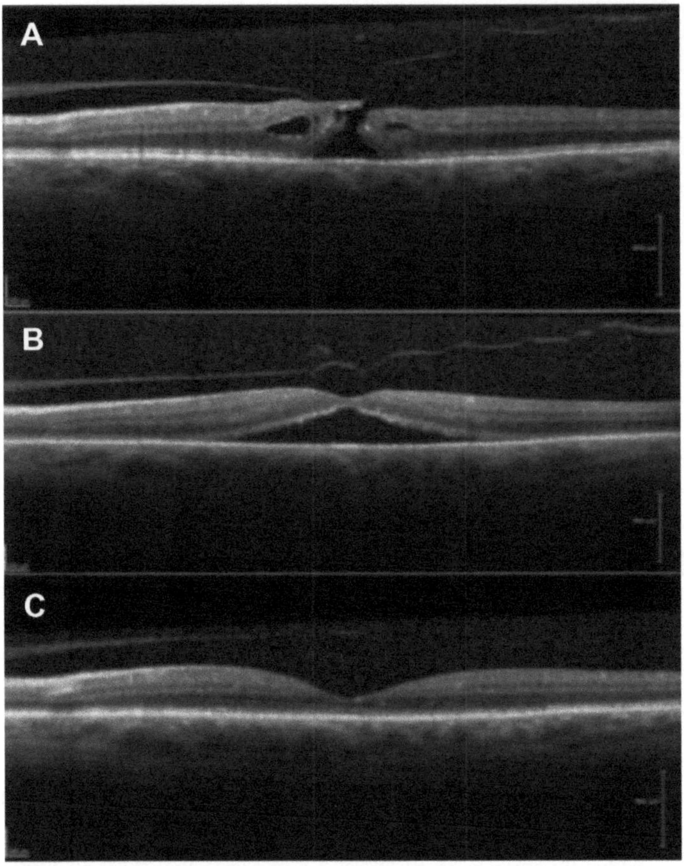


**Fig. 6.** Macular hole before (*A*) and after ocriplasmin injection at 5 days (*B*) and 1 month (*C*) postprocedure.

*Treatments for large (>400 μm) macular holes*

Larger MHs create a surgical challenge with lower closure rates, and often will require additional surgical maneuvers to ensure success (Box 1).

*Temporal macular arcuate retinotomy.* A temporal macular arcuate retinotomy can augment the increase in retinal compliance attained with ILM peel. A semicircular retinotomy is created with intraocular scissors 500 to 700 μm temporal to the MH followed by an air-fluid exchange and drainage of subretinal fluid while the temporal retinal bridge is repositioned inward. MH closure occurred in 83% of eyes with VA improvement in 50%. Despite the small sample size of 6 eyes, the results make additional studies compelling [11].

*Inverted internal limiting membrane flap.* An inverted ILM flap can be used to improve outcomes in large stage 4 and myopic MHs. The technique involves a circumferential ILM peel that preserves a cuff of ILM at the rim of the MH.

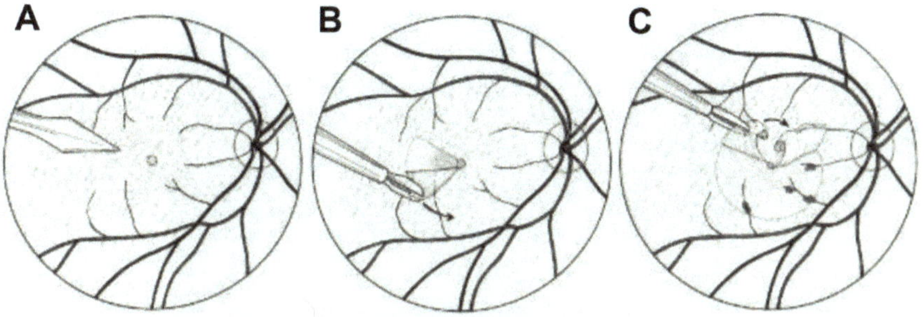


**Fig. 7.** Steps of an internal limiting membrane peel. Incision using a bent microvitreoretinal blade ~1500 μm from the hole edge (*A*). ILM forceps are used to perform the circular ILM rhexis (*B*). ILM is pulled directly over the hole to release traction from umbo (*C*). (*From* Brooks HL Jr. Macular hole surgery with and without internal limiting membrane peeling. Ophthalmology 2000;107(10):1939–48 [discussion 1948-9].)

This ILM "frill" is inverted into the hole using forceps (Video 1). The inverted flap acts as a scaffold for proliferation, migration, and activation of Muller cells. Neurotrophic factors and basic fibroblast growth factor released by activated Muller cells may facilitate MH closure [12].

*Adjuvant therapy.* Transforming growth factor-β2 injection has been shown to improve closure rates but is associated with limited gains in VA [13]. An RCT evaluated the adjuvant use of autologous platelet concentrate with stage 3 and 4 MHs, confirming a higher closure rate of 98% compared with 82% in the PPV-only group, although with no difference in final VA [14].

*Laser photocoagulation.* Laser for FTMH closure promotes cytokine production by RPE and induces formation of a glial plug. One study applied three 100-μm argon green spots at a slit lamp for patients with FTMHs greater than 400 um before PPV with ILM removal. Closure rate was 94% in the laser plus surgery group compared with 77% in the surgery-only group, but there was no concomitant improvement in postoperative VA [15].

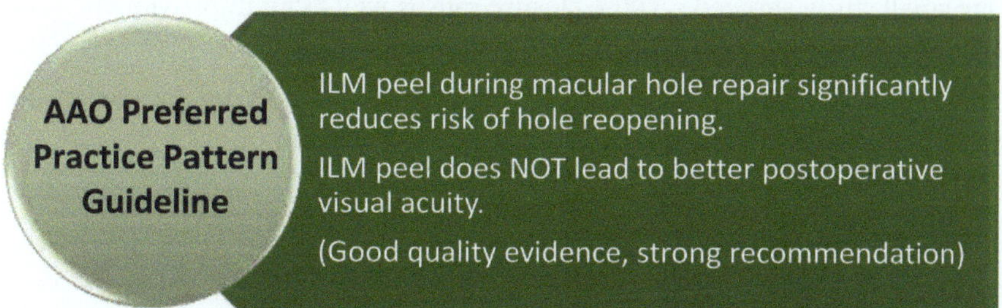


**Fig. 8.** ILM peel during macular hole repair surgery. (*Data from* Flaxel CJ, Adelman RA, Bailey ST, et al. Idiopathic macular hole Preferred Practice Pattern®. Ophthalmology. 2020;127(2):P184–222.)

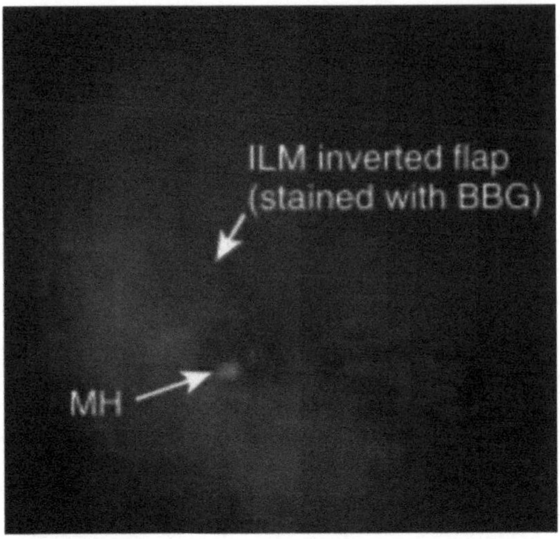


**Fig. 9.** Brilliant blue G (BBG) dye is used to stain ILM for improved visualization during MH repair. (*From* Ikuno Y, Ohji M. Chapter 117: High myopia and the vitreoretinal complications. In: Schachat AP, editor. Ryan's retina. 6th edition. Elsevier; 2018. p. 2146–154.)

*Treatments for recurrent/recalcitrant macular holes*

Box 2 lists various methods for recurrent and recalcitrant MHs.

*Repeat surgery with internal limiting membrane repeel.* Several methods exist for treatment of MHs that fail to close or that reopen after initial surgery. Repeat PPV and ILM repeel is the most common method used. Closure rates vary between 47% and 70% with improved postoperative VA, but earlier reoperation is correlated with better outcomes [16].

*Radial retinal incisions.* Radial retinal incisions relax traction on perifoveal tissue and stimulate glial cell proliferation, migration, and activation. In this technique, 5 radial incisions are made to the level of RPE beginning 1 MH diameter from the edge of the MH. Incisions are extended centripetally toward the hole. One small study showed a 100% closure rate as well as an improvement in final VA [17].

*Heavy silicone oil.* Repeat PPV with heavy silicone oil injection may be used for failed MH surgery. Oxane HD is a mixture of silicone oil (SO) and partially

**Box 1: Treatments for large (>400 μm) macular holes**

- Temporal macular arcuate retinotomy
- Inverted ILM flap technique
- Adjuvant therapy (eg, transforming growth factor-β2, serum, thrombin, whole blood, platelet concentrate, gluconated blood clumps)
- Laser photocoagulation

**Box 2: Treatments for recurrent/persistent macular holes**

- Repeat PPV with ILM repeel/rhexis enlargement
- Radial retinal incisions
- Heavy silicone oil
- Cryopreserved human amniotic membrane transplant

fluorinated alkanes conferring higher density (HDSO) and consequent better contact angle with the retina compared with standard hydrophobic SO. Use of Oxane HD was associated with an 85% closure rate and a median improvement in VA from 20/800 to 20/600 after HDSO removal [18]. Another HDSO is Densiron-68, a mixture of 69.5% SO and 30.5% perfluorohexyloctane. Reports suggest an 85% closure rate for recalcitrant FTMH using Densiron-68 [19].

*Cryopreserved human amniotic membrane transplant.* Human amniotic membrane (hAM) transplants have been tested during repeat PPV for persistent/recurrent MH. A hAM plug is inserted under the edges of the MH using vitreoretinal forceps to cover the entire defect. The initial study found a 100% closure rate, with fully stratified retina over the patch. Mean VA was noted to improve from 20/800 to 20/50 at 6 months after surgery. No adverse events were observed [20].

*Retinal tamponade*

At the conclusion of MH surgery, a retinal tamponade agent is injected. An effective agent facilitates absorption of subretinal fluid and serves as a scaffold for proliferating cells. No differences exist in outcomes comparing air, SF6, C3F8, and SO. SO should be considered for patients who are unable to lie face down, are monocular, or need to fly soon after surgery. However, a second operation is required for SO removal generally after 2 to 3 months [21].

*Postoperative positioning*

Originally, patients were instructed to remain face-down for 10 to 14 days, which was challenging. Later studies with 1 to 3 days of prone positioning also showed excellent anatomic and visual outcomes. Because prone positioning may minimize posterior pressure on the lens, it was theorized that shorter positioning would be associated with greater cataract progression. Formal trials, however, have not found any difference. More recent reviews of "no face-down" upright positioning found closure rates similar to those in patients with face-down positioning [22]. Despite these findings, longer periods are still recommended for large holes or for those cases with inadequate gas fill. Fig. 10 lists the AAO PPP recommendation for positioning.

*Surgical outcomes*

*Efficacy.* The Moorfields Macular Hole Study showed 81% of eyes with stage 2 to 4 MHs undergoing surgery closed by 24 months compared with 12% of

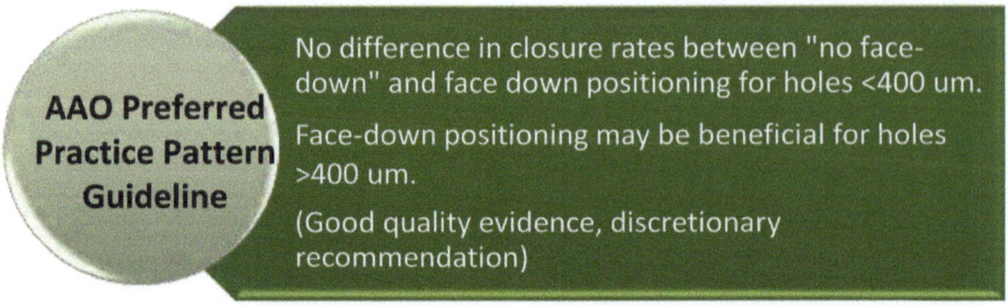


**Fig. 10.** Postoperative positioning after macular hole surgery. (*Data from* Flaxel CJ, Adelman RA, Bailey ST, et al. Idiopathic Macular Hole Preferred Practice Pattern®. Ophthalmology 2020;127(2):P184–222.)

observed eyes. Mean VA at 24 months was 20/60 after surgery in contrast to 20/200 after observation [23]. The Vitrectomy for Macular Hole Study found 69% of eyes undergoing surgery for Stage 2 MH closed by 6 months versus 4% of observed eyes. Mean VA at 12 months was 20/62 after surgery compared with 20/80 after observation [24]. With an overall closure rate of 91% to 98% and a median postoperative VA 20/40, combined with the low risk profile of small-gauge vitrectomy, the argument for early surgical intervention is quite compelling [1]. Although later studies found less benefit with vitrectomy for Stage 2 MHs, current practice most commonly uses surgery for stage 2 to reduce additional vision loss from progression to stage 3.

*Prognostic factors for successful surgery.* Case series suggest higher rates of MH closure and better postoperative VA for surgery within 6 months of symptom onset. MHs present for greater than 2 years have lower closure rates and worse final VA. Factors that predict MH surgical failure include MHs that occurred after retinal detachment surgery and traumatic MHs that fail to close spontaneously [21]. For MHs that fail to close after initial surgery, repeat surgery has a 41% to 70% closure rate, although VA improvement is often limited to 20/100. Reoperation for recurrent MHs that closed initially seems to yield better visual outcomes than for recalcitrant MHs [25].

*Surgical complications.* Box 3 lists surgical complications of MH repair surgery.

*Cataract.* Visually significant cataract formation occurs in 80% of phakic eyes within the first few years after surgery. The presence of postoperative CME increases the risk of cataract formation 7-fold. Some surgeons perform combined cataract extraction and MH repair. Advantages include consolidating 2 operations and possibly allowing for greater gas fill. Complications of this combined technique include hypotony, intraocular lens-iris capture, and increased risk of CME [26].

*Retinal tears and detachments.* MH surgery confers a 3% to 17% risk of retinal tears, most of which form inferiorly. Also a 1% to 5% risk of retinal detachment exists. Retinal detachments typically occur inferiorly and are usually secondary to flap tears at the posterior vitreous base. Fortunately, most surgeries for post-

**Box 3: Complications of macular hole surgery**

- Cataract
- Retinal tear/detachment
- Visual field constriction
- Endophthalmitis
- Intraocular pressure increase at high altitude
- Hypotony and retinal detachment at low altitude
- Intraocular pressure increase with nitrous oxide

MH repair retinal detachments do not lead to reopening of successfully closed holes [1].

*Visual field constriction.* Permanent postoperative temporal visual field constriction is reported in up to 20% of patients. One possible reason is mechanical damage to the peripapillary retinal vasculature or retinal nerve fiber layer. Another theory is that dehydration injury occurs due to air flow from the temporal infusion cannula during air-fluid exchange. Box 4 details the intraoperative maneuvers that have been suggested to obviate or minimize visual field loss [27].

*Endophthalmitis.* Endophthalmitis is exceedingly rare after MH repair surgery with an incidence of less than 0.05%. Treatment should follow the standard of care that has been described extensively for other causes of postoperative endophthalmitis [1].

*Complications related to gas fill.* Acute elevation of intraocular pressure (IOP) can occur secondary to gas expansion at altitudes greater than 1000 feet above sea level. Wound dehiscence, gas leakage, retinal arterial occlusion, and glaucomatous changes may result. On the other hand, very low altitudes may decrease gas volume and subsequently cause hypotony and postoperative retinal detachments. Use of nitrous oxide for general anesthesia and air travel can precipitate dangerous IOP elevations and loss of vision. Patients must be warned of these risks and given wrist bands that highlight these concerns [28].

## PRESENT RELEVANCE AND FUTURE AVENUES

As discussed, a variety of treatments exist for MH repair. Important considerations exist for each form of management, and multiple future directions for research.

### Topical agents

Topical agents are appealing due to their noninvasive nature. However, comparison of results from case series is difficult to interpret because most patients received more than 1 medication simultaneously. Also, no trial exists comparing same or different classes of medications, and there is no RCT comparing any medication to observation alone. This fact raises the possibility

**Box 4: Methods to reduce visual field loss after macular hole surgery**

- Limit direct contact between instruments and optic nerve head during air-fluid exchange
- Limit duration of air flow at high pressure
- Suture sclerotomies to minimize air flow through the eye during air-fluid exchange
- Allow a thin layer of fluid posteriorly to remain until final part of aspiration during air-fluid exchange
- Humidify the air
- Use low infusion pressure during air-fluid exchange
- Reduce air circulation with small-gauge vitrectomy or valved cannulae

that some MHs observed to have closed with topical therapy may have closed spontaneously [6]. Future studies are necessary to better determine the effect of each medication on MH closure to delineate how topical agents fit into the armamentarium of MH treatment tools.

### Ocriplasmin

Ocriplasmin has not been widely adopted due to reports of serious complications. Adverse events included acute vision loss, electroretinogram changes, retinal tears/detachments, color vision abnormalities, photopsias, visual field defects, and zonular fiber weakening with risk of lens subluxation. In response, the drug manufacturer developed the Ocriplasmin for Treatment for Symptomatic Vitreomacular Adhesion Including Macula Hole (OASIS) trial, which revealed ocriplasmin was indeed efficacious and safe [29]. Even so, the availability of smaller-gauge vitrectomy with a high safety profile and ~90% closure rate has made it quite appealing compared with the idiosyncratic risks reported with ocriplasmin. In addition, given the 4% to 11.5% spontaneous closure rate in the same subgroup of eyes demonstrating the highest ocriplasmin success rate, use of this agent remained limited and it is currently is not available [1].

### Pneumatic vitreolysis

The DRCR Retina Network Protocol AH was performed as a single-arm exploratory study of MHs $\leq$ 250 μm using C3F8 injection. Closure without rescue PPV was observed in 29% of eyes by 8 weeks after PVL, but rescue PPV was eventually required in 68% of eyes by 24 weeks. More concerning was that 14% of eyes developed rRD. In addition, 7% of eyes undergoing PVL developed traumatic cataracts from anterior chamber paracentesis. Although no patient experienced endophthalmitis or severe loss of vision, the aforementioned complications contributed to early discontinuation of the protocol [8]. Future studies would need to provide convincing safety data for this technique to be used clinically.

### Internal limiting membrane staining

Although ILM staining is widely performed, it is not without risk. Electroretinogram (ERG) photopic negative responses were decreased in some eyes that were treated intraoperatively with ICG, but not in eyes treated with other dyes, suggesting possible subclinical retinal ganglion cell layer impairments. However, another study showed no difference in macular ERG among various dyes [30]. Also of note is that direct ICG exposure to RPE cells in FTMH surgery can cause apoptosis secondary to phototoxicity from intraoperative illumination. Such phototoxicity has not been observed with BB [31]. Limited ICG concentration and exposure time is suggested to prevent this complication.

### Glial plug after internal limiting membrane manipulation

A hyperreflective foveal "plug" found on OCT after surgery has been observed in both traditional ILM peeling and patients with inverted flap. This plug may represent glial tissue, suggesting that even ILM removal may trigger proliferation and migration of Muller cells by damaging the ILM. Interestingly, eyes that experience postoperative resolution of the plug are more likely to recover the ellipsoid zone (EZ) than eyes with persistent plugs at 1 year after surgery. If plugs represent activated glial cells that are crucial for MH closure, persistence may interfere with normalization of the EZ [32]. An optimal solution and future line of study could focus on developing a way to maximize glial cell proliferation/activation without interfering in EZ recovery.

### Intraoperative optical coherence tomography

A newer technology now permits OCT imaging during surgery. The Determination of Feasibility of Intraoperative Spectral Domain Microscope Combined/Integrated OCT Visualization During En face Retinal and Ophthalmic Surgery (DISCOVER) study examined surgical repair with intraoperative optical coherence tomography (iOCT). In 12% of cases, iOCT changed surgical decision making [33]. Current advantages of iOCT for FTMH repair are listed in Box 5. A future direction involves using high-resolution data from iOCT to develop automated computer algorithms to quantify MH covariates to predict time until MH closure and assist in deciding which adjuvant surgical techniques would be most beneficial to improve surgical outcomes.

### Autologous mesenchymal stem cell transplantation

One trial examined injection of mesenchymal stem cells (MSCs) in phosphate-buffered saline after PPV/ILM peel/air-fluid exchange. A different trial arm tested injections of MSC exosomes, microvesicle-containing proteins, and ribonucleic acid. Exosomes have lower immunogenicity and risk of proliferation than MSCs. The trial examined chronic idiopathic FTMH and found an 86% closure rate, with 71% of eyes exhibiting VA improvement. Complications included a fibrotic ERM formed secondary to injected MSCs in 1 eye. There was 1 moderate but temporary anterior chamber inflammation in 1 eye with high-dose exosome injection [34]. Such work is very promising, and additional

**Box 5: Utility of intraoperative optical coherence tomography for full-thickness macular hole repair**

- Estimating hole size after membrane peel
- Confirming VMT release
- Identifying flap location
- Confirming membrane peel completion
- Identifying occult residual membranes
- Avoiding dyes and risks of dye toxicity

studies already are being performed on photoreceptor rescue by RPE derived from induced pluripotent stem cells in murine models [35].

### Autologous retinal transplantation

A recent retrospective study explored harvested autologous retina for treatment of very large FTMHs (Video 2). In this technique, endodiathermy and barrier endolaser are performed to demarcate and prevent RD of the harvest site, respectively. The graft is placed preretinally over the MH, at the level of the retina, or inserted into the subretinal plane. Overall, this method yielded an 89% closure rate and at least a 3-line VA improvement in 43% of eyes. Complications included 3.8% rate of graft dislocation, 3.8% rate of postoperative rRD, and a 0.77% rate of endophthalmitis [36].

## SUMMARY

This article provides a detailed overview regarding diagnosis and treatment of MHs. The AAO PPP provided a well-researched document with guidelines for treatment of MHs [1]. This article expanded on the AAO PPP by supplementing with one of the most up-to-date discussions of newer treatment modalities. Table 1 provides a summary of treatment recommendations stratified using Gass stage nomenclature.

MHs are defects in the foveal portion of the neurosensory retina. MHs more commonly affect women and patients older than 55 years. Once a diagnosis is made, the unaffected fellow eye must also be examined and followed because there is a 10% to 15% rate of MH formation in the fellow eye within 5 years [1].

Gass staging currently is used to stratify management. Stage 1A and 1B MHs should be observed, because no evidence exists that treatment affects prognosis. Patients should be followed in 2- to 4-month intervals or more frequently if new visual symptoms arise. Patients also should be provided with a home Amsler grid to evaluate for metamorphopsia and given strict return precautions [1].

Gass Stage 2 MHs may be treated in a variety of ways. Cystoid dehydration using topical agents looks promising, but more studies are required to isolate effects of individual agents to determine the best medication or combinations, dosing, and duration of treatment.

**Table 1**
Treatments for each stage of macular hole

| Macular Hole Stage (Gass) | Recommended Treatment |
|---|---|
| 1A and 1B | Observation |
| 2 | a. Vitreopharmacolysis within 1–2 wk of diagnosis<br>b. PVL within 1–2 wk of diagnosis<br>c. Surgery within 1 mo of diagnosis |
| 3 | Surgery within 1 mo of diagnosis |
| 4 | Surgery within 1 mo of diagnosis |

Vitreopharmacolysis with agents such as ocriplamsin is another option for stage 2 MHs. Follow-up should occur at 1 week and 4 weeks after injection, or sooner if new visual symptoms develop [29]. Although extensive testing debunked the initial concern for unacceptably high complication rates, success is variable and notably less than that of surgery.

PVL is an option for stage 2 MHs, with follow-up 1 to 2 days and 1 week after injection, or sooner for new ocular symptoms. Multiple small case series have shown encouraging results for smaller MHs, but the larger DRCR.net Protocol AH was discontinued early due to a 14% rate of rRD [8]. The high complication rate, combined with a lower success rate than surgery, has led to a low overall adoption rate.

In fact, the 2018 American Society of Retina Specialists Preferences and Trends survey revealed that for patients with VMT, small MHs, and 20/50 vision, ocriplasmin was used as an initial treatment by 7.4% of US specialists (5.3% international), compared with PVL by 9.6% of US specialists (10.2% international), and to vitrectomy by 70.4% US retinal surgeons (72.4% international) [37]. Accordingly, small-gauge surgery is still the most common treatment of stage 2 MHs, particularly given the significant rate of progression to stage 3 or 4 without surgery. Regardless of specific surgical technique, follow-up should occur at 1 to 2 days and 1 to 2 weeks afterward. Stage 3 and 4 MHs definitely require surgery, with the same recommended follow-up schedule as for stage 2.

ILM removal improves closure rate and reduces reopening rate without negatively affecting final VA. As such, ILM peeling should be a staple in surgical management, particularly for large, chronic (>6–12 months), and myopic holes. To assist in ILM identification, the ILM can be safely stained with BB to improve its visualization, without the inherent risks of phototoxicity from ICG use.

Various techniques have been discussed in this article for treatment of large MHs in particular. All the techniques feature promising results from small studies, although larger prospective RCTs are required to confirm their utility. Inverted ILM flap shows particular promise for very large MHs > 650 μm and for those secondary to high myopia.

For recurrent or recalcitrant MHs, a myriad of strategies exist. hAM has shown remarkable success with no specific adverse events in small trials, but more rigorous testing is warranted. Moreover, current work with stem cell injection has offered a glimpse of promising future treatments. Even more recent work with autologous retinal transplants is equally encouraging, particularly for extremely large MHs.

Overall, this is an exciting age for MH management. An increasingly large toolbox of treatments offers a collective closure rate surpassing 90% with improved visual outcomes in most cases. Treatment should be tailored according to multiple characteristics, with careful attention paid to accurate staging for proper management.

## CLINICAL CARE POINTS

- Patients with an MH in one eye should be monitored closely for development of an MH in the contralateral eye, because this can occur in 10% to 15% of cases.
- Multiple staging systems have been developed to classify MHs: Gass stage 1 and 2 holes should be watched closely for progression to stage 3, because surgical intervention is indicated for closure if the MH progresses to stage 3.
- Stage 1 holes can be observed for spontaneous closure. Although nonsurgical interventions exist for later stages, success is variable and surgical closure remains the gold standard for large macular holes (stages 3 and 4).
- A large toolbox exists for clinicians managing MHs, and a tailored approach is recommended. Larger RCTs are required to confirm usefulness of new techniques discussed.

## DISCLOSURE

None of the authors report any financial disclosures.

## SUPPLEMENTARY DATA

Supplementary data related to this article can be found online at https://doi.org/10.1016/j.yaoo.2022.03.018.

## References

[1] Flaxel CJ, Adelman RA, Bailey ST, et al. Idiopathic macular hole Preferred practice pattern. Ophthalmology 2020;127(2):P184–222.
[2] Feldman B, Shah VA, Weng CY, et al. Macular hole. USA: EyeWiki; 2021.
[3] Gass JD. Idiopathic senile macular hole. Its early stages and pathogenesis. Arch Ophthalmol 1988;106(5):629–39.
[4] Majumdar T, Tripathy K. Macular hole. Treasure Island, FL: StatPearls; 2021.
[5] Freund KB, Serraf D, Mieler WF, et al. The retinal Atlas E-book. USA: Elsevier Health Sciences; 2016.
[6] Sokol JT, Schechet SA, Komati R, et al. Macular hole closure with medical treatment. Ophthalmol Retina 2021;5(7):711–3.

[7] Stalmans P, Benz MS, Gandorfer A, et al. MIVI-TRUST Study Group. Enzymatic vitreolysis with ocriplasmin for vitreomacular traction and macular holes. N Engl J Med 2012;367(7):606–15.
[8] Chan CK, Mein CE, Glassman AR, et al. Pneumatic Vitreolysis with C3F8 for Vitreomacular Traction with and without Macular Hole: DRCR Retina Network Protocols AG and AH. Ophthalmology 2021;128(11):1592–603.
[9] Chatziralli IP, Theodossiadis PG, Steel DH. Internal limiting membrane peeling in macular hole surgery; why, when, and how? Retina 2018;38(5):870–82.
[10] Spiteri CK, Lois N, Scott N, et al. Vitrectomy with internal limiting membrane (ILM) peeling versus vitrectomy with no peeling for idiopathic full-thickness macular hole (FTMH). Cochrane Database Syst Rev 2013;6:CD009306.
[11] Charles S, Randolph JC, Neekhra A, et al. Arcuate retinotomy for the repair of large macular holes. Ophthalmic Surg Lasers Imaging Retina 2013;44(1):69–72.
[12] Michalewska Z, Michalewska J, Adelman RA, et al. Inverted internal limiting membrane flap technique for large macular holes. Ophthalmology 2010;117:2018–25.
[13] Glaser BM, Michels RG, Kuppermann BD, et al. Transforming growth factor-β2 for the treatment of full-thickness macular holes: a prospective randomized study. Ophthalmology 1992;99(7):1162–73.
[14] Paques M, Chastang C, Mathis A, et al. Effect of autologous platelet concentrate in surgery for idiopathic macular hole: results of a multicenter, double-masked, randomized trial. Platelets in Macular Hole Surgery Group. Ophthalmology 1999;106(5):932–8.
[15] Cho HY, Kim YT, Kang SW, et al. Laser photocoagulation as adjuvant therapy to surgery for large macular holes. Korean J Ophthalmol 2006;20(2):93–8.
[16] D'Souza MJ, Chaudhary V, Devenyi R, et al. Re-operation of idiopathic full-thickness macular holes after initial surgery with internal limiting membrane peel. Br J Ophthalmol 2011;95(11):1564–7.
[17] Reis R, Ferreira N, Meireles A, et al. Management of stage IV macular holes: when standard surgery fails. Case Rep Ophthalmol 2012;3:240–50.
[18] Cheung BT, Lai TY, Yuen CY, et al. Results of high-density silicone oil as a tamponade agent in macular hole retinal detachment in patients with high myopia. Br J Ophthalmol 2007;91(6): 719–21.
[19] Cillino S, Cillino G, Ferraro LL, et al. Treatment of persistently open macular holes with heavy silicone oil (Densiron 68) versus C2F6. A prospective randomized study. Retina 2016;36(4):688–94.
[20] Rizzo S, Caporossi T, Tartaro R, et al. A human amniotic membrane plug to promote retinal breaks repair and recurrent macular hole closure. Retina 2019;39:S95–103.
[21] Tam A, Yan P, Gan NY, et al. The current surgical management of large, recurrent, or persistent macular holes. Retina 2018;38(7):1263–75.
[22] Pasu S, Bell L, Zenasni Z, et al. Facedown positioning following surgery for large full-thickness macular hole: a multicenter randomized clinical trial. JAMA Ophthalmol 2020;138(7):725–30.
[23] Ezra E, Gregor ZJ, Moorfields Macular Hole Study Group. Surgery for idiopathic full-thickness macular hole: two-year results of a randomized clinical trial comparing natural history, vitrectomy, and vitrectomy plus autologous serum: moorfields macular hole study group report no. 1. Arch Ophthalmol 2004;122(2):224–36.
[24] Kim JW, Freeman WR, Azen SP, et al. Vitrectomy for Macular Hole Study Group. Prospective randomized trial of vitrectomy or observation for stage 2 macular holes. Am J Ophthalmol 1996;121(6):605–14.
[25] Valldeperas X, Wong D. Is it worth reoperating on macular holes? Ophthalmology 2008;115(1):158–63.
[26] Haritoglou C, Gass CA, Schaumberger M, et al. Long-term follow-up after macular hole surgery with internal limiting membrane peeling. Am J Ophthalmol 2002;134:661–666f.

[27] Pendergast SD, McCuen BW, II. Visual field loss after macular hole surgery. Ophthalmology 1996;103(7):1069–77.
[28] Gsellman L, Amini R. Patients with intravitreal gas bubbles at risk of high intraocular pressure without exceeding elevation of surgery: theoretical analysis. Invest Ophthalmol Vis Sci 2016;57(7):3340–7.
[29] Dugel PU, Tolentino M, Feiner L, et al. Results of the 2-year Ocriplasmin for Treatment for Symptomatic Vitreomacular Adhesion Including Macular Hole (OASIS) randomized trial. Ophthalmology 2016;123(10):2232–47.
[30] Machida S, Nishimura T, Ohzeki T, et al. Comparisons of focal macular electroretinograms after indocyanine green-, brilliant blue G-, or triamcinolone acetonide-assisted macular hole surgery. Graefes Arch Clin Exp Ophthalmol 2017;255(3):485–92.
[31] Charles S. Illumination and Phototoxicity Issues in Vitreoretinal Surgery. Retina 2008;28(1): 1–4.
[32] Bottoni F, Parrulli S, Mete M, et al. Large idiopathic macular hole surgery: remodelling of outer retinal layers after traditional internal limiting membrane peeling or inverted flap technique. Ophthalmologica 2020;243(5):334–41.
[33] Yee P, Sevgi DD, Abraham J, et al. iOCT-assisted macular hole surgery: outcomes and utility from the DISCOVER study. Br J Ophthalmol 2021;105(3):403–9.
[34] Zhang X, Liu J, Yu B, et al. Effects of mesenchymal stem cells and their exosomes on the healing of large and refractory macular holes. Graefe's Archive Clin Exp Ophthalmol 2018;256(11):2041–52.
[35] Sun Y, Williams A, Waisbourd M, et al. Stem cell therapy for glaucoma: science or snake oil? Surv Ophthalmol 2015;60(2):93–105.
[36] Moysidis SN, Koulisis N, Adrean SD, et al. Autologous retinal transplantation for primary and refractory macular holes and macular hole retinal detachments: The global consortium. Ophthalmology 2021;128(5):672–85.
[37] PAT survey editors. 2018 Preferences and trends 20th annual membership survey: American Society of Retina Specialists (ASRS) Congress Proceedings; Vancouver (BC); 2018.

Advances in Ophthalmology and Optometry 7 (2022) 219–235

ADVANCES IN OPHTHALMOLOGY AND OPTOMETRY

# Peripheral Retinal Degenerations and Treatment Options

George Jiao, MD[a], Marib Akanda, MD[a], Ronni M. Lieberman, MD[b,*]

[a]Department of Ophthalmology, Northwell Health Eye Institute, 600 Northern Boulevard, Suite 214, Great Neck, NY 11021, USA; [b]Department of Ophthalmology, Mount Sinai Health Systems, New York, NY, USA

**Keywords**

• Peripheral retinal degeneration • Retinal detachment • Retinal tears • Benign lesions • Predisposing lesions

**Key points**

- The incidence of many peripheral retinal degenerations increases with age and myopia.
- Optical coherence tomography (OCT) can be used to elucidate the underlying pathology of uncertain lesions.
- Based on the current evidence available, most asymptomatic peripheral retinal degenerations should not be treated.
- Acute symptomatic horseshoe tears, dialysis, and traumatic breaks should be treated promptly.
- Risk factors for retinal detachments, including high myopia, lattice degeneration, cataract surgery and others, should be considered when evaluating the peripheral retina.

## INTRODUCTION

The peripheral retina is defined as the area from the equator to the ora serrata and can harbor many different types of degenerations and developmental variations. They can be classified based on risk for retinal detachment, prognosis, location, depth, and morphology. Because these lesions can take on similar

*Corresponding author. 82-68 164th Street Pavilion, 452, Jamaica, NY 11432. *E-mail address:* liebermr@nychhc.org

https://doi.org/10.1016/j.yaoo.2022.03.007

appearances during an indirect ophthalmoscopy examination, scleral depression and ancillary testing, such as optical coherence tomography (OCT) and widefield fundus photography, can be useful in elucidating the underlying condition.

Benign lesions must be distinguished from lesions that predispose a patient to retinal detachments. In certain cases, evolution of predisposing lesions can be treated prophylactically to avoid future complications. Retinal tears in symptomatic patients must be accurately and swiftly identified, as they usually require prompt treatment. Laser photocoagulation and cryotherapy are the treatment of choice for inducing strong chorioretinal adhesions, which act as a barrier to prevent progression of subretinal fluid in detaching the retina. To recognize cases that warrant prophylactic or interventional treatment, one must first be able to accurately identify the benign lesions, predisposing lesions, and retinal tears that exist in the peripheral retina.

## BENIGN LESIONS

### Peripheral retinal drusen

Retinal drusen are extracellular deposits of various lipids, polysaccharides, and proteins between the Bruch's membrane and the basement membrane of retinal pigment epithelium (RPE), seen clinically as small yellow spots under the retina. They are thought to be the result of normal age-related processes arising from accumulated light damage at the RPE and Bruch's membrane interface, from oxidative damage and reactive oxygen species formation, leading to immune-mediated inflammatory responses [1]. When confined in the peripheral retina, drusen are benign findings and do not lead to any visual symptoms or warrant any treatment [2].

### Paving-stone (cobblestone) degeneration

Paving-stone degenerations are age-related atrophy of the choriocapillaris and outer retinal layers, resulting in adherence of the remaining retina with the Bruch's membrane. Most commonly found in the inferior retina anterior to the equator, they appear as discrete, round, pale-yellow areas of hypopigmentation with exposed underlying choroidal vessels. These lesions confer no predisposition to break formation and may actually prevent further extension of an existing retinal detachment due to fusion of the neurosensory retina to Bruch's membrane, preventing liquid vitreous from further advances.

### Retinal pigment epithelium hyperplasia

Hyperplasia of the RPE is a process induced by chronic low-grade traction, either idiopathic or from inflammation or trauma. These reactive processes occur typically near the vitreous base or on the pars plana. Although it can be associated with lattice degeneration and vitreoretinal tufts, which are predisposing retinal lesions, RPE hyperplasia by itself does not lead to increased risk of retinal detachment.

## Retinal pigment epithelium hypertrophy

Congenital or acquired hypertrophy of RPE is characterized by large, round macromelanosomes, giving it its typical hyperpigmented appearance. No active intervention is indicated for classic solitary or grouped lesions. Careful examination and documentation at the time of the initial finding is important as hypopigmentation may occur with time and may give it the appearance of a retinal hole. Atypical congenital hypertrophy of the RPE (CHRPE) lesions have been associated with Gardner syndrome. Nodular adenocarcinoma has been documented to arise from CHRPE [3] and may lead to serous retinal detachment.

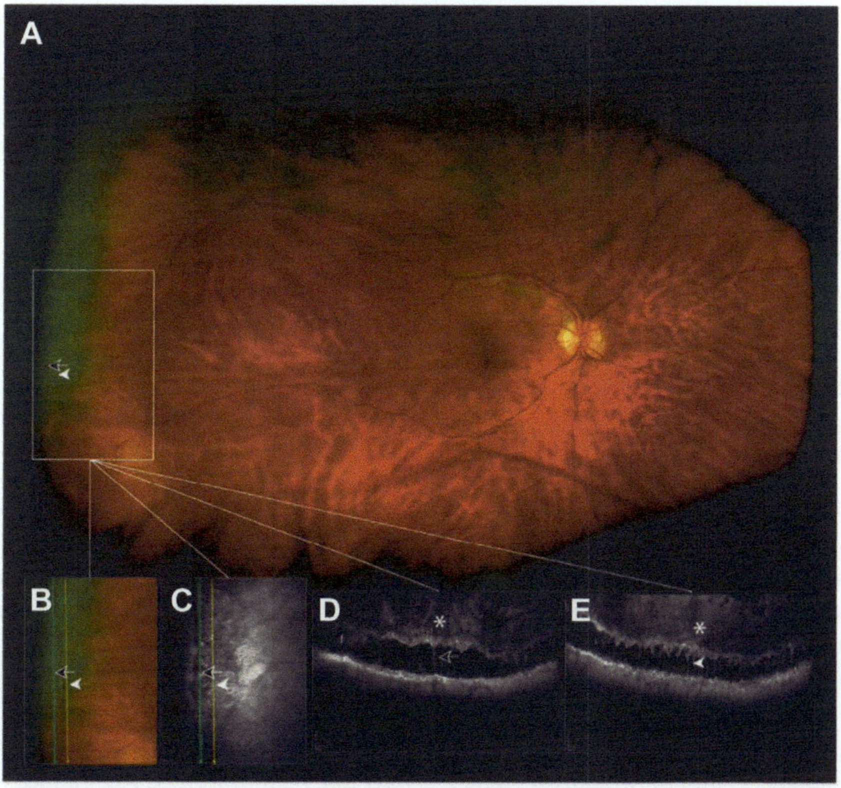


**Fig. 1.** (A) Color fundus photo with typical cystoid degeneration (inset) (B) Color and (C) near-infrared scanning laser ophthalmoscopy photos with green and yellow lines indicating the raster scans of peripheral OCT cross sections (D, E respectively). Black and white arrows indicate saw-tooth patterns formed by hyporeflective cystoid cavities and broad columns at the locations in each panel. Asterisks demonstrate condensed cortical vitreous (D,E, asterisks) (*From* Choudhry N, Golding J, Manry MW, Rao RC. Ultra-Widefield Steering-Based Spectral-Domain Optical Coherence Tomography Imaging of the Retinal Periphery. Ophthalmology. 2016;123(6):1368-1374.)

### Peripheral cystoid degeneration

Typical peripheral cystoid degeneration (Fig. 1) is almost universal over the age of 20 years and appears as clusters of tiny vesicles in the far periphery. Histologically it represents splitting of the outer retina layers with cystoid spaces, and if extended deeper into the retina, it will very rarely lead to retinal holes. Reticular peripheral cystoid degeneration is found posterior to the typical type and presents with a linear or reticular pattern bordered by retinal vessels. In these cases, the cystoid spaces are in the inner nerve fiber layer and may develop into reticular degenerative retinoschisis.

### Snowflake degeneration

Snowflake degeneration is an autosomal dominant condition that appears as yellow-white granular deposits in the periphery retina. These deposits are often numerous, bilateral, and extend toward the equator. This rare condition has been associated with a multitude of degenerative ocular pathologies [4,5], including predisposing retinal lesions such as lattice degeneration, retinal tears, and holes, and even retinal detachment. However, in the absence of any co-existing pathologies, it most likely represents a stable and benign condition that nevertheless requires regular monitoring.

### Pars plana cysts

Pars plana cysts are clear, smooth, cystoid cavities between the pigmented and nonpigmented epithelial layers of the pars plana. The prevalence of these cysts is about 16% in the general population and increases with age [6]. Schepens and colleagues described pars plana cysts as histologically equivalent to retinal detachment, as the nonpigmented epithelium at the pars plana is a continuation of the sensory retina [7]. No evidence currently exists that pars plana cysts, when found in isolation, confer any increased risk of retinal detachment. However, they are associated with predisposing retinal pathology such as degenerative retinoschisis, peripheral cystoid degeneration, and traction. Larger and more numerous cysts have been found in areas where retinoschisis is adjacently present, and the same substance, hyaluronic acid, is found in these cysts, schisis, and cystoid spaces. Ultrasound biomicroscopy can aid in the diagnosis by elucidating the size, pattern, and shapes of these cysts [8].

### Pearl degeneration

Ora serrata pearls are drusen-like deposits that appear as white beads at the ora serrata or pars plana. Initially thought to be congenital in nature, these pearls contain calcium phosphate [9], which is the same composition of calcium found in age-related drusens. Morphologically, they are found between the RPE and Bruch's membrane, consistent with basal laminar drusen. They may appear as a single pearl or as a confluence of pearls. Ora pearls are incidental findings, cause no symptoms, and do not require prophylactic treatment.

### White-with-pressure and white-without-pressure

White-with-pressure (WWP) is a phenomenon seen in the peripheral retina where there is sharply demarcated retinal opacification seen only with scleral indentation. White-without-pressure (WWOP) is an advanced form of WWP that can be appreciated without indentation and can involve the entire circumference of the retina. The incidence of these phenomena is 15% to 32% in normal eyes [10] and increases with myopia and axial length. The pathogenesis of WWP is unknown. Theories range from optical phenomenon due to vitreous traction [11] to abnormal light reflex from normal vitreoretinal interface [12]. OCT findings have shown that the white areas correspond to areas of hyperreflectivity of the outer retinal areas [12]. WWOP may be misdiagnosed as shallow retinal detachment or retinoschisis, but upon scleral indentation, the retina is shown to be attached to the underlying RPE. Localized adhesions of the posterior hyaloid membrane of the vitreous have been documented in areas of WWOP [12] although it has not been associated with retinal detachments [13]. Lattice degeneration is more commonly found in myopic eyes with WWOP than in myopic eyes without WWOP [14]. Areas of WWOP increasing over time is a risk factor for giant retinal tears [15]. WWP by itself does not indicate any pathologic disease states in the retina and does not warrant prophylactic treatment.

## LESIONS PREDISPOSING TO RETINAL DETACHMENT

### Lattice degeneration

Lattice degeneration (Fig. 2) is a vitreoretinal degenerative process that leads to retinal thinning, vitreous liquefaction, and strong vitreoretinal adhesions at the margins. Ultimately, these changes predispose the eye to retinal tears and detachments. Risk factors include myopia and hereditary vitreopathies such as Stickler syndrome. It is present in 6% to 10% of the population; the incidence is higher in myopes. Lattice degeneration may manifest a variety of

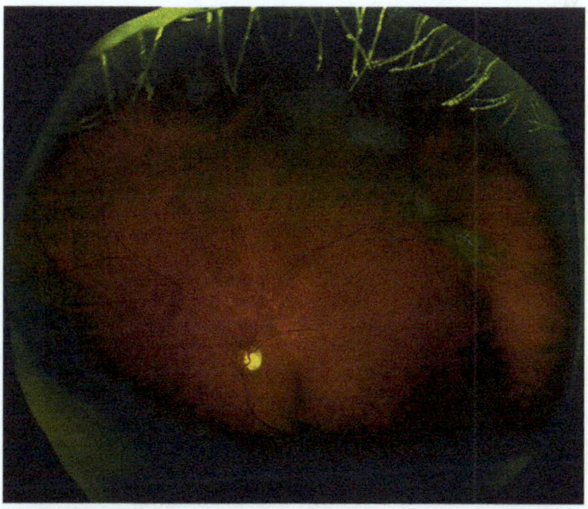

**Fig. 2.** Fundus photograph of lattice degeneration. (*From* Quinn N, Csincsik L, Flynn E, et al. The clinical relevance of visualising the peripheral retina. Prog Retin Eye Res. 2019;68:83-109.)

morphologic features. Most often, it appears as linear or ovoid areas of retinal thinning with or without surrounding pigmentation. It also may be seen as whitish-yellow surface flecks, white patches, red craters, branching white lines, and yellow atrophic spots [16]. Atrophic holes can be seen in lattice in up to 35% of eyes, and approximately 20% to 30% of patients with rhegmatogenous retinal detachments have associated lattice [17]. If no other risk factors exist, the risk of lattice degeneration progressing into a clinical retinal detachment is less than 1%; it usually does not require treatment even if retinal holes or minimal subretinal fluid is identified. Associated symptomatic posterior vitreous detachment, an increase in the size of subretinal fluid (Fig. 3), or retinal detachment in the fellow eye can be an indication for prophylactic or interventional treatment. The most common cause of retinal detachment in eyes with lattice is PVD-induced horseshoe tear, for which prophylactic treatment is indicated. Laser photocoagulation is the preferred treatment, and prognosis for lattice degeneration in itself is good.

## Senile retinoschisis

Senile retinoschisis (Fig. 4) is the splitting of the outer plexiform layer, presenting as a transparent, smooth, dome-shaped elevation typically in the inferotemporal quadrant. It occurs in up to 4% of individuals older than 40 years, is typically asymptomatic, and often is bilateral and more common in hyperopic eyes. It can be the result of progressive typical cystoid degeneration coalescing into a single cavity. Although it can be difficult to distinguish from retinal detachments, retinoschisis cavities will be displaced equally during a scleral depression examination, while retinal detachments will only shift the subretinal fluid leading to a flattened cavity over the area of scleral depression. OCT can also be used to visualize the split in the outer plexiform layer. Furthermore, laser photocoagulation can be used to blanch the area of retinoschisis, whereas

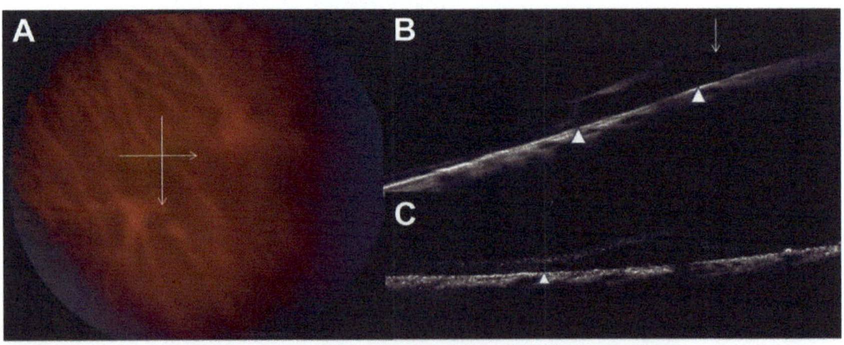


**Fig. 3.** Photograph of lattice degeneration (*A*) with vertical (*B*) and horizontal (*C*) SD-OCT images demonstrating subretinal fluid. (*From* Tsai CY, Hung KC, Wang SW, Chen MS, Ho TC. Spectral-domain optical coherence tomography of peripheral lattice degeneration of myopic eyes before and after laser photocoagulation. J Formos Med Assoc. 2019;118(3):679-685.)

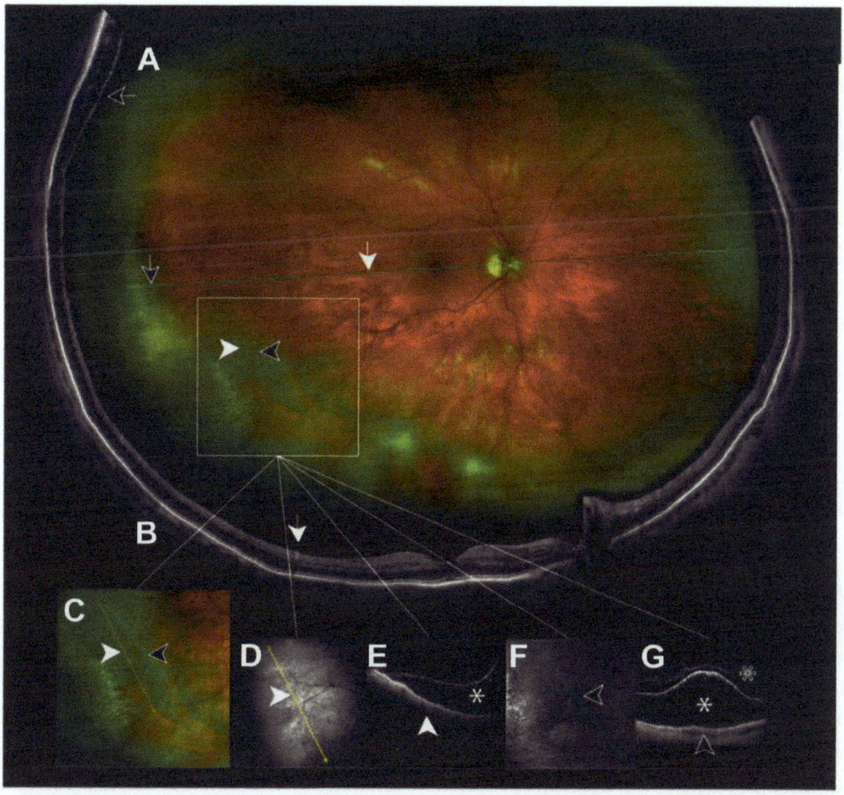


**Fig. 4.** (A) Color fundus photo of senile retinoschisis. (Inset) Junction of unaffected and schitic retina. (B) Montaged OCT cross-section from nasal to temporal temporal periphery obtained along the green line in the fundus photo. The white arrow indicates the posterior extent of schisis extending to the indicated area anteriorly by the black arrow. (C) Color and (D, F) near-infrared scanning laser ophthalmoscopy images with overlaid raster scans (yellow and green lines) demonstrate the position of OCT cross sections (E, G). Arrowheads correspond to the inferotemporal portion analyzed by OCT. White asterisks demonstrate splitting along the inner nuclear and outer plexiform layers (E, G). The black asterisk demonstrates the vitreous interface (G, black asterisk). (*From* Choudhry N, Golding J, Manry MW, Rao RC. Ultra-Widefield Steering-Based Spectral-Domain Optical Coherence Tomography Imaging of the Retinal Periphery. Ophthalmology. 2016;123(6):1368-1374.)

rhegmatogenous retinal detachments will not blanch due to the underlying fluid. Most cases of posterior retinoschisis will not progress beyond where it is first observed and usually is seen beyond 3 disc diameters from the macula [18]. No treatment has been shown to halt the progression of retinoschisis. Schisis with outer wall breaks are typically greater than 3 disc diameters and can contain subretinal fluid. Although they typically remain stable, outer wall breaks can lead to schisis detachment in over 50% of cases. The subretinal fluid does not typically extend beyond the borders of the schisis cavity. Very rarely, breaks in both inner and outer layers allow vitreous fluid to enter the subretinal space and lead to retinal detachment associated with retinoschisis. The outer wall breaks should be closed, and treating the inner wall breaks is optional, as the schisis cavity will likely recur and treatment will not reverse the associated scotoma [19]. Pars plana vitrectomy is preferred in cases of posterior outer wall breaks and presence of posterior vitreous detachments. Scleral buckle is preferred in all other cases [20].

### Vitreoretinal tufts

Peripheral retinal tufts are congenital focal lesions of vitreoretinal adhesions due to glial hyperplasia, seen in 5% to 7% of the general population [21]. Areas of RPE hyperplasia may surround the tuft, giving it a pigmented surrounding. These tufts can be classified as cystic, noncystic, or zonular, where the retina is projected anteriorly and attaches to the zonules. Cystic and zonular tractional tufts have strong vitreoretinal adhesions and therefore predispose the eye to flap tears, operculated holes, and retinal detachments. However, the risk of cystic retinal tuft leading to retinal detachment is less than 1% and given the high incidence in the population, prophylactic treatment is not advised [22].

### Meridional folds

Meridional folds are considered a developmental variation of the peripheral retina, along with enclosed ora bays and peripheral retinal excavations [23]. They are present in about 20% of eyes, are present at birth, and tend to occur symmetrically and bilaterally. Clinically they present as a radially oriented, elevated redundancy of the neurosensory retina that originates at the ora serrata, extends posteriorly, and projects into the vitreous. A meridional complex consists of a large dentate process, a meridional fold, and peripheral retinal excavations in the same meridian. Posterior vitreous detachments and retinal breaks have identified posterior to meridional folds in eyes with rhegmatogenous retinal detachments [24].

### Enclosed ora bays

Enclosed and partially enclosed ora bays are oval islands of nonpigmented pars plana epithelium located posterior to the ora serrata and surrounded by the peripheral neurosensory retina. It may appear depressed and give the appearance of a retinal hole but can be distinguished from a true tear by a thin epithelial layer extending across the base and the absence of any elevation surrounding the retina [24]. Retinal tears are associated with 17% of either type of ora bays, occur posterior to and meridionally aligned with the bays, and are secondary to posterior vitreous detachments [25].

### Peripheral retinal excavations

Peripheral retinal excavations are small oval depressions aligned with meridional folds posterior to the ora serrata and are thought to be a mild form of lattice degeneration. Microscopic examination reveals focal loss of inner retinal tissue with intact surrounding tissue. Because of its circular and focal appearance, it may be mistaken as a retinal hole or round tear. Tears and rhegmatogenous retinal detachments may occur at sites of excavation as strong surrounding vitreoretinal adhesions may occur [24].

### Chorioretinal atrophy

Diffuse chorioretinal atrophy is characterized by ill-defined yellow-white areas of choroidal depigmentation with thinning of the surrounding retina. Patchy chorioretinal atrophy is a well-defined gray-white area of atrophy. The prevalence of these atrophic degenerations increases with age, longer axial length, and higher myopia. Although myopic chorioretinal atrophy typically occurs at the posterior pole, it may enlarge over time and can extend to the equator and the peripheral retina. A significant correlation exists between highly myopic eyes and retinoschisis and foveal retinal detachment [26]. In the periphery, atrophic retinal holes may develop in areas of atrophy. Cases of paravascular linear retinal breaks overlying patchy chorioretinal atrophy leading to rhegmatogenous retinal detachment have been documented in the literature as well [27].

### Dark-without-pressure

Dark without pressure lesions are typically seen as flat, hypopigmented, well-demarcated lesions in the peripheral retina. These may represent altered reflexes at the RPE or outer retinal level, as photopigments are present in varying densities within these lesions compared with normal-appearing retina. Enhanced visibility on red-free photography suggests that they absorb short-wavelength light more effectively. Hyporeflectivity in the ellipsoid zone and outer segments of the photoreceptor has been demonstrated by spectral-domain OCT [28]. No histologic correlations or functional deficits have been found in relation with dark-without-pressure lesions. Patients usually are asymptomatic; therefore, no treatment is indicated. It has been documented to enlarge, regress, and change in shape [29]; however, the clinical significance is still unclear. Recently, evidence shows that it may be associated with viral infection leading to ongoing intraretinal stimulus [30].

### Snail track degeneration

Snail track degenerations are sharply demarcated, elongated groups of white dots in the far periphery. They are typically bilateral, in the superotemporal quadrant, and more commonly seen in myopic patients. These lesions are thought to be a variant or early stages of lattice degeneration [31] because of these similarities and the fact that they are often found together. Histologically, these elongated areas contain degeneration and atrophy of the retina. Vitreoretinal adhesion can occur at the margins and cause traction, resulting in retinal holes and tears. Findings of holes or tears associated with snail track degeneration should be treated accordingly with barrier laser. Lesions without holes or tears can be monitored for progression.

## RETINAL TEARS AND HOLES

### Dialysis

Retinal dialysis is a type of retinal break that occurs circumferentially at the ora serrata, with its posterior edge attached to the vitreous base. Avulsion of the vitreous base may be seen with dialysis and is considered pathognomonic for ocular contusion. The incidence of rhegmatogenous retinal detachment from retinal dialysis is 8% to 17%, and it is the most frequent type of retinal break seen after blunt trauma [32]. Other causes of dialysis include proliferative vascular disorders, old vitreous membranes, and chorioretinitis [32]. Oftentimes patients do not present with any symptoms until it has progressed to a retinal detachment. Hagler [32] reported that 61% of those with nontraumatic dialysis and 58% with traumatic dialysis complained of no symptoms. The most common symptoms patients experienced were photopsias, floaters, decreased vision, or loss of peripheral visual field. In acute, symptomatic retinal dialysis with minimal subretinal fluid, prompt prophylactic treatment with photocoagulation or cryotherapy is recommended. In asymptomatic dialysis, no consensus currently exists regarding prophylactic treatment; however, these patients have a high risk of progression to retinal detachment. Treatment should be strongly considered, especially in eyes with other risk factors such as myopia, lattice degeneration, cataract surgery, trauma, and rhegmatogenous retinal detachment in the fellow eye. Scleral buckling alone has been proven to be effective in patients with retinal detachment due to retinal dialysis [33,34] and can spare patients the complications related to vitrectomy. Pneumatic retinopexy also has been shown to be effective for superior retinal dialysis [35].

### Horseshoe tear

Horseshoe tears (Fig. 5b; see Fig. 7B) are U-shaped full-thickness breaks in the retina that most commonly occur secondary to posterior vitreous detachment. This classic shape is the result of vitreoretinal traction directed toward the vitreous, while the base remains firmly attached. About 30% to 50% of untreated horseshoe tears result in rhegmatogenous retinal detachment [36]. Patients typically experience symptoms such as photopsias and floaters from the ongoing traction. New-onset symptoms with visual field loss are suggestive of a new tear or retinal detachment. Prophylactic treatment always is indicated for acute symptomatic horseshoe tears, as the risk of progression is unacceptably high. Cryotherapy or laser photocoagulation is used to create chorioretinal adhesion around the tear so that vitreous is unable to push through the subretinal space and create a retinal detachment. Treatment of peripheral horseshoe tears should extend to the ora serrata if the tear cannot be surrounded adequately with cryotherapy or laser [37], as an inadequately treated tear at the anterior border is the most common cause of treatment failure. Asymptomatic horseshoe tears have about a 5% chance of progressing to retinal detachments. Observation without treatment can be considered when the tear is chronic, demarcated by pigmentation, or lacks evidence of ongoing vitreoretinal traction.

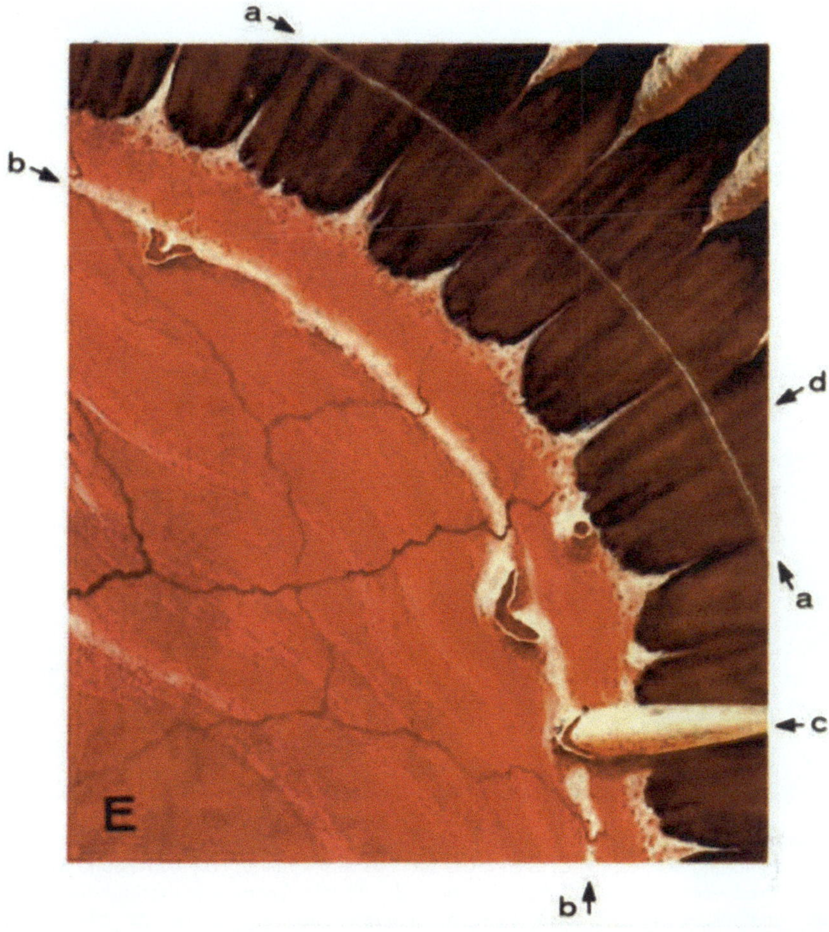


**Fig. 5.** Findings surrounding the ora serrata. (a) Anterior limit of the vitreous base. (b) Posterior limit of the vitreous base with 2 small horseshoe breaks. (c) Meridional fold with retinal break. (d) Cystoid degeneration with a round hole. (*From* Dumas J, Schepens CL. Chorioretinal lesions predisposing to retinal breaks. *Am J Ophthalmol* 1966;61:620-630.)

## Operculated round tear

Operculated retinal holes are the result of strong vitreoretinal traction that pulls a piece of round retinal tissue, termed an operculum, into the vitreous. If resulting from a posterior vitreous detachment, which is the most common cause, then traction surrounding the area of the tear should be relieved. Asymptomatic operculated holes rarely lead to retinal detachments [38,39]. Symptomatic operculated retinal tears, when discovered without ongoing vitreoretinal traction at the edges, do not typically progress to retinal detachments either. Treatment can be considered if evidence of ongoing traction exists, the hole large or

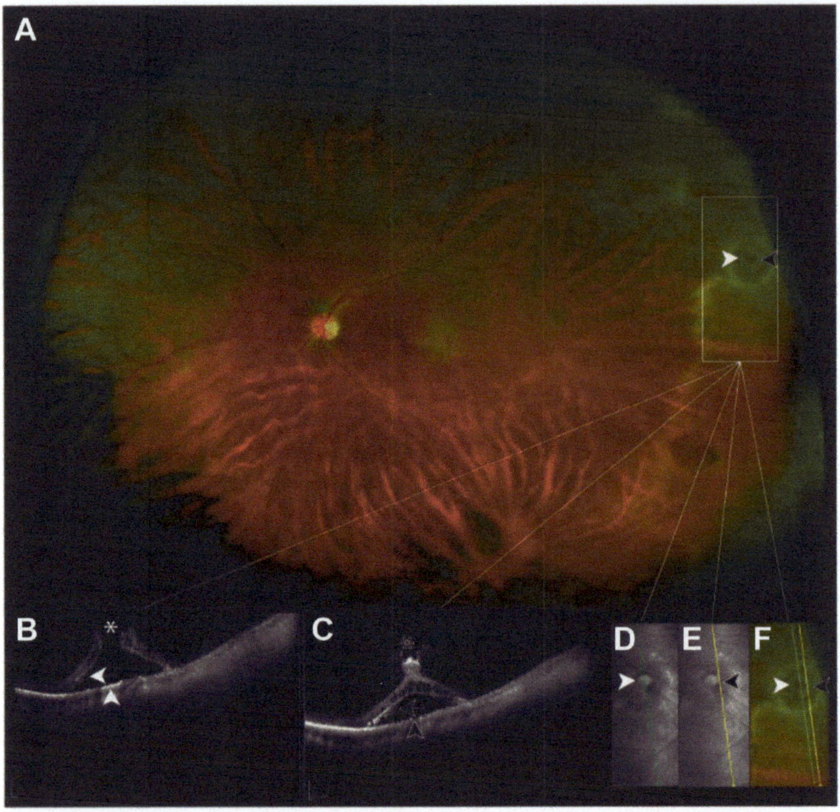


**Fig. 6.** (A) Color fundus photo with retinal holes. (Inset) one hole corresponding to the included imaging studies. (B, C) OCT cross sections of the retinal hole correspond to (D, E) near-infrared scanning laser ophthalmoscopy and a (F) color image with overlaid raster scans (green and yellow lines). (B, C, arrowheads) subretinal fluid. (C, asterisk) partially attached operculum. (C, asterisk) Vitreous hyper-reflectivity and attachment to the inner retina, contrasted with (B, asterisks) where no such adhesion is seen. (B, C, arrows) variable regions of cystoid degeneration and the subretinal space around the hole contained hyperreflective material. Arrowheads in A-F represent corresponding locations in each panel. (*From* Choudhry N, Golding J, Manry MW, Rao RC. Ultra-Widefield Steering-Based Spectral-Domain Optical Coherence Tomography Imaging of the Retinal Periphery. Ophthalmology. 2016;123(6):1368-1374.)

located superiorly, or if there is associated vitreous hemorrhage. Untreated, asymptomatic subclinical retinal detachment, defined as a retinal break with subretinal fluid extending at least 1 disc diameter away from the break, have a 11% to 31% chance of progressing into clinical retinal detachment [36,40].

## Atrophic round hole

Atrophic holes (Fig. 6) found in the peripheral retina are formed from chronic retinal atrophy, more commonly found in myopic patients, and not associated

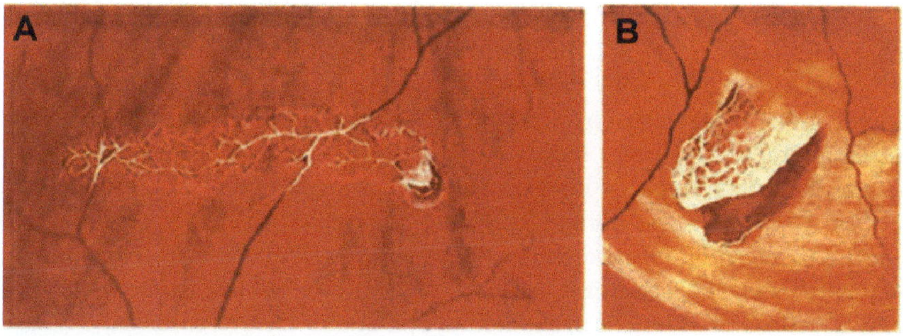


**Fig. 7.** (*A*) Incomplete retinal tear at the edge of lattice degeneration. (*B*) Large horseshoe tear with associated lattice. (*From* Dumas J, Schepens CL. Chorioretinal lesions predisposing to retinal breaks. *Am J Ophthalmol* 1966;61:620-630.)

with vitreoretinal traction. It is important to differentiate an atrophic round hole from an operculated round tear by evaluating the surrounding area of the break for an operculum. These full-thickness retinal breaks can occur within areas of lattice degeneration or within normal-appearing retina. Patients will generally be asymptomatic. If a patient presents with acute symptoms of posterior vitreous detachment, atrophic holes are generally incidental, pre-existing lesions, and not the cause of the patient's symptoms. Atrophic holes within lattice lesions, with minimal subretinal fluid, or without evidence of posterior vitreous detachment do not warrant treatment [41]. Closer follow-up is recommended if the fellow eye has had a previous retinal detachment or if the fluid increases. If atrophic holes are the primary cause of a macula-threatening or macula-off retinal detachment in a young, phakic patient without evidence of posterior vitreous detachment, scleral buckling may be the treatment of choice over pars plana vitrectomy [42].

## TREATMENT OPTIONS FOR LATTICE PERIPHERAL DEGENERATION

The question of treatment for select peripheral degenerations has been explored in the literature and is an important clinical topic that arises when patients with such findings present. Lattice degeneration, a predisposing peripheral degeneration, is present in 6% to 8% of the population and may progress into a clinical retinal detachment in less than 1% of cases when no other risk factors exist [41]. Simple cases thus do not require treatment, but if symptoms occur with associated posterior vitreous detachment, or increased subretinal fluid (see Fig. 3) or retinal detachment develops, laser photocoagulation treatment is recommended [41]. Treatment of asymptomatic lattice degeneration with laser photocoagulation is not strongly supported by the current literature. In the absence of randomized control trial data, some physicians may follow anecdotal or experiential patterns of management for lattice degeneration, which may include treatment when eyes are significantly myopic, the fellow eye has a history of retinal degeneration, or there is an absence of posterior vitreous detachment before planned cataract surgery [43]. However, prior studies of eyes with more than 6 diopters of myopia or more than 6 clock-hours of degeneration did not support prophylactic treatment [43,44]. Additionally, some studies have noted that retinal detachment still may occur despite treatment and may be due to development of breaks in areas that were previously noted to be normal and thus not treated prophylactically [41,45]. The most recent published preferred practice pattern does not recommend treatment of stable lattice degeneration, regardless of extent of myopia or presence of retinal detachment in the fellow eye due to lack of sufficient evidence, and solely recommends treatment when associated posterior vitreous detachment results in a horseshoe tear (Fig. 7) [41]. Eyes with lattice degeneration should thus be monitored carefully over time to monitor for progression, and better-quality data from prospective randomized trials may help further elucidate which cases may benefit from treatment.

## SUMMARY

Many different types of degenerations and developmental variations occur in the peripheral retinal, with variations in risk for retinal detachment, prognosis, location, depth, and morphology. Thorough examination and ancillary imaging studies may help elucidate the underlying condition. After identification of the lesion, the patient should be monitored with frequency determined by the potential for complications to develop. Progression of predisposing peripheral lesions on follow-up examinations should be treated with laser photocoagulation or cryotherapy, especially when retinal breaks or detachment are incipient. In cases of lattice degeneration where the lesion is strongly associated with development of tears or detachments, additional studies are still needed to determine which cases would most benefit from treatment as current evidence does not warrant prophylactic management. Identification and prompt management of these cases are essential to not only prevent retinal detachments and associated vision loss or surgical comorbidity but also reassure patients who may have been referred for a peripheral finding that happens to be benign.

## CLINICS CARE POINTS

- Of the benign degenerations, cases of congenital hypertrophy of the RPE (CHRPE) should be carefully monitored and documented due to the association with Gardner syndrome and reports of adenocarcinoma arising from the lesions.
- Progression of predisposing peripheral lesions or retinal tears on follow-up examinations usually warrants prophylactic treatment with laser photocoagulation or cryotherapy.
- Laser photocoagulation treatment is recommended for lattice degeneration associated with symptomatic posterior vitreous detachment or increased subretinal fluid.

- Prophylactic treatment is always indicated for acute symptomatic horseshoe tears and acute symptomatic retinal dialysis.
- Treatment of peripheral horseshoe tears should extend to the ora serrata if the tear cannot be surrounded adequately with cryotherapy or laser

## Disclosure

The authors have nothing to disclose.

## References

[1] Crabb JW. The proteomics of drusen. Cold Spring Harb Perspect Med 2014;4(7): a017194.
[2] Egbu E, Ihemedu C, Eze UR, et al. Atypical bilateral peripheral drusen in a forty-year-old man: case report and review of literature. Int J Ophthalmol Clin Res 2020;7:119.
[3] Trichopoulos N, Augsburger JJ, Schneider S. Adenocarcinoma arising from congenital hypertrophy of the retinal pigment epithelium. Graefes Arch Clin Exp Ophthalmol 2006;244(1):125–8.
[4] Edwards AO, Robertson JE. Hereditary vitreoretinal degenerations. In: Ryan SJ, et al, editors. Retina. Philadelphia: Elsevier Inc.; 2006. p. 519–38.
[5] Robertson DM, Link TP, Rostvold JA. Snowflake degeneration of the retina. Ophthalmology 1982;89(12):1513–7.
[6] OKUN E. Gross and microscopic pathology in autopsy eyes. IV. Pars plana cysts. Am J Ophthalmol 1961;51:1221–8.
[7] Grignolo A, Schepens CL, Heath P. Cysts of the pars plana ciliaris: ophthalmoscopic appearance and pathological description. AMA Arch Ophthalmol 1957;58(4):530–43; https://doi.org/10.1001/archopht.1957.00940010548008.
[8] Mannino G, Malagola R, Abdolrahimzadeh S, et al. Ultrasound biomicroscopy of the peripheral retina and the ciliary body in degenerative retinoschisis associated with pars plana cysts. Br J Ophthalmol 2001;85(8):976–82.
[9] Wright L, Eagle RE, Abraham JL, et al. Elemental composition of ora serrata pearls—a form of focal nodular drusen. JAMA Ophthalmol 2016;134(5):601–3.
[10] Shukla M, Anuja OP. White with pressure (WWP) and white without pressure (WWOP) lesions. Indian J Ophthalmol 1982;30:129–32.
[11] WATZKE RC. The ophthalmoscopic sign "white with pressure". A clinicopathologic correlation. Arch Ophthalmol 1961;66:812–23.
[12] Diaz RI, Sigler EJ, Randolph JC, et al. Spectral domain optical coherence tomography characteristics of white-without-pressure. Retina 2014;34(5):1020–1.
[13] Bedi N, Shah M. Association of peripheral retinal degeneration with retinal detachment in myopia. Int J Med Sci Educ 2019;6(4):92–5.
[14] Dhull VK, Manisha Nada, Sood Sundan, et al. Analysis of white without pressure retinal lesions in myopia and hypermetropia. Int J Adv Case Rep 2019;6(2):17–25.
[15] Freeman HM. Fellow eyes of giant retinal breaks. Trans Am Ophthalmol Soc 1978;76: 343–82.
[16] Byer NE. Lattice degeneration of the retina. Surv Ophthalmol 1979;23(4):213–48.
[17] Byer NE. Long-term natural history of lattice degeneration of the retina. Ophthalmology 1989;96(9):1396–401 [discussion: 1401-2].
[18] Byer NE. Long-term natural history study of senile retinoschisis with implications for management. Ophthalmology 1986;93:1127–36.
[19] Byer NE. Spontaneous regression of senile retinoschisis. Arch Ophthalmol 1972;88(2): 207–9.
[20] Gotzaridis EV, Georgalas I, Petrou P, et al. Surgical treatment of retinal detachment associated with degenerative retinoschisis. Semin Ophthalmol 2014;29(3):136–41.

[21] Suzuki CR, Farah ME. Retinal peripheral changes after laser in situ keratomileusis in patients with high myopia. Can J Ophthalmol 2004;39(1):69–73.
[22] Byer NE. Cystic retinal tufts and their relationship to retinal detachment. Arch Ophthalmol 1981;99(10):1788–90.
[23] Engstrom RE Jr, Glasgow BJ, Foos RY, et al. Degenerative diseases of the peripheral retina. In: Tasman W, Jaeger EA, editors. Duane's clinical ophthalmology on DVD-ROM, 3. Philadelphia: Lippincott Williams & Wilkins; 2013 chap 26.
[24] Dumas J, Schepens CL. Chorioretinal lesions predisposing to retinal breaks. Am J Ophthalmol 1966;61:620–30.
[25] Spencer LM, Foos RY, Straatsma BR. Enclosed bays of the ora serrata: relationship to retina tears. Arch Ophthalmol 1970;83(4):421–5.
[26] Takano M, Kishi S. Foveal retinoschisis and retinal detachment in severely myopic eyes with posterior staphyloma. Am J Ophthalmol 1999;128:472–6.
[27] Chen L, Wang K, Esmaili DD, et al. Rhegmatogenous Retinal Detachment Due to Paravascular Linear Retinal Breaks Over Patchy Chorioretinal Atrophy in Pathologic Myopia. Arch Ophthalmol 2010;128(12):1551–4.
[28] Flores Pimentel MA, Duncan JL, de Alba Campomanes AG, et al. Dark without pressure retinal changes in a paediatric age group. Eye (Lond) 2021;35(4):1221–7.
[29] Fawzi AA, Nielsen JS, Mateo-Montoya A, et al. Multimodal imaging of white and dark without pressure fundus lesions. Retina 2014;34(12):2376–87; https://doi.org/10.1097/IAE.0000000000000388.
[30] Steptoe PJ, Momorie F, Fornah AD, et al. Evolving longitudinal retinal observations in a cohort of survivors of ebola virus disease. JAMA Ophthalmol 2020;138(4):395–403.
[31] Shukla M, Ahuja OP. A possible relationship between lattice and snail track degenerations of the retina. Am J Ophthalmol 1981;92(4):482–5.
[32] Hagler WS. Retinal dialysis: a statistical and genetic study to determine pathogenic factors. Trans Am Ophthalmol Soc 1980;78:686–733.
[33] Chang JS, Marra K, Flynn HW Jr, et al. Scleral buckling in the treatment of retinal detachment due to retinal dialysis. Ophthalmic Surg Lasers Imaging Retina 2016;47(4):336–40.
[34] Qiang Kwong T, Shunmugam M, Williamson TH. Characteristics of rhegmatogenous retinal detachments secondary to retinal dialyses. Can J Ophthalmol 2014;49(2):196–9.
[35] Melgen SE, Michels M. Pneumatic retinopexy for the treatment of giant retinal dialyses. Am J Ophthalmol 1994;118(6):762–5.
[36] Davis MD. The natural history of retinal breaks without detachment. Trans Am Ophthalmol Soc 1973;71:343–72.
[37] Delaney WV Jr. Retinal tear extension through the cryosurgical scar. Br J Ophthalmol 1971;55(3):205–9.
[38] Byer NE. What happens to untreated asymptomatic retinal breaks, and are they affected by posterior vitreous detachment? Ophthalmology 1998;105(6):1045–9 [discussion: 1049-50].
[39] Byer NE. Rethinking prophylactic treatment of retinal detachment. In: Stirpe M, editor. Advances in vitreoretinal surgery. Acta third international congress on vitreoretinal surgery. Rome, 12–14 september 1991. New York: Ophthalmic Communications Society; 1992. p. 399–411.
[40] Byer NE. Subclinical retinal detachment resulting from asymptomatic retinal breaks: prognosis for progression and regression. Ophthalmology 2001;108(8):1499–503 [discussion: 1503-4].
[41] Flaxel CJ, Adelman RA, Bailey ST, et al. Posterior vitreous detachment, retinal breaks, and lattice degeneration preferred practice pattern®. Ophthalmology 2020;127(1):P146–81.
[42] Park SW, Lee JJ, Lee JE. Scleral buckling in the management of rhegmatogenous retinal detachment: patient selection and perspectives. Clin Ophthalmol 2018;12:1605–15.

[43] P Wilkinson C. Evidence-based analysis of prophylactic treatment of asymptomatic retinal breaks and lattice degeneration. Ophthalmology 2000;107(Issue 1):12–5; https://doi.org/10.1016/S0161-6420(99)00049-4.
[44] Folk JC, Arrindell EL, Klugman MR. The fellow eye of patients with phakic lattice retinal detachment. Ophthalmology 1989;96:72–9, (II).
[45] Mastropasqua L, Carpineto P, Ciancaglini M, et al. Treatment of retinal tears and lattice degenerations in fellow eyes in high risk patients suffering retinal detachment: a prospective studyBritish. J Ophthalmol 1999;83:1046–9.

Advances in Ophthalmology and Optometry 7 (2022) 237–251

ADVANCES IN OPHTHALMOLOGY AND OPTOMETRY

# Update on Retinal and Ocular Imaging

Samuel Gelnick, MD[a,*], Minh Trinh, MD[a],
Ronni M. Lieberman, MD[b]

[a]Northwell Health Eye Institute, 600 Northern Boulevard Suite 214, Great Neck, NY 11021, USA; [b]Department of Ophthalmology, Mt Sinai Medical Center, Icahn School of Medicine, 1 Gustave L. Levy Place, New York, NY 10029-5674, USA

**Keywords**

• Optical coherence tomography (OCT)
• Optical coherence tomography angiography (OCT-A)
• Fluorescein angiography (FA) • Retcam • Optos • Fundus photography
• Artificial intelligence • Teleophthalmology

**Key points**

- Fundus photography has progressed rapidly over the past 2 decades, now capable of capturing high resolution 200° ultra-widefield images.
- Although fluorescein angiography remains the gold standard for evaluating retinal perfusion, optical coherence tomography angiography is emerging as an alternative, noninvasive, technology.
- Fundus photography is a powerful tool that addresses the growing need for teleophthalmology, especially for screening diabetic patients for evidence of retinopathy.

## BACKGROUND AND INTRODUCTION

The first commercially available fundus camera was produced by Carl Zeiss in 1926 [1]. This fundus camera was limited to a 10° field of view, the same field of view as direct ophthalmoscopy. For reference, indirect ophthalmoscopy, depending on the condensing lens, typically has a field of view of approximately 30°. As optics technology and image processing technology improved, the idea of taking multiple fundus photos over different areas to build a complete image

*Corresponding author. *E-mail address:* sgelnick@northwell.edu

https://doi.org/10.1016/j.yaoo.2022.03.009

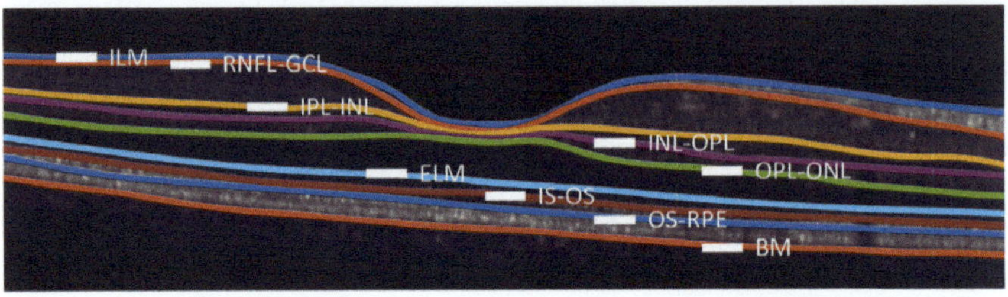


**Fig. 1.** OCT imaging with highlighted layers as follows: retinal nerve fiber layer (RNFL), ganglion cell layer (GCL), inner plexiform layer (IPL), inner nuclear layer (INL), outer plexiform layer (OPL), outer nuclear layer (ONL), inner segment (IS), outer segment (OS), retinal pigment epithelium (RPE), inner limiting membrane (ILM), external limiting membrane (ELM), and Bruch's membrane (BM). (*From* He Y, Carass A, Liu Y, Jedynak BM, Solomon SD, Saidha S, Calabresi PA, Prince JL. Structured layer surface segmentation for retina OCT using fully convolutional regression networks. Med Image Anal. 2021 Feb;68:101856.)

was investigated. This technology continued to progress to today, where we are able to capture a single image with a large field of view.

In addition to the advancement of fundus photography, the introduction of optical coherence tomography (OCT) in the 1980s and 1990s revolutionized ophthalmologists' ability to diagnose, characterize, and monitor pathology. This fairly recent development in the field of ophthalmic imaging not only has impacted the field of retina, but also glaucoma and comprehensive ophthalmologists.

Previous time periods struggled with the problem of a limited ability to image the retina. It was limited to expensive technology and highly trained photographers. Over the last 20 years, retinal imaging has become more accessible. This progress is in part due to moving to digital imaging, as well as near-infrared focusing, nonmydriatic imaging, wide-field imaging, and deep learning technology, to name a few advances. In addition, teleophthalmology as a whole, and specifically in the post-coronavirus disease-2019 (COVID) era will play a big role in furthering the progress of retinal imaging in ophthalmology. As technology progresses, the limit of ophthalmic and retinal imaging has yet to be seen.

## OPTICAL COHERENCE TOMOGRAPHY

OCT is an imaging technology used primarily in ophthalmology for the visualization and differentiation of the different layers of the retina (Fig. 1) [2]. Although a relatively new technology, over the past 30 years it has become standard of care in the retinal field, specifically in regard to macular pathology. It is used commonly to assess the thickness of a patient's macula as well as the presence or absence of fluid in diseases such as diabetic retinopathy and macular degeneration. The imaging results are followed closely, and the treatment plan is adjusted based on findings and clinical correlations.

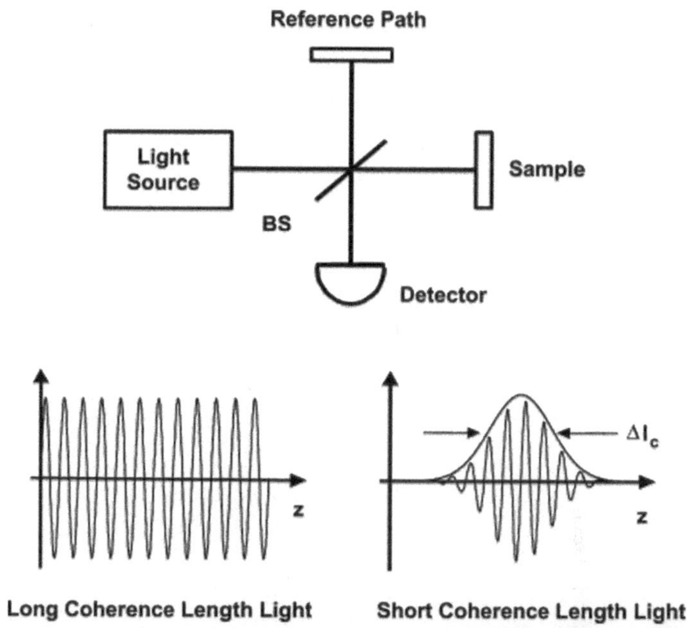


**Fig. 2.** Cartoon schematic of an OCT machine. (*From* Fujimoto JG, Pitris C, Boppart SA, Brezinski ME. Optical coherence tomography: an emerging technology for biomedical imaging and optical biopsy. Neoplasia. 2000 Jan-Apr;2(1-2):9-25.)

Since its inception, the fundamental principles have remained the same. In essence, tissue layers, on the order of microns, are differentiated based on the specific backscatter or reflection of light produced by each individual layer, as compared with a reference beam (Fig. 2) [3]. Because light, as opposed to sound, literally travels at the speed of light, a low coherence light source is used, and the time of flight is measured with interferometry to be able to differentiate the layers, and ultimately produce an image with clinically relevant information. Therefore, at the proper frequencies, deeper tissues can be differentiated from superficial tissues based on the time of flight of the specific tissue backscatter. Based on the wavelength of light used, the different layers of tissues can be identified and portrayed as varying intensities to create a set of A-scans. As the light beam goes across the retina in 2 directions, a 3-dimensional image, or a B-scan, can be created. To maximize the resolution, decrease artifacts, and minimize time, the goal is to maximize the number of A-scans per unit time.

As opposed to time domain, OCT creates A-scans based on time of flight at varying distance of the reference mirror as representative of varying depths of tissue, Fourier domain OCT has been developed, which adjusts the wavelength of the light (with a constant reference beam) to acquire data from the different layers of the retina. The reliance on wavelength as opposed to distance of reference

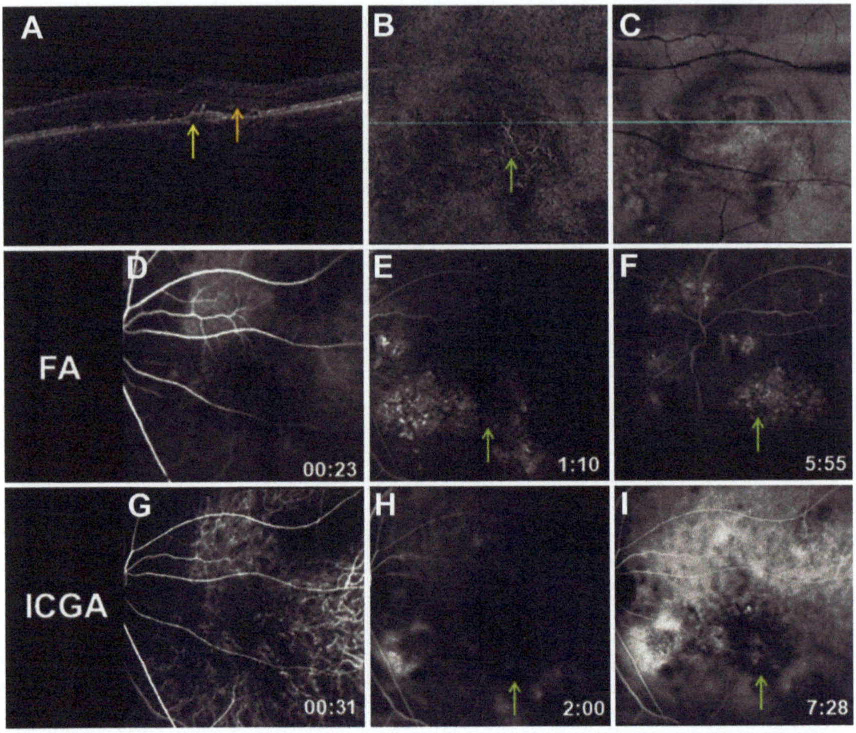


**Fig. 3.** Example of a left eye with occult or type 1 choroidal neovascularization (CNV). (*A*) OCT image of foveal region with subfoveal retinal pigment epithelium (RPE) changes (yellow arrow) with subretinal fluid (orange arrow). (*B*) OCTA angiography of the outer retina to choriocapillaris (ORCC), highlighting the areas of CNV (green arrow) underlying the RPE changes shown in A. (*C*) OCTA structural image of the ORCC. (*D–F*) Fluorescein angiography (FA) showing a type 1 CNV (green arrow) with late leakage. (*G–I*) Indocyanine green angiography (ICGA) showing the presence of a type 1 CNV (green arrow) with late leakage. (*From* Laíns I, Wang JC, Cui Y, Katz R, Vingopoulos F, Staurenghi G, Vavvas DG, Miller JW, Miller JB. Retinal applications of swept source optical coherence tomography (OCT) and optical coherence tomography angiography (OCTA). Prog Retin Eye Res. 2021 Sep;84:100951.)

beam has allowed a much faster time of acquisition, enabling a significant increase in number of A-scans in one session and increased resolution and quality of imaging. Fourier domain can be split up into spectral domain, which uses a broadband of light, which is made up of varying wavelengths and allows for high resolution, and swept source, which uses a tunable laser as its source, allowing for quick high-frequency image acquisition and for increased depth of imaging (somewhat sacrificing resolution). Low coherence swept source lasers with 1000 to 1300 μm wavelengths have even been able to visualize larger areas and deeper tissue such as choroidal neovascularization (Fig. 3) [4–6]. Through the development of this technology, efficient, accurate, and detailed imaging of the retina has been made accessible to eye care providers across the globe.

OCT angiography (OCTA) is an additional development in the OCT arena that enables the visualization of blood vessel perfusion without dye insertion. The fundamental principle of OCTA bases the difference in backscattering between A-scans in a series based solely on the flow of red blood cells in a vessel. The difference in flow then produces images at varying depths in the retina, representing the perfusion in retinal and choroidal vessels at varying depths [6]. Swept source OCTA, given its ability to visualize deeper tissue, has been compared with indocyanine green in identifying choroidal lesions. When considering clinical applications, OCTA imaging becomes beneficial in the diagnosis of choroidal and retinal lesion because it eliminates the need for dye injection and the potential adverse events associated with that. Studies have identified pathologic differences in the foveal avascular zone between normal and diabetic eyes, especially in deeper vascular zones with OCTA [7]. Similarly, recent studies have identified signs on wide-field OCTA of patients that are more likely to develop vitreous hemorrhages [8]. Although fluorescein angiography remains the gold standard in terms of identifying flow-related disease, specifically ischemia and leakage, the advantage of OCTA in the realm of depth differentiation and visualization of pathology beneath leakage provide OCTA a strong potential advantage [9]. However, its dependence on red blood cell flow to create the images opens a lot of room for artifact error. For example, the overlying of vessels in different layers may produce artifactual differences in vessel flow that may not be representative of actual changes in perfusion. Patient movement also may alter image capture. In addition, although poor perfusion can be identified, areas of leakage cannot be seen on OCTA (Fig. 4) [6]. In addition, cost may be a limiting factor in generalizing this technology [5,9].

Finally, another recent advancement in the OCT world is the intraoperative OCT. Developed in multiple stages, the concept that started as a hand-held OCT brought into an operating room setting, has since been set up as a microscope-mounted combination, and ultimately a microscope-integrated system. Given the pervasive use of OCT imaging both preoperatively and postoperatively in management of retinal diseases, the natural progression is to have an intraoperative OCT. Mounted and, more so, integrated intraoperative OCT, has overcome much of the practical issues surrounding obtaining reliable images during retinal surgery. This practice has allowed studies such as PIONEER and DISCOVER to use these devices on a large number of patients. Both studies reported beneficial usefulness with imaging affecting surgical management of macular peeling surgeries 43% of the time in the former, and posterior surgeries 29% of the time in the latter [10,11]. Other studies have reported clinical usefulness by the retinal surgeons in areas such as retinal traction, membrane peeling and placement of intraocular treatments. It currently is limited due to the cost of machinery, need for specific instruments, and image quality. Additionally, future clinical trials are still needed to assess its clinical effectiveness on patient outcomes before its generalization to patient care [12].

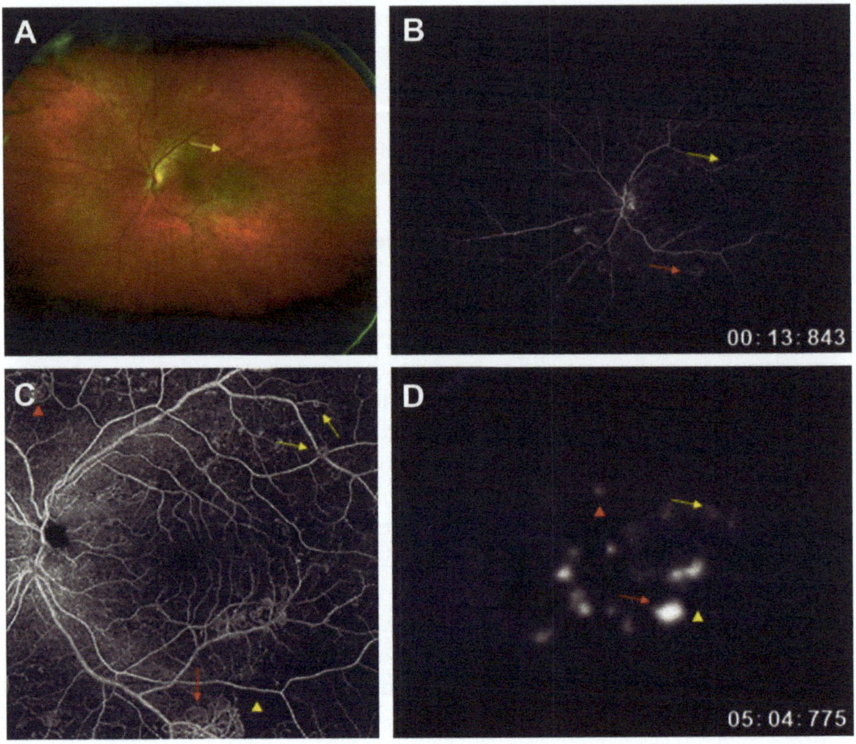


**Fig. 4.** Swept source OCTA imaging of neovascularization in proliferative diabetic retinopathy (PDR). (*A*) Widefield image of a left eye with PDR (yellow arrow). (*B*) Early fluorescein angiography (FA) image highlighting areas of nonperfusion (yellow arrow), venous looping, and neovascularization elsewhere (NVE) (red arrow). (*C*) Swept source-OCTA showing venous looping (yellow arrow) and NVE (red arrow)in greater detail, with clear identification of areas of poor perfusion (yellow arrowhead). (*D*) FA with late leakage (arrows) from areas of NVE and areas of non-perfusion (arrowheads). Of note, this late leakage cannot be seen on OCTA. (*From* Laíns I, Wang JC, Cui Y, Katz R, Vingopoulos F, Staurenghi G, Vavvas DG, Miller JW, Miller JB. Retinal applications of swept source optical coherence tomography (OCT) and optical coherence tomography angiography (OCTA). Prog Retin Eye Res. 2021 Sep;84:100951.)

## FUNDUS PHOTOGRAPHY

Fundus photography began in 1926 with a 20° Carl Zeiss fundus camera. Soon, as technology advanced and imaging improved, a 30° image providing adequate imaging of the nerve and posterior pole was produced. By placing 7 of these photos together, a composite with a width of 75° was created. This 7-field composite became the standard for the initial diabetic retinopathy studies. This classic field was expanded to include 9 photos for many studies concerning cytomegalovirus retinitis. Composites, however, are limited for many reasons, including alignment issues, focusing irregularities, astigmatism, poor fixation, and light reflex artifacts [13,14].

This limitation led to the development of wide and ultrawidefield (UWF) photography, which coincided with the advent of digital photography. The combination of the 2 modalities has further pushed the limits of ophthalmic fundus photography. A number of systems exists that can capture between 100° and 200°. All differ somewhat from each other, but all enjoy a fast acquisition time, coupled with enhanced resolution, short processing times, and, importantly, the acquisition of both posterior pole and far retinal peripheral images. In addition, as the images are digitalized, they can be easily transmitted to the electronic medical record and storage systems.

A number of systems are in use today (Table 1). These include OPTOS (Optos PLC, Dunfermline, UK), Claris 500 (Carl Zeiss Meditec, Jena, Germany), RetCam (Clarity Medical Systems, Inc., Pleasanton, CA), and the Heidelberg Spectralis with the Staurenghi lens (Ocular Staurenghi 230 SLO Retina Lens; Ocular Instruments Inc, Bellevue, WA), among others.

The Optos camera produces a 200° view (82% of surface area) using scanning laser ophthalmoscopy and an ellipsoidal mirror. It is a noncontact lens camera and can function without mydriasis. It has capabilities for red and green reflectance imaging, as well as autofluorescence and fluorescein angiography/indocyanine green angiography (Fig. 5) [15].

Zeiss has in production the CLARUS 500- UWF imaging device. This device produces images in true color, producing images most closely resembling the view seen on indirect fundoscopy. Some investigators feel it can enable more accurate diagnosis of disease processes. Additionally, although its image produces 133° images, it has a montage mode that can stitch 6 images to create 267° images in a single display [16].

Retcam, a contact-based camera, gives a 130° view and is used primarily for neonatal and pediatric patients. It is handheld and, therefore, not limited by patient positioning. It is mainly used for retinopathy of prematurity (ROP) and patients who are otherwise unable to sit upright.

The Equator Plus camera is a contact lens camera and obtains a 148° capture anterior to the equator. However, its drawbacks include a lack of good resolution in addition to significant artifact in the periphery.

The Heidelberg Spectralis uses the Staurenghi lens system; although quite cumbersome, it produces high-resolution 150° images with the scanning laser ophthalmoscopy system. It is both noncontact for the central 105° and contact for 150° and produces pseudocolor images.

Confocal scanning laser ophthalmoscopy imaging systems use laser to produce images, rather than flash, reducing light scatter. This image then is integrated with an OCT image, producing the OCT ophthalmoscope, which can image the fundus using a point-to-point correlation. Both OPTOS and Heidelberg (Sepctralis) have products available.

The clinical ramifications of UWF photography are tremendous. In diabetic retinopathy, for instance, UWF imaging and angiography of up to 200° of retina can be captured with 1 photo, enabling the assessment of peripheral areas of ischemia. This process then allows targeted retinal photocoagulation.

**Table 1**
Table 1 deliniates the multiple systems availble for retinal fundoscopic photography. These systems vary in Lens type, basic fundemental priciple, and field of view.

| | Available platforms | Type of lens system | Principle | Field of view | Facilities available |
|---|---|---|---|---|---|
| WFI | Heidelberg Spectralis | Noncontact | SD-OCT with CSLO | $55^\circ$ ($\leq 105^\circ$ with HRA 2) | FFA, ICGA, FAF |
| | | Contact | SD-COT with CSLO using Staurenghi Lens | $150^\circ$ | FFA, ICGA, FAF |
| | RetCam 3 | Contact | Optical light source to obtain high resolution | Field depends on lens used among the 5 changeable lens systems: $-130^\circ$ (pediatric retain and adult anterior chamber), $-120^\circ$ (pediatric and young adult), $-80^\circ$ (high contrast pediatric and adult), $-30^\circ$ (high magnification) and Portrait (external imaging) | FFA, ICGA |
| | Clarus 500 | Noncontact | Slit scanning ophthalmoscope also referred to as broad line fundus imaging | $133^\circ$–wide field–1 image<br>$200^\circ$–UWF–2 images<br>$267^\circ$–montage–6 images | FAF |
| UWFI | Optos Optomap | Noncontact | CSLO based | 200 | FFA, FAF |

*Abbreviations*: CSLO, confocal scanning laser ophthalmoscopy; FAF, fundus autofluorescence; FFA, fundus fluorescein angiography; ICGA, indocyanine green angiography; SD, spectral domain.

*Reproduced with permission from* Kumar A, Gupta, Y. EyeWiki, "Wide Field Retinal Imaging Systems". Accessed November 3, 2021.

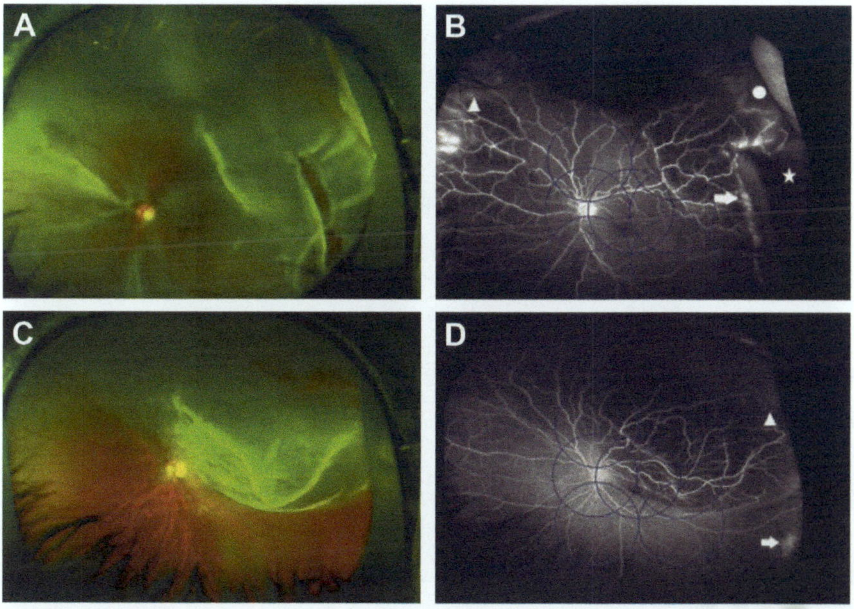


**Fig. 5.** (*A*) UWF image demonstrating a large retinal tear with detachment (*B*). UWFA demonstrates of image (*A*), which highlights areas of capillary nonperfusion (*round dot, arrow head*) and posterior flap of the retinal break (*arrow*). Note that the anterior flap, marked by the star, shows no dye transit. (*C*) UWF image showing a superotemporal retinal detachment. (*D*) UWFA helps to highlight area suspect NVE, (arrowhead), and the inferotemporal area of lattice degeneration (arrow). (*From* Tripathy K, Chawla R, Wadekar BR, Venkatesh P, Sharma YR. Evaluation of rhegmatogenous retinal detachments using Optos ultrawide field fundus fluorescein angiography and comparison with ETDRS 7 field overlay. J Curr Ophthalmol. 2018 Jul 3;30(3):263-267.)

Several studies have shown that UWF angiography demonstrated nonperfusion and neovascularization in eyes that with standard fluorescein angiography would have been undetected [17–19] (Fig. 6). Similarly, areas of nonperfusion in RVO's can be identified with peripheral imaging using UWF photography. It is postulated that by targeting these peripheral areas of ischemia, which would otherwise not be able to be seen, can possibly prevent neovascularization and macular edema, without damaging other areas of perfused retina [20].

It must be acknowledged that with increased use of UFW imaging (UWFI), a system to diagnose and guide treatment based on these images needs to be in place. It has been noted that the use of UWFI in the Early Treatment Diabetic Retinopathy Study would have increased the severity of many subjects [17,21].

UWF has been studied in further evaluation of patients with wet age-related macular degeneration and whether peripheral ischemia plays a role or not. Other diseases that UWF imaging has been used in aiding in diagnosis include

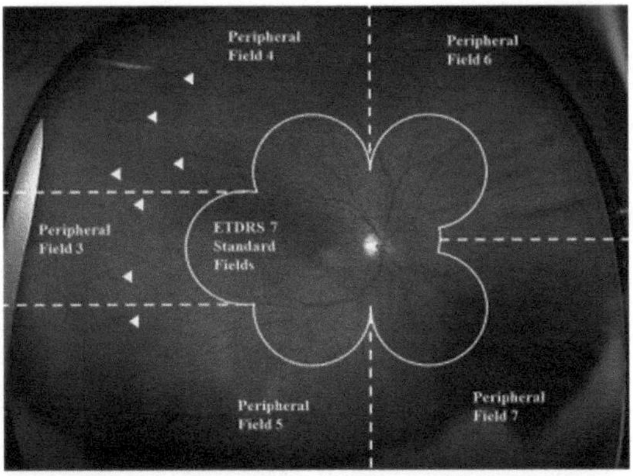


**Fig. 6.** An UWF image with an Early Treatment Diabetic Retinopathy Study (ETDRS) field overlay. This image highlighting the ability of UWFI to detect retinopathy (arrow heads) in the peripheral fields, which would be missed by the ETDRS images. (*From* Silva PS, Cavallerano JD, Haddad NM, Kwak H, Dyer KH, Omar AF, Shikari H, Aiello LM, Sun JK, Aiello LP. Peripheral Lesions Identified on Ultrawide Field Imaging Predict Increased Risk of Diabetic Retinopathy Progression over 4 Years. Ophthalmology. 2015 May;122(5):949-56).

ROP, choroidal melanoma, Coats disease, von Hippel–Lindau disease, pathologic myopia, and retinal detachments [13]. UWF imaging used to clearly identify retinal lesions in uveitis as well.

## ARTIFICIAL INTELLIGENCE–DEEP LEARNING

Although not strictly an imaging technique, this promising emerging image processing tool may prove to be pivotal in the diagnosis or monitoring of common retinal pathologies.

Artificial intelligence (AI) and deep learning algorithms have been shown to be able to detect diseases such as ROP, age-related macular degeneration, and diabetic retinopathy, with high sensitivity and specificity [22]. These algorithms can perform at the same level as a trained retina specialist.

AI deep learning algorithms are built using complex computer code, which essentially functions as a highly specialized brain. These so-called neural networks require large training datasets before they can be used in any practical applications. These training datasets are a set of images, accompanied by "answers." For instance, if the algorithm were designed to identify monkeys, then 1 conceivable training dataset may contain thousands of images of monkeys, but also contain images of other animals. Through each iteration of these training datasets, the neural network makes small adjustments to its parameters randomly when it gets an answer wrong. Through these random corrections, the machine fine tunes its parameters. In this example, the end result would be an algorithm that may be able to identify monkeys with incredibly high reliability.

These algorithms, however, are not without their own limitations. To start, they do require a large training dataset. Although this factor may not be a problem if training the machine to identify common diseases such as diabetic retinopathy or age-related macular degeneration, we would struggle to provide the machine with a large enough training dataset to identify rare retinal pathologies. Additionally, the quality of images provided to the machine may greatly affect how it adjusts its parameters and limit the performance of our algorithm. Another issue with these algorithms is the so-called black box phenomenon, which is the inability to provide an explanation for why the algorithm is able to use certain features to arrive at its conclusion. For instance, using OCT macular images, 1 deep learning algorithm identified areas in the ganglion cell layer and retinal pigmented epithelium to identify sex with an accuracy of 91% [23]. No known anatomic or physiologic explanation exists for how these features differ between males and females.

Despite these variables, multiple groups have shown that deep learning algorithms have performed exceptionally well to identify retinal pathology. Retinal grids have been created for the purpose of deep learning (Fig. 7) [16]. For ROP, deep learning algorithms have been able to identify severe ROP with plus disease with a sensitivity of 100% and specificity of 94% [22]. Multiple algorithms have been created to detect referrable diabetic retinopathy, defined as moderate nonproliferative diabetic retinopathy or worse, with sensitivities and specificities as high as 100% and 98%, respectively. For age-related macular degeneration, algorithms have been able to achieve sensitivities of greater than 90% [22].

Although AI and deep learning algorithms may become widespread in the future, the issue of acquiring large training datasets and gaining a better understanding of the black box phenomena must first be addressed.

## ADAPTIVE OPTICS

Adaptive optics is not a standalone imaging device; rather, it can be thought of as a modification to existing retinal imaging technologies. In its simplest form, the principle of adaptive optics is to correct for the optical aberrations induced by the anterior structures of the eye. The corrective element is commonly a deformable mirror coupled with actuators. By negating the optical aberrations, it is possible to achieve higher resolution imaging down to the cellular level [24]. At this imaging resolution, it is possible to measure cell density and even vessel wall thickness.

Currently, this technology is used primarily in the research setting to better understand retinal pathologies on the cellular level. The only adaptive optics device currently approved for clinical use is the Imagine Eyes RTX1 Adaptive Optics Retinal Camera. Because the level of detail is so high, it is possible to detect changes in the retina that may be missed on conventional imaging or examination. Zaleska-Zmijewska and colleagues [25] compared the cone density in the central 2° among 56 patients, 36 with mild or moderate nonproliferative diabetic retinopathy and 20 healthy patients. They found that the cone density

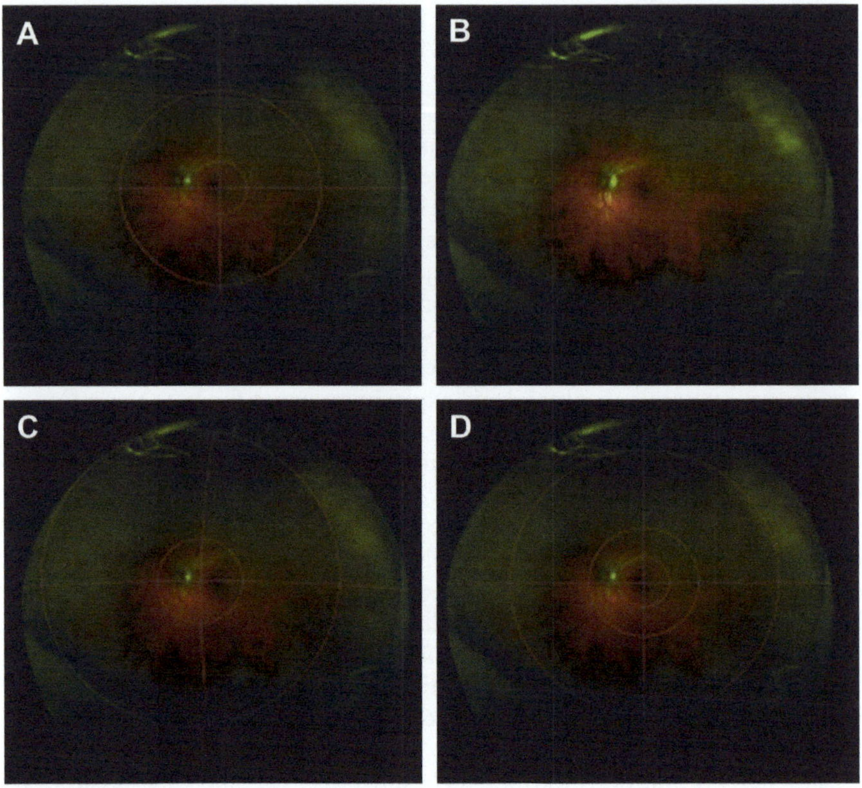


**Fig. 7.** Moorfield's grid (*A*), Manchester grid (*B*), Opera grid (*C*), and Boston grid (*D*) for AI/deep learning systems. (*From* Quinn N, Csincsik L, Flynn E, Curcio CA, Kiss S, Sadda SR, Hogg R, Peto T, Lengyel I. The clinical relevance of visualising the peripheral retina. Prog Retin Eye Res. 2019 Jan;68:83-109.)

was significantly lower in the nonproliferative group as compared with the control group [25]. Although this tool may be excellent for detecting early changes in the photoreceptors, it is unclear if a clinical correlation occurs to this loss of cell density.

Because this technology remains in its infancy, it is unclear how it may be incorporated into future clinical practice.

## TELEOPHTHALMOLOGY

Teleophthalmology uses both imaging techniques and digital communication to bring patients and providers together across physical space. It is best used to bring care to patients in remote areas and to provide screening for multiple ophthalmic conditions, and is helping to level health care disparities in underserved communities. In addition, it is very efficient, both as a physician time saver and as a cost saver as well. It has been especially useful during the

COVID pandemic, because many patients were unable to personally be seen by an eye care provider. Because there is theoretically no limit to the geographic distance between patient and reader, it is hoped it can play a role in ultimately decreasing global blindness.

### Types of teleophthalmology

Synchronous teleophthalmology allows the ophthalmologist to interact in real time with either another provider (direct them in examination and management of the patient) or the patient directly. The COVID pandemic has pushed the boundaries of this method, which is in its early stages.

Asynchronous teleophthalmology refers to the capturing of an image, its storage and then transmission to a qualified reader. Using a predetermined algorithm, the reader than makes an appropriate disposition for the patient. Although any part of the examination can be transmitted, it is most commonly seen with fundus photos, in diabetic and ROP screening. This is the more common type of teleophthalmology.

## DIABETIC SCREENING

An image is taken using a nonmydriatic camera, usually by an allied health professional in low light conditions, when the patient is seen by a primary care provider [26]. The image is then stored, encryption used to protect patient confidentiality, and then transmitted to a trained reader. The reader can, if needed, manipulate the image. As noted elsewhere in this article, the reader, using a predetermined algorithm, then makes an appropriate determination as to referral, need for management or follow-up. Although originally created for diabetic retinopathy screening, it has been found that ARMD, glaucoma, and other ophthalmic diseases can be detected [27]. A 97% predictive value has been found, and the sensitivity for remote grading is noted to be 98.2%.

## RETINOPATHY OF PREMATURITY

Screening for ROP is another example of an excellent use for teleophthalmology. The dearth of trained ophthalmologists to perform the screening, combined with the large geographic areas that 1 provider may need to cover, makes teleophthalmology the perfect tool for ROP screening. In the United States alone, approximately 16,000 premature infants may be effected by ROP annually [28]. An allied health professional, usually nursing in the NICU, are trained to take fundus photos, using the Retcam (Clarity). Images are then read within 24 hours. The e-ROP study compared evaluation of wide-field images with in-person examination [29]. Remote grading was found to have 90% for ROP.

## FUTURE DIRECTIONS

Teleophthalmology is a remarkable combination of advances in imaging, electronic storage, and communication and medicine. Challenges remain however, including patient follow-up, cost and continued recruitment and training of staff. In addition, ophthalmology must work with government to create fair and appropriate policies regulating its use.

## CLINICS CARE POINTS

- OCT imaging is a powerful and established means of assessing retinal pathology. OCTA, although not a replacement for fluorescein angiography, allows physicians to noninvasively image and assess retinal vasculature.
- UWFI fundus photography can pick up diseases in the far periphery, although not a replacement for a dilated fundus examination, this tool may be a useful adjunct for monitoring retinal pathology overtime.
- AI and deep learning technologies have the potential to identify retinal diseases with high accuracy and precision.
- Ophthalmic telemedicine has seen rapid growth, particularly with the onset of the COVID-19 pandemic. However, the uncertainty of examination accuracy, patient satisfaction, and reimbursement makes in office visits the preferred method of ophthalmologic assessment.

## Disclosure

The authors have no relevant financial disclosures.

## References

[1] Panwar N, Huang P, Lee J, et al. Fundus photography in the 21st century–a review of recent technological advances and their implications for worldwide healthcare. Telemed J E Health 2016;22(3):198–208.
[2] He Y, Carass A, Liu Y, et al. Structured layer surface segmentation for retina OCT using fully convolutional regression networks. Med Image Anal 2021;68:101856.
[3] Fujimoto JG, Pitris C, Boppart SA, et al. Optical coherence tomography: an emerging technology for biomedical imaging and optical biopsy. Neoplasia 2000;2(1–2):9–25.
[4] Abràmoff MD, Garvin MK, Sonka M. Retinal imaging and image analysis. IEEE Rev Biomed Eng 2010;3:169–208.
[5] Miller AR, Roisman L, Zhang Q, et al. Comparison between spectral-domain and swept-source optical coherence tomography angiographic imaging of choroidal neovascularization. Invest Ophthalmol Vis Sci 2017;58(3):1499–505.
[6] Laíns I, Wang JC, Cui Y, et al. Retinal applications of swept source optical coherence tomography (OCT) and optical coherence tomography angiography (OCTA). Prog Retin Eye Res 2021;84:100951.
[7] Sun Z, Yang D, Tang Z, et al. Optical coherence tomography angiography in diabetic retinopathy: an updated review. Eye (Lond) 2021;35(1):149–61.
[8] Cui Y, Zhu Y, Lu ES, et al. Widefield swept-source OCT angiography metrics associated with the development of diabetic vitreous hemorrhage: a prospective study. Ophthalmology 2021;128(9):1312–24.
[9] Morgan JI. The fundus photo has met its match: optical coherence tomography and adaptive optics ophthalmoscopy are here to stay. Ophthalmic Physiol Opt 2016;36(3):218–39.
[10] Ehlers JP, Dupps WJ, Kaiser PK, et al. The prospective intraoperative and perioperative ophthalmic imaging with optical coherence tomogRaphy (PIONEER) study: 2-year results. Am J Ophthalmol 2014;158(5):999–1007.

[11] Ehlers JP, Goshe J, Dupps WJ, et al. Determination of feasibility and utility of microscope-integrated optical coherence tomography during ophthalmic surgery: the DISCOVER Study RESCAN Results. JAMA Ophthalmol 2015;133(10):1124–32.
[12] Steinkerchner, Megan S, Justis P Ehlers. "The Ins and Outs of Intraoperative Oct." Retina Today, Bryn Mawr Communications, https://retinatoday.com/articles/2021-apr/the-ins-and-outs-of-intraoperative-oct.
[13] Shoughy SS, Arevalo JF, Kozak I. Update on wide- and ultra-widefield retinal imaging. Indian J Ophthalmol 2015;63(7):575–81.
[14] Silva PS, Cavallerano JD, Haddad NM, et al. Peripheral lesions identified on ultrawide field imaging predict increased risk of diabetic retinopathy progression over 4 Years. Ophthalmology 2015;122(5):949–56.
[15] Tripathy K, Chawla R, Wadekar BR, et al. Evaluation of rhegmatogenous retinal detachments using Optos ultrawide field fundus fluorescein angiography and comparison with ETDRS 7 field overlay. J Curr Ophthalmol 2018;30(3):263–7.
[16] Quinn N, Csincsik L, Flynn E, et al. The clinical relevance of visualising the peripheral retina. Prog Retin Eye Res 2019;68:83–109.
[17] Wessel MM, Aaker GD, Parlitsis G, et al. Ultra-wide-field angiography improves the detection and classification of diabetic retinopathy. Retina 2012;32(4):785–91.
[18] Arora R, Goel R, Kumar S, et al. Evaluation of SARS-CoV-2 in tears of patients with moderate to severe COVID-19. Ophthalmology 2020; https://doi.org/10.1016/j.ophtha.2020.08.029.
[19] Kong M, Lee MY, Ham DI. Ultrawide-field fluorescein angiography for evaluation of diabetic retinopathy. Korean J Ophthalmol 2012;26(6):428–31.
[20] Tsui I, Williams BK, Kok YO, et al. Reliability of ischemic index grading in common retinal vascular diseases. Ophthalmic Surg Lasers Imaging Retina 2015;46(6):618–25.
[21] Talks SJ, Manjunath V, Steel DH, et al. New vessels detected on wide-field imaging compared to two-field and seven-field imaging: implications for diabetic retinopathy screening image analysis. Br J Ophthalmol 2015;99(12):1606–9.
[22] Ting DSW, Pasquale LR, Peng L, et al. Artificial intelligence and deep learning in ophthalmology. Br J Ophthalmol 2019;103(2):167–75.
[23] Chueh KM, Hsieh YT, Chen HH, et al. Identification of sex and age from macular optical coherence tomography and feature analysis using deep learning. Am J Ophthalmol 2021;235:221–8.
[24] Godara P, Dubis AM, Roorda A, et al. Adaptive optics retinal imaging: emerging clinical applications. Optom Vis Sci 2010;87(12):930–41.
[25] Zaleska-Żmijewska A, Wawrzyniak ZM, Dąbrowska A, et al. Adaptive Optics (rtx1) high-resolution imaging of photoreceptors and retinal arteries in patients with diabetic retinopathy. J Diabetes Res 2019;2019:9548324.
[26] Shahid K, Kolomeyer AM, Nayak NV, et al. Ocular telehealth screenings in an urban community. Telemed J E Health 2012;18(2):95–100.
[27] Kolomeyer AM, Baumrind BR, Szirth BC, et al. Fundus autofluorescence and colour fundus imaging compared during telemedicine screening in patients with diabetes. J Telemed Telecare 2013;19(4):209–12.
[28] "Retinopathy of Prematurity." National Eye Institute, U.S. Department of Health and Human Services, 10 July 2019, https://www.nei.nih.gov/learn-about-eye-health/eye-conditions-and-diseases/retinopathy-prematurity.
[29] Quinn GE, Ying GS, Daniel E, et al. Validity of a telemedicine system for the evaluation of acute-phase retinopathy of prematurity. JAMA Ophthalmol 2014;132(10):1178–84.

# Glaucoma

Advances in Ophthalmology and Optometry 7 (2022) 253–261

ADVANCES IN OPHTHALMOLOGY AND OPTOMETRY

# 30-Gauge Needle in Glaucoma/ Anterior Segment Management

Ramesh Ayyala, MD, Alireza Baradaran-Rafii, MD*, Jacob Liechty, MD

Department of Ophthalmology, University of South Florida College of Medicine, 13330 USF Laurel Drive, Tampa, FL 33612, USA

**Keywords**

• 30-Gauge • Needle • Glaucoma • Anterior segment • Slit lamp • Needling • Bleb

**Key points**

- As a surgeon, many procedures can be carried out at the slit lamp.
- An opportunity exists for cost savings and better patient care by optimizing slit lamp-based procedures.
- Numerous glaucoma and anterior segment-related complications can be managed via the use of a 30-gauge needle at the slit lamp.
- Sterility should be well maintained outside of a controlled operating room setting to ensure adequate patient outcomes.

**Video content accompanies this article at http://www.advancesinophthalmology.com.**

## INTRODUCTION

Many clinical presentations of acute glaucoma and complications of glaucoma exist, whether acute or chronic, along with anterior segment surgery (bleb fibrosis, encapsulation, and so forth) that can be managed at the slit lamp with the help of a 30 gauge (G) needle. This article presents the indications and techniques involved in the use of a 30G needle at the slit lamp in the management of a myriad of ophthalmologic presentations and complications.

*Corresponding author. *E-mail address:* alirezab@usf.edu

https://doi.org/10.1016/j.yaoo.2022.05.001

## PREPARATION OF THE PATIENT

Any manipulation on the ocular surface, especially manipulation within the eye itself, should be performed in a sterile fashion. Typically, after instilling topical anesthetic drops, an eyelid speculum is placed to allow for adequate exposure of the ocular surface. Betadine 5.0% to 7.5% is applied on the ocular surface for 3 to 5 minutes. Sterile gloves are then donned, and the relevant manipulation is performed (Video 1).

## FOLLOW-UP AFTER SLIT LAMP PROCEDURES

Infection is a concern after any ocular surface or intraocular procedure, so special care should be taken when performing these manipulations outside of a more controlled operating room environment. These patients should be followed up closely especially in the first week after manipulation. Patients should be educated regarding the signs and symptoms of infection or any other potential complication that may happen including choroidal effusion or choroidal hemorrhage. Of note, the entry site into the subconjunctival space should be cauterized to prevent leakage from that area.

## INDICATIONS AND PROCEDURE DESCRIPTION

### Bleb needling revision for scarred, fibrosed blebs

Glaucoma surgeries that divert the aqueous into the subconjunctival space include trabeculectomy, Express shunt, Xen implant, and the various glaucoma drainage devices (GDDs). The leading cause for failure of these surgeries is over fibrosis (either subconjunctival or subscleral) in the process of healing. The degree of fibrosis usually is worse in patients who are young, of African heritage, and in eyes with underlying inflammation. This heightened fibrosis can be addressed via a simple 3-minute procedure performed at the slit lamp using a 30G needle. Dissection of the subconjunctival fibrosis and lifting of the scleral flap often leads to successful bleb formation and intraocular pressure (IOP) reduction.

Procedure: Following Betadine and Lidogel (2.8% lidocaine hydrochloride) preparation, the patient is positioned at the slit lamp with a lid speculum to aid in keeping the lids apart. Using high magnification, the area in question is studied carefully to identify the edges of the scleral flap. I like to move the overlying conjunctiva with a cotton tip applicator to help differentiate subscleral fibrosis from subconjunctival fibrosis. If the overlying conjunctiva moves freely, then the failure is from subscleral fibrosis. If the conjunctive is immobile and firmly attached to the flap area, then failure could be from both the subconjunctival scar tissue formation along with subscleral fibrosis. In some situations, the overlying conjunctiva is so injected that the flap may not be readily identified. In these instances, I recommend applying a drop of 10% phenylephrine in order to blanch the superficial blood vessels. Another helpful tip when hunting for the scleral flap is to use the location of the iridectomy as a guide. The scleral flap should lie within 1 to 2 mm on either side of the iridectomy.

A bent 30G needle is entered into the subconjunctival space usually 10 mm away from the filtering bleb. Areas with large blood vessels should be avoided because it can lead to subconjunctival hemorrhage. The needle is gently advanced into the area of fibrosis and adhesions are removed via sweeping movements. Once the conjunctiva has been freed up, attention is paid to the scleral flap. The needle tip is advanced to lift the edge of the scleral flap and, sometimes, the anterior chamber may be entered as well. It is at this stage that bleb formation should be appreciated. I prefer to inject antifibrosing agents such as Mitomycin C (MMC) subconjunctivally and superiorly to the bleb in order to reduce the likelihood of recurrent fibrosis. This procedure may be repeated several times with a 50% success rate at 2 years [1]. This rate of success leads many to think that this simple, in-office procedure should at least be attempted before taking the patient back to the operating room. Technique is not the only factor at play because the timing of needling also plays an important role in whether or not you will have a successful outcome. It is thought that needling a failing bleb has a higher likelihood for success as compared with needling a bleb that has already failed completely. Therefore, bleb surveillance after trabeculectomy or GDD surgery is very important. In the case of an established, thick subconjunctival scar, the chance of success may be less than a thin, early fibrosing membrane. Of note, the entrance area of the needle should be cauterized after needling; otherwise, leakage from that area may continue [1].

Published literature: Although the procedure seems to be effective, inconsistencies exist in IOP reduction and complication occurrence among the published literature. In a meta-analysis including 37 studies with a total of 2182 patients, the overall effect of bleb needling at the last visit revealed a reduction in IOP of 9.74 mm Hg (95% confidence interval [CI] [8.85, 10.63]), a complete success rate of 45.9% (95% CI [39.0%, 53.0%]), and a qualified success rate of 70.4% (95% CI [63.5%, 77.0%]) [2]. Application of MMC and 5-fluorouracil (5-FU) during the procedure was efficacious for IOP control during the follow-up. Their metaregression revealed that the possible origination of heterogeneity was baseline IOP before bleb needling, which revealed a trend that higher baseline IOP correlated with a greater IOP reduction result ($P < .001$). The procedure seems to be safe although conjunctival hemorrhage (5.7%, 95% CI [2.5%, 10.1%]), hyphema (5.5%, 95% CI [3.0%, 8.7%]) and bleb leakage (5.0%, 95% CI [3.2%, 7.3%]) had the highest estimated incidence [2]. A relationship seemed to exist between the number of times that needling was performed and the overall risk of needling failure, although it is unclear whether this is correlation or causation. Overall, it seems that bleb needling with antimetabolites should be considered an effective and safe procedure after trabeculectomy failure. After the process, patients will gain IOP reduction and reduce antiglaucoma medications for at least 6 months with MMC or 5-FU (Video 2) [2].

Role of MMC injection during bleb revision: It is important to not allow the MMC to enter the anterior chamber. This can lead to severe iritis/iris pigment shedding and corneal decompensation from MMC induced toxicity.

Therefore, when we inject MMC at the same time as bleb needling, we opt to inject less than 0.1 cc of 0.4 mg/cc MMC superior to the revised bleb. The other option that one has is to perform the MMC injection first followed a week later by the actual bleb revision [3].

### Bleb needling revision for encapsulating/encapsulated blebs following Ahmed glaucoma valve implantation

In addition to needling of fibrosed trabeculectomy blebs, needling with or without subconjunctival injection of antifibrosing agents can be done for encapsulating/encapsulated blebs after GDD implantation. Bleb encapsulation is most prominent after Ahmed glaucoma valve (AGV) implantation during or following the hypertensive phase. In this situation, a 30G needle is used to puncture the conjunctiva nearly 1 cm away from the bleb (usually from the 12 o'clock position) and then advanced toward and ultimately into the encapsulated bleb. Sweeping movements are then used to disrupt the encapsulated collagen bleb.

Bleb reformation should be appreciated if the encapsulation has been adequately disrupted. This then is followed by injection of MMC into the subconjunctival space. In the case of valved plates such as AGV, MMC (0.4 mg/cc) can be safely injected into the bleb space because the valve mechanism will prevent the MMC from migrating into the anterior chamber. However, in non-valved drainage devices such as a Baerveldt implant, these substances should only be injected into the subconjunctival space but not the bleb space. Injecting MMC into the bleb space may lead to migration into the anterior chamber, which, as already detailed, is highly toxic and detrimental to the structures of the anterior chamber. Again, after this manipulation, the conjunctival entrance site should be cauterized (Video 3). If the size of the bleb fails to enlarge following the needling procedure, especially in eyes where the bleb is flat to begin with, it may indicate that the valve mechanism itself has been obstructed with fibrous tissue. This situation will not respond to needling and needs blebectomy and revision of the AGV. In a retrospective study on 27 eyes of 27 patients who underwent needling bleb revision with adjuvant MMC performed at the slit lamp, there were 12 eyes with encapsulated blebs and 15 eyes with flat blebs. The mean interval between index filtering surgery and bleb revision was 32.74 ± 15.36 months. Mean IOP was 25.07 ± 4.80 mm Hg before surgery and 19.66 ± 4.97 mm Hg at last postoperative follow-up. The mean follow-up was 20.31 ± 15.63 months. Complete and qualified successes were 7.4% and 51.9%, respectively. Cumulative rates of success at 1, 2, 3, and 4 years were 76%, 65%, 49%, and 37%, respectively. The mean number of antiglaucoma medications was reduced from 3.15 ± 0.36 preoperatively to 2.33 ± 1.21 postoperatively ($P$<.001) [4].

Furthermore, in a prospective, observational study on consecutive patients with medically uncontrolled primary open-angle glaucoma (POAG) with AGV encapsulation or fibrosis and inadequate IOP control, bleb needling with 5-FU injection (0.1 cc of 50 mg/cc) was performed at the slit-lamp.

Thirty-six patients with an encapsulated or fibrotic AGV underwent 67 procedures (mean 1.86 ± 0.83). Complete success, defined as IOP $\leq$ 18 mm Hg without medications, was obtained in 25% at 24 months of observation. The cumulative proportion of cases achieving either qualified (IOP $\leq$ 18 mm Hg with medications) or complete success at 24 months of observation was 72.2%. The authors concluded that needling over the plate of an AGV supplemented with 5-FU is an effective and safe choice in a significant proportion of POAG patients with elevated IOP due to encapsulation or fibrosis [5,6].

## Paracentesis to decrease intraocular pressure

### *Acute angle-closure glaucoma*

Acute angle-closure glaucoma is an ophthalmic emergency and should be treated promptly with eye pressure reduction. Standard teaching suggests YAG peripheral iridotomy (PI) along with topical, oral, and intravenous pressure lowering agents. Oftentimes, the eyes may be slow to respond or may not respond at all to this line of treatment. All the while, the patient is sick from elevated eye pressure, and the optic nerve will continue to be damaged. The quickest way to reduce the eye pressure and break the attack is this simple 3-step procedure:

Step 1: Prepare and position the patient at the slit lamp. A 30 g needle with an open hub is used to enter the anterior chamber via clear cornea as close to the limbus as possible. Once entered, the needle is held in place long enough for a few drops of aqueous to escape. This is followed by the removal of the needle. In some instances, one can perform an iridotomy with the needle tip. Moreover, should the patient have a pupillary membrane or pupillary block mechanism, synechial adhesions and the pupillary membrane can be broken with the needle, thus helping to resolve the attack. At the end of the procedure, the IOP is invariably reduced to low teens and the attack is broken. From the patient's perspective, the pain is resolved, and the cornea clears immediately.

Step 2: Peripheral argon laser iridoplasty is performed to peel the iris from the angle structures. YAG-laser peripheral iridectomy can be performed at the same time if desired or during a follow-up visit.

Step 3: Two to 4 weeks after the eye is quiet, cataract extraction with intraocular lens (IOL) placement and gonio synechiolysis then is performed (Video 4).

Acute glaucoma may also arise from secondary causes such as post cataract surgery, neovascular glaucoma, uveitic glaucoma, and sometimes following laser procedures (YAG capsulotomy), laser trabeculoplasty (argon laser trabeculoplasty or selective laser trabeculoplasty). In all these situations, the IOP can be temporally controlled via paracentesis using the 30G needle. It is important that this is followed by procedures that can lead to permanent pressure reduction.

## Anterior chamber reformation

One of the most common procedures at the slit lamp is anterior chamber reformation. This may be needed after trabeculectomy or GDD implantation due to over filtration of the bleb resulting in a flat anterior chamber. In these cases, the anterior chamber may be reformed using ophthalmic viscosurgical devices or an air bubble. This can be repeated several times before definitive measures, such as tube ligation or scleral flap suturing, can be done (Video 5).

## Suturing at the slit lamp

Suturing the bleb can be performed easily at the slit lamp when indicated. This requires proper instruments (2 jeweler's forceps, small needle driver, Vannes scissors, and 10-0 nylon), good anesthesia (Lidogel application 5 minutes before procedure), and understanding from the patient that they will stay still and remain calm during the procedure. While suturing, hand stability can be achieved by resting the surgeon's surgical hand edge or fingers on the patient's cheek. There are times when the patient's nose or the slit lamp headrest belt may prove to be a better alternative. The slit beam should be fully opened, and the magnification set at its lowest to get the widest field of view. An assistant should be available to hand over the required instruments during the procedure.

Hypotony from over filtering bleb: This condition requires closure of the scleral flap with a mattress suture (or individual sutures). The necessary technique for correction involves the placement of transconjunctival scleral bites 2 mm temporal to the scleral flap in such a way that it will exit through the middle of the scleral flap. A second bite is taken through the middle of the scleral flap to exit on the medial aspect of the flap. The direction is then reversed, and the exact same process is repeated in the opposite direction such that the needle ends up next to the original scleral bite. The tightness of the mattress suture is adjusted gently to regulate the IOP [7].

Eye pain from large over hanging bleb: On occasion a bleb can grow large enough to begin trapping air every time the patient blinks, leading to eye pain and tearing. This can be controlled with the placement of mattress suture as described above with the exception that I prefer to place the sutures in the figure of 8 formation to maximize the compression effect in this situation versus a mattress suture that is placed parallel to the limbus in the case of hypotony.

Leaky blebs: Leaky blebs can sometimes be repaired at the slit lamp. This is especially true if the leak is at the limbus and is discovered in the immediate postoperative period.

## Suture removal

As a routine procedure, suture removal is done at the slit lamp. Some surgeons even use releasable sutures during trabeculectomy or GDD implantation. In these cases, sutures can be initially cut using 30G needle followed by removal using a jeweler's forceps.

## Injections

Subconjunctival, subtenon, and intraocular injections are among different procedures that can be performed via a 30G needle. Of note, MMC, 5-FU, bevacizumab, and other substances can be injected once or multiple times subconjunctivally before or after trabeculectomy in order to increase the chance of success. Typically, these substances are injected close to the filtering bleb. Extended-release steroids including methylprednisolone and triamcinolone also can be injected into the subtenon's space. For the treatment of infectious blebitis or suture abscess, antibiotics can be injected subconjunctivally via a 30G needle (Video 6).

### Ahmed glaucoma valve removal

Sometimes, after GDD surgeries, the tube or plate can become exposed. If these GDD implants are still working, then they typically will be repaired in the operating room by repositioning of the tube or plate, scleral/pericardial patch graft, and rotational/advancement conjunctival flap or free conjunctival graft. However, in some cases, GDD is no longer effective and severe foreign body sensation, irritation, redness, and the risk of endophthalmitis leads the surgeon to remove them. In these cases, using scissors and appropriate forceps, the tube or plate or both can be removed at the slit lamp. If the conjunctival wound is large enough, conjunctival suturing then can be performed at the slit lamp (Video 7).

### Unplugging sclerotomy

Iris tissue sometimes can block the trabeculectomy site or opening of the GDD and lead to acute pressure spikes. This easily can be addressed at the slit lamp using a 30G needle. The iris tissue can be swept away from the clogged site with a gentle tugging motion.

Before initiating the procedure, have the nurse or technician hold the patient's head firmly against the slit lamp head band and warn the patient to expect some degree of pain during the procedure. I oftentimes reassure the patient while doing the procedure.

## CORNEAL PROCEDURES

### DSEAK-related issues and 30G needle

Descemet Stripping Automated Endothelial Keratoplasty (DSAEK) graft dehiscence is not uncommon in eyes with prior glaucoma surgery, especially, GDDs. Surgeons can prevent the air bubble from escaping out of the GDD tube by simply ligating the tube in the anterior chamber (AC) via a clear cornea paracentesis and a 10-0 Prolene suture. If that fails or if graft dehiscence occurs in spite of tube ligation, then the graft can be refloated at the slit lamp using the 30G needle on a 3 cc syringe with an air bubble or an air bubble trapped in Healon. The technique involves priming the 30G needle, and then detaching the needle followed by gentle withdrawal of the plunger and then reattachment of the needle. This allows for air to be trapped in the middle of Healon syringe. The patient is then prepped with betadine and topical anesthetic drops (avoid Lidogel here because it obscures the surgeon's view of the anterior chamber details), the lid speculum is placed, and the patient is positioned at the slit lamp. Study the anterior chamber and locate the graft edge. The needle is then introduced through clear cornea close to the limbus (preferably from the superotemporal side) and the AC is entered in such a way that the needle tip is behind the detached graft. Using the needle tip, the graft is centered, and then the Healon-air-Healon combo is injected into the AC. The patient should be warned that they will experience a sudden increase in eye pressure, and their head should be supported to prevent head movement. Before the needle is withdrawn, be sure to center the graft. As the needle is withdrawn, it is important to apply pressure with a cotton tip applicator to the corneal entry site to prevent air escape. The procedure is followed by placing the patient in a supine position for 30 minutes before discharge. The patient should be instructed to lie flat in bed as much as possible for 3 to 4 days before reexamination in the clinic. The procedure can be repeated as many times as is needed until the graft is nicely attached. One should monitor the eye pressure during the follow-up period.

Angle-closure glaucoma following DSAEK: Sometimes, after DSAEK or DMEK surgery, patients can present with severe pain due to pupillary block from the air bubble migrating behind the pupil, leading to angle-closure glaucoma and iris bombe. In this situation, a 30G needle may be used to resolve the attack in one of 3 ways:

1. Depress the iris/pupillary margin with the needle to help migrate the air bubble into the anterior chamber.
2. Create a PI.
3. Tap some of the air bubble to break the attack of glaucoma (Video 8).

### Vitreous strand release

Sometimes, after cataract or glaucoma surgery, especially in complicated cases, there may be a vitreous strand that may attach to the wound. It also is possible for a vitreous strand to migrate anteriorly and occlude the drainage tube of a GDD. In these cases, especially when YAG laser is not available, these vitreous strands can be released using a 30G needle. The bent 30G needle should be introduced into the AC via clear cornea from the opposite direction of the vitreous strands. Using the cutting edge of the needle, the vitreous strands are cut and tucked under the pupillary margin (Video 9).

### Astigmatic keratotomy

Significant astigmatism can result from glaucoma surgery. This can be corrected in some cases with astigmatic keratotomy (AK). Generally, trabeculectomy surgery can induce about 0.5 to 1 D of cylinder along the 12 o'clock axis (assuming the surgery was done at 12). The degree of astigmatism is significantly higher in a myopic eye following trabeculectomy surgery. Note that AK should not be attempted on patients with low IOP (<7 mm Hg) because it can result in a gaping incision.

Procedure: The astigmatic axis and degree are measured using corneal topography. One or 2 paired incisions are performed 2 mm inside the limbus measuring 4 to 6 mm in an arcuate fashion. The nomogram is as follows: paired incisions 2 mm inside the limbus for astigmatism up to 1.5 D and 2 paired incisions for greater than 1.5 D. I prefer the 15 D sharp blade for the procedure. It gives me the option to deepen the cut to 90% depth by simply examining the incision depth, which easily can be appreciated at the slit lamp.

Other indications: Rotating a toric IOL is another procedure that can be done at the slit lamp. Postoperative rotation is a known, potential complication when implanting a toric IOL. These IOLs can be rotated and repositioned at the slit lamp in the early postoperative period in order to decrease the residual astigmatism (Video 10).

## SUMMARY

In conclusion, many procedures exist that can be performed economically and safely at the slit lamp. This article has demonstrated the different indications for these procedures and how to properly perform them with the use of a 30G needle. Care should always be taken to maintain sterility when performing procedures outside of a more controlled operating room environment.

### Disclosure

The authors have nothing to disclose.

## SUPPLEMENTARY DATA

Supplementary data related to this article can be found online at https://doi.org/10.1016/j.yaoo.2022.05.001.

### References

[1] Feyi-Waboso A, Ejere HO. Needling for encapsulated trabeculectomy filtering blebs. Cochrane Database Syst Rev 2012;2012(8):CD003658.

[2] Chen X, Suo L, Hong Y, et al. Safety and Efficacy of Bleb Needling with Antimetabolite after Trabeculectomy Failure in Glaucoma Patients: A Systemic Review and Meta-Analysis. J Ophthalmol 2020;2020:4310258.

[3] Halili A, Kessel L, Subhi Y, et al. Needling after trabeculectomy - does augmentation by antimetabolites provide better outcomes and is Mitomycin C better than 5-Fluoruracil? A systematic review with network meta-analyses. Acta Ophthalmol 2020;98(7):643–53.

[4] Amini H, Esmaili A, Zarei R, et al. Office-based slit-lamp needle revision with adjunctive mitomycin-C for late failed or encapsulated filtering blebs. Middle East Afr J Ophthalmol 2012;19(2):216–21.

[5] Erdem B, Imamoglu S, Ercalik NY. Needling with 5-fluorouracil for encapsulated blebs after Ahmed glaucoma valve implantation. Cutan Ocul Toxicol 2019;38(4):395–400.

[6] Thomas M, Boese EA, Lieu P, et al. Slit-lamp Pars Plana Needle Hyaloidotomy-Zonulotomy-Iridotomy for the Treatment of Spontaneous Malignant Glaucoma. J Glaucoma 2020;29(5):e31–2.

[7] Letartre L, Basheikh A, Anctil JL, et al. Transconjunctival suturing of the scleral flap for overfiltration with hypotony maculopathy after trabeculectomy. Can J Ophthalmol 2009;44(5):567–70.

# Neuro-ophthalmology

Advances in Ophthalmology and Optometry 7 (2022) 263–278

ADVANCES IN OPHTHALMOLOGY AND OPTOMETRY

# Screening for Plaquenil

Pushpinder Kanda, MD, PhD[a,*],
Stuart Coupland, PhD[a,b], Chloe Gottlieb, MD[a,b],
Lynca Kantungane, COMT[a], Rustum Karanjia, MD[a,b,c,d]

[a]Department of Ophthalmology, Faculty of Medicine, University of Ottawa, Ottawa, Ontario, Canada; [b]Ottawa Hospital Research Institute, The Ottawa Hospital, Ottawa, Ontario, Canada; [c]Doheny Eye Institute, Los Angeles, CA, USA; [d]Doheny Eye Centers UCLA, Department of Ophthalmology, David Geffen School of Medicine at UCLA, Los Angeles, CA, USA

**Keywords**

• Automated visual fields • Bull's eye maculopathy • Fundus autofluorescence
• Hydroxychloroquine • Multifocal electroretinogram
• Optical coherence tomography • Plaquenil screening • Retinopathy

**Key points**

- Retinal function abnormalities from Plaquenil toxicity precedes structural damage.
- Structural metrics like spectral-domain optical coherence tomography (sdOCT) are less sensitive for detecting early retinopathy compared with functional metrics like multifocal electroretinograms (mfERGs) or automated visual fields (AVFs).
- AVF is an objective test and provides unreliable results for detecting early retinopathy. The 2020 Royal College of Ophthalmologists (United Kingdom) guideline does not recommend AVF as the primary screening modality.
- Clinically, mfERG is the only objective test available to measure retinal function but has been used as an ancillary test primarily due to limited accessibility.
- mfERG should be considered as one of the primary screening tools as innovation continues to make the test faster, more reliable, and accessible.

## INTRODUCTION

Chloroquine (CQ) and hydroxychloroquine (HCQ, or Plaquenil; a less toxic metabolite of CQ) were initially introduced as an antimalarial treatment, but the anti-inflammatory and immunomodulatory properties have expanded their

*Corresponding author. University of Ottawa Eye Institute, The Ottawa Hospital, General Campus, 501 Smyth Road, Ottawa, Ontario K1H 8L6, Canada. *E-mail address:* pkanda@toh.ca

https://doi.org/10.1016/j.yaoo.2022.03.013

use in treating various rheumatological and dermatologic diseases including systemic lupus erythematosus, rheumatoid arthritis, Sjögren syndrome, and porphyria cutanea tarda [1]. Compared with other disease-modifying immunomodulatory drugs, HCQ has become the mainstay treatment for these rheumatological conditions because of its low cost and favorable side-effect profile. Despite its therapeutic benefits, retinal toxicity is a clinically significant side effect that must be carefully monitored by physicians [2]. The pathophysiology of HCQ/CQ-induced retinal toxicity remains unclear and is summarized in Fig. 1 [3,4]. Although pathogenesis is thought to begin at the level of retinal pigment epithelium (RPE), animal histopathological studies suggest that early degeneration starts in ganglion and photoreceptor cells followed by secondary RPE atrophy [5]. Overall, the sequelae of toxicity results in the characteristic fundus appearance of bilateral bull's eye maculopathy, which appears as a parafoveal depigmented ring lesion (Fig. 2).

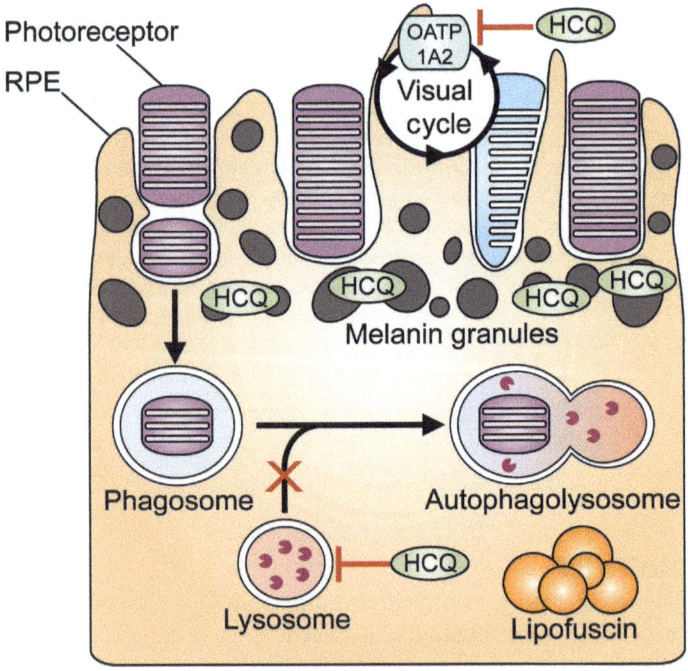


**Fig. 1.** Mechanism of HCQ-induced retinopathy. HCQ (or CQ) binds to melanin and accumulates within the retinal pigment epithelium (RPE). HCQ causes increased lysosome pH, which inhibits lysosomal enzyme activity and fusion with phagosomes. This inhibition of autophagy prevents the degeneration of phagocytosed outer-photoreceptor segments resulting in the accumulation of toxic cellular byproducts like lipofuscin. HCQ/CQ also inhibits the organic anion transporting polypeptide (OATP) 1A2 causing extracellular accumulation of all-trans-retinol, which may disrupt the visual cycle pathway and cause cellular toxicity.

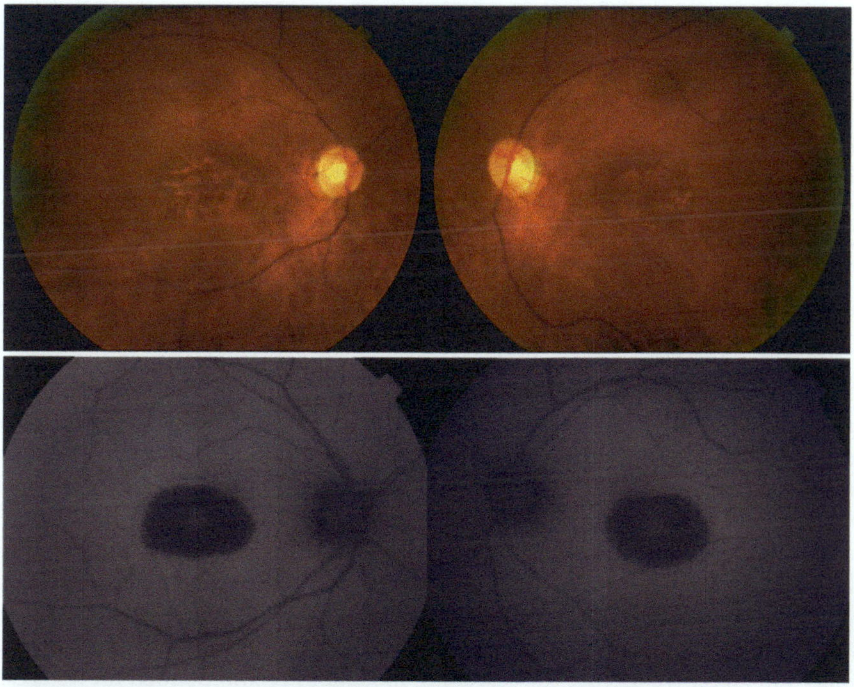

**Fig. 2.** Severe HCQ retinopathy. Top panels show the fundus photograph of bilateral bull's eye maculopathy in an advanced case of HCQ toxicity. Bottom panels are the corresponding FAF images showing ring of reduced autofluorescence in the parafoveal region.

Population studies show that the risk of HCQ retinopathy has an overall prevalence of 7.5% but varies depending on the dose and duration of therapy [2]. When the dose exceeds 5.0 mg/kg, the prevalence can reach 20% after 10 years or 50% after 20 years [2]. Even patients on HCQ $\leq$5 mg/kg (real body weight) are at risk for toxicity with the prevalence increasing from less than 1% risk within the first 5 years, to 2% risk at 10 years, and increasing to almost 20% after 20 years [2]. Although a true safe dose for long-term use may not exist, the American Academy of Ophthalmology (AAO) statement outlines risk factors for developing retinal toxicity as summarized in Table 1 [6].

Patients with early retinopathy (before visible RPE structural damage) may be asymptomatic or present with paracentral scotoma, but continuous exposure can involve the central fovea causing decreased visual acuity. Interestingly, progression of retinopathy can continue up to 3 to 20 years after cessation of drug in part due to the accumulation of drug within melanin [7,8]. As such, the earliest possible detection of HCQ retinopathy and cessation of therapy is essential to preventing vision loss. The 2016 AAO guidelines have provided recommendations for screening timelines as is summarized in Fig. 3. The primary modality recommended for screening includes both automated visual

**Table 1**
Major risk factors for developing Plaquenil-related retinal toxicity

| | |
|---|---|
| Dose | HCQ >5.0 mg/kg real body weight<br>CQ >2.3 mg/kg real body weight |
| Duration of therapy | >5 y (with no other risk factors) |
| Comorbidities | Renal disease |
| Concomitant medications | Tamoxifen (increases risk of toxicity by 5 folds) |
| Ocular disease | Macular disease |

*Abbreviations:* CQ, chloroquine; HCQ, hydroxychloroquine.

*Adapted from* Marmor MF, Kellner U, Lai TY, Melles RB, Mieler WF; American Academy of Ophthalmology. Recommendations on Screening for Chloroquine and Hydroxychloroquine Retinopathy (2016 Revision). Ophthalmology. 2016 Jun;123(6):1386-94.

field (AVF) and spectral-domain optical coherence tomography (sdOCT). Although sdOCT can provide objective measures of definitive structural changes, this often occurs at a late stage of retinal toxicity. As such, structural metrics are not as sensitive as functional metrics such as AVF or multifocal electroretinogram (mfERG) at detecting early retinopathy [6]. Unlike AVF, which is a subjective test, mfERG provides an objective functional metric of retinal function and some studies suggest it is more sensitive at detecting early toxicity [9]. Despite its clinical utility, the use of mfERG was only recommended as an ancillary test by the AAO, largely due to what was felt to be limited accessibility [6]. Here, we discuss the screening modalities recommended for detecting HCQ retinopathy and explore the utility of using mfERG as a primary screening test while highlighting future trends and avenues for research.

## PLAQUENIL SCREENING MODALITIES

The landscape for HCQ retinopathy screening has evolved over the years because of the improved understanding of pathophysiology, disease prevalence, and the advent of newer technologies to detect structural or functional changes. In 2011, the AAO guideline recommended using AVF as the primary subjective test for screening that should be confirmed with an objective test like sdOCT or mfERG. However, the 2016 AAO guideline (see Fig. 3) demoted mfERG as an adjunct test based on limited accessibility, lack of data on test sensitivity/specificity, and in part due to a landmark case-control study that assessed HCQ prevalence and risk factors using primarily AVF and sdOCT [2]. In contrast, the recent Royal College of Ophthalmologist (UK) guidelines include mfERG as the confirmatory test for definite toxicity (Fig. 4). mfERG was deemed especially useful in patients with ambiguous structural changes seen on sdOCT or fundus autofluorescence (FAF) in these updated guidelines [10]. In the absence of a universally accepted gold standard, there remains an ongoing debate regarding which test is the best for confirming early toxicity. As such, a multimodal approach is often required to accurately diagnose HCQ retinopathy. This is especially important when trying to balance the diagnosis of HCQ retinopathy in early stages to prevent vision loss while avoiding premature cessation of a beneficial therapy.

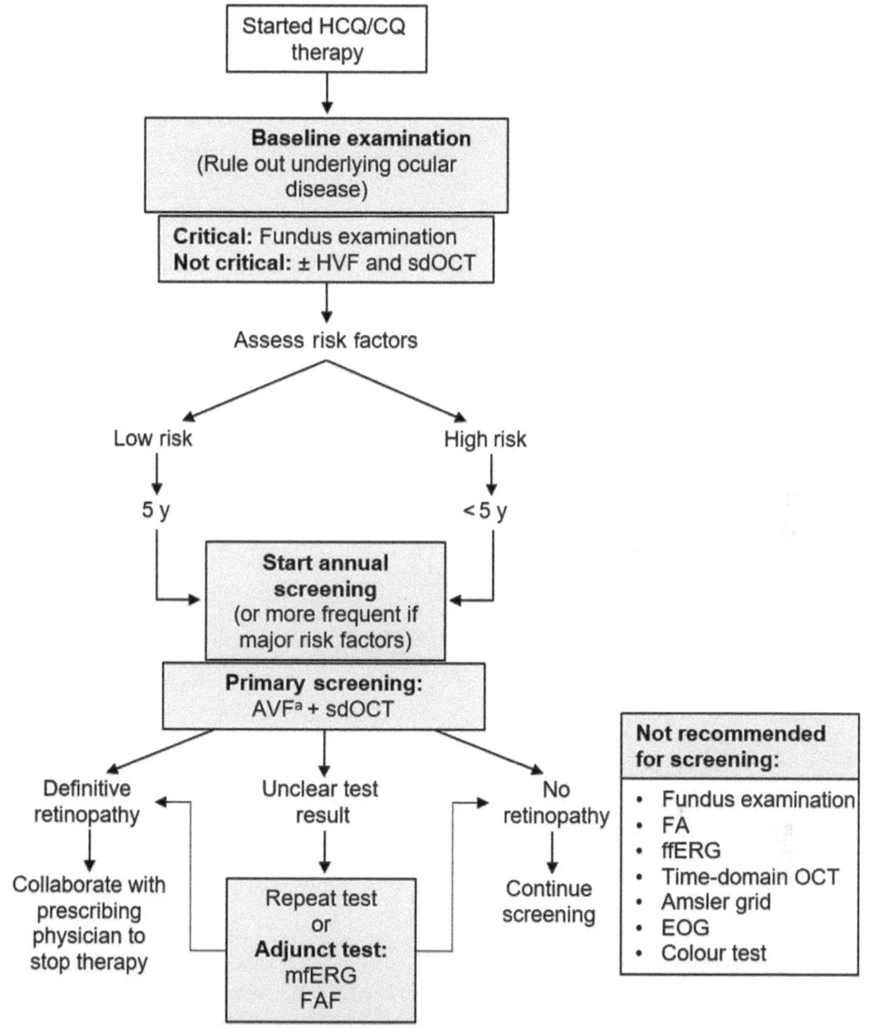


**Fig. 3.** The American Academy of Ophthalmology 2016 Plaquenil screening guideline. [a]10-2 AVF but test should be appropriate for race (24-2 or 30-2 for Asian population). AVF, automated visual fields; CQ, chloroquine; EOG, electrooculogram; FA, fluorescein angiography; FAF, fundus autofluorescence; ffERG, full-field electroretinogram; HCQ, hydroxychloroquine; HVF, humphrey visual field; mfERG, multifocal electroretinogram; OCT, optical coherence tomography; sdOCT, spectral-domain optical coherence tomography.

## AUTOMATED VISUAL FIELDS

AVF is a functional test that can detect retinopathy earlier than structural changes; however, results can be unreliable in 17% to 33% of cases, and no specific definition for HCQ-related field defects especially for early toxicity exists

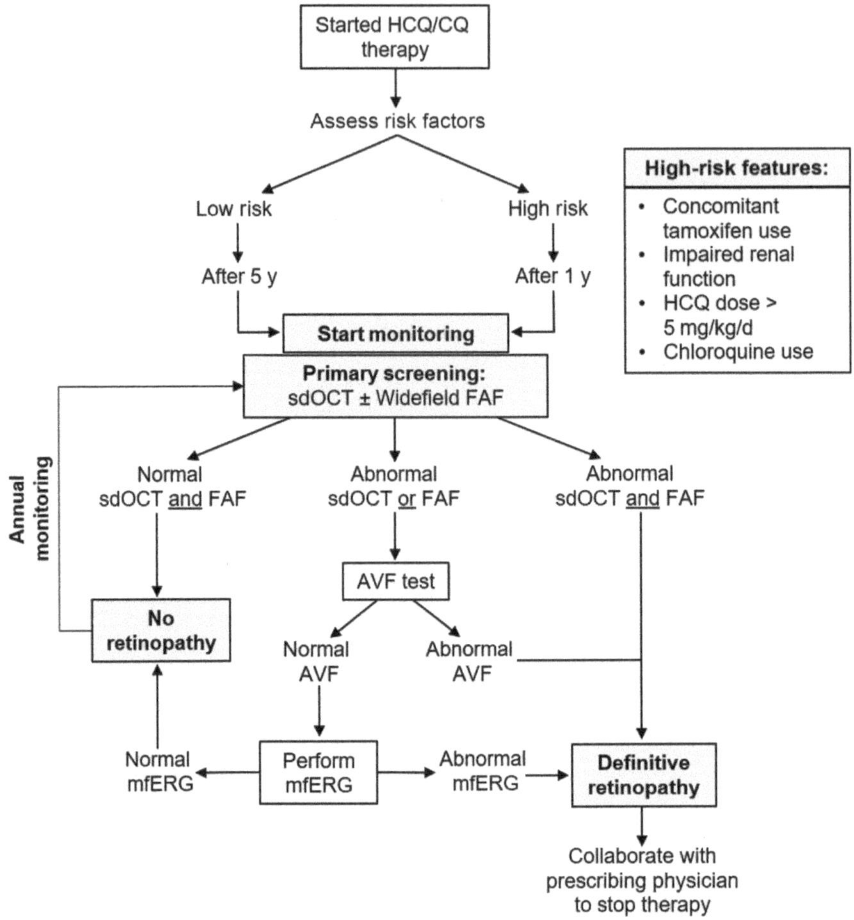


**Fig. 4.** Royal College of Ophthalmologists hydroxychloroquine and chloroquine retinopathy monitoring algorithm (2020). AVF, automated visual fields; CQ, chloroquine; EOG, electrooculogram; FAF, fundus autofluorescence; HCQ, hydroxychloroquine; mfERG, multifocal electroretinogram; sdOCT, spectral-domain optical coherence tomography. (*Adapted from* Yusuf IH, Foot B, Lotery AJ. The Royal College of Ophthalmologists recommendations on monitoring for hydroxychloroquine and chloroquine users in the United Kingdom (2020 revision): executive summary. Eye (Lond). 2021 Jun;35(6):1532-1537.)

[11,12]. Definitive toxicity on 10-2 AVF is classically characterized by parafoveal ring or partial ring scotoma with early damage appearing as patchy parafoveal depression or nonspecific scattered defects that are persistent on repeat testing (Fig. 5) [7,13]. For the Asian population, wider field tests (ie, 24-2 or 30-2) are required to capture more peripheral pericentral toxicity [14]. Some authors suggest using a dimmer red-target over a white-target stimuli to improve sensitivity for early retinopathy but this comes at the expense of diminishing specificity and consistency [15]. Current guidelines recommend that nonspecific

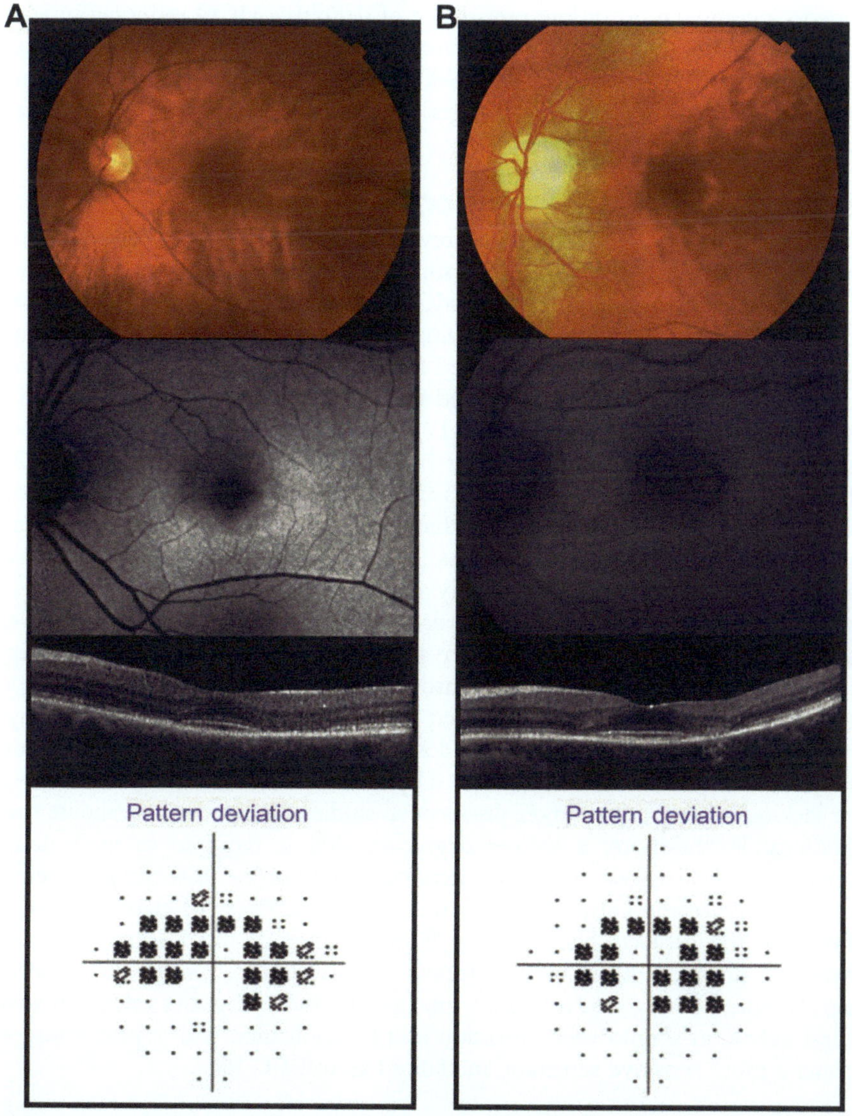


**Fig. 5.** Early to mild HCQ retinopathy. (*A*) Patient with early HCQ toxicity with subtle bull's eye maculopathy on fundus photo, early FAF changes (increased parafoveal autofluorescence), flying saucer sign on sdOCT, and partial ring scotoma on HVF (10-2). (*B*) Patient with a more evident maculopathy on fundus photo, decreased autofluorescence on FAF, flying saucer sign on sdOCT, and a complete ring scotoma on HVF.

visual field defects should prompt either repeat visual field testing, or usage of another objective functional test like mfERG to confirm retinopathy [6]. Conversely, the Royal College of Ophthalmologists 2020 guidelines (based on UK data) no longer recommend AVF as the primary screening test partially due to a combination of low prevalence of definitive HCQ retinopathy (1.6% UK population), low risk of retinopathy in the first 5 years, increasing health care costs due to repeating unreliable AVF tests, and needing adjunct confirmatory tests [10]. Whether these changes are adopted by future AAO guidelines remains to be seen.

## SPECTRAL-DOMAIN OPTICAL COHERENCE TOMOGRAPHY

sdOCT is an objective test that has revolutionized screening by providing reliable and definitive morphologic distinction between normal and abnormal retina. The characteristic finding on sdOCT includes bilateral loss of parafoveal ellipsoid zone, which appears as a flying saucer sign (see Fig. 5) [16]. Although specificity of 98.1% has been reported for sdOCT, its sensitivity to detect retinopathy is significantly less compared with AVF and mfERG (78.6% sdOCT vs 85.7% AVF vs 92.9% mfERG) [17]. As such, many studies have demonstrated that functional deficits occur before structural alterations [7,9,18–20]. By using mfERG as a sensitive measure for early retinopathy, a few studies have characterized early structural changes on sdOCT that precede clinically visible retinopathy or visual field loss [21–23]. Borrelli and colleagues demonstrated that patient without clinically detectable retinopathy has significantly thinner outer and inner nuclear layer and these morphologic changes were significantly associated with electrophysiological changes on mfERG [21]. Similarly, Garrity and colleagues demonstrated that attenuation of ellipsoid zone (ie, thinning, depression, or increased granularity) represented early changes on sdOCT that preceded visual field loss but corroborated with mfERG testing [22]. However, these studies are limited by either small size, retrospective design, or lacking controls, thus larger prospective studies are needed to validate these findings. Furthermore, a greater degree of skill is required to meticulously analyze subtle changes on sdOCT, making it more prone to subjective interpretation. Interpretation also is limited by intratest variability of ellipsoid band reflectivity and artifacts like scanning fragmentation or tilted scans of myopic eyes that produce altered band reflectivity not related to toxicity [22]. Independently, sdOCT may not recognize subclinical retinopathy, but uncertain structural alteration should raise suspicion and be confirmed with repeat testing or using a more sensitive screening modality like mfERG [6].

## FUNDUS AUTOFLUORESCENCE

FAF is a noninvasive imaging modality that measures the endogenous autofluorescence from the RPE, emitted mainly by lipofuscin pigment, and provides functional information regarding cell metabolism and health [24]. Like sdOCT, FAF allows physicians to visualize morphologic abnormalities and allow definitive diagnosis of HCQ retinopathy [7,24]. Earlier changes are characterized by increased parafoveal autofluorescence that is thought to result from accumulation of lipofuscin in RPE due to abnormalities in phagocytosis of outer-photoreceptors or photo-receptor degeneration causing increased phagocytotic activity [7,24]. In later stages of the disease, RPE loss is seen as either a mottled pattern or a complete/partial ring of decreased autofluorescence in the parafoveal region (see Fig. 5); in more severe disease, the fovea and more peripheral rings can be involved [7]. Although FAF is more sensitive than fundoscopy to detect retinopathy, it is considered less sensitive compared with AVF and mfERG and, therefore, recommended as an ancillary test to assist in diagnosis [6,25].

## MULTIFOCAL ELECTRORETINOGRAM

mfERG is an objective functional test, which produces a topographic map of electrophysiological signals generated by photoreceptors, bipolar cells, and to a lesser extent other inner retinal cells (Müller and amacrine cells) [26,27]. It is thought that cellular stress from HCQ produces altered electrophysiological responses that occur before morphologic changes [9]. Toxicity produces depressed signal amplitude and prolonged implicit time in the parafoveal region in early disease while sparing the fovea [9,28]. Signal responses are averaged as concentric rings around central fovea, which is useful for measuring para-perifoveal retinal dysfunction occurring in a concentric fashion while improving the signal-to-noise ratio. The single central hexagon is called ring 1 (R1), and the consecutive concentric hexagon rings are called rings 2 to 5 (R2 to R5) (Fig. 6) [27]. Lyons and colleagues demonstrated that

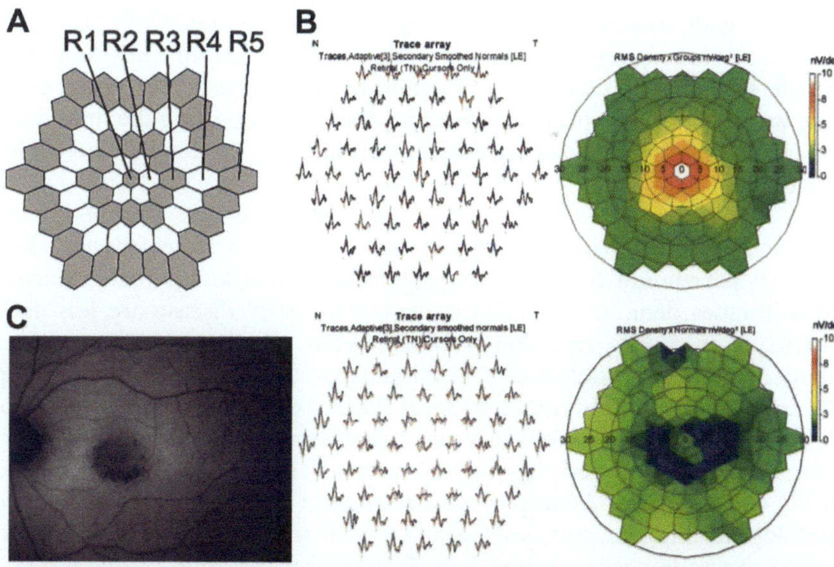


**Fig. 6.** mfERG for HCQ screening. (*A*) Schematic diagram showing the different rings (R1–R5) in a 61-hexagon mfERG stimulus. (*B*) mfERG response waveforms and the corresponding density map of a healthy eye. (*C*) Mottled hypoautofluorescence pattern on FAF with the mfERG showing depressed parafoveal waveforms and response density in a patient with HCQ retinopathy.

age-corrected central hexagon (R1) normalized to concentric hexagon rings (eg, R1/R2, R1/R3, etc) further improved sensitivity, variability, and confidence for interpreting mfERG results [29]. The study also showed that mfERG detects early HCQ retinopathy as most patients with abnormal ring ratios displayed a nonspecific or scattered visual field defect pattern and only a few had characteristic paracentral field defects. mfERG abnormalities were seen in patients with as little as 400g of cumulative HCQ dose [19]. Similarly, multiple studies support the utility of mfERG for detecting early toxicity with an estimated sensitivity ranging from 90% (when compared to AVF as a reference test) to nearly 100% (when compared to 2–3 tests including AVF, FAF, or sdOCT); the sensitivity improves with increased duration of therapy or cumulative dose [9,17–19,25,30,31]. When directly comparing the use of mfERG to the AAO 2016 screening guidelines (ie, using sdOCT + AVF as primary screening tests), mfERG demonstrated a remarkable sensitivity of 100% with a specificity of 78% [31]. In addition, 23 eyes with normal sdOCT or AVF had abnormal mfERG and were likely to represent early retinopathy. These results corroborated with a systematic review that analyzed 23 studies and demonstrated that mfERG had the greatest proportion of positive results with robust sensitivity [9]. The report also showed high rates of "false-positive" cases (mfERG positive but AVF negative) and was proposed to represent subclinical toxicity rather than testing error, because these false-positive cases received higher cumulative HCQ dose compared with true-negative cases (negative mfERG and AVF). Likewise, Bertoli and colleagues showed progressive depression of ring amplitude with increasing HCQ cumulative dose and worsening disease stage (ie, correlating with sdOCT morphologic changes), thereby supporting the notion that false-positive mfERG cases should be considered as having subclinical toxicity [28].

Given that even after drug cessation the degree of disease progression depends on the stage at which retinopathy was detected, early detection of HCQ toxicity is paramount for preventing significant vision loss [7,8,30]. Marmor and colleagues demonstrated that patients with early disease are less likely to progress after drug cessation and have better visual prognosis compared to patients with morphologically visible disease (visible bull's eye maculopathy or significant RPE damage on sdOCT) that can have foveal progression [7]. Some have demonstrated that early detection and cessation of drug (or decreased dose) resulted in the recovery of mfERG signal amplitudes [30,32]. For example, Adamptey and colleagues demonstrated that electrophysiological abnormalities can appear earlier than sdOCT and that recovery of ring amplitude occurred over 3 to 4 years after cessation of therapy [32]. The degree of improvement depended on the stage (or severity) of the disease at which therapy was stopped. Taken together, these studies stress the importance of longitudinal assessment with mfERG for identifying early disease and allow for timely cessation of HCQ therapy to prevent vision loss. As such, mfERG should be considered as one of the primary screening tools for retinopathy and efforts should be directed to technical innovation to improve accessibility.

Similar to AVF, test variability can limit mfERG reliability while the need for specialized equipment, highly qualified personnel to interpret results, and local institute normative data precludes its accessibility [27]. Researchers have started to address some of these limitations to improve test efficacy and bring mfERG one step closer to becoming the ideal screening test. For example, it is well known that the central hexagon (R1) produces a more variable signal amplitude compared with other peripheral rings. As such, some authors have reported improved mfERG reliability and decreased dependency on age correction by normalizing the parafoveal ring (ring 2) amplitude to the peripheral ring 5 [31,33]. Ongoing research continues to optimize factors like decreasing test time and improving signal-to-noise ratio, thereby improving intratest reliability and accessibility [34].

## CURRENT TRENDS AND FUTURE RESEARCH

Exploration of new technologies or modification of existing imaging modalities provides exciting new avenues for diagnosing early HCQ retinopathy with robust sensitivity and specificity. For instance, Tsang and colleagues developed novel 5-ring stimuli, which projected concentric rings onto the retina to precisely match the parafoveal region to improve the signal-to-noise ratio [34]. The 5-ring stimuli performed similar to the traditional 61-hexagon stimuli to detect HCQ-induced electrophysiological abnormalities, but the simplicity of the 5-ring design significantly shortened the test duration to just under 2 minutes. A shorter test duration improves reliability by minimizing the patient fatigue that is responsible for generating signal artifacts via patient movement or fixation loss [26]. Since AVF also is complicated by long test duration, the 5-ring mfERG has the potential to become a good alternative for primary screening, especially for patients who are more prone to fatigue.

Microperimetry (MP) is another type of visual field test but with the additional ability to track the retina for fixation stability and precisely correlate the function with fundus location. Iftikhar and colleagues demonstrated that MP has comparable specificity to mfERG but is less sensitive (73%) for detecting HCQ retinopathy [35]. In contrast, another study demonstrated that MP was in fact more sensitive compared with mfERG but less specific [36]. Moving forward, large-scale prospective studies are needed to establish the role of MP in screening HCQ retinopathy.

Optical coherence tomography angiography is a noninvasive method to characterize retinal vasculature at different retinal depths [37]. Few studies have reported decreased retinal thickness and altered retinal vessel density within the para/perifoveal region after using HCQ; however, some studies presented opposing conclusions [37–39]. Given that some animal studies show that the earliest HCQ-related toxicity occurs within the ganglion cell or photoreceptor layer [5], alterations in superficial and deep capillary plexus may prove useful in detecting early HCQ toxicity but requires further clarification.

The qualitative nature of FAF limits its ability to monitor the subtle progression of retinal disease and is prone to subjective interpretation. As such, quantitative FAF was introduced to measure the intensity of retinal autofluorescence and allow comparison of serial images [40]. A few studies show that this technique may prove useful in HCQ screening by providing a more sensitive longitudinal assessment of early retinopathy [40,41]. An alternative technique called fluorescence lifetime imaging ophthalmoscopy (FLIO) quantifies the average time a fluorophore stays in the excited state and can be used to reflect metabolic changes within retinal tissue [42]. Prolonged FLIO lifetime in parafoveal regions was seen in patients with definitive HCQ retinopathy and also in some patients with no clinically visible disease [42]. Thus, screening with FLIO may provide useful information about early metabolic dysfunction before irreversible structural changes.

Adaptive optics (AO) allows in vivo visualization of cone-cell density and morphology with an optical resolution of less than 2 μm [43]. AO may prove to be another sensitive and subjective method for detecting early HCQ toxicity. One study demonstrated a negative correlation between parafoveal cone cell density and HCQ dose with changes occurring before clinically detectable disease [43]. However, technical advancements still are required as the method is artifact-prone and can produce high number of uninterpretable images or fail to recognize cones in areas of retinal degeneration [43,44].

Retromode imaging of the fundus with an infrared laser is a method for visualizing deep retinal structures including changes occurring within the RPE layer [45]. This imaging modality has been used to clearly visualize pathologies like cystic macular edema, myopic retinoschisis, or drusen in age-related macular degeneration [45]. In patients with HCQ retinopathy, ring-shaped or round-shaped decreased reflectance with prominent deep choroidal vessels can be seen in the para/perifoveal regions [46]. Ahn and colleagues demonstrated that retromode imaging had greater sensitivity compared with FAF in detecting retinopathy, thus it may serve as a useful tool to screen for HCQ toxicity but is limited by its moderate specificity [46].

Artificial intelligence (AI) is an attractive avenue for future research as it has the potential to automate the analysis of a large volume of data, identify subtle test abnormalities, and decrease the dependency on skilled personnel to interpret results. Although AI has proven to be useful in various diagnostic applications in Ophthalmology [47], its application for HCQ screening is lagging. For example, De Silva and colleagues reported that AI can be a powerful tool for objectively and rapidly quantifying ellipsoid zone loss on OCT, especially for subtle cases in early retinopathy that can be easily missed with human interpretation [48]. The use of AI also could directly enhance mfERG reliability and availability by using algorithms to automatically eliminate signal artifact while decreasing the need for subjective human interpretation. At the time of writing this article, only one published abstract reported the use of AI for recognizing HCQ-related electrophysiological changes on mfERG [49].

Identifying genetic variants with either protective effects or increasing susceptibility to HCQ retinopathy may influence future screening protocols. Patients with "risk alleles" may require more frequent screening or have a lower test threshold for diagnosing retinopathy. Early work by Shroyer and colleagues proposed that ABCA4 mutations may predispose patients to HCQ retinopathy, whereas Grassmann and colleagues suggested that some ABCA4 variants may reduce susceptibility to retinopathy [50,51]. In addition to genetics, Petri and colleagues demonstrated that higher serum levels of HCQ were correlated with developing retinopathy and suggested its potential use in risk stratifying patients, monitoring dose, or guiding frequency of screening [52]. Although these studies are intriguing, more research is required to establish their clinical utility.

As screening technologies continue to push the boundaries for identifying early HCQ retinopathy, a few key studies need to be performed:

- Unifying classification of different stages of HCQ retinopathy that is, suspected, subclinical (or early), and definitive retinopathy while establishing prevalence of each stage.
- Need large-scaled prospective studies to establish the relative sensitivity and specificity of different screening modalities with cost-benefit analysis. Also, identifying patient risk factors for which certain modalities would be more appropriate
- Require longitudinal studies to understand if subclinical disease predicts future disease stage and whether these patients would benefit from stopping HCQ therapy.

## SUMMARY

HCQ is commonly used to treat various rheumatological and dermatologic disorders; however, the development of retinopathy needs to be carefully monitored to prevent severe visual impairment. Significant evidence has been published to suggest that abnormalities in retinal function precede structural damage. As such, an objective functional test would constitute the ideal screening tool for detecting early HCQ toxicity. Of the various screening modalities, mfERG is the only clinically available test in this category. sdOCT is an objective test measuring structural changes but is less sensitive for detecting early toxicity. AVF used as the primary functional screening modality has limited utility as it is becoming increasingly evident that it is subjective and unreliable. More recent evidence considered in the UK guidelines no longer recommend AVF as the primary screening test and uses mfERG as the adjudicating test when ambiguity exists regarding possible retinal toxicity, in effect making it the gold standard test. As such, mfERG should be considered a primary screening test as technological advances in this field are making it faster, more reliable, and accessible.

## CLINICS CARE POINTS

- It is important to regularly update patient's real body weight, hydroxychloroquine dose, and assess for systemic or ocular risk factors associated with developing Plaquenil retinopathy.
- Physicians should not solely rely on fundus examination or fundus autofluorescence to diagnose Plaquenil retinopathy.
- In addition to automated visual field and sdOCT tests, mfERG should be considered for screening early retinopathy.
- Visual fields that demonstrate possible early retinopathy should be confirmed using an objective test like mfERG.

### Disclosure

The authors have nothing to disclose.

### References

[1] Plantone D, Koudriavtseva T. Current and Future Use of Chloroquine and Hydroxychloroquine in Infectious, Immune, Neoplastic, and Neurological Diseases: A Mini-Review. Clin Drug Investig 2018;38(8):653–71.

[2] Melles RB, Marmor MF. The risk of toxic retinopathy in patients on long-term hydroxychloroquine therapy. JAMA Ophthalmol 2014;132(12):1453–60.

[3] Jorge A, Ung C, Young LH, et al. Hydroxychloroquine retinopathy - implications of research advances for rheumatology care. Nat Rev Rheumatol 2018;14(12):693–703.

[4] Xu C, Zhu L, Chan T, et al. Chloroquine and Hydroxychloroquine Are Novel Inhibitors of Human Organic Anion Transporting Polypeptide 1A2. J Pharm Sci 2016;105(2):884–90.

[5] Rosenthal AR, Kolb H, Bergsma D, et al. Chloroquine retinopathy in the rhesus monkey. Invest Ophthalmol Vis Sci 1978;17(12):1158–75.

[6] Marmor MF, Kellner U, Lai TY, et al. Recommendations on Screening for Chloroquine and Hydroxychloroquine Retinopathy (2016 Revision). Ophthalmology 2016;123(6): 1386–94.

[7] Marmor MF, Hu J. Effect of disease stage on progression of hydroxychloroquine retinopathy. JAMA Ophthalmol 2014;132(9):1105–12.

[8] Pham BH, Marmor MF. Sequential changes in hydroxychloroquine retinopathy up to 20 years after stopping the drug: implications for mild versus severe Toxicity. Retina 2019;39(3):492–501.

[9] Tsang AC, Ahmadi Pirshahid S, Virgili G, et al. Hydroxychloroquine and chloroquine retinopathy: a systematic review evaluating the multifocal electroretinogram as a screening test. Ophthalmology 2015;122(6):1239–51.e4.

[10] Yusuf IH, Foot B, Lotery AJ. The Royal College of Ophthalmologists recommendations on monitoring for hydroxychloroquine and chloroquine users in the United Kingdom (2020 revision): executive summary. Eye (Lond) 2021;35(6):1532–7.

[11] Marshall E, Robertson M, Kam S, et al. Prevalence of hydroxychloroquine retinopathy using 2018 Royal College of Ophthalmologists diagnostic criteria. Eye (Lond) 2021;35(1): 343–8.

[12] Gobbett A, Kotagiri A, Bracewell C, et al. Two years' experience of screening for hydroxychloroquine retinopathy. Eye (Lond) 2021;35(4):1171–7.

[13] Marmor MF. Comparison of screening procedures in hydroxychloroquine toxicity. Arch Ophthalmol 2012;130(4):461–9.

[14] Melles RB, Marmor MF. Pericentral retinopathy and racial differences in hydroxychloroquine toxicity. Ophthalmology 2015;122(1):110–6.
[15] Marmor MF, Chien FY, Johnson MW. Value of red targets and pattern deviation plots in visual field screening for hydroxychloroquine retinopathy. JAMA Ophthalmol 2013;131(4): 476–80.
[16] Chen E, Brown DM, Benz MS, et al. Spectral domain optical coherence tomography as an effective screening test for hydroxychloroquine retinopathy (the "flying saucer" sign). Clin Ophthalmol 2010;4:1151–8.
[17] Browning DJ, Lee C. Relative sensitivity and specificity of 10-2 visual fields, multifocal electroretinography, and spectral domain optical coherence tomography in detecting hydroxychloroquine and chloroquine retinopathy. Clin Ophthalmol 2014;8:1389–99.
[18] Greenstein VC, Amaro-Quireza L, Abraham ES, et al. A comparison of structural and functional changes in patients screened for hydroxychloroquine retinopathy. Doc Ophthalmol 2015;130(1):13–23.
[19] Lyons JS, Severns ML. Detection of early hydroxychloroquine retinal toxicity enhanced by ring ratio analysis of multifocal electroretinography. Am J Ophthalmol 2007;143(5): 801–9.
[20] Marmor MF, Melles RB. Disparity between visual fields and optical coherence tomography in hydroxychloroquine retinopathy. Ophthalmology 2014;121(6):1257–62.
[21] Borrelli E, Battista M, Cascavilla ML, et al. Impact of Structural Changes on Multifocal Electroretinography in Patients With Use of Hydroxychloroquine. Invest Ophthalmol Vis Sci 2021;62(12):28.
[22] Garrity ST, Jung JY, Zambrowski O, et al. Early hydroxychloroquine retinopathy: optical coherence tomography abnormalities preceding Humphrey visual field defects. Br J Ophthalmol 2019;103(11):1600–4.
[23] Ruberto G, Bruttini C, Tinelli C, et al. Early morpho-functional changes in patients treated with hydroxychloroquine: a prospective cohort study. Graefes Arch Clin Exp Ophthalmol 2018;256(11):2201–10.
[24] Kellner U, Kellner S, Weinitz S. Chloroquine retinopathy: lipofuscin- and melanin-related fundus autofluorescence, optical coherence tomography and multifocal electroretinography. Doc Ophthalmol 2008;116(2):119–27.
[25] Kellner U, Renner AB, Tillack H. Fundus autofluorescence and mfERG for early detection of retinal alterations in patients using chloroquine/hydroxychloroquine. Invest Ophthalmol Vis Sci 2006;47(8):3531–8.
[26] Asanad S, Karanjia R. Multifocal electroretinogram. Treasure Island (FL): StatPearls Publishing; 2021.
[27] Hoffmann MB, Bach M, Kondo M, et al. ISCEV standard for clinical multifocal electroretinography (mfERG) (2021 update). Doc Ophthalmol 2021;142(1):5–16.
[28] Bertoli F, Sustar M, Jarc Vidmar M, et al. Electrophysiological and SD-OCT findings in patients receiving chloroquine therapy in relation to cumulative dosage and duration of treatment. Doc Ophthalmol 2020;141(1):1–14.
[29] Lyons JS, Severns ML. Using multifocal ERG ring ratios to detect and follow Plaquenil retinal toxicity: a review : Review of mfERG ring ratios in Plaquenil toxicity. Doc Ophthalmol 2009;118(1):29–36.
[30] Saez-Moreno JA, Dominguez-Hidalgo C, Rodriguez-Ferrer JM. Multifocal ERG Guiding Therapy in a Case of Hydroxychloroquine Premaculopathy. Case Rep Ophthalmol Med 2015;2015:656928.
[31] Tsang AC, Ahmadi S, Hamilton J, et al. The Diagnostic Utility of Multifocal Electroretinography in Detecting Chloroquine and Hydroxychloroquine Retinal Toxicity. Am J Ophthalmol 2019;206:132–9.
[32] Adamptey B, Rudnisky CJ, MacDonald IM. Effect of stopping hydroxychloroquine therapy on the multifocal electroretinogram in patients with rheumatic disorders. Can J Ophthalmol 2020;55(1):38–44.

[33] Adam MK, Covert DJ, Stepien KE, et al. Quantitative assessment of the 103-hexagon multifocal electroretinogram in detection of hydroxychloroquine retinal toxicity. Br J Ophthalmol 2012;96(5):723–9.
[34] Tsang A, Kanda P, Gottlieb C, et al. A novel 5-ring multifocal electroretinography stimulus for detecting hydroxychloroquine retinal toxicity. Doc Ophthalmol 2021; https://doi.org/10.1007/s10633-021-09858-4.
[35] Iftikhar M, Kaur R, Nefalar A, et al. Microperimetry as a screening test for hydroxychloroquine retinopathy: the hard-Risk-1 Study. Retina 2019;39(3):485–91.
[36] Alghanem H, Padhi TR, Chen A, et al. Comparison of Fundus-Guided Microperimetry and Multifocal Electroretinography for Evaluating Hydroxychloroquine Maculopathy. Transl Vis Sci Technol 2019;8(5):19.
[37] Tarakcioglu HN, Ozkaya A, Yigit U. Is optical coherence tomography angiography a useful tool in the screening of hydroxychloroquine retinopathy? Int Ophthalmol 2021;41(1): 27–33.
[38] Goker YS, Ucgul Atilgan C, Tekin K, et al. The Validity of Optical Coherence Tomography Angiography as a Screening Test for the Early Detection of Retinal Changes in Patients with Hydroxychloroquine Therapy. Curr Eye Res 2019;44(3):311–5.
[39] Bulut M, Akidan M, Gozkaya O, et al. Optical coherence tomography angiography for screening of hydroxychloroquine-induced retinal alterations. Graefes Arch Clin Exp Ophthalmol 2018;256(11):2075–81.
[40] Reichel C, Berlin A, Radun V, et al. Quantitative Fundus Autofluorescence in Systemic Chloroquine/Hydroxychloroquine Therapy. Transl Vis Sci Technol 2020;9(9):42.
[41] Greenstein VC, Lima de Carvalho JR Jr, Parmann R, et al. Quantitative Fundus Autofluorescence in HCQ Retinopathy. Invest Ophthalmol Vis Sci 2020;61(11):41.
[42] Sauer L, Calvo CM, Vitale AS, et al. Imaging of Hydroxychloroquine Toxicity with Fluorescence Lifetime Imaging Ophthalmoscopy. Ophthalmol Retina 2019;3(10):814–25.
[43] Debellemaniere G, Flores M, Tumahai P, et al. Assessment of parafoveal cone density in patients taking hydroxychloroquine in the absence of clinically documented retinal toxicity. Acta Ophthalmol 2015;93(7):e534–40.
[44] Babeau F, Busetto T, Hamel C, et al. Adaptive optics: a tool for screening hydroxychloroquine-induced maculopathy? Acta Ophthalmol 2017;95(5):e424–5.
[45] Lee WJ, Lee BR, Shin YU. Retromode imaging: Review and perspectives. Saudi J Ophthalmol Apr 2014;28(2):88–94.
[46] Ahn SJ, Lee SU, Lee SH, et al. Evaluation of Retromode Imaging for Use in Hydroxychloroquine Retinopathy. Am J Ophthalmol 2018;196:44–52.
[47] Nuzzi R, Boscia G, Marolo P, et al. The Impact of Artificial Intelligence and Deep Learning in Eye Diseases: A Review. Front Med (Lausanne) 2021;8:710329.
[48] De Silva T, Jayakar G, Grisso P, et al. Deep Learning-Based Automatic Detection of Ellipsoid Zone Loss in Spectral-Domain OCT for Hydroxychloroquine Retinal Toxicity Screening. Ophthalmol Sci 2021;1(4):100060.
[49] Wright T, Yan P, Easterbrook M. Machine learning to identify multifocal ERG deficits in patients taking hydroxychloroquine. Invest Ophthalmol Vis Sci 2019;60:5959.
[50] Shroyer NF, Lewis RA, Lupski JR. Analysis of the ABCR (ABCA4) gene in 4-aminoquinoline retinopathy: is retinal toxicity by chloroquine and hydroxychloroquine related to Stargardt disease? Am J Ophthalmol 2001;131(6):761–6.
[51] Grassmann F, Bergholz R, Mandl J, et al. Common synonymous variants in ABCA4 are protective for chloroquine induced maculopathy (toxic maculopathy). BMC Ophthalmol 2015;15:18.
[52] Petri M, Elkhalifa M, Li J, et al. Hydroxychloroquine Blood Levels Predict Hydroxychloroquine Retinopathy. Arthritis Rheumatol 2020;72(3):448–53.

Advances in Ophthalmology and Optometry 7 (2022) 279–293

ADVANCES IN OPHTHALMOLOGY AND OPTOMETRY

# Update on Optic Neuritis in Adults

## Multiple Sclerosis, Neuromyelitis Optica Spectrum Disorder, and Myelin Oligodendrocyte Glycoprotein Antibody–Associated Disease

Serena Li, BA[a,c], Rahul A. Sharma, MD, MPH, FRCSC[d,e], Benson S. Chen, MBChB, MSc, FRACP[a,b,c,*]

[a]Department of Clinical Neurosciences, University of Cambridge, Cambridge, United Kingdom; [b]Cambridge Eye Unit, Addenbrooke's Hospital, CUH-NHS, Cambridge, United Kingdom; [c]Gonville and Caius College, University of Cambridge, Trinity Street, Cambridge, CB2 1TA, United Kingdom; [d]Department of Ophthalmology and Vision Sciences, University of Toronto, Toronto, Ontario, Canada; [e]Prism Eye Institute, 2201 Bristol Circle Suite 100, Oakville, Ontario, L6H 0J8, Canada

**Keywords**

• Optic neuritis • Multiple sclerosis • Neuromyelitis optica spectrum disorder • Aquaporin-4 • Myelin oligodendrocyte glycoprotein–associated disorder

**Key points**

- The diagnosis of neuromyelitis optica spectrum disorder (NMOSD) and myelin oligodendrocyte glycoprotein antibody–associated disease (MOGAD) require identification of specific autoantibodies, which may be challenging when patients present acutely with optic neuritis (ON).
- Recognizing clinical clues that distinguish ON associated with multiple sclerosis, NMOSD, and MOGAD is crucial, given the variability in their natural histories and visual prognosis.
- Increasing evidence exists that early and aggressive management of ON is associated with better visual prognosis in individuals with NMOSD and MOGAD.
- Long-term immunosuppression needs to be considered, particularly in patients with NMOSD and for some with MOGAD, to reduce risk of recurrent ON.

*Corresponding author. Gonville and Caius College, University of Cambridge, Trinity Street, Cambridge, CB2 1TA, United Kingdom. *E-mail address:* bsc33@cam.ac.uk

https://doi.org/10.1016/j.yaoo.2022.04.001
2452-1760/22/

## INTRODUCTION

Although the term "optic neuritis" (ON) is technically nonspecific and may refer to any inflammation of one or both optic nerves, its use implies an inflammatory demyelinating cause. In its typical form, acute inflammatory demyelinating ON may occur as a clinically isolated syndrome (CIS) or as the initial manifestation of a central nervous system (CNS) disorder, such as multiple sclerosis (MS). Historically, it was recognized that different types of ON existed and could be classified based on clinical features including severity of vision loss, associated neurologic symptoms, response to treatment, and recurrence. This led to clinical descriptors, such as "typical ON," "atypical ON," and, for individuals with recurrent ON that seemed to be steroid-responsive, "chronic recurrent inflammatory optic neuropathy" (CRION).

In the last 20 years, significant progress has been made in the understanding of the immunopathogenic basis of inflammatory demyelinating ON. This includes the identification of the antibodies aquaporin-4 IgG (AQP4-IgG) and myelin oligodendrocyte glycoprotein (MOG) IgG (MOG-IgG), associated with neuromyelitis optica spectrum disorder (NMOSD) and MOG-IgG-associated diseases (MOGAD), respectively. It is now recognized that most patients who were previously described as having CRION were, in fact, positive for the MOG-IgG antibody.

Acute ON has a high rate of misdiagnosis. Even when ON is appropriately identified and distinguished from other causes of acute optic neuropathy, it may be difficult to identify any underlying disease, such as MS, NMOSD, or MOGAD. This distinction is crucial, because these disorders vary in their natural history, visual prognosis, and potential treatment options; a delay in diagnosis and initiating appropriate treatment, therefore, may contribute to a worse visual outcome. This review provides an up-to-date overview of the diagnosis and management of ON associated with MS (MS-ON), NMOSD (NMOSD-ON), and MOGAD (MOG-ON), with a focus on clinical and paraclinical features, acute and long-term management, and prognosis.

## DIAGNOSIS

Although most ON cases are idiopathic or associated with MS, acute ON also is a common presentation of NMOSD and MOGAD. Early identification of NMOSD-ON and MOG-ON is essential to guide acute management and optimize long-term outcomes. However, timely detection of serum AQP4-IgG or MOG-IgG, to make a diagnosis of NMOSD or MOGAD (Table 1), may not be possible. The CNS disorders associated with ON may be differentiated based on patient demographics, clinical, and neuroimaging features (Table 2). Although such features may be highly suggestive of a particular diagnosis, they are not exclusive nor absolute.

### Demographics

- Age: Idiopathic and MS-ON most often occurs in the third or fourth decades of life (mean age at onset, 30) [1]. Patients with MOG-ON have a mean age of

**Table 1**
Diagnostic criteria for MS, NMOSD, and MOGAD in the setting of optic neuritis

| 2017 Revised McDonald Criteria for MS [25] | 2015 International Consensus Diagnostic Criteria for NMOSD with AQP4-IgG [10] | 2018 Proposed Diagnostic Criteria for MOGAD [16] |
|---|---|---|
| Following an attack of optic neuritis, the diagnosis of MS is made with evidence of:<br>• Dissemination in space demonstrated by an additional clinical attack implicating a different CNS site or by MRI[a]; AND<br>• Dissemination in time demonstrated by an additional clinical attack or by MRI[b] OR demonstration of CSF-specific oligoclonal bands | • At least 1 core clinical characteristic (optic neuritis); AND<br>• Positive test for AQP4-IgG using best available detection method (cell-based assay strongly recommended);[c] AND<br>• Exclusion of alternative diagnosis[d] | • Clinical finding (monophasic or relapsing optic neuritis); AND<br>• Laboratory finding: serum positive for MOG-IgG by cell-based assay; AND<br>• MRI or electrophysiologic findings compatible with CNS demyelination; AND<br>• Exclusion of alternative diagnosis[d] |

*Abbreviation:* CSF, cerebrospinal fluid.

[a]MRI criteria for dissemination in space: the presence of one or more T2-hyperintense lesions that are characteristic of MS in two or more of four areas of the CNS: periventricular, cortical or juxtacortical, infratentorial brain regions, and spinal cord.

[b]MRI criteria for dissemination in time: the simultaneous presence of gadolinium-enhancing and nonenhancing lesions at any time or by new T2-hyperintense or gadolinium-enhancing lesion on follow-up MRI, with reference to a baseline scan, irrespective of the timing of the baseline MRI.

[c]Diagnostic criteria for NMOSD without AQP4-IgG or unknown AQP4-IgG status require at least two different core clinical characteristics in addition to fulfilment of additional MRI requirements. Patients presenting with acute ON without any other associated neurologic syndromes (eg, transverse myelitis, area postrema syndrome, or acute brainstem syndrome) are unlikely to meet the criteria for NMOSD without AQP4-IgG.

[d]Alternative diagnoses include: neurosarcoidosis, cancer, lymphoma, paraneoplastic disease, chronic infection including HIV and syphilis, Leber hereditary optic neuropathy, nonarteritic ischemic optic neuropathy, MS, NMOSD, and MOGAD.

approximately 30, although MOGAD can occur throughout the life span including in childhood, when it more commonly presents as acute disseminated encephalomyelitis (ADEM) [1,2]. Patients with NMOSD-ON generally are older with a mean age of onset of 40 years [1].

- Sex: In idiopathic or MS-ON and NMOSD-ON, a strong female bias occurs. In the Optic Neuritis Treatment Trial (ONTT), a 3:1 female-to-male ratio exists in patients with idiopathic and MS-ON [3]. In NMOSD-ON, the female-to-male ratio is more significant, up to 9:1 [1]. Conversely, in an observational case series of 87 patients with MOG-ON, only a slight female predilection (57%; female-to-male ratio of 1.3:1) occurred [4]. However, MOGAD does not have a predilection for a particular sex [1].
- Ethnicity: The prevalence of idiopathic and MS-ON is highest in White populations, with the highest risk in populations living at higher northern latitudes [3,5]. Patients with NMOSD often are of African or Asian ethnicity [1,6]. A recent systematic review and meta-analysis found that the seroprevalence of

**Table 2**
Comparison of the clinical and radiologic features of ON associated with MS, AQP4-IgG-positive NMOSD, and MOGAD

| | MS | NMOSD | MOGAD |
|---|---|---|---|
| Sex (female/male) | 3:1 | 9:1 | No predilection |
| Age (y) | Any, although generally young adults (mean age, 32) | Any, although generally slightly older than patients with MS (mean age, 41) | Any, including children (mean age, 30) |
| Ethnicity | Higher risk in White populations | Higher risk in African, Afro-Caribbean, and Asian populations | No known predisposition |
| Bilateral | Very rare | Infrequent | Frequent |
| Optic disk edema | Rare | Infrequent | Frequent, often severe |
| Visual acuity at nadir | Often better than 20/200 | Often worse than <20/200 | Variable; mean acuity count fingers |
| Visual field loss | Diffuse or central scotoma | Variable, including bitemporal hemianopia and homonymous hemianopia | Variable |
| Recurrence | Rare | Frequent | Frequent |
| Visual prognosis | Good | Poor | Fair |
| MRI characteristics | Unilateral, short, segmented, anteriorly located lesion without OPN | Long posteriorly located lesion with frequent optic chiasm or tract involvement; OPN infrequent | Bilateral long anteriorly located lesion with disk swelling and very frequent OPN |

*Abbreviation:* OPN, optic perineuritis.

AQP4-IgG in adults with isolated ON was 4% in non-Asian and 27% in Asian populations, whereas MOG-IgG seroprevalence was 8% and 20% respectively [6]. However, epidemiologic studies have not found a significant racial preponderance for MOGAD [1].

## Clinical features

*Laterality and recurrence*

- ON almost always is unilateral in idiopathic and MS-ON [3], whereas nearly 50% of MOG-ON cases are bilateral [2].
- Bilateral ON also occurs in NMOSD-ON, but less frequently than in MOG-ON.
- Recurrent ON is more common in MOG-ON and NMOSD-ON compared with MS-ON [6–8].

*Visual acuity and visual field*

- The presenting visual acuity of patients with MS-ON is highly variable. In the ONTT, 35% of patients had a best-corrected visual acuity (BCVA) of better than

20/40, whereas 35% had 20/200 or worse [3]. In NMOSD-ON and MOG-ON, visual acuity is variable at onset, although BCVA is often worse than 20/400 [4].
- In MOG-ON, BCVA at nadir ranges from 20/25 to no light perception, with the mean and median BCVA at nadir of the most severe ON attack being count fingers and hand motion vision respectively [4]. Similarly, in NMOSD-ON, most patients have vision worse than 20/200 at nadir.
- The subtypes of ON also may present with differences in the pattern of visual field loss. In the ONTT, visual field loss was most often diffuse or central [9]. In NMOSD-ON, visual field loss may be diffuse or focal, or as a bitemporal or homonymous hemianopic field defect, indicating involvement of the optic chiasm or tract. In MOG-ON, visual field loss is highly variable and also may occur in a pattern that suggests either optic nerve or chiasmal involvement.

*Optic disk appearance*
- In the ONTT, two-thirds of patients with idiopathic and MS-ON had normal optic disk appearance [3]. The remaining one-third of patients showed mild disk edema.
- Similarly, patients with NMOSD-ON do not tend to have disk edema [2].
- In MOG-ON, up to 86% of cases show disk edema at onset, which can be severe and associated with peripapillary hemorrhages [2].

*Associated symptoms*
- In MOGAD, prodromal or viral symptoms, such as fever, rhinorrhea, malaise, and cough, may precede the ON [2]. Around 50% of patients with MOGAD have other CNS involvement that may precede, occur during, or after a flare of ON. Such syndromes as ADEM or brainstem encephalitis occur more frequently in MOGAD compared with NMOSD and MS [2].
- In NMOSD, patients may experience ON with accompanying longitudinal transverse myelitis (characterized by paraparesis or tetraparesis, gait alteration, sexual dysfunction, and changes in the bladder and bowels) or area postrema syndrome (nausea, hiccups, and vomiting). Patients may have other brainstem syndromes including brainstem encephalitis, symptomatic narcolepsy, and neuroendocrine dysfunction [10].

## Radiologic features

The preferred imaging modality for ON is MRI with T1-weighted sequences of the orbits with fat suppression and contrast, and T2-weighted sequences of the orbits and brain. The typical MRI findings are swelling of the optic nerve with high T2 signal, and contrast enhancement best seen on T1-weighted sequences with fat suppression [11]. Acute ON is associated with optic perineuritis (OPN), inflammation of the optic nerve sheath, which appears on MRI as contrast enhancement and circumferential thickening of the optic nerve sheath and peribulbar structures [12].

In idiopathic and MS-ON, the optic nerve lesion is short and segmented, and contrast enhancement is usually only seen in the anterior orbit [13]. Optic chiasm and tract involvement is rare, as is OPN [12].

In NMOSD-ON, optic nerve lesions typically involve more than 50% of the optic nerve length and usually are posterior, with the intracranial segment of the optic nerve commonly affected and frequent involvement of the optic chiasm and tract (Fig. 1) [12,13].

In MOG-ON, optic nerve lesions frequently are bilateral and long (Fig. 2) [12]. In contrast to NMOSD-ON, most lesions involve the anterior optic nerve, in particular the retrobulbar segment of the optic nerve, and frequent optic nerve head swelling occurs [12,13]. OPN is frequent in MOG-ON, occurring in up to 50% of cases [2].

## ACUTE MANAGEMENT

The approach to patients with ON differs based on the initial classification of the presentation as either typical (young patients with subacute, painful vision loss) or atypical. Atypical features include (1) severe unilateral or bilateral vision loss, (2) severe disk edema with exudates or peripapillary hemorrhages, (3) vitritis, (4) progression of vision loss after 1 to 2 weeks, (5) lack of partial recovery within 4 weeks of the onset of vision loss, and (6) persistent pain. Patients with atypical ON are more likely to have ON related to either MOG-ON or NMO-ON. As outlined previously, additional clinical clues and radiographic findings contribute to a clinical suspicion for either NMOSD-ON or MOG-ON.

The ONTT demonstrated that in patients with typical features, no tests (serologic studies, lumbar puncture, MRI) were helpful in diagnosis of ON. Thus, the diagnosis of typical ON remains clinical. Applying clinical criteria for typical ON has a high degree of specificity for idiopathic or MS-ON; in fact, 177 of the 448 patients enrolled in the ONTT were tested for AQP4-IgG and MOG-IgG 20 years after initial enrollment, with zero patients seropositive for AQP4-IgG and only three showing MOG-IgG seropositivity [14]. In atypical cases, clinicians should have a low threshold to obtain additional serologic studies, recognizing the limitations of even the most sensitive assays: a quarter of patients meeting clinical diagnostic criteria for NMOSD test negative for AQP4-IgG [10], and a quarter of MOG-IgG-positive patients were designed as false-positives in a large retrospective study [15].

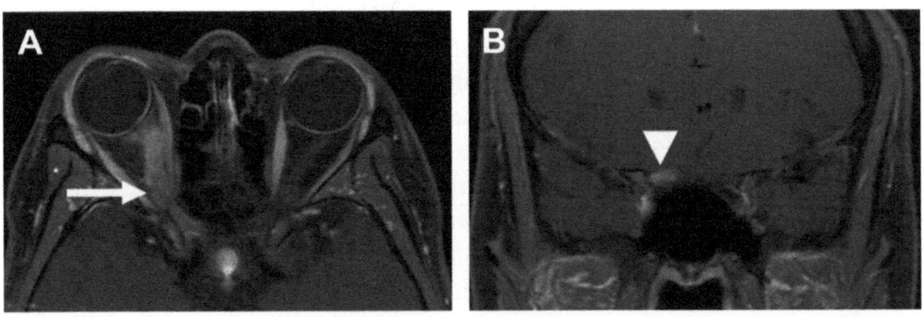


**Fig. 1.** MRI signs of optic neuritis associated with NMOSD. (*A*) Long-segment right optic neuritis (*arrow*) with significant swelling and gadolinium enhancement on T1 fat-suppressed sequence. (*B*) Same patient demonstrating gadolinium enhancement of intracranial optic nerve (*arrowhead*), extending into the chiasm.

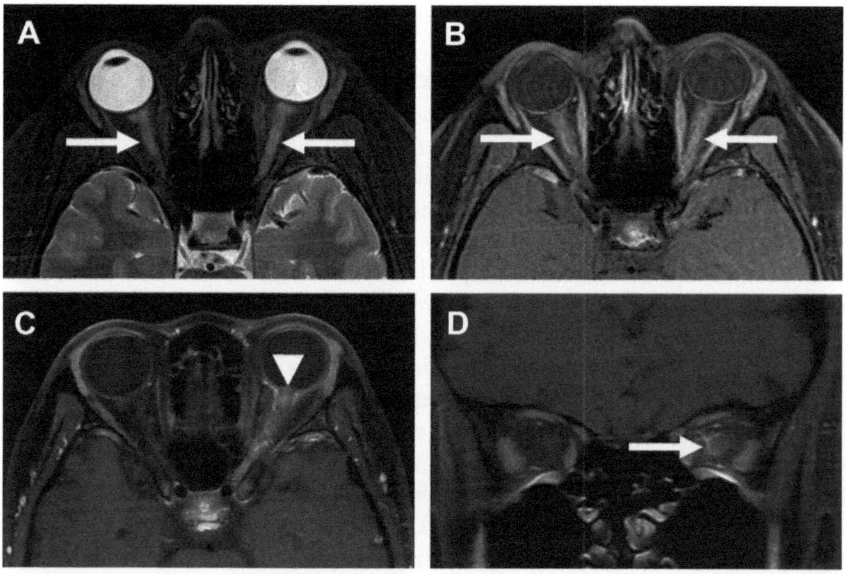


**Fig. 2.** MRI signs of optic neuritis associated with MOGAD. (*A*) Bilateral optic neuritis with long-segment high T2 signal on T2-weighted sequence without gadolinium (*arrows*), and (*B*) extensive gadolinium enhancement on T1 fat-suppressed sequence (*arrows*). (*C*) Long-segment left optic neuritis associated with edema of the optic nerve head (*arrowhead*), and (*D*) optic perineuritis (*arrow*).

Although no consensus exists to support routine testing in typical ON cases, AQP4-IgG should be obtained in all patients with severe or bilateral visual loss, transverse myelitis or other neurologic manifestations of NMOSD, or involvement of greater than half of the optic nerve and/or involvement of the optic chiasm on MRI [10]. The anti-AQP4 assay has high specificity and is inexpensive, with significant implications for clinical decision-making [10]. NMOSD may coexist with other autoimmune conditions and should especially be considered in patients with systemic lupus erythematosus, Sjögren syndrome, or myasthenia gravis. Evaluation of MOG-IgG also should be considered in patients with clinically atypical ON, ADEM, APQ4-seronegative NMOSD, or demyelinating disease atypical for MS [16]. The need for additional serologic studies or lumbar puncture depends on the particular clinical scenario and usually is determined in consultation with a neurologist or neuro-ophthalmologist.

The ONTT provides class I clinical trial evidence for the acute treatment of typical ON. The ONTT involves three treatment arms [3]. One group received high-dose intravenous methylprednisolone (IVMP) (1 g daily in divided doses) for 3 days followed by oral prednisolone (1 mg/kg/d) for days 4–14, then 20 mg of prednisone on day 15 and 10 mg on days 16 and 18. A second group received oral prednisone (1 mg/kg/d for 14 days). The third group received placebo. Patients treated with IVMP showed hastened visual recovery compared with patients receiving either low-dose steroid or placebo. Visual outcome at

12 months did not differ among the three treatment arms. A 2015 Cochrane review confirmed these results [17].

A careful discussion of risks and benefits should be undertaken in all patients with typical ON to allow for individualized decision-making. Low-dose oral steroid should not be used in patients with ON. Patients should be aware that high-dose steroids is administered safely (and often as an outpatient therapy, either orally or intravenously) in young, healthy patients without relative contraindications, such as coronary artery disease, diabetes, and peptic ulcer disease. The use of oral, high-dose prednisone is supported by a randomized controlled trial (RCT) of 55 patients who showed no significant difference in visual recovery between typical patients with ON treated with IVMP (1000 mg) and oral bioequivalent prednisone (1250 mg) [5].

Treatment of atypical ON should begin immediately and more aggressively than in typical cases. Whereas patients with MS-ON experience a similar visual prognosis whether or not treatment is pursued, patients with NMOSD-ON and MOG-ON have an improved chance for good visual recovery if treatment is commenced on a hyperacute basis [18,19]. Treatment should therefore be initiated based on clinical suspicion of the diagnosis, because serologic confirmation may take a week or more.

For patients with suspected or confirmed NMOSD-ON, the general consensus has been to treat patients with high-dose IVMP, and then initiate plasmapheresis or plasma exchange (PLEX) if no improvement occurs. However, the paradigm for the acute management of NMOSD-ON is changing. Recent studies have demonstrated that rapid initiation of high-dose IVMP affects eventual visual prognosis, independent of the severity of ON [19]. Retrospective studies also have shown that initiation of PLEX within 48 hours of onset of vision loss leads to the best recovery [20]. PLEX seems to confer functionally important visual recovery in more than half the patients with severe, steroid-refractory ON, whether related to NMOSD-ON or MS-ON. Thus, empiric treatment seems beneficial even while antibody tests are pending [21]. Intravenous immunoglobulin (IVIG) may have a role in treatment of acute relapses of NMOSD, particularly in cases where PLEX is unavailable, although its impact is less well-studied [22].

Similarly, in MOGAD, most experts suggest 3 to 5 days of IVMP followed by an oral prednisone taper over 1 to 3 months [2]. If vision loss is severe or no improvement in vision occurs after 1 to 2 weeks of treatment with corticosteroids, PLEX is an option [2]. The efficacy of IVIG in the management of acute MOG-ON in adults is yet to be determined.

## LONG-TERM MANAGEMENT

Long-term management after ON is focused on preventing recurrent attacks of inflammatory demyelination in the optic nerve and elsewhere in the CNS. Recurrent attacks of ON can hasten the loss of retinal ganglion cells, resulting in incomplete recovery after each subsequent attack and poor long-term visual prognosis. Patients are best managed by a neurologist with experience managing neuroimmunologic conditions, in conjunction with a neuro-ophthalmologist. The management strategy differs depending on the condition associated with the initial acute attack of ON. For patients who have atypical ON and are seronegative for AQP4-IgG and MOG-IgG, assessment by a neuro-ophthalmologist is vital to confirm the diagnosis of an inflammatory demyelinating ON and rule out other causes of optic neuropathy. A proportion of patients with NMOSD or MOGAD initially test negative and subsequently become positive, so reassessment of antibody status is essential. Long-term management of double seronegative patients is challenging and is beyond the scope of this review.

### Clinically isolated syndrome and multiple sclerosis

In typical ON, additional treatment usually is not required after the initial course of corticosteroids. In a patient without fever, infection, or a previous diagnosis of MS, an attack of unilateral idiopathic ON lasting 24 hours or more, with or without recovery, is classified as CIS. Individuals who experience CIS may or may not go on to develop clinically definite MS. However, the presence of MRI-detected brain lesions suggestive of MS at the time of the CIS increases the risk of a second neurologic event and diagnosis of clinically definite MS over a 15-year period from 25% to 72% [23].

The diagnosis of CIS should be made by a neurologist, taking into consideration any historical neurologic symptoms or clinical signs suspicious for previous CNS demyelination, and accurate review of neuroimaging for CNS lesions of MS by an experienced neuroradiologist. Clinical trials of individuals with CIS have focused on delaying the progression of CIS to clinically definite MS. However, the benefits of initiating disease-modifying therapy have only been established in individuals with CIS and MRI-detected brain lesions consistent with MS. Current practice guidelines only recommend disease-modifying therapy in individuals with CIS who have two or more brain imaging characteristics consistent with MS (level B recommendation, American Academy of Neurology Practice Guideline) [24]. Individuals with CIS and no evidence of MS lesions on MRI should be followed closely, with consideration for serial imaging [23].

After an attack of unilateral idiopathic ON or CIS, the diagnostic criteria for MS should be applied carefully to avoid misdiagnosis (see Table 1). Using the 2017 revision of the McDonald Criteria for MS [25], the diagnosis of MS is made when CIS is accompanied by clinical or MRI findings that confirm dissemination in space and dissemination in time. In contrast to earlier diagnostic criteria, the 2017 revision of the McDonald Criteria excludes optic nerve involvement as an anatomic location for dissemination in space. Thus, a diagnosis of MS only is made in a patient presenting with acute ON if clinical or MRI evidence exists of an attack involving another CNS region (demonstrating dissemination in space) and evidence that this second attack occurred at a different time (demonstrating dissemination in time). Specific MRI criteria also set out what can be used as evidence of dissemination in space and dissemination in time (see Table 1) [25]. Additionally, the presence of oligoclonal bands in cerebrospinal fluid can aid in the diagnosis of MS in lieu of dissemination in time.

Misdiagnosis of MS because of erroneous application of MS clinical and MRI criteria can lead to patient distress and potentially harmful risks, such as initiation of unnecessary treatments. However, a delayed diagnosis of MS and subsequent delay in initiating disease-modifying therapy potentially can lead to further neurologic disability.

### Neuromyelitis optica spectrum disorder

Patients with NMOSD require long-term immunosuppression because each attack of NMOSD can contribute to severe, permanent neurologic disability [26,27]. Seropositivity for AQP4-IgG is associated with a high risk of relapse in those with single or recurrent ON [8]. An indefinite long-term immunosuppressive regimen is recommended even after a single attack of ON in individuals who are AQP4-IgG positive [26]. The goal of treatment is to prevent relapses while limiting side effects of immunosuppressive agents.

Before 2019, the three most commonly used steroid-sparing medications (with or without oral corticosteroids) were azathioprine, mycophenolate mofetil, and rituximab. A relapse-free rate of 30% to 80% was observed at last follow-up with these treatments [26]. Oral corticosteroids without any other immunosuppressive medications have been used, but rarely prescribed long-term because of systemic adverse effects.

Data from observational studies suggest that azathioprine is not as effective as rituximab and mycophenolate mofetil in preventing relapses in patients with antibody-positive NMOSD [27]. Retrospective studies also indicate that rituximab seems to be more effective than mycophenolate mofetil in suppressing clinical activity and reducing the risk of relapse [28]. A recent meta-analysis found rituximab to be more effective than mycophenolate mofetil as a first-line therapy [29]. However, when only AQP4-IgG-positive patients were included, no difference was observed between patients on azathioprine, mycophenolate mofetil, or rituximab.

The US Food and Drug Administration has approved three treatments for patients with AQP4-IgG NMOSD: eculizumab, satralizumab, and inebilizumab. Both eculizumab and satralizumab have been approved in Australia, Canada, and by the European Medicine Agency, with inebilizumab granted "initial authorization" status by the European Medicine Agency. In the United Kingdom, the National Institute for Clinical Excellence has not made a recommendation on any of the three medications.

Eculizumab, satralizumab, and inebilizumab were studied in four RCTs, with a relapse risk reduction of 74% to 94% observed across the four trials [26]. Comparison of the trials is difficult because of differences in trial design. Nevertheless, all three medications have demonstrated significant efficacy in preventing disabling NMOSD attacks and should be considered as preventative treatment following an acute attack of NMOSD-ON.

### Myelin oligodendrocyte glycoprotein antibody–associated diseases

In MOGAD, decisions regarding whether to treat a patient with long-term immunosuppression are guided by risk of relapse and degree of recovery from an event. Although patients with MOG-ON generally experience a more favorable recovery after the initial episode, recurrent attacks can lead to accumulation of disability and morbidity not only from recurrent ON but also from involvement of other CNS regions. If a patient has significant residual vision impairment following an attack of MOG-ON, long-term immunosuppression should be considered [2]. Although 30% to 50% of adult patients have a relapsing course of MOGAD [2], consensus shows that a second event is required to warrant long-term immunosuppression [30]. These decisions are further complicated by challenges of differentiating true relapses from disease rebound (during steroid wean or discontinuation of steroids) and pseudorelapses (secondary to intercurrent illness) [30]. Other factors that need to be taken into consideration include the age of the patient and the infectious risks of current immunosuppressive medications.

Unlike MS and NMOSD, evidence for the efficacy of currently used immunosuppressive treatments in MOGAD is not obtained from clinical trials, but from real-world clinical data. A recent review examined data for 291 adult and pediatric patients receiving immunosuppressive medication, from the six largest retrospective studies on treatment of relapsing MOGAD [30]. At a median of 9 to 16 months after the start of treatment, the number of relapse-free patients was 20 (69%) of 29 patients on IVIG, 47 (50%) of 94 on rituximab, 30 (47%) of 63 on mycophenolate mofetil, and 21 (39%) of 55 on azathioprine. The remainder of patients who were treated with other immunosuppressive treatments including medications for MS tended to have a higher relapse rate.

There has also been interest in the use of tocilizumab, an interleukin-6 inhibitor, in the treatment of relapsing MOGAD. A recent retrospective observational study found that 79% of 14 patients with MOGAD remained relapse-free during treatment with tocilizumab (mean duration, 23.8 months) [31]. Future prospective RCTs are required to determine the best long-term immunotherapy for relapsing MOGAD.

## PROGNOSIS

The visual prognosis of ON differs depending on the underlying condition, emphasizing the importance of making the correct diagnosis and using the most appropriate management strategy, acutely and in the long-term. Alongside traditional measures of visual function, such as BCVA, structural changes to the retinal architecture that occur after acute ON are quantified using optical coherence tomography. Optic nerve injury results in irreversible thinning of the retinal nerve fiber layer (RNFL), which is mainly composed of the axons of the retinal ganglion cells, and the ganglion cell–inner plexiform layers (GCIPL), which contains the cell bodies and dendrites of the retinal ganglion cells. After ON, lower peripapillary RNFL (pRNFL) and macular GCIPL (mGCIPL) values are generally associated with worse deficits in visual acuity, visual field, and color vision. A pRNFL of 75 μm after ON has previously been identified as a cutoff below which RNFL measurements predicted persistent visual dysfunction (BCVA and visual field deficits) [32].

Direct comparison of long-term visual outcomes after ON is challenging because of differences in the management strategy used. A systematic literature review and meta-analysis of 65 studies of patients presenting with isolated ON found that eyes affected by NMOSD-ON and MOG-ON exhibited similarly severely decreased pRNFL and mGCIPL thickness, which was greater than that observed in MS-ON eyes [6]. Despite similar pRNFL and mGCIPL thinning in NMOSD-ON and MOG-ON eyes, visual outcomes were significantly better in MOG-ON. High-contrast BCVA of eyes affected by MOG-ON were preserved and did not differ from MS-ON, indicating a discordance between structural and functional outcomes in MOG-ON-affected eyes.

A recent study of a Japanese cohort of patients followed at one tertiary center for at least 5 years found NMOSD-ON eyes had the worst visual prognosis [7]. At 5-year follow-up, the median logMAR BCVA of NMOSD-ON eyes was 1.00 (equivalent to 6/60; interquartile range, 0.47–1.78), compared with 0.00 (equivalent to 6/6; interquartile range, 0.00–0.00) in eyes affected by MS-ON and MOG-ON. All patients had received similar acute management for ON, consisting of high-dose IVMP, followed by PLEX in patients who did not respond to IVMP. Almost all MOG-ON-affected eyes had fully recovered shortly after initiating acute treatment. Administration of IVMP further facilitated early recovery of visual acuity. However, patients with MOG-ON with extensive optic nerve lesions involving the chiasm irreversibly experienced several visual impairments despite appropriate acute treatment [7]. Similarly, lesion length also was an important predictor of visual prognosis in patients with NMOSD, particularly involvement of the intraorbital and canalicular segments of the optic nerve [33].

Serum antibody titer level has been investigated as a prognostic factor. In NMOSD, studies have demonstrated that AQP4-IgG titer level does not reflect disease activity or correlate with visual prognosis [34]. Although in MOGAD, the MOG-IgG titer is highest during an acute attack and, in some patients with monophasic disease, has been reported to disappear with time [16]. Disappearance of the MOG-IgG may confer a better prognosis, but decisions regarding long-term management should not be made solely on antibody serostatus alone [2,16].

## FUTURE AVENUES

With the identification of NMOSD and MOGAD, the treatment paradigm of acute ON must be revisited; specifically the dose, duration, and mode of administration of steroid therapy, and when to initiate long-term immunosuppressive treatments. The challenge for clinicians managing acute ON is determining whether the initiated treatment is working or needs to be escalated. Bedside and clinic-based measures of visual function are subjective. Further research is required to identify structural and functional biomarkers that will help with clinical decision-making regarding escalation of therapy.

Much of the evidence for the widely used immunosuppressive therapies in NMOSD and MOGAD are from real-world clinical data, which limits assessment and comparison of therapeutic efficacy. Prospective RCTs are required to provide high-quality evidence of the treatments that are currently prescribed, in particular azathioprine and mycophenolate mofetil for NMOSD, and confirm the observations from real-world clinical data (eg, maintenance IVIG for MOGAD). The impact of long-term immunosuppressive therapy still needs to be clarified, especially because some patients remain on these treatments indefinitely.

Lastly, patients who present with atypical ON and who are seronegative for AQP4-IgG and MOG-IgG present a diagnostic and management dilemma. Like the patients who were initially described as having CRION and later discovered to have MOG-IgG, it is possible that these patients may have an unidentified autoantibody based on the response to immunosuppressive therapies. Further research is required to clarify the management of these patients, because the evidence to-date suggests that individuals with this condition have a high rate of treatment failure, high relapse rate, and significant disability.

## SUMMARY

Ophthalmologists and optometrists are first-line care providers for patients with acute or subacute vision loss and must be familiar with the clinical presentations of patients with ON, which has a high rate of misdiagnosis and can cause significant visual morbidity. ON may be a harbinger of CNS demyelinating disorders including MS, NMO, and MOG. Acute treatment of ON most often is necessary before serologic confirmation of a CNS disorder, and delay in diagnosis and initiating appropriate treatment may contribute to a worse visual outcome. Thus, an understanding of the clinical features that differentiate the ON subtypes allows clinicians to promptly pursue the work-up and treatments that are necessary to optimize visual outcomes.

## CLINICS CARE POINTS

(1) Features suggestive of an atypical inflammatory ON, which should raise clinical suspicion for NMOSD and MOGAD and prompt testing for AQP4-IgG and MOG-IgG, include severe unilateral or bilateral ON in non-White patients, with significant vision loss at presentation and nadir. Other clinical clues include hemianopic or bitemporal visual field defects and lack of response to high-dose intravenous methylprednisolone (NMOSD); or significant disk edema (MOGAD).

(2) MRI features suggestive of NMOSD include long segment optic nerve lesion (often greater than half the length of the optic nerve) with involvement of the intracranial optic nerve, optic chiasm, or optic tract. Optic nerve lesions in MOGAD are also long segment and involve the retrobulbar and intraorbital optic nerve, usually accompanied by significant perineural enhancement and swelling (optic perineuritis).

(3) Acute treatment of atypical inflammatory ON, where NMOSD or MOGAD are suspected, should be initiated early after onset of vision loss. Treatment with high-dose intravenous methylprednisolone and early commencement of plasma exchange are associated with better visual prognosis after an attack of NMOSD-ON or MOG-ON.

(4) Long-term management after ON should focus on preventing recurrent attacks. Long-term immunosuppression should be started after the first attack of AQP4-IgG-seropositive NMOSD. Decisions regarding long-term immunosuppression in MOGAD need to take into consideration the degree of recovery from the initial attack and risk of further relapses.

## Disclosure

Dr Chen is supported by the Cambridge-Rutherford Memorial Scholarship awarded by the Royal Society Te Apārangi - Rutherford Foundation and the Cambridge Commonwealth, European & International Trust, and also the Aotearoa New Zealand Fellows Research Entry Scholarship awarded by the Royal Australasian College of Physicians (RACP). The remaining authors have no disclosures.

## References

[1] Hor JY, Asgari N, Nakashima I, et al. Epidemiology of neuromyelitis optica spectrum disorder and its prevalence and incidence worldwide. Front Neurol 2020;11:501.

[2] Chen JJ, Bhatti MT. Clinical phenotype, radiological features, and treatment of myelin oligodendrocyte glycoprotein-immunoglobulin G (MOG-IgG) optic neuritis. Curr Opin Neurol 2020;33:47–54.

[3] Optic Neuritis Study Group. The clinical profile of optic neuritis. Experience of the Optic Neuritis Treatment Trial. Arch Ophthalmol 1991;109:1673–8.

[4] Chen JJ, Flanagan EP, Jitprapaikulsan J, et al. Myelin oligodendrocyte glycoprotein antibody-positive optic neuritis: clinical characteristics, radiologic clues, and outcome. Am J Ophthalmol 2018;195:8–15.

[5] Morrow SA, Fraser JA, Day C, et al. Effect of treating acute optic neuritis with bioequivalent oral vs intravenous corticosteroids: a randomized clinical trial. JAMA Neurol 2018;75:690–6.

[6] Filippatou AG, Mukharesh L, Saidha S, et al. AQP4-IgG and MOG-IgG related optic neuritis-prevalence, optical coherence tomography findings, and visual outcomes: a systematic review and meta-analysis. Front Neurol 2020;11:540156.

[7] Akaishi T, Himori N, Takeshita T, et al. Five-year visual outcomes after optic neuritis in anti-MOG antibody-associated disease. Mult Scler Relat Disord 2021;56:103222.

[8] Matiello M, Lennon VA, Jacob A, et al. NMO-IgG predicts the outcome of recurrent optic neuritis. Neurology 2008;70:2197–200.

[9] Keltner JL, Johnson CA, Cello KE, et al. Visual field profile of optic neuritis: a final follow-up report from the optic neuritis treatment trial from baseline through 15 years. Arch Ophthalmol 2010;128:330–7.

[10] Wingerchuk DM, Banwell B, Bennett JL, et al. International consensus diagnostic criteria for neuromyelitis optica spectrum disorders. Neurology 2015;85:177–89.

[11] Kupersmith MJ, Alban T, Zeiffer B, et al. Contrast-enhanced MRI in acute optic neuritis: relationship to visual performance. Brain 2002;125:812–22.

[12] Shor N, Deschamps R, Cobo Calvo A, et al. MRI characteristics of MOG-Ab associated disease in adults: an update. Rev Neurol (Paris) 2021;177:39–50.

[13] Ramanathan S, Prelog K, Barnes EH, et al. Radiological differentiation of optic neuritis with myelin oligodendrocyte glycoprotein antibodies, aquaporin-4 antibodies, and multiple sclerosis. Mult Scler 2016;22:470–82.

[14] Chen JJ, Tobin WO, Majed M, et al. Prevalence of myelin oligodendrocyte glycoprotein and aquaporin-4-IgG in patients in the optic neuritis treatment trial. JAMA Ophthalmol 2018;136:419–22.
[15] Sechi E, Buciuc M, Pittock SJ, et al. Positive predictive value of myelin oligodendrocyte glycoprotein autoantibody testing. JAMA Neurol 2021;78:741–6.
[16] Jarius S, Paul F, Aktas O, et al. MOG encephalomyelitis: international recommendations on diagnosis and antibody testing. J Neuroinflammation 2018;15:134.
[17] Gal RL, Vedula SS, Beck R. Corticosteroids for treating optic neuritis. Cochrane Database Syst Rev 2015;8:CD001430.
[18] Stiebel-Kalish H, Hellmann MA, Mimouni M, et al. Does time equal vision in the acute treatment of a cohort of AQP4 and MOG optic neuritis? Neurol Neuroimmunol Neuroinflamm 2019;6:e572.
[19] Akaishi T, Takeshita T, Himori N, et al. Rapid administration of high-dose intravenous methylprednisolone improves visual outcomes after optic neuritis in patients with AQP4-IgG-positive NMOSD. Front Neurol 2020;11:932.
[20] Bonnan M, Valentino R, Debeugny S, et al. Short delay to initiate plasma exchange is the strongest predictor of outcome in severe attacks of NMO spectrum disorders. J Neurol Neurosurg Psychiatry 2018;89:346–51.
[21] Deschamps R, Gueguen A, Parquet N, et al. Plasma exchange response in 34 patients with severe optic neuritis. J Neurol 2016;263:883–7.
[22] Elsone L, Panicker J, Mutch K, et al. Role of intravenous immunoglobulin in the treatment of acute relapses of neuromyelitis optica: experience in 10 patients. Mult Scler 2014;20:501–4.
[23] Optic Neuritis Study G. Multiple sclerosis risk after optic neuritis: final optic neuritis treatment trial follow-up. Arch Neurol 2008;65:727–32.
[24] Rae-Grant A, Day GS, Marrie RA, et al. Practice guideline recommendations summary: disease-modifying therapies for adults with multiple sclerosis: report of the guideline development, dissemination, and implementation subcommittee of the American Academy of Neurology. Neurology 2018;90:777–88.
[25] Thompson AJ, Banwell BL, Barkhof F, et al. Diagnosis of multiple sclerosis: 2017 revisions of the McDonald criteria. Lancet Neurol 2018;17:162–73.
[26] Pittock SJ, Zekeridou A, Weinshenker BG. Hope for patients with neuromyelitis optica spectrum disorders: from mechanisms to trials. Nat Rev Neurol 2021;17:759–73.
[27] Weinshenker BG, Wingerchuk DM. Neuromyelitis spectrum disorders. Mayo Clin Proc 2017;9:663–79.
[28] Poupart J, Giovannelli J, Deschamps R, et al. Evaluation of efficacy and tolerability of first-line therapies in NMOSD. Neurology 2020;94:e1645–56.
[29] Giovannelli J, Ciron J, Cohen M, et al. A meta-analysis comparing first-line immunosuppressants in neuromyelitis optica. Ann Clin Transl Neurol 2021;8:2025–37.
[30] Marignier R, Hacohen Y, Cobo-Calvo A, et al. Myelin-oligodendrocyte glycoprotein antibody-associated disease. Lancet Neurol 2021;20:762–72.
[31] Ringelstein M, Ayzenberg I, Lindenblatt G, et al. Interleukin-6 receptor blockade in treatment-refractory MOG-IgG-associated disease and neuromyelitis optica spectrum disorders. Neurol Neuroimmunol Neuroinflamm 2022;9:e1100.
[32] Costello F, Coupland S, Hodge W, et al. Quantifying axonal loss after optic neuritis with optical coherence tomography. Ann Neurol 2006;59:963–9.
[33] Akaishi T, Nakashima I, Takeshita T, et al. Lesion length of optic neuritis impacts visual prognosis in neuromyelitis optica. J Neuroimmunol 2016;293:28–33.
[34] Akaishi T, Takahashi T, Nakashima I, et al. Repeated follow-up of AQP4-IgG titer by cell-based assay in neuromyelitis optica spectrum disorders (NMOSD). J Neurol Sci 2020;410:116671.

Advances in Ophthalmology and Optometry 7 (2022) 295–309

ADVANCES IN OPHTHALMOLOGY AND OPTOMETRY

# Efficacy and Safety of Tocilizumab in the Treatment of Ocular Manifestations in Giant Cell Arteritis

Nooran Badeeb, MBBS[a,*], Rustum Karanjia, MD, PhD[b,c,d]

[a]Department of Ophthalmology, University of Jeddah, Jeddah, Saudi Arabia; [b]Doheny Eye Centers, Department of Ophthalmology, David Geffen School of Medicine at UCLA, UCLA Stein Eye Institute, 100 Stein Plaza UCLA, Los Angeles, CA 90095-7000, USA; [c]Ottawa Hospital Research Institute, The Ottawa Hospital, Ottawa, Canada; [d]Doheny Eye Institute, Los Angeles, CA, USA

**Keywords**

• Actemra • Giant cell arteritis • Anterior ischemic optic neuropathy

**Key points**

- Tocilizumab is able to control giant cell arteritis progression in patients with ocular symptoms.
- Ocular complications and side effects of giant cell arteritis are mitigated with early Tocilizumab treatment and rapid tapering of glucocorticoids.
- The optimal time to remission on Tocilizumab and glucocorticoids is around 3 months.
- Tocilizumab should be considered early in the treatment of giant cell arteritis, especially in refractory cases and patients who experience toxicity or have flare-ups while on optimal glucocorticoids.
- Tocilizumab has a good safety profile with the greatest risk related to opportunistic infections.

## INTRODUCTION

Giant cell arteritis (GCA) is the most common autoimmune vasculitis of medium to large vessels in people aged over 50 years. Incidence varies between 1 in 100,000 and 30 in 100,000 and depends on several factors, including racial background and major histocompatibility complex genes. For example, Caucasian patients or subjects living in northern latitudes who carry the HLA-DRB1*04

*Corresponding author. University of Jeddah, Hamzah Ibn Al Qasim St, Al Sharafeyah dist, Jeddah 23218, Saudi Arabia. *E-mail address:* nooran.badeeb@gmail.com

https://doi.org/10.1016/j.yaoo.2022.03.010

allele have a higher incidence [1–3]. A predilection exists for women who have a 1% lifetime risk of getting GCA versus men who have a 0.5% lifetime risk of GCA [3]. Sight-threatening and life-threatening complications occur in GCA as a result of ischemic injury, aneurysms, and systemic inflammation. Patients can complain of polymyalgia rheumatica symptoms, such as neck, shoulder, and hip myalgias with movement, and jaw claudication. Furthermore, constitutional symptoms, such as fever, chills, night sweats, weight loss, and loss of appetite, have been reported [3]. Patients with GCA can present to the ophthalmology clinic with either afferent or efferent pathway disease [4]. Afferent issues primarily present as episodes of transient vision loss, amaurosis fugax (AF), which is a harbinger for potential permanent vision loss from ischemic optic neuropathy (ION). ION can take many forms including anterior ischemic optic neuropathy (AION), posterior ischemic optic neuropathy (PION), central retinal artery occlusion (CRAO), or cilioretinal artery occlusion. In patients with AION, 8% to 28% of them reported having AF before the episode of permanent vision loss [4–6]. Retrochiasmal visual field defects (VFDs) such as homonymous hemianopia or quadrantanopia are uncommon in GCA (0.76/100,000 per year) and occur more commonly in men [7]. On the efferent side patients typically present with diplopia. Causes for this include ischemic insult to the cranial nerves; most commonly a sixth nerve palsy, ischemia of the extraocular muscles, and brain stem strokes, which can produce cranial neuropathies or a skew deviation [5].

If vision-related complications are not recognized and treated early in the disease, they can lead to permanent vision loss, with reports of up to a quarter of patients suffering from permanent vision loss [8]. Some of these patients will experience visual hallucinations with Charles Bonnet syndrome [4].

GCA is a T-cell–mediated immune disease of medium to large vessels. Three layers compromise the arterial wall in these vessels (adventitia, media, and intima), which are separated by the external and internal elastic lamina [1,2]. In GCA, the internal elastic lamina is damaged and the smooth muscle cells within the media are degraded by matrix metalloproteinase, which is secreted by macrophages. This promotes the passage and proliferation of myofibroblast within the intima causing intimal hyperplasia leading to lumen occlusion and subsequent end-organ ischemia [1,2].

Given the autoimmune nature of GCA, visual complications typically are treated with glucocorticoid (GC) therapy; however, GC can cause other health issues with its own morbidity and mortality, especially in an elderly population [9,10]. Trials to reduce iatrogenic side effects of GC treatments have looked at several GC-sparing agents. This review looks at the role of these GC-sparing agents, specifically Tocilizumab (TCZ) for the treatment of ocular manifestations of GCA.

## METHODOLOGY

The following electronic databases were searched on October 27, 2021: EMBASE, Ovid MEDLINE, Cochrane central library from 1947 to 2021 October

26. The search terms included different keywords and abbreviations of the following: GCA, tocilizumab, and ocular manifestations. All studies published in English were included.

### Selection criteria

We screened the titles and abstracts to identify studies that looked at GCA patients with visual manifestations treated with TCZ. Studies with no mention of the ocular manifestations and outcomes were excluded. Data were extracted from eligible articles and summarized in a table (see supplementary materials; Table S1). The primary measure was TCZ in the management and/or control of ocular manifestations of GCA, secondary measures included the indication for TCZ use, treatment-related side effects, and treatment failures, were also captured.

## RESULTS

From the literature search, we identified 607 studies that involved information about GCA and TCZ. Of these only 65 studies were compatible with our objectives. After reading the full text, 10 were included because they evaluated the use of TCZ in the management and/or the control of ocular manifestations of GCA (Fig. 1)—Three case reports, 3 randomized and nonrandomized clinical trials (RCTs), and 4 retrospective studies.

## SIGNIFICANCE

Systemic and ocular side effects of GC are well known, and although the dose and modality of administration for GC varies depending on the treating location, typically IV methylprednisolone or dexamethasone and oral prednisone, the dose is typically high and for a long duration. This high dose is required to halt disease progression, and the long duration of treatment is due to the high rate of disease reactivation in patients who are rapidly tapered off GC. This increases the risk of these iatrogenic side effects, particularly in patients with ocular involvement [10–12]. Furthermore, this elderly population has other comorbidities exacerbated by GC, increasing the risk of myocardial infarction, stroke, cardiac arrhythmias, hypertensive crisis, hyperosmolar hyperglycemic nonketotic syndrome, psychosis, and sudden death [12]. Ocular side effects such as cataract, glaucoma, and central serous chorioretinopathy also can develop [10]. As such, reducing the iatrogenic burden of GCs is an important consideration when treating patients with GCA.

Several GC sparing agents exist, which have been tried to reduce the iatrogenic adverse events in GCA. Most like methotrexate (MTX) have shown inconsistent results in the studies [13,14], although a meta-analysis reported a benefit from MTX in reducing relapses and GC requirement [15]. Trials of anti-TNF agents, again, have had conflicting results for infliximab, adalimumab was found to be not effective while etanercept showed promising results; no difference in the number or type of adverse events occurred [9]. The dihydroorotate dehydrogenase inhibitor Leflunomide had some benefit in an

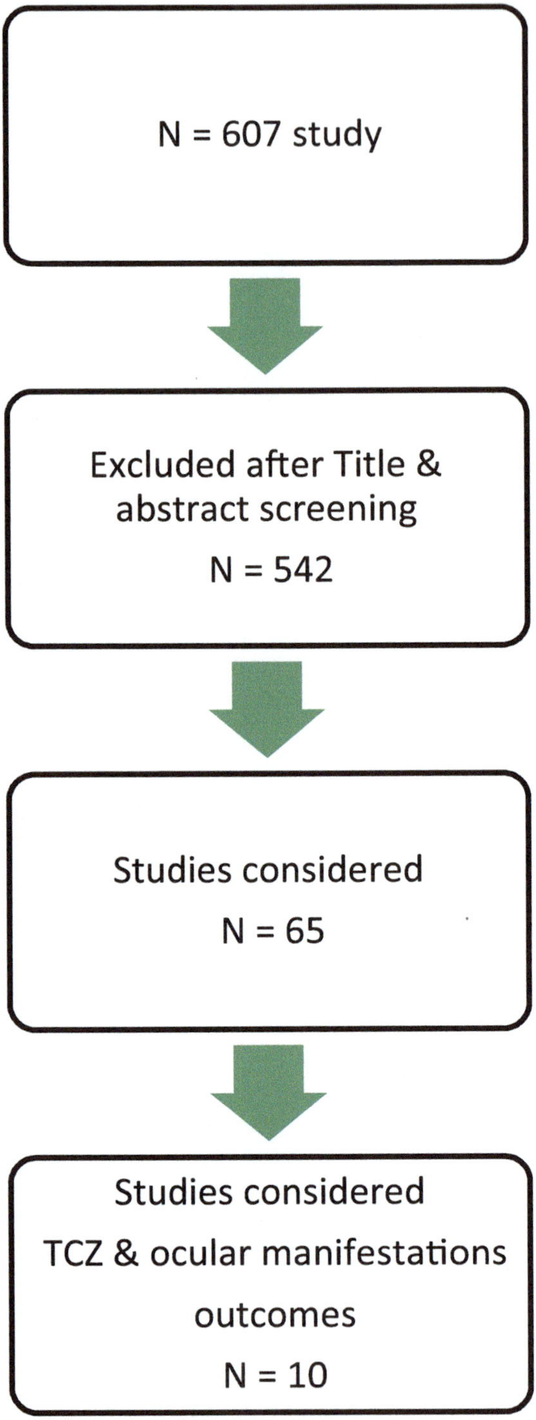


**Fig. 1.** Flow diagram of the study selection process.

uncontrolled retrospective study, but further data are needed. Other cytotoxic drugs such as azathioprine, cyclosporine A, cyclophosphamide, and dapsone have weak evidence for controlling disease activity, and the risks of major side effects mean that these medications are not recommended [9]. Medications targeting cytokines have been tried in GCA, and the IL-1 inhibitor Anakinra showed some promise in a small case series [9]. Subsequent understanding of the pathophysiology of GCA highlighted the importance of the cytokine IL-6 in the disease pathogenesis [1,2]. IL-6 is produced by macrophages, endothelial cells, and T and B cells. This cytokine causes a strong proinflammatory reaction and is needed for TH17 cell differentiation [2,3]. The IL-6 inhibitor, Tocilizumab (TCZ, monoclonal antibody against IL-6 receptor), was first approved by the United States Food and Drug Administration (FDA) in 2010 to treat moderate to severe rheumatoid arthritis, and is used in other autoimmune diseases like polyarticular juvenile idiopathic arthritis, systemic juvenile arthritis, and idiopathic cytokine release syndrome [2,3].

TCZ blocks both the soluble and the membrane-bound forms of IL-6 receptors [16], thus it had potentially been used as a treatment for GCA [17]. TCZ was shown to be effective in controlling GCA disease activity and preventing relapses in a multicentre phase III randomized control clinical trial–the Giant-Cell Arteritis Actemra (GiACTA) trial. GiACTA is a cornerstone study that compared TCZ to steroids. GCA patients were randomized into 4 groups, 2 groups received TCZ 162 mg subcutaneous (SC), one group was dosed weekly, and another group received TCZ every other week along with a 26-week GC taper. The other 2 groups received placebo and a GC taper, one group was tapered over 26 weeks and the other group was tapered over 52 weeks. In their results, TCZ groups had superior outcomes in maintaining remission and reducing the cumulative dose of GC [18]. TCZ received FDA approval for the treatment of GCA in 2017.

Since then, the Swedish Society of Rheumatology published guidelines to treat GCA with TCZ: (1) relapse with GC during or after the treatment is done, (2) involvement of large vessels evident by imaging or biopsy, (3) clinically active GCA, (4) high erythrocyte sedimentation rate (ESR) and C-reactive protein (CRP), and (5) side effects or anticipated severe side effects from GC [19]. The optimal time to treat a patient with ocular symptoms from GCA, however, is not covered by this guidance.

## Visual outcomes reported with Tocilizumab

The initial case reports of TCZ use in GCA was in patients who were suffering severe side effects from GC. In some cases, TCZ was started early in the course of the disease with short course of intravenous (IV) GC [20]. In other reports, TCZ was used in refractory GCA patients with evidence of clinical progression [21]. The effects of adding TCZ on vision varied and are reviewed in the following.

Svasti-Salee et al reported a case of a 72-year-old man with systemic symptoms of GCA, diplopia, and AF that progressed to afferent vision disturbance

**Table S1**
Studies demonstrating the visual outcome with the use of TCZ

| Study | Type | N | Indication of TCZ | Objectives | Results | Conclusion | Safety Data |
|---|---|---|---|---|---|---|---|
| Amsler et al, [25] 2021 | Retrospective<br>Observational monocentric | 186<br>(12%) vision loss at presentation | GC sparing | To study the occurrence of new vision loss in GCA treated with TCZ.<br>Efficacy of TCZ (8 g/kg every month) with short course IV GC x3 days. | New vision loss in 2 patients (1.1%). Both with AION.<br>Vision outcome on TCZ for patients presenting with vision loss:<br>15/28 eyes (54%) had stabilization.<br>8/28 eyes (29%) had improvement. | Both cases presented at the initiation of TCZ, likely that structural changes were too advanced. | No data |
| Khanna et al, [23] 2021 | Case report | 1<br>Unilateral AION | Sensitivity to steroids by allergy test | | Vision and visual field defects remained the same. | TCZ with short course of IV GC could be effective in GCA with ophthalmic involvement. | No data |
| Christ et al, [20] 2021 | Clinical trial | 18<br>6/18 presented with visual symptoms. | - | To assess IVMP 500 mg × 3 days followed by TCZ IV 8 mg/kg then weekly sc 162 mg) | 13/18 sustained remission at 52 wk.<br>1 new onset of AION. | Early weaning of GC is feasible.<br>Good control of GCA with TCZ monotherapy. | 2 cases had withdrawal from the study due to Hepatopathy and the other with diverticulitis. |
| Unizony et al, [26] 2021 | Retrospective | 60<br>22/60 (36.7%) with vision manifestations<br>(AION, CRAO, AF, diplopia, transient blurry vision) | Multiple flares on GC.<br>Side effects from GC. | Assess GCA flare-up as visual manifestations occurring while on TCZ. | Before TCZ:<br>(71.7%) had ≥ 1 flare. | TCZ reduced the occurrence of new GCA-related visual manifestations, and no new cases of AION or permanent vision loss occurred. | Rate of complications after TCZ 53.3% (44.4% from GC, 35.9% from TCZ, and 67.9% were either due to CG or TCZ or both)<br>Common side effects were cataract and pneumonia. |

| | | | | | | | |
|---|---|---|---|---|---|---|---|
| | | | | | (15%) had visual manifestations<br>2 with AION.<br>After TCZ:<br>(30%) $\geq$ 1 flare.<br>(8.1%) had visual manifestations.<br>None with AION.<br>2 patients had AF. | | (8.3%) discontinued TCZ:<br>1 pneumonia,<br>1 sepsis<br>1 bowel perforation<br>1 severe leukopenia<br><br>1 allergic reaction<br>1 malignancy (leiomyosarcoma)<br>1 diverticulitis.<br>No deaths occurred |
| Regola et al, [27] 2020 | Retrospective observational monocentric | 32<br><br>Visual manifestations at presentation: 9/32 (78%) blurred vision or AF 4/32, permanent unilateral or bilateral blindness 5/32. | 1) Relapsing disease refractory to previous GC treatment and/or conventional DMARDs (6 with MTX, 1 with AZA)<br>2) Side effects from GC.<br><br>3) Contraindications to prolonged high-dose GC. | Analyze the efficacy and safety of long-term TCZ treatment. | 92% sustained remission after tapering of TCZ which was used >1 y. | Efficacy of long-term treatment prevents relapse of GCA.<br><br>TCZ treatment for >52 weeks should be considered. | 10 with infections<br><br>1 pneumonia, 1 urinary infection, 1 gastrointestinal infection, 1 esophageal candidiasis, 1 dental abscess, 2 cutaneous herpes zoster, and 3 cutaneous infections.<br>1 severe urinary sepsis<br><br>High liver function test |

(*continued on next page*)

**Table S1**
**(*continued*)**

| Study | Type | N | Indication of TCZ | Objectives | Results | Conclusion | Safety Data |
|---|---|---|---|---|---|---|---|
| Svasti-Salee et al, [21] 2019 | Case report | 1 | | Role of TCZ in acute steroids refractory GCA | TCZ IV 8 mg/kg + 1 mg/kg PO steroids stopped the progression and prevented bilateral blindness. | TCZ may represent a new early effective second-line treatment option in GC resistant anterior ischemic optic neuropathy | Most of these infections (73%) occurred in the first 6 months of treatment. |
| | | Diplopia, AF then progressed to unilateral AION + CRAO | Refractory to steroids after 2 wk of IV GC and PO GC. | Role of TCZ in acute steroid refractory GCA. | Vision recovery from HM to 6/9 ph 6/6 5 d postinitiation of TCZ IV 8 mg/kg + prednisolone 1 mg/kg | IV TCZ improved vision in AION and CRAO from GCA in the acute stage. | No data |
| Vionnet et al, [22] 2017 | Case report | 1 Bilateral AION | Steroid resistance after 5 d IVMP | Role of TCZ in acute steroid refractory GCA | TCZ IV 8 mg/kg +1 mg/kg PO steroids stopped the progression and prevented bilateral blindness. | TCZ may represent a new early effective second-line treatment option in GC resistant anterior i schemic optic neuropathy | Pneumonia and Pulmonary embolism. |
| Stone et al, [18] 2017 | RCT | 251 | - | The effect TCZ on the rates of relapse during GC taper. | 1 AION in disease group of TCZ every other week. Vision resolved with GC. | TCZ received weekly or every other week, combined with a 26-wk prednisone taper was superior to either 26-wk or 52-wk prednisone tapering plus placebo with regard to sustained glucocorticoid-free remission | TCZ received weekly or every other week, combined with a 26-wk prednisone taper was superior to either 26-wk or 52-wk prednisone tapering plus placebo with regard to sustained glucocorticoid-free remission |
| | 4 groups: | | | | Flare and median GC dose over 52 wk | | 7% TCZ weekly serious infections. |
| | 1) Group of TCZ every week | | | | 1) Group TCZ every week 23% –1862 mg | | 4% in TCZ every other week group. |

| | | | | | | | |
|---|---|---|---|---|---|---|---|
| | 2) Group of TCZ every other week<br>3) Group of placebo + GC taper 26 wk<br>4) Group of placebo + GC taper 52 wk | | | | 2) Group TCZ every other week' 26%- 1862 mg<br>3) Group Placebo + GC taper 26 wk 68%- 3296<br>4) Placebo + GC taper 52 wk 55%- 3818 mg. | | neutropenia in 4% in both the groups.<br>high alanine aminotransferase level 2% both groups. |
| Peña et al, [19] 2016 | Retrospective multicenter | 30 | - | Assess the evolution of visual manifestations in patients with GCA treated TCZ and GC or TCZ with MTX. | 7/30 with complete blindness had no recovery.<br>2/30 with unilateral VFD recovered.<br>1 patient with bilateral VFD and 1 with bilateral vision blurring had partial improvement.<br>The rest of the patients achieved a complete recovery. | TCZ is useful in the treatment of visual manifestations of GCA but seems not to be effective when blindness has occurred. | No data |
| Villiger et al, [24] 2016 | RCT | 30<br>5/30 with ocular manifestations. | - | Efficacy and safety of TCZ in patients with newly diagnosed or recurrent giant cell arteritis. | No ocular relapse.<br>Remission 85% in TCZ group by 3 mo.<br>Remission 40% in GC group by 3 mo. | Efficacy of TCZ in the induction and maintenance of remission in patients with GCA. | GI perforations<br>GI bleeding<br>Hepatopathy<br>Infections<br>Eye infection (Moraxella catarrhalis and herpes) |

OD with reduced color vision and a relative afferent pupillary defect. Initially, he was treated with methylprednisolone 500 mg IV (IVMP) for 3 days followed by 60 mg PO prednisolone. After 2 weeks, the vision progressively worsened and another 3 days of IVMP 1000 mg was given, this time the vision continued to worsen and on day 16, a clinical picture of AION and CRAO was apparent, and TCZ 8 mg/kg IV was given along with prednisolone 1 mg/kg a day PO. Five days after the start of TCZ, the vision improved from HM to 6/9 (back to his baseline vision). In the subsequent 6 months with monthly TCZ administration, the GC was weaned from 60 mg to 5 mg, he remained in remission and his vision was 6/9 in the affected eye [21]. The authors concluded that early IV TCZ with GC treatment worked to improve vision despite the severity of his vision loss from a combined CRAO and AION.

Vionnet and colleagues reported a case of a 73-year-old woman who presented with systemic symptoms of GCA and bilateral AION. She had high inflammatory markers ESR 75 mm/h (0–29 mm/h) and CRP 67 mg/L (<10 mg/L) and temporal artery biopsy positive. She was treated with 1000 mg IVMP daily. Subsequently, the patient had a worsening headache with progressive vision loss to NLP in the right eye and a new inferior VFD in the left eye. TCZ 8 mg/kg IV was started on day 6 with prednisone PO 1 mg/kg daily. TCZ was given for a total of 12 doses every 4 weeks along with a slow tapering dose of PO GC. Eight months after stopping immunosuppressant medications, the patient remained in ophthalmologic and systemic remission with preservation of remaining vision in her left eye [22].

Khanna and colleagues reported another case of a 71-year-old Caucasian man with a previously documented allergy from GC. He presented with a right AION evident on the examination by pallid disc swelling and a ring scotoma. His temporal artery biopsy was positive and CRP was elevated at 83 mg/L (<10 mg/L). The patient received IVMP 120 mg on day 1, 240 mg on day 2, followed by 70 mg PO prednisone on day 3; subsequently, the patient developed a severe rash from GC. TCZ was initiated on day 3 with a dose of 8 mg/kg IV once monthly as a monotherapy. Treatment continued for 2 years with an increasing interval from 4 to 8 weeks. TCZ had disease control with no relapse, and the visual field was reported to have improved slightly [23].

Larger clinical studies include Villiger and colleagues report of a phase II randomized double-blinded, placebo-controlled trial with one arm assigned to TCZ and GC and the other arm received placebo and GC. They had no ocular flare-ups in the control group [24]. This success was followed by the GiACTA trial where only 1 patient receiving TCZ every other week had an ocular flare-up manifesting as AION. The visual loss resolved with GC treatment, and the patient was considered to have treatment failure on TCZ with regard to the primary outcome [18].

In another observational study, Amsler and colleagues had 186 GCA patients who were treated with pulse IVMP 500 to 1000 mg for 3 days followed by PO prednisone 1 mg/kg a day, along with TCZ 8 mg/kg IV every 4 weeks or at a dosage of 162 mg subcutaneously at weekly or biweekly intervals. Twenty-two (12%; 28 eyes) of these patients presented with vision loss and among these patients, the vision stabilized in 15 of 28 eyes (54%), whereas 8 of 28 eyes (29%) showed improvement (defined as a gain of 2 or more Snellen lines on the visual acuity chart). Unfortunately, 2 patients (1.1%) developed new ocular complications while on the TCZ and GC therapy; both had AION. The first patient was a 69-year-old man with an initial presentation of AF with progression to AION 2 days after he received a pulse IVMP for 6 days and TCZ IV with no improvement. Then 2 weeks later while on the optimal dose of GC 75 mg PO daily, he developed AION in the other eye. The other patient was a 78-year-old woman who received 3 doses of 500 mg IVMP followed by TCZ monotherapy. She lost vision 15 days afterward and despite another round of 1g IVMP followed by prednisone 1 mg/kg PO she did not improve. In these two cases, the vision loss happened early in the treatment course within the first month, possibly they already had advanced disease at presentation with vessel remodeling and inflammation that was difficult to control. Risk factors for vision loss on TCZ from this study were older age and positive temporal artery biopsy. While lower risk for vision loss was found in patients with high CRP levels and patients with aortitis [25].

Unizony and colleagues reported retrospective data on 60 patients, of which 36.7% had visual symptoms at baseline. In a comparison between patients without visual manifestations at presentation and the patients with visual manifestations at the presentation, disease flare manifesting in the form of visual symptoms occurred in 15% of patients before the TCZ treatment and only in 8% of patients after the initiation of TCZ treatment. In the first group, 2 of the patients had flare-ups in the form of AION, and none in the latter group had AION. Their study results showed a significant increase in the time to flare-up and a reduction in the number of flare-ups while on TCZ. The rate of $\geq 1$ disease flare-ups went from 71.7% before TCZ to 30% after TCZ [26].

### Duration of treatment with Tocilizumab

The Gusto study by Christ and colleagues tested the notion of giving short-term IVMP 500 mg for 3 days followed by 1 dose of TCZ 8 mg/kg IV, then a maintenance dose of TCZ 126 mg SC. At presentation, 33.3% of the study patients had visual symptoms. Of their patients, one had new-onset AION. Of the total GCA patients in this study, 25% achieved complete remission in the first 31 days. The mean duration of remission was 11.1 weeks on TCZ monotherapy [20]. A similar observation was found in the study by Regola and colleagues [27], where 90% of their patients had remission at 3 months while on a combination of GC and TCZ. Together these studies support the early weaning of GC as both studies had almost the same time to remission [20,27]. The RCT by Villiger and colleagues [24] compared time to remission between the groups with GC alone and the group with combined TCZ 8 mg/kg every 4 weeks and GC, they found that 85% of the latter group are in remission and were tapered fast as they were only on 7 mg adjunctive GC at

3 months post-TCZ use. In the GC monotherapy group, only 40% were in remission by 3 months.

### Administration of Tocilizumab

Guidelines for prescribing TCZ for GCA recommend a dose of 162 mg SC for adult patients once every week, in combination with a tapering course of GC. A more spaced dose of 162 mg once every other week with GC tapering may be prescribed based on clinical considerations. There are no specific additional recommendations for patients with vision loss associated with GCA [28].

Importantly it should be noted that the IV form of TCZ is not FDA approved for the treatment of GCA [28]. A pharmacokinetic study from a trial examining TCZ therapy in rheumatoid arthritis found that IV TCZ achieved a peak concentration quicker in comparison to the subcutaneous delivery (6 vs 74 hours). Although no evidence correlates the time to peak of the TCZ in the serum with the speed of efficacy in GCA, these data only provide a rationale for a possible benefit of IV over SC TCZ [29].

Monitoring disease remission in GCA is typically done through clinical symptoms, signs, and serologic markers. TCZ treatment makes the serologic markers, in particular CRP, less reliable as an acute phase reactant, because its formation is blocked by TCZ in the liver. Hence, monitoring of disease activity is mainly through clinical signs and symptoms [27].

### Safety and side effects of Tocilizumab

Known major and minor side effects that occur with the use of TCZ, most concerning is opportunistic infections [18,22,24,26,27]. It is important to note that most of the patients were on concurrent GC at the same time, so the side effects are not solely from TCZ use [18].

In a long-term safety study by Regola and colleagues [27], the rate of infections was observed to be at its highest where 73% of the documented infections in this study were at the first 6 months when on both GC high dose and TCZ. In the GiACTA trial, a higher rate of infection was seen in the group with the 52-week GC taper (12%), followed by the TCZ every week group (7%); finally, both the TCZ every other week and 26-week GC-taper groups had the lowest rate of infections (4%) [18]. Another important metric from the GiACTA trail to consider is the rate of withdrawal. The highest rate was in the TCZ groups at 6%, and 4% for the 26-week GC group. Surprisingly, all patients in the 52 weeks GC group completed the trial. In a separate study, Unizony and colleagues [26] reported 8.3% of patients had to stop the TCZ because of the side effects; only 2 were attributed to severe infections. Other reported side effects were injection site reaction and altered levels of white blood cells including neutropenia and elevated liver enzymes [18].

Gastrointestinal side effects have been reported, including some serious adverse effects such as gastrointestinal bleeding and bowel perforations [24,26]. In the Gusto study, 2 subjects had to withdraw from the study because of diverticulitis and hepatopathy [20]. In the RCT by Villiger and colleagues,[24] a patient suffered from hepatopathy and an unknown viral infection. In the same study, a case of Stevens-Johnson syndrome was reported 3 days after the third infusion but a causal relationship was not possible as multiple drugs were started at the same time [24].

Other rare side effects include a case report of a patient who developed pulmonary embolism and pneumonia 1 week after the TCZ infusion [22]. The pulmonary embolus occurred despite being on acetylsalicylic acid, and the patient was anticoagulated with acenocoumarol for 4 months. The pneumonia was diagnosed on radiography, but no causative agent was found by polymerase chain reaction testing of pulmonary secretions. The respiratory symptoms resolved under inhaled GC and long-acting bronchodilators. The same patient also suffered from a post-traumatic leg cellulitis that required systemic antibiotics [22].

## SUMMARY

Most GCA patients present with severe vision loss with little chance of improvement. Thus, it is imperative to look for treatment options that halt the progression of the disease and maximize the possibility of vision improvement. A role exists for TCZ in stabilizing or improving vision, especially if it is introduced early in the disease process before vascular remodeling has occurred. TCZ can be used as an initial treatment option in GCA patients with visual manifestations especially if the GCA is refractory to GC, or the patient is having a flare-up while on GC, or even to mitigate the risk of potential iatrogenic side effects from GC. TCZ appears most effective when used with short-term GC therapy, with therapeutic immunosuppressant effect and clinical remission observed at around 3 months after TCZ initiation. Rarely, a progression of eye problems occurs, specifically, AION when on TCZ. The major concerns when using TCZ are increased risk of infections, neutropenia, and GI perforations. Physicians' awareness and monitoring are important throughout the disease course and must rely on a combination of clinical and serologic markers of disease activity.

## CLINICS CARE POINTS

- When faced with a case of GCA with ocular involvement that is progressing despite the optimal treatment with glucocorticoids, Tocilizumab has a potential benefit in stopping the disease activity especially if considered at an early stage.
- Caution is warranted when treating GCA patients with TCZ as there are reported ocular relapses on the medication.
- If TCZ is initiated in GCA patients, it is best to keep them on the glucocorticoids treatment for at least 3 months from the start of the TCZ.
- It is important to have interdisciplinary teamwork when managing patients with GCA on TCZ and glucocorticoids to monitor for complications like opportunistic infections.

## Acknowledgments

The authors would like to acknowledge Ms Risa Shorr, our librarian, for her collaboration and help in the literature review.

## Disclosure

The authors have nothing to disclose.

## References

[1] Yoshifuji H. Pathophysiology of large vessel vasculitis and utility of interleukin-6 inhibition therapy. Mod Rheumatol 2019;29(2):287–93.
[2] Al-Mousawi AZ, Gurney SP, Lorenzi AR, et al. Reviewing the pathophysiology behind the advances in the management of giant cell arteritis. Ophthalmol Ther 2019; https://doi.org/10.6084/m9.figshare.7673285.
[3] Weyand CM M, Goronzy JJ M. Giant cell arteritis and Polymyalgia Rheumatica. Ann Intern Med 2003;139(6):505.
[4] Vodopivec I, Rizzo JF. Ophthalmic manifestations of giant cell arteritis. Rheumatology (United Kingdom) 2018;57:ii63–72.
[5] Hayreh SS, Podhajsky PA, Zimmerman B. Ocular manifestations of giant cell arteritis. Am J Ophthalmol. 1998;125(4):509–20.
[6] Hayreh SS. Giant cell arteritis: Its ophthalmic manifestations. Indian J Ophthalmol 2021;69(2):227–35.
[7] Kleindorfer DO, Khoury J, Moomaw CJ, et al. Stroke incidence is decreasing in whites but not in blacks: a population-based estimate of temporal trends in stroke incidence from the greater cincinnati/northern kentucky stroke study. Stroke 2010;41(7):1326–31.
[8] Patil P, Achilleos K, Williams M, et al. Fast track pathway reduces sight loss in giant cell arteritis: results of a longitudinal observational cohort study. Clin Exp Rheumatol 2015;35(3): 246–53. Available at: https://academic.oup.com/rheumatology/article/53/suppl_2/i5/1819986. Accessed November 22, 2013.
[9] Almarzouqi SJ, Morgan ML, Lee AG. Treatment of giant cell arteritis. Curr Opin Ophthalmol 2015;26(6):469–75.
[10] Oray M, Abu Samra K, Ebrahimiadib N, et al. Long-term side effects of glucocorticoids. Expert Opin Drug Saf 2016;15(4):457–65.
[11] Stanbury RM, Graham EM. Systemic corticosteroid therapy - Side effects and their management. Br J Ophthalmol 1998;82(6):704–8.
[12] Chan CCK, Paine M, O'Day J. Steroid management in giant cell arteritis. Br J Ophthalmol 2001;85(9):1061–4.
[13] Hoffman GS, Cid MC, Hellmann DB, et al. A multicenter, randomized, double-blind, placebo-controlled trial of adjuvant methotrexate treatment for giant cell arteritis. Arthritis Rheum 2002;46(5):1309–18.
[14] Jover JA, Cé Sar Herná Ndez-García, Morado IC, Vargas E, et al. Combined Treatment of giant-cell arteritis with methotrexate and prednisone a randomized, double-blind, Placebo-Controlled Trial Background: Corticosteroids Remain the Cornerstone of Therapy.; 2001.Availble at: www.annals.org. Accessed January 16, 2001
[15] Mahr AD, Jover JA, Spiera RF, et al. Adjunctive methotrexate for treatment of giant cell arteritis: an individual patient data meta-analysis. Arthritis Rheum 2007;56(8):2789–97.
[16] Al-Homood IA. Tocilizumab: a new therapy for large vessel vasculitis. Clin Exp Med 2014;14(4):355–60.
[17] Rubio-Rivas M, Forero CG, Mora-Luján JM, et al. Beneficial and harmful outcomes of tocilizumab in severe COVID-19: a systematic review and meta-analysis. Pharmacotherapy 2021;41(11):884–906.
[18] Stone JH, Tuckwell K, Dimonaco S, et al. Trial of Tocilizumab in Giant-Cell Arteritis. N Engl J Med 2017;377(4):317–28.

[19] Turesson C, Börjesson O, Larsson K, et al. Swedish Society of Rheumatology 2018 guidelines for investigation, treatment, and follow-up of giant cell arteritis. Scand J Rheumatol 2019;48(4):259–65.
[20] Christ L, Seitz L, Scholz G, et al. OP0061 a proof-of-concept study to assess the efficacy of tocilizumab monotherapy after ultra-short glucocorticoid administration to treat giant cell arteritis - the gusto trial. Ann Rheum Dis 2021;80(Suppl 1):33.2-33.
[21] Svasti-Salee CR, Mollan SP, Morgan AW, et al. Rapid visual recovery following intravenous tocilizumab in glucocorticoid resistant refractory giant cell arteritis. BMJ Case Rep 2019;12(10); https://doi.org/10.1136/bcr-2019-229236.
[22] Vionnet J, Buss G, Mayer C, et al. Tocilizumab for giant cell arteritis with corticosteroid-resistant progressive anterior ischemic optic neuropathy. Joint Bone Spine 2017;84(5): 615–9.
[23] Khanna RK, Hage R, Lecler A, et al. Giant cell arteritis with ocular involvement successfully treated with tocilizumab and very short-course glucocorticoids: a case report. J Francais d'Ophtalmologie 2021;44(4):481–4.
[24] Villiger PM, Adler S, Kuchen S, et al. Tocilizumab for induction and maintenance of remission in giant cell arteritis: a phase 2, randomised, double-blind, placebo-controlled trial. Lancet 2016;387(10031):1921–7.
[25] Amsler J, Kysela I, Tappeiner C, et al. Vision loss in patients with giant cell arteritis treated with tocilizumab. Arthritis Res Ther 2021;23(1); https://doi.org/10.1186/s13075-021-02480-4.
[26] Unizony S, McCulley TJ, Spiera R, et al. Clinical outcomes of patients with giant cell arteritis treated with tocilizumab in real-world clinical practice: decreased incidence of new visual manifestations. Arthritis Res Ther 2021;23(1); https://doi.org/10.1186/s13075-020-02377-8.
[27] Regola F, Cerudelli E, Bosio G, et al. Long-term treatment with tocilizumab in giant cell arteritis: Efficacy and safety in a monocentric cohort of patients. Rheumatol Adv Pract 2020;4(2); https://doi.org/10.1093/rap/rkaa017.
[28] Genentech, Inc. Highlights of prescribing information. Available at: www.fda.gov/medwatch. Accessed March 3, 2021.
[29] Abdallah H, Hsu JC, Lu P, et al. Pharmacokinetic and Pharmacodynamic analysis of subcutaneous tocilizumab in patients with rheumatoid arthritis from 2 randomized, controlled trials: SUMMACTA and BREVACTA. J Clin Pharmacol 2017;57(4):459–68.

Advances in Ophthalmology and Optometry 7 (2022) 311–323

ADVANCES IN OPHTHALMOLOGY AND OPTOMETRY

# Coronavirus Disease 2019–Related Health Disparities in Ophthalmology with a Retrospective Analysis at a Large Academic Public Hospital

Y. Grace Chung, BS[a], Christie M. Person, OD[b], Jacquelyn O'Banion, MD, MSc[c,d], Susan A. Primo, OD, MPH[c,d,*]

[a]Emory University School of Medicine, 201 Dowman Drive, Atlanta, GA 30322, USA; [b]Grady Health System, Eye Clinic, 80 Jesse Hill Jr Drive, SE, Atlanta, GA 30303, USA; [c]Emory Eye Center, 1365B Clifton Road, NE Suite B1100, Atlanta, GA 30322, USA; [d]Department of Ophthalmology, Emory University School of Medicine

**Keywords**

• COVID-19 • Ophthalmic findings • Public U.S. hospital • Health care disparities

**Key points**

- Coronavirus disease 2019 has disproportionately affected racial and ethnic minorities in the United States, in particular Black, Latinx, and Native American populations.
- Significant health care disparities within ophthalmology owing to coronavirus disease 2019 also have been discovered.
- Ophthalmic manifestations of coronavirus disease 2019 are prevalent; common findings include dryness, redness, and increased discharge, and may be the initial symptoms of a coronavirus disease 2019 infection.
- There is a lack of data of ophthalmic findings from coronavirus disease 2019 specifically in underrepresented minorities, and public hospitals have a unique opportunity to research presentation of disease in these populations.
- Ocular findings in patients with coronavirus disease 2019 potentially will support health care providers in managing these cases.

*Corresponding author. Emory Eye Center, 1365B Clifton Road, NE Suite B1100, Atlanta, GA 30322. *E-mail address:* sprimo@emory.edu

https://doi.org/10.1016/j.yaoo.2022.04.005
2452-1760/22/

## INTRODUCTION

Initially detected and identified in Wuhan, China in late 2019, severe acute respiratory syndrome coronavirus 2 has rapidly progressed to the coronavirus disease 2019 (COVID-19) pandemic, officially declared on March 22, 2020 [1]. The severity of this disease has had devastating fatality rates globally [2] and has had an extensive range of presentations, not solely limited to the respiratory system [3]. Asymptomatic transmission of the virus was discovered early on, with ophthalmic care being limited in most practices across the world to primarily emergency services, particularly owing to the close physical proximity needed to properly conduct a diagnostic eye examination [4–6]. Ultimately, ocular manifestations were found to be prevalent among patients with COVID-19, most commonly dry eye or foreign body sensation, redness, tearing, itching, eye pain, and discharge [7]. These manifestations may be the initial symptoms of a COVID-19 infection; a greater understanding of COVID-19–related ocular signs may lead to earlier diagnosis and improved ophthalmic care [8].

COVID-19 has disproportionately affected racial and ethnic minority groups, specifically resulting in much higher rates of death from disease in Black, Latinx, and Native American communities [9]. Alongside the impact of COVID-19 on patients, the pandemic has drastically impacted health care delivery, particularly at the beginning of the pandemic, with an increase in the use of telemedicine and a large decrease in outpatient visits [10–12]. Although access to telemedicine had been shown to alleviate the disruptions in outpatient care [13,14], racial and socioeconomic disparities have been prevalent in patient engagement to telemedicine and in outpatient visits, disproportionately affecting Black, Latinx, and Native American ethnic groups and patients with fewer socioeconomic resources [15–19]. These disparities in access to telemedicine have also been studied specifically within ophthalmology [20]. In 1 study, Black patients were less likely to be seen in a retina clinic, despite no increase in telemedicine visits [21].

Even with the disproportionate impact on Black, Latinx, and Native American populations of COVID-19, the ophthalmic manifestations of this virus have not specifically been studied in these communities. Large public hospitals may serve as a unique opportunity to study COVID-19 ocular disease presentation in underrepresented minorities. To further elucidate the effects of COVID-19 on patient demographics and health disparities in ophthalmology, the authors performed an analysis of patient demographics and ocular findings among COVID-19 positive patients at a public academic tertiary health care center primarily serving underserved populations during the height of the first wave of the COVID-19 pandemic. A retrospective chart review of ambulatory ophthalmology outpatient visits, as well as inpatient consultations, during this initial surge of the virus was undertaken because there is a dearth of research of COVID-19–related ocular manifestations in underserved populations to better define its impact on currently present health disparities.

## SIGNIFICANCE

### COVID-19 disproportionate impact

COVID-19 has disproportionately impacted all minority racial and ethnic groups, including Black, Latinx, Asian, Native Hawaiian and Pacific Islanders, and American Indian and Alaska Native communities in both infection and mortality rates [22]. A systematic review found that Black and Latinx individuals also have disproportionately higher rates of hospitalization with moderate to high-strength evidence [23]. Most studies attribute poverty, low household income, housing insecurity, education level, and language barriers as risk factors for higher rates of infection, death, and hospitalization [23]. With multivariable analyses, the excess burden of COVID-19 infections is not fully explained by other variables, such as underlying comorbidities and socioeconomic factors [24]. Other studies also have identified higher rates of infection for Black and Latinx patients compared with White patients; however, once hospitalized, lower rates of critical illness and death, indicating the presence of previously known existing structural barriers in accessing care [25]. These disparities are compounded by racial and ethnic minority communities also experiencing lower vaccination rates; Black and Latinx vaccination rates were shown to be approximately 2.1 and 2.9 times lower, respectively, compared with non-Hispanic White population across the United States [26]. Lower vaccination rates are not fully attributable to vaccine hesitancy from mistrust resulting from systemic injustices, but rather underlying structural inequities and vaccine accessibility are major contributing factors [27]. Moreover, Black and Latinx populations are underrepresented in vaccine clinical trials and for COVID-19 treatment trials [28,29].

### COVID-19–related health care disparities in ophthalmology

Barriers to care exist for underserved patients and racial and ethnic minorities, particularly around the constructs of social determinants of health. Factors like cost, transportation, language, and health literacy, to name a few, remain as barriers in normal times, only to be magnified during times of medical crisis, like the COVID-19 pandemic. Eye care delivery is no exception, and, although alternative methods of evaluation have been attempted, such as telemedicine, missed clinic visits have dramatically increased among elderly and non-White patients [12], particularly in the first wave of the pandemic. Timely interventions for ophthalmic diseases like diabetic retinopathy and macular degeneration can stave off preventable vision loss, whereas glaucoma requires continuous monitoring in most cases. Generally speaking, deviation and delay in eye care can be both tragic and insurmountable when urgent ocular diseases either are not identified or when chronic ones miss periodic and appropriate follow-up.

Many medical disciplines have been able to pivot to telemedicine through incorporating virtual, video, and/or phone visits into their daily practices [30]. Innovative hybrid care has allowed for medication check-ins, follow-ups, and even diagnostic capabilities, in many instances leading to improved compliance and continuity of care. Those specialties that are technology driven have been able to order tests, scans, images, and so on, allowing patients to undergo a procedure and then have a consultation with their provider regarding the results and management. In many cases, patients can defer in-person care, particularly if anxious about physically visiting health care facilities.

For ophthalmologic care, although it is technology driven in many instances, a face-to-face in-person visit is needed to accurately measure and monitor things like vision and eye pressure, although innovative solutions have been proposed and implemented, even circumventing the need for the traditional delivery model [31]. However, treatment for retinal diseases such as diabetic retinopathy and age-related macular degeneration rely on periodic intravitreal injections with the significant potential for vision loss if delayed [32]. Retina and glaucoma also require the use of specialized equipment that limit telemedicine use. A study found that, during COVID-19, cataracts saw a more than 60% decrease in visits, with only approximately 1% telemedicine use; glaucoma saw a more than 50% decrease in visits with only approximately 3% telemedicine use [30]. Telemedicine remains a less prevalent form of delivering eye care in most facilities, unlike other areas of medicine, and has significant limitations. Sudden painful or painless loss of vision, especially in monocular patients, new cases of retinal tumors or cancers, retinopathy of prematurity, recent surgical patients, and more all require physical examination of the eye [33]. Ophthalmic disparities will prevail when barriers to care from social determinants of health exist.

## COVID-19–related ophthalmic manifestations

The ocular findings associated with COVID-19 are varied and have affected both the anterior and posterior structures of the eye. A meta-analysis of 38 studies found that the most common diagnoses from December 2019 through August 2020 were foreign body sensation, redness, tearing, itching, eye pain, and discharge [7]. Another meta-analysis of 20 studies determined that one of the earliest ocular symptoms associated with COVID-19 is viral conjunctivitis and is associated with more severe disease, requiring hospitalization [34]. Microvascular alterations were also noted in the SERPICO-19 study, which cited findings of retinal hemorrhages, cotton wool spots, dilated veins, and tortuous vessels in patients with COVID-19 [35]. Cranial nerve abnormalities also have been noted in a few cases, specifically with oculomotor, trochlear, and abducens nerve palsies in patients with COVID-19. Other neuro-ophthalmic findings include Guillain Barre syndrome and Miller Fisher syndrome, with cases that improved with intravenous immunoglobulin treatment. Optic neuritis and intracranial hypertension have been observed in patients with COVID-19 as well, with angiotensin-converting enzyme 2 receptor cells postulated as the method of entry; they are present in the aqueous humor, retina, retinal pigment epithelium, choroid, and conjunctival epithelium [36,37].

The authors performed a retrospective, cross-sectional, observational study at a large public hospital serving primarily underrepresented minorities seen during the first surge of the COVID-19. A total of 7022 ambulatory patients seen in the ophthalmology clinic were identified between March 1 and November 30, 2020. Of these patients, 192 ambulatory patients had COVID-19–positive tests within this time frame, with a prevalence rate of 2.73%. An additional 10 inpatient ophthalmology consults also were identified. Of the ambulatory patients included in this study, 116 patients had a positive COVID-19 test before or within 1 week of their ambulatory visit. The average time to visit–the length of time from a positive COVID-19 test to the patient's next ambulatory visit–was 85.0 ± 39.6 days.

The demographics of ambulatory and inpatient consultation patients were examined (Table 1). The mean age of ambulatory and inpatients was 56.4 ± 12.5 and 51.0 ± 17.2 years, respectively. The majority of patients in both settings were female (65.6% for ambulatory patients, 70.0% for inpatient consultations). Black or African American and Latinx patients constituted the predominant ethnicity in both settings (78.6% Black or African American and 16.1% Hispanic ambulatory patients, 60% Black or African American and 20% Latinx inpatients), which is consistent with the overall patient population within the large, urban, academic hospital from which this subset was taken.

All 10 inpatients had at least 2 comorbidities, with hypertension (70%) and tobacco use (30%) being the most common. No inpatients had ocular symptoms directly related to COVID-19. Comorbidities were analyzed for all 192 ambulatory patients. The average number of comorbidities for all ambulatory patients was 3.4 ± 2.1, and 157 of 192 (81.8%) patients had at least 2 comorbidities. The most common comorbidities were tobacco use (70.8%), hypertension (70.3%), diabetes mellitus (47.4%), dyslipidemia (40.6%), and overweight and obesity (34.9%).

The most common *International Classification of Diseases*, 10th edition, diagnosis for ambulatory and inpatients were examined (Tables 2 and 3) with age-related nuclear cataracts, presbyopia, and type 2 diabetes mellitus with ophthalmic complications being the most common for ambulatory patients and viral pneumonia, severe sepsis, and mixed disorder of acid–base balance being the most common for inpatients. Two ambulatory patients had ocular manifestations of COVID-19, including dry eye and conjunctivitis.

Within the ambulatory patient population who tested positive from March 1, 2020, to November 30, 2020, 63.8% were diagnosed with age-related nuclear cataracts, 63.8% with presbyopia, and 52.6% with diabetic-related ophthalmic complications. Diabetic ophthalmic complications included retinal hemorrhage, vitreous hemorrhage, retinal vein occlusion, and nonproliferative and proliferative diabetic retinopathy. These findings were the top 4 diagnoses prevalent within our patient population during this 8-month time period and are consistent with ocular conditions that presented in our clinic before the pandemic. Retinal vaso-occlusion, often in the form of a central retinal vein occlusion, is an ophthalmic COVID-19 finding, which may occur as a result of immune-mediated pathogenesis after infection [38,39]. COVID-19 should be suspected in any patient who presents with retinal vaso-occlusion, but without

**Table 1**
Ambulatory and inpatient patient demographics

| | Ambulatory | Inpatient |
|---|---|---|
| Total number | 116 | 10 |
| Age, years | | |
| Mean | 55.1 ± 13.2 | 51.0 ± 17.2 |
| Median (range) | 56.5 (26–87) | 50.0 (20–72) |
| Sex, proportion (%) | | |
| Female | 76/116 (65.5) | 7/10 (70.0) |
| Male | 40/116 (34.5) | 3/10 (30.0) |
| Ethnicity, no. (%) | | |
| Asian | 2/116 (1.7) | 0/10 (0.0) |
| Black | 88/116 (75.9) | 6/10 (60.0) |
| Hispanic | 21/116 (18.1) | 2/10 (20.0) |
| White | 4/116 (3.4) | 1/10 (10.0) |
| Other | 1/116 (0.9) | 1/10 (10.0) |

known vascular disease risk factors; vasculitis in patients with COVID-19 has been identified in the lung, liver, kidney, and skin [40].

A study done in a medical center with similar demographics during the same time period revealed that patients who tested positive for COVID-19 had

**Table 2**
Ambulatory most common ICD-10 codes

| ICD-10 Code | Description | Frequency, proportion (%) |
|---|---|---|
| H25.1 | Age-related nuclear cataract | 74/116 (63.8) |
| H52.4 | Presbyopia | 74/116 (63.8) |
| E11.3 | Type 2 diabetes mellitus with ophthalmic complications | 61/116 (52.6) |
| H52.2 | Astigmatism | 60/116 (51.7) |
| H40.0 | Glaucoma suspect | 43/116 (37.1) |
| H52.1 | Myopia | 38/116 (32.8) |
| H04.1 | Other disorders of lacrimal gland | 37/116 (31.9) |
| Z96.1 | Presence of intraocular lens | 37/116 (31.9) |
| E11.9 | Type 2 diabetes mellitus without complications | 33/116 (28.4) |
| I10 | Essential (primary) hypertension | 32/116 (27.6) |
| Z79.8 | Other long term (current) drug therapy | 32/116 (27.6) |
| H25.8 | Other age-related cataract | 25/116 (21.6) |
| H52.0 | Hypermetropia | 23/116 (19.8) |
| Z79.4 | Long term (current) use of insulin | 21/116 (18.1) |
| H40.1 | Open-angle glaucoma | 20/116 (17.2) |
| Z98.4 | Cataract extraction status | 19/116 (16.3) |
| Z48.8 | Encounter for other specified postprocedural aftercare | 17/116 (14.7) |
| E78.5 | Hyperlipidemia, unspecified | 15/116 (12.9) |
| H2.8 | Other specified disorders of eyelid | 14/116 (12.1) |

*Abbreviations*: ICD-10, *International Classification of Diseases*, 10th edition.

outcomes comparable with their White counterparts when controlled for age, sex, and comorbidities [41]. A more recent study found that Black inpatients had a higher mortality rate than White patients, which was due to the different hospitals where each group of patients was admitted. This study adjusted for age, sex, income, and comorbidities. It also included a much larger and more diverse patient sample of 44,217 compared with 5902 in the earlier study [42]. When reviewing hospitalized patients within our patient population, the 2 most prevalent in-patient diagnoses include viral pneumonia (60%) and severe sepsis (50%). A similar study at Oschner Health in New Orleans from March to April 2020 reported that a diagnosis of pneumonia along with a coinfection of hypoxic respiratory failure were more commonly observed [43]. The patient demographics were comparable with those of our inpatient population with 70.4% of the COVID-19 positive patients in the study identifying as Black non-Hispanic.

The most common comorbidities identified in this study were tobacco use, hypertension, diabetes mellitus, dyslipidemia, and overweight and obesity. Hypertension and diabetes reflect the most common comorbidities found in meta-analysis pertaining to COVID-19; however, the prevalence found in this demographic was much higher than found in the literature [44]. The high rate of comorbidities found is especially important to take note in this population, in which the majority of the demographic are minorities disproportionately impacted by COVID-19, because comorbidities have been associated with higher rates of mortality owing to COVID-19 [45].

Although an estimated 1 in 10 patients with COVID-19 had at least 1 ocular manifestation [7], only 2 of 116 ambulatory patients with positive COVID-19 tests had ocular complaints directly related to COVID-19. The 2 symptoms seen in this study were dry eye and conjunctivitis, 2 of the most common eye concerns related to COVID-19, as discussed elsewhere in this article. The low prevalence of COVID-19 ocular manifestations in comparison with previously described meta-analyses may be a result of several factors, including hospital restrictions for ambulatory visits for patients with a positive COVID-19 tests, symptoms not correctly identified as related to COVID-19, or ocular symptoms overlooked owing to other COVID-19 symptoms. This finding highlights the importance of an awareness of COVID-19 ocular symptoms, because the prevalence of COVID-19–related ocular symptoms identified may be low, even in large institutions.

Our findings present the ocular diagnoses observed during the onset of the COVID-19 pandemic and one of a few studies with patients from an urban, academic hospital. There are limitations to our study, including a relatively small sample size. Additionally, COVID-19 tests included in the study were only those performed at our institution; patients with positive COVID-19 tests performed elsewhere may exist who were not included in our analysis. Another limitation to consider is that the COVID-19 vaccine was not approved during the study time period; therefore, the observed diagnoses may differ from those in breakthrough cases among vaccinated patients. A point-prevalence survey of

**Table 3**
Inpatient most common ICD-10 codes

| ICD-10 Code | Description | Frequency, proportion (%) |
|---|---|---|
| J12.8 | Other viral pneumonia | 6/10 (60.0) |
| R65.2 | Severe sepsis | 5/10 (50.0) |
| E87.4 | Mixed disorder of acid-base balance | 4/10 (40.0) |
| G93.4 | Other and unspecified encephalopathy | 4/10 (40.0) |
| J80 | Acute respiratory distress syndrome | 4/10 (40.0) |
| D68.8 | Other specified coagulation defects | 3/10 (30.0) |
| J95.8 | Other intraoperative and postprocedural complications and disorders of respiratory system, not elsewhere classified | 3/10 (30.0) |
| D62 | Acute posthemorrhagic anemia | 3/10 (30.0) |
| I10 | Essential (primary) hypertension | 3/10 (30.0) |
| A41.5 | Sepsis owing to other gram-negative organisms | 3/10 (30.0) |

*Abbreviations*: ICD-10, *International Classification of Diseases*, 10th edition.

100,000 people in England and a randomized trial of the Moderna vaccine both found that fully vaccinated individuals were two-thirds less likely to be asymptomatic COVID-19 carriers than the unvaccinated [46]. There is little in the literature documenting ocular symptoms in these breakthrough cases. It would be beneficial to compare the ocular findings in COVID-19–positive patients before vaccinations were available with those of COVID-19–positive breakthrough cases. This work may provide insight on the effectiveness of the current messenger RNA vaccines in preventing ocular symptoms in patients who test positive for COVID-19. Our retrospective study in an academic setting also was limited by the need to rely on the accuracy of the data entered in the electronic medical record.

## RELEVANCE AND FUTURE AVENUES

Ophthalmic practice requires close physical contact with patients along with proper understanding of potential ocular findings from COVID-19 within various settings and among different populations. COVID-19–related ocular manifestations may not be seen as commonly in an outpatient setting, further underscoring the importance of identifying ocular findings from this virus. The information from our study underscores the importance of local demographic evaluation, particularly from large, urban settings with a predominance of underrepresented minorities who have been disproportionately affected by COVID-19.

The disparities in COVID-19–related diagnoses are due to numerous factors, including socioeconomic status, increased incidence of comorbidities, and a lack of access to quality health care, all resulting in poor outcomes [47,48]. Black and Latinx patients are more likely to work in jobs requiring frontline exposure to COVID-19; however, the positions often provide inadequate or no health insurance. These individuals also are more likely to live in crowded housing, thus putting them at risk of COVID-19 infection [47,48]. Reduced access to quality care was examined in a recent study involving telemedicine practices during the early phase of the pandemic. Older non-White patients were less likely to access care, largely owing to a preference for in-person visits as opposed to video visits or phone calls. Non-White patients also were less likely to have access to internet service to facilitate a video visit [21]. As a result, ophthalmic and other COVID-19–related findings may not be detected at the same rate as White patients or are diagnosed at later stages of the viral process, with little to no correlation between the findings and the patient's COVID-19 testing status.

Future research directions should concentrate efforts at both further elucidating the impact of COVID-19 on racial and ethnic disparities and interventions for eliminating systemic barriers, both broadly and specifically within ophthalmology. Our study observed the average time for follow-up for patients during the initial surge of COVID-19 at an academic center; the impact of COVID-19 on access to ophthalmic care should continue to be studied. Several studies have identified the changes in ophthalmic care, from decreases in the number of in-person visits to increases in telemedicine use, and the impact on vision [32,49,50]. One retrospective analysis of medical retina patients in Australia found an average delay of 8 weeks or more in 40% of patients, with patients with neovascular macular degeneration experiencing the greatest vision loss from treatment delay [32]. Another study in Brazil found a decrease in the mean number of visits and medications for glaucoma patients before and during the pandemic [51]. There remains a lack of research on follow-up delay owing to COVID-19 in the United States and racial and ethnic disparities in regards to follow-up care in ophthalmology during COVID-19. Because the pandemic continues and telemedicine remains as a greater part of patient care, ensuring adequate follow-up care to prevent vision loss must be a priority. The burden of canceled visits remains on patients, whether the patient or the provider cancels [52], and racial and ethnic minorities may be disproportionately affected in follow-up care as seen with other disparities related to COVID-19. Current systemic reviews of racial and ethnic health disparities primarily identify these disparities; however, other articles expand on strategies for addressing them. Such strategies involve multipronged policy approaches, including accessible testing, contact tracing, and vaccination [48,53,54]. Evaluating the intersectionality between racial and ethnic health disparities with socioeconomic, environmental, and disability status is crucial for developing effective interventions for equitable access to care.

## CONCLUSION

Studies that present findings from large public hospitals and large urban medical centers are integral in examining gaps in health care for Black and Latinx patients and ensure that future management and treatment options during the pandemic will be focused on identifying areas for improvement during ophthalmic examination. Eye care professionals and providers from all disciplines should be aware of the common ocular diagnoses found in all patient populations, particularly minority patients, when working in similar settings as the one in our study. Our study serves to inform assessing ocular findings for patients with COVID-19–positive tests, expanding on and adding to our current body of literature to date and perhaps for future variants or pandemics.

The question remains as to how this information can be applied during ophthalmic examinations. The common diagnoses of age-related nuclear cataracts and diabetes-related ophthalmic complications are found in many patients and may not prompt much concern for possible COVID-19 infection. Diabetes-related ophthalmic findings should however cause us to further examine the likelihood that these findings may be due to COVID-19, especially if the patient has a known recent positive test result. The vaso-occlusive retinal findings discussed in other studies supports the necessity of comprehensive examinations with a careful history focused on a positive COVID-19 diagnosis in the past. The history should include questioning patients on any recent dry eye or conjunctivitis-related symptoms around the time of COVID-19 diagnosis. Breakthrough cases also must be studied more closely to determine if ophthalmic findings are present in these patients at the same or lower rates. Some patients may be asymptomatic and present to their eye examination with symptoms that prompt COVID-19 testing, further contributing to the identification of these individuals who otherwise would have no awareness of their status.

## SUMMARY

Opportunities exist in both eye care delivery and implementation of observational studies with intervention-based strategies to examine and evaluate the past, current, and ongoing effects COVID-19 has on our patients. In particular, investigational research in underserved populations should remain a cornerstone for reducing health disparities and improving access to care for those patients most vulnerable. Public hospitals and urban academic medicals must seize this opportunity and are uniquely positioned to do so.

### Disclosure

The authors declare there are no conflicts or competing interests.

### References

[1] Khalili M, Karamouzian M, Nasiri N, et al. Epidemiological characteristics of COVID-19: a systematic review and meta-analysis. Epidemiol Infect 2020;148:e130.
[2] Matta S, Chopra KK, Arora VK. Morbidity and mortality trends of Covid 19 in top 10 countries. Indian J Tuberc 2020;67(4):S167–72.
[3] Mahajan R, Paul G, Mahajan R, et al. Systemic manifestations of COVID-19. J Anaesthesiol Clin Pharmacol 2020;36(4):435.
[4] Nair A, Gandhi R, Natarajan S. Effect of COVID-19 related lockdown on ophthalmic practice and patient care in India: results of a survey. Indian J Ophthalmol 2020;68(5):725.

[5] Wan KH, Huang SS, Young AL, et al. Precautionary measures needed for ophthalmologists during pandemic of the coronavirus disease 2019 (COVID-19). Acta Ophthalmol 2020;98(3):221–2.
[6] Lai THT, Tang EWH, Chau SKY, et al. Stepping up infection control measures in ophthalmology during the novel coronavirus outbreak: an experience from Hong Kong. Graefe's Arch Clin Exp Ophthalmol 2020;258(5):1049–55.
[7] Nasiri N, Sharifi H, Bazrafshan A, et al. Ocular manifestations of COVID-19: a systematic review and meta-analysis. J Ophthalmic Vis Res 2021;16(1):103–12.
[8] Zhong Y, Wang K, Zhu Y, et al. Ocular manifestations in COVID-19 patients: a systematic review and meta-analysis. Trav Med Infect Dis 2021;44:102191.
[9] Tai DBG, Shah A, Doubeni CA, et al. The disproportionate impact of COVID-19 on racial and ethnic minorities in the United States. Clin Infect Dis 2021;72(4):703–6.
[10] Chatterji P, Li Y. Effects of the COVID-19 pandemic on outpatient providers in the United States. Med Care 2021;59(1):58–61.
[11] Ohannessian R, Duong TA, Odone A. Global telemedicine implementation and integration within health systems to fight the COVID-19 pandemic: a call to action. JMIR Public Heal Surveill 2020;6(2):e18810.
[12] Brant AR, Pershing S, Hess O, et al. The impact of COVID-19 on missed ophthalmology clinic visits. Clin Ophthalmol 2021;15:4645–57.
[13] Patel SY, Mehrotra A, Huskamp HA, et al. Trends in outpatient care delivery and telemedicine during the COVID-19 pandemic in the US. JAMA Intern Med 2021;181(3):388.
[14] Koonin LM, Hoots B, Tsang CA, et al. Trends in the use of telehealth during the emergence of the COVID-19 pandemic — United States, January–March 2020. MMWR Morb Mortal Wkly Rep 2020;69(43):1595–9.
[15] Yang J, Landrum MB, Zhou L, et al. Disparities in outpatient visits for mental health and/or substance use disorders during the COVID surge and partial reopening in Massachusetts. Gen Hosp Psychiatry 2020;67:100–6.
[16] Eberly LA, Kallan MJ, Julien HM, et al. Patient characteristics associated with telemedicine access for primary and specialty ambulatory care during the COVID-19 pandemic. JAMA Netw Open 2020;3(12):e2031640.
[17] Differences in the use of telephone and video telemedicine visits during the COVID-19 pandemic. Am J Manag Care 2021;27(1):21–6.
[18] Ye S, Kronish I, Fleck E, et al. Telemedicine expansion during the COVID-19 pandemic and the potential for technology-driven disparities. J Gen Intern Med 2021;36(1):256–8.
[19] Cao YJ, Chen D, Liu Y, et al. Disparities in the use of in-person and telehealth outpatient visits among Medicare beneficiaries in an accountable care organization during COVID-19. Health Serv Res 2021;56(S2):5.
[20] Aziz K, Moon JY, Parikh R, et al. Association of patient characteristics with delivery of ophthalmic telemedicine during the COVID-19 pandemic. JAMA Ophthalmol 2021;139(11):1174.
[21] Elam AR, Sidhom D, Ugoh P, et al. Disparities in eye care utilization during the COVID-19 pandemic. Am J Ophthalmol 2022;233:163–70.
[22] Boserup B, McKenney M, Elkbuli A. Disproportionate impact of COVID-19 pandemic on racial and ethnic minorities. Am Surg 2020;86(12):1615–22.
[23] Mackey K, Ayers CK, Kondo KK, et al. Racial and ethnic disparities in COVID-19–related infections, hospitalizations, and deaths. Ann Intern Med 2021;174(3):362–73.
[24] Rentsch CT, Kidwai-Khan F, Tate JP, et al. Patterns of COVID-19 testing and mortality by race and ethnicity among United States veterans: a nationwide cohort study. In: Zelner J, editor. PLoS Med 2020;17(9):e1003379.
[25] Ogedegbe G, Ravenell J, Adhikari S, et al. Assessment of racial/ethnic disparities in hospitalization and mortality in patients with COVID-19 in New York City. JAMA Netw Open 2020;3(12):e2026881.

[26] Disparities in COVID-19 vaccination rates across racial and ethnic minority groups in the United States. ASPE Off Sci Data Policy; 2021 (Issue Brief). Available at: https://aspe.hhs.-gov/reports/disparities-covid-19-vaccination-rates-across-racial-ethnic-minority-groups-united-states. Accessed May 18, 2022.
[27] Nguyen LH, Joshi AD, Drew DA, et al. Self-reported COVID-19 vaccine hesitancy and uptake among participants from different racial and ethnic groups in the United States and United Kingdom. Nat Commun 2022;13(1):636.
[28] Flores LE, Frontera WR, Andrasik MP, et al. Assessment of the inclusion of racial/ethnic minority, female, and older individuals in vaccine clinical trials. JAMA Netw Open 2021;4(2): e2037640.
[29] Chastain DB, Osae SP, Henao-Martínez AF, et al. Racial disproportionality in Covid clinical trials. N Engl J Med 2020;383(9):e59.
[30] Patel SY, Mehrotra A, Huskamp HA, et al. Variation in telemedicine use and outpatient care during the COVID-19 Pandemic in the United States. Health Aff 2021;40(2):349–58.
[31] Parikh D, Armstrong G, Liou V, et al. Advances in telemedicine in ophthalmology. Semin Ophthalmol 2020;35(4):210–5.
[32] Stone LG, Grinton ME, Talks JS. Delayed follow-up of medical retina patients due to COVID-19: impact on disease activity and visual acuity. Graefe's Arch Clin Exp Ophthalmol 2021;259(7):1773–80.
[33] Gelnick S, Akanda M, Lieberman R. Retina in the age of COVID-19. Adv Ophthalmol Optom 2021;6:187–200.
[34] Al-Namaeh M. COVID-19 and conjunctivitis: a meta-analysis. Ther Adv Ophthalmol 2021;13:251584142110033.
[35] Invernizzi A, Torre A, Parrulli S, et al. Retinal findings in patients with COVID-19: results from the SERPICO-19 study. EClinicalMedicine 2020;27:100550.
[36] Betsch D, Freund PR. Neuro-ophthalmologic manifestations of novel coronavirus. Adv Ophthalmol Optom 2021;6:275–88.
[37] Bypareddy R, Rathod BS, Shilpa Y, et al. Fundus evaluation in COVID-19 positives with non-severe disease. Indian J Ophthalmol 2021;69(5):1271.
[38] Venkatesh R, Reddy NG, Agrawal S, et al. COVID-19-associated central retinal vein occlusion treated with oral aspirin. BMJ Case Rep 2021;14(5):e242987.
[39] Walinjkar J, Makhija S, Sharma H, et al. Central retinal vein occlusion with COVID-19 infection as the presumptive etiology. Indian J Ophthalmol 2020;68(11):2572.
[40] Sheth J, Narayanan R, Goyal J, et al. Retinal vein occlusion in COVID-19: a novel entity. Indian J Ophthalmol 2020;68(10):2291.
[41] Kabarriti R, Brodin NP, Maron MI, et al. Association of race and ethnicity with comorbidities and survival among patients with COVID-19 at an urban medical center in New York. JAMA Netw Open 2020;3(9):e2019795.
[42] Asch DA, Islam MN, Sheils NE, et al. Patient and hospital factors associated with differences in mortality rates among Black and White US Medicare beneficiaries hospitalized with COVID-19 Infection. JAMA Netw Open 2021;4(6):e2112842.
[43] Price-Haywood EG, Burton J, Fort D, et al. Hospitalization and mortality among black patients and white patients with Covid-19. N Engl J Med 2020;382(26):2534–43.
[44] Paudel S. A meta-analysis of 2019 novel corona virus patient clinical characteristics and comorbidities. Res Sq 2020; https://doi.org/10.21203/rs.3.rs-21831/v1.
[45] Ejaz H, Alsrhani A, Zafar A, et al. COVID-19 and comorbidities: deleterious impact on infected patients. J Infect Public Health 2020;13(12):1833–9.
[46] Klompas M. Understanding breakthrough infections following mRNA SARS-CoV-2 vaccination. JAMA 2021;326(20):2018.
[47] Dalsania AK, Fastiggi MJ, Kahlam A, et al. The relationship between social determinants of health and racial disparities in COVID-19 mortality. J Racial Ethn Heal Disparities 2022;9(1):288–95.

[48] Lopez L, Hart LH, Katz MH. Racial and ethnic health disparities related to COVID-19. JAMA 2021;325(8):719.
[49] Subathra G, Rajendrababu S, Senthilkumar V, et al. Impact of COVID-19 on follow-up and medication adherence in patients with glaucoma in a tertiary eye care centre in south India. Indian J Ophthalmol 2021;69(5):1264.
[50] Valentim CCS, Muste JC, Iyer AI, et al. Characterization of ophthalmology virtual visits during the COVID-19 pandemic. Eye 2022; https://doi.org/10.1038/s41433-022-01938-2.
[51] Ayub G, Vasconcellos JPC de, Costa VP. The impact of Covid-19 in the follow-up of glaucoma patients in a tertiary center: a comparison between pre-pandemic and pandemic periods. Clin Ophthalmol 2021;15:4381–7.
[52] Morse AR. The Importance of patients' perspectives in providing ophthalmic care—lessons from the COVID-19 pandemic. JAMA Ophthalmol 2021;139(5):516.
[53] White A, Liburd LC, Coronado F. Addressing racial and ethnic disparities in COVID-19 among school-aged children: are we doing enough? Prev Chronic Dis 2021;18:210084.
[54] Wen LS, Sadeghi NB. Addressing Racial Health Disparities In The COVID-19 Pandemic: Immediate And Long-Term Policy Solutions. Health Aff Forefront 2020; https://doi.org/10.1377/forefront.20200716.620294.

# Cornea and External Diseases

Advances in Ophthalmology and Optometry 7 (2022) 325–344

ADVANCES IN OPHTHALMOLOGY AND OPTOMETRY

# Stepwise Approach to the Diagnosis and Management of Dry Eye and Ocular Surface Disease

Jennifer B. Nadelmann, MD*, Angela Gupta, MD, PhD, Caroline W. Chung, MD, Stephen E. Orlin, MD

Scheie Eye Institute, 51 North 39th Street, Philadelphia, PA 19104, USA

**Keywords**

• Dry eye disease • Aqueous deficiency • Evaporative dry eye disease • Meibomian gland dysfunction • Inflammatory dry eye disease

**Key points**

- Dry eye disease (DED) is a multifactorial disorder caused by abnormalities of the tear film causing damage to the ocular surface.
- Dry eye can be broadly categorized into aqueous-deficient and evaporative dry eye.
- Appropriate diagnosis, classification, and treatment of DED in a timely manner are crucial.
- A stepwise approach is critical to ensure that patients receive appropriate treatment based on the severity of their disease and symptoms.

## INTRODUCTION

Dry eye disease (DED) is a multifactorial disorder caused by abnormalities of the tear film causing damage to the ocular surface. In epidemiologic studies, the prevalence of DED varies widely, and DED has become an evolving public health concern because of its high prevalence and socioeconomic impact [1].

Symptoms of patients with DED include burning, irritation, foreign body sensation, pain, photophobia, tearing, redness, and fluctuating blurred vision. DED affects quality of life, interfering with activities of daily living. DED can be categorized into aqueous-deficient and evaporative dry eye [2]. (Fig. 1). Patients with aqueous deficiency primarily have failure of the lacrimal system, whereas patients with evaporative DED typically have an unstable tear film

*Corresponding author. *E-mail address:* Jennifer.nadelmann@gmail.com

https://doi.org/10.1016/j.yaoo.2022.03.011

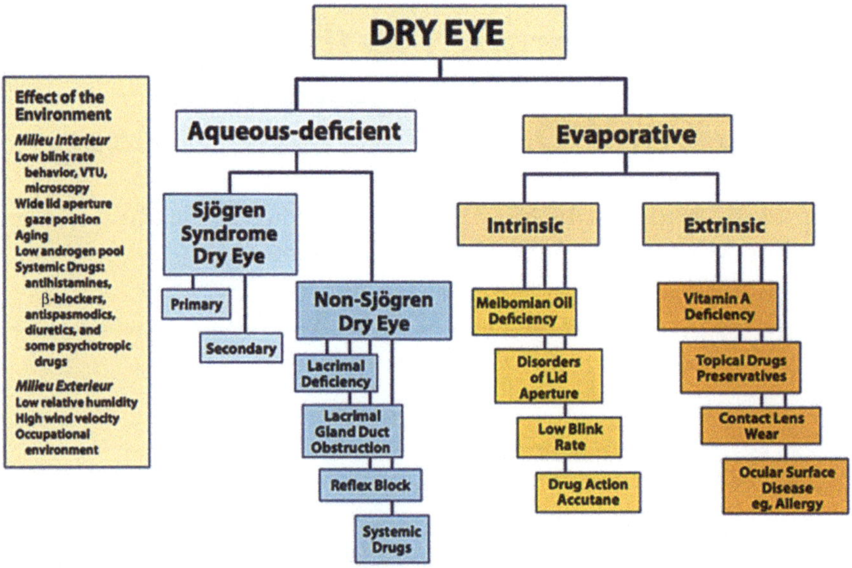


**Fig. 1.** Diagnostic classification of DED from the 2007 Dry Eye Workshop report. (*From* The definition and classification of dry eye disease: report of the Definition and Classification Subcommittee of the International Dry Eye WorkShop (2007). Ocul Surf. 2007 Apr;5(2):75-92; *with permission.* Please see cited paper for full figure description.)

caused by lipid deficiency. These two subtypes can often coexist in the same patient.

A stepwise approach is critical to ensure that patients receive appropriate treatment based on the severity of their disease and symptoms. In 2017, the Tear Film and Ocular Surface Society (TFOS) Dry Eye Workshop II (DEWS II) Management and Therapy report outlined an algorithm for a staged treatment [3]. (Box 1).

Appropriate diagnosis, classification, and treatment of DED are crucial. This article provides a stepwise approach to diagnosis and treatment for clinicians to be able to use in their practice.

## SIGNIFICANCE

### Approach to diagnosis

#### *Subjective evaluation*

*Symptoms.* A detailed history is crucial to appropriately diagnose DED and should include the timing and nature of symptoms, and environmental factors. Screening for symptoms of Sjögren syndrome, including dry mouth and fatigue, should be performed.

*Patient history and epidemiology.* Underlying systemic diseases, including seasonal allergies, thyroid disease, autoimmune conditions, collagen vascular disease,

**Box 1: Staged management and treatment recommendations for dry eye disease**

Step 1:

- Education regarding the condition and its management, treatment, and prognosis
- Modification of local environment
- Education regarding potential dietary modifications (including oral essential fatty acid supplementation)
- Identification and potential modification/elimination of offending systemic and topical medications
- Ocular lubricants of various types (if MGD is present, then consider lipid-containing supplements)
- Lid hygiene and warm compress of various types

Step 2:

If above options are inadequate consider:

- Nonpreserved ocular lubricants to minimize preservative-induced toxicity
- Tea tree oil treatment of *Demodex* (if present)
- Tear conservation
  - Punctal occlusion
  - Moisture chamber spectacles/goggles
- Overnight treatments (such as ointment or moisture chamber devices)
- In-office, physical heating and expression of the meibomian glands (including device-assisted therapies, such as LipiFlow)
- In-office intense pulsed light therapy for MGD
- Prescription drugs to manage DED
  - Topical antibiotic or antibiotic/steroid combination applied to the lid margins for anterior blepharitis (if present)
  - Topical corticosteroid (limited duration)
  - Topical secretagogues
  - Topical nonglucocorticoid immunomodulatory drugs (such as cyclosporine)
  - Topical lymphocyte functional associated antigen-1 antagonist drugs (such as lifitegrast)
  - Oral macrolide or tetracycline antibiotics

Step 3:

If above options are inadequate, consider:

- Oral secretagogues
- Autologous/allogeneic serum eye drops
- Therapeutic contact lens options

- Soft bandage lenses
- Rigid scleral lenses

Step 4:

If above options are inadequate consider:

- Topical corticosteroid for longer duration
- Amniotic membrane grafts
- Surgical punctal occlusion
- Other surgical approaches (eg, tarsorrhaphy, salivary gland transplant)

*Abbreviation:* MGD, meibomian gland dysfunction.
*From* Jones L, Downie LE, Korb D, Benitez-Del-Castillo JM, Dana R, Deng SX, Dong PN, Geerling G, Hida RY, Liu Y, Seo KY, Tauber J, Wakamatsu TH, Xu J, Wolffsohn JS, Craig JP. TFOS DEWS II Management and Therapy Report. Ocul Surf. 2017 Jul;15(3):575-628; *with permission*. Please see cited paper for full figure description.

neurologic conditions (stroke, Bell palsy, Parkinson), and diabetes may predispose patients to DED. Dry eye also can be associated with several iatrogenic interventions, such as refractive surgery and contact lens wear, in addition to preservative-containing glaucoma drops [4] and other systemic medications [5].

*Questionnaires.* Several questionnaires exist that can be useful tools to standardize symptomatic evaluation of dry eye and to monitor patients. This article focuses on the most common and validated questionnaires.

NEI-VFQ25 is a 25-item questionnaire developed by the National Eye Institute (NEI) that focuses on quality of life and symptoms [6]. The questionnaire's subcategories evaluate the patients' perceptions of their general health and vision, symptoms (pain and discomfort), and difficulty with daily activities and functioning.

The Ocular Surface Disease Index (OSDI) was developed by Allergan to assess symptoms of dry eye and how they affect functioning. It is a 12-item survey with three subsections: ocular symptoms, vision related function, and environmental triggers. The OSDI has a high internal consistency, excellent validity, and good sensitivity and specificity [7].

The Dry Eye Questionnaire-5 (DEQ-5) consists of five questions to evaluate the frequency of watery eye, discomfort and dryness, and late day discomfort and dryness intensity [8]. The DEQ-5 has been validated to identify patients with dry eye and is comparable with the OSDI questionnaire [9].

The Standard Patient Evaluation of Eye Dryness (SPEED) questionnaire was designed to offer a quick method to track symptoms [10]. The questionnaire gives a score from 0 to 28 to assess frequency and severity of symptoms. SPEED scores have been found to be repeatable and valid, correlating well to ocular surface staining and meibomian gland dysfunction (MGD) [11].

*Diagnostic criteria*

*Dry Eye Workshop II.* The TFOS DEWS published the second DEWS report (DEWS II) in 2017, which proposed a diagnostic algorithm for DED (Fig. 2)

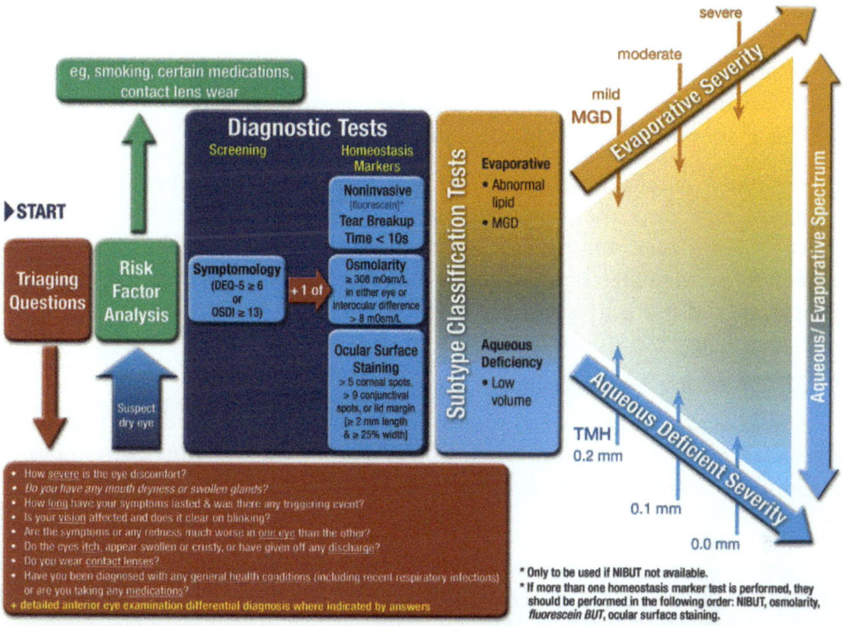


**Fig. 2.** Approach to diagnosis of DED. (*From* Wolffsohn JS, Arita R, Chalmers R, Djalilian A, Dogru M, Dumbleton K, Gupta PK, Karpecki P, Lazreg S, Pult H, Sullivan BD, Tomlinson A, Tong L, Villani E, Yoon KC, Jones L, Craig JP. TFOS DEWS II Diagnostic Methodology report. Ocul Surf. 2017 Jul;15(3):539-574; *with permission.* Abbreviations: NIBUT,non-invasive break up time, TMH tear meniscus height

[12]. The first step to diagnosis was triage questions that asked about DED symptoms and helped screen out patients with other conditions, including ocular infection and allergy. They then needed to demonstrate both (1) DED symptoms on the DEQ-5 or OSDI, and (2) signs of tear film instability by measuring either tear breakup time (TBUT), osmolarity, or positive ocular surface staining.

*Japan Dry Eye Society.* The Japan Dry Eye Society proposed the first definition and diagnostic criteria of DED in 1995. In this report, the diagnosis required abnormalities of the tear film and ocular surface epithelial damage identified by staining. An update was published in 2006, which described that patients also needed to have subjective symptoms for diagnosis [13].

*Ocular Dryness Disease Severity European Consensus Group.* The Ocular Dryness Disease Severity European Consensus Group (ODISSEY) diagnostic criteria take into account that patients may have discordant signs and symptoms [14]. If the patient's OSDI is more than 33 and corneal fluorescein staining (CFS) Oxford scale for surface staining is more than 3, then the patient automatically meets the criteria for severe dry eye. If discordance exists between the OSDI and CFS, then the presence of additional determinant data is used to confirm the diagnosis.

## Clinical examination

### *Eyelids*

*Lid closure.* Lid incongruity caused by ectropion or entropion, floppy eyelid syndrome, or lagophthalmos can lead to ocular surface irritation and exposure, disturbing the integrity of the tear film.

*Lid margins.* A careful examination of the eyelid margin can provide useful information regarding the meibomian glands. Expression of thickened, turbid, and/or creamy meibum may be seen in patients with MGD. In blepharitis, debris may be visualized on the lashes and erythema, telangiectasias, and thickening of the lid margins also may occur. Collarettes along the base of the eyelashes can help identify *Demodex.*

### *Conjunctiva*

*Lid-parallel conjunctival folds.* Lid-parallel conjunctival folds result from increased friction of the lid and conjunctiva and can be seen on slit lamp examination or with optical coherence tomography (OCT) [15].

### *Tear film*

*Tear film meniscus.* Measurement of the height of the tear meniscus can help identify a hyposecretory process. A height of less than 0.2 cm is considered pathologic [16]. A foamy tear film can indicate an altered lipid layer.

*Tear breakup time.* TBUT measures stability of the tear film and is quantified by measuring the time interval to the first appearance of a dry spot after the patient blinks. A TBUT of less than 10 seconds is considered pathologic [17].

*Schirmer test.* Schirmer test quantifies tear production from the lacrimal gland. The basic test is performed by instillation of a topical anesthetic using a strip of filter paper folded in the inferior cul de sac for five minutes. Saturation of the filter paper of less than 3 mm is suggestive of aqueous tear deficiency. The Schirmer I test also accounts for reflex tearing and is performed without a topical anesthetic. Wetting of less than 5 mm in five minutes is diagnostic of aqueous tear deficiency. The Schirmer II test accounts for reflex tearing by using a cotton-tipped applicator to irritate the nasal mucosa. Wetting of less than 15 mm after two minutes is considered abnormal.

*Tear film osmolarity.* Tear osmolarity increases with the severity of dry eye. The exact cutoff threshold value is variable in the literature; however, the currently agreed-on value is 308 mOsm/L [18].

*Tear fluid protein immunoassays.* Matrix-metalloproteinase 9 (MMP-9) is an inflammatory cytokine secreted by distressed epithelial cells. Increased MMP-9 level (>40 ng/mL) correlates well to OSDI scores, TBUT, Schirmer testing, and corneal staining [19]. Lactoferrin is secreted by the acinar cells, correlates to the function of the lacrimal gland, and is significantly decreased in patients with dry eye [20].

*Tear normalization test.* A trial of nonviscous artificial tears in patients in clinic can be a useful tool. Improvement of vision by two lines after instillation of

0.5% carboxymethylcellulose drops has been found to be 82.5% sensitive and 100% specific for dry eye [21].

*Cornea*

*Staining.* Ocular surface stains to evaluate for corneal and conjunctival disease include fluorescein, rose bengal, and lissamine green. (Fig. 3). Fluorescein is a nontoxic, water-soluble dye that stains the precorneal tear film and disruption cell junctions and erosions. Rose bengal and lissamine green stain devitalized cells on the conjunctiva. Rose bengal can cause direct toxicity to epithelial cells and is no longer used frequently in clinical practice.

These tests can be subjective with respect to intensity and staining patterns, and the use of grading systems such as the Oxford, Van Bijsterveld, NEI scale, and Collaborative Longitudinal Evaluation of Keratoconus (CLEK) scale can aid in more consistent evaluation [22].

## Approach to treatment

*Nonpharmacologic treatments*

*Patient education.* Conservative measures to treat DED include eliminating factors that can worsen patients' symptoms (eg, medications and environmental

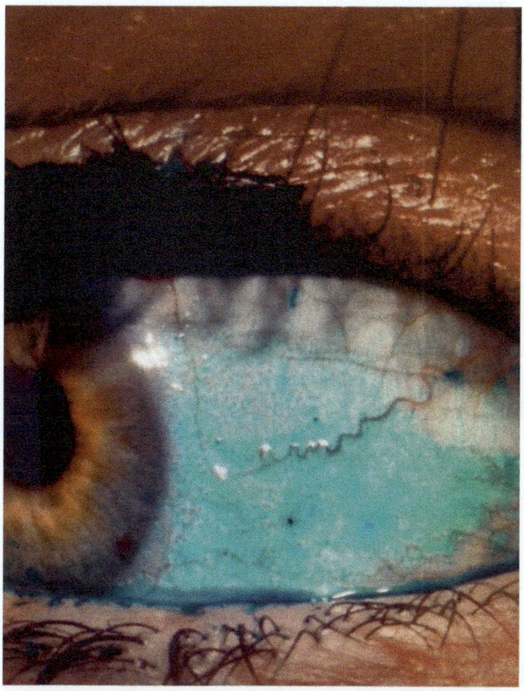

**Fig. 3.** Lissamine green staining in a patient with DED. (*Courtesy of* Dr. Mina Massaro-Giordano, Philadelphia, PA.)

factors) [23]. Protective eyewear and limiting screen time may be beneficial in reducing symptoms.

*Dietary supplementation.* Patients with DED may benefit from dietary or nutritional supplementation with essential fatty acids such as omega-3 and linoleic acid [24].

The Dry Eye Assessment and Management (DREAM) trial, a large, multicenter, double-blind clinical trial that compared a daily oral dose of fish-derived n-3 eicosapentaenoic and docosahexaenoic acids with olive oil placebo in subjects with moderate to severe DED did not show significantly better outcomes in the treatment group [25].

Vitamin D deficiency may be a risk factor for DED because it is associated with worse symptoms, tear film dysfunction, and decreased tear production [26].

*Eyelid hygiene.*

1. Warm compresses
   In patients with MGD, the application of heat and physical manipulation to the eyelids with warm compresses with a towel or commercially available micro-waveable masks should be considered. Heat liquefies the lipids that can be expressed from the meibomian glands with gentle pressure [27].
2. Cleaning eyelids
   Cleansing scrubs, foams, premedicated wipes, or tear-free baby shampoo can help clean eyelashes and loosen debris and oil from the eyelids. Tea tree oil and terpinen-4-ol is effective against *Demodex* [28].

*Lubrication.* First-line pharmacotherapy for treating mild to moderate DED includes over-the-counter artificial tear substitutes, such as drops, gels, or ointments. Artificial tears mimic the different layers of the tear film and supplement the patient's tears. Numerous formulations exist with various ingredients, including cellulose and polyvinyl derivatives, chondroitin sulfate, and sodium hyaluronate, which contribute to the product's viscosity, retention time, and adhesion to the ocular surface [29]. Preservative-free artificial tears are preferable because preservatives, such as benzalkonium chloride, are associated with ocular allergies and toxicities [30].

*Punctal plugs.* Punctal plugs can be inserted into the tear ducts (puncta) of the upper and lower eyelids in order to decrease drainage of tears from the ocular surface in DED refractory to topical lubricants. Punctal plugs can either be placed at the level of the punctal opening or deeper within the canaliculus [3,31].

*Prescription drugs*

*Cyclosporine.* Topical cyclosporine A (CsA) 0.05% (Restasis) is a fungal antimetabolite with antiinflammatory mechanisms to decrease interleukin (IL)-2–mediated T-cell activation approved by the US Food and Drug Administration (FDA) in 2003 for treatment of aqueous production–deficient DED. Multiple studies have shown it is effective in improving symptoms; side effects include burning, conjunctival hyperemia, and blurry vision [32,33].

Cequa (cyclosporine ophthalmic solution 0.09%) (Sun Pharmaceuticals, Cranbury, NJ) was approved by the FDA in 2018 to increase tear production in patients with DED. Cequa is a nanomicellar solution that enhances bioavailability to ocular tissues [34].

Compounded cyclosporine-based formulations include Klarity-C (Imprimis Pharmaceuticals, San Diego, CA), which is a 0.1% CsA in a chondroitin sulfate emulsion that may have antiinflammatory properties and reduce corneal edema [35].

CsA may have maximal effect at 3 months; therefore, topical steroids are often used before starting CsA as an induction agent and can be used as an early maintenance agent [36].

*Lifitegrast.* Lifitegrast 5% (Xiidra) became the second FDA-approved topical ocular antiinflammatory medication for the treatment of DED in 2016. The drug blocks T-cell activation and migration by mimicking intercellular adhesion molecule-1 (ICAM-1) and blocking its interaction with lymphocyte function-associated antigen-1 (LFA-1) [37]. Advantages include a rapid effect compared with CsA, and long-term safety; however, side effects include ocular irritation, pain, metallic taste, and blurry vision.

*Topical steroids.* A course of topical corticosteroids such as loteprednol etabonate, dexamethasone, prednisolone, and fluorometholone instilled over two to four weeks can be used in moderate to severe DED. Their efficacy is limited to short-term usage to prevent the development of complications such as increased intraocular pressure or cataracts [38].

*Antibiotics*

*Topical azithromycin and erythromycin.* Topical azithromycin 1% has been shown to improve meibomian gland function and symptoms of dry eye. A reduction in bacterial colonization of the eyelid margins and normalization of the meibomian gland secretion lipid profile were found [39].

Erythromycin ointment can be used in blepharoconjunctivitis.

*Oral antibiotics: azithromycin and tetracyclines.* Tetracyclines are antibiotics that have antiinflammatory effects by reducing the activity of matrix metalloproteinases, the production of IL-1, and B-cell activation. Low doses have been shown to improve tear film stability, tear production, and dry eye symptoms [40]. Tetracyclines can be used to treat blepharitis, MGD, and acne rosacea, which are associated with DED [41].

However, gastrointestinal and skin problems can occur at higher doses.

*Blood products*

*Autologous and/or allogenic serum drops.* The use of blood-derived products, such as serum, has the potential to stimulate and accelerate wound healing and tissue regeneration [42]. Human serum composition resembles that of tears, including the lipid, proteins, antimicrobial elements, and growth factors. Autologous and/or allogenic serum drops have been shown to improve both symptoms and objective signs of DED [42,43]. However, serum drops contain leukocytes and proinflammatory cytokines that may affect the ocular surface [44]. Serum is usually administered at a 20% concentration; however, higher concentrations from 50% to 100% have been used.

*Platelet-rich plasma and plasma rich in growth factors.* Platelet-rich plasma (PRP) and plasma rich in growth factors contain higher platelet concentrations and are intended to maximize the concentration of growth factors, cell adhesion molecules, and cytokines, which may result in therapeutic effects on the ocular surface. Importantly, they do not contain leukocytes [43]. These products have shown promising results in the treatment of DED, persistent epithelial defects, Sjögren syndrome, neurotrophic keratitis, and graft-versus-host disease (GVHD) [44,45]. An interventional study showed a clinically beneficial impact of autologous PRP in clinical signs and symptoms in patients with moderate to severe DED [45].

*Surgical procedures*

*Punctal cautery.* Permanent surgical closure of the punctum can be performed for those who cannot retain or tolerate punctal plugs, such as those with GVHD and SJS [46].

*Eyelid procedures, including tarsorrhaphy and ectropion/entropion repair.* Corneal exposure may result from eyelid malpositions, including lagophthalmos, cicatricial scarring, ectropion, and entropion, which often require an eyelid surgical procedure. This procedure includes the implantation of upper lid weights, lid springs, eyelid reconstruction, or partial/complete tarsorrhaphy to reduce the mechanistic cause of corneal exposure. Tightening of the canthal tendons and removal of scar tissue or other mechanical reasons for eyelid malpositions may be helpful [3].

*Surgical treatment of conjunctivochalasis.* Conjunctivochalasis is an age-related ocular disorder characterized by loose, redundant, nonedematous inferior bulbar conjunctiva, which is a common cause of ocular surface irritation and tearing. In severe cases of conjunctivochalasis, resection, electrocoagulation, or thermal cauterization of excessive conjunctival tissue can be considered [47].

*Eyelid procedures for evaporative dry eye disease*

*Intense pulsed light.* Intense pulsed light (IPL) uses high-intensity light that is absorbed by the skin and then converted to destructive heat with wavelengths customized based on various targets. Several studies have shown periocular IPL improving DED [48].

*Vectored thermal pulsation (LipiFlow).* LipiFlow vectored thermal pulsation system (TearScience, Morrisville, NC) is a 12-minute procedure that heats the meibomian glands to clear blockages by applying localized heat to both inner eyelid surfaces to 42.5 C while pulsating pressure is applied to the outer eyelids through an inflatable air bladder. Subjective and objective improvements in DED have been reported [27,49].

*iLux.* The Systane iLux MGD Treatment System (Alcon, Fort Worth, TX) is a handheld battery-powered instrument that applies localized heat and compression in a procedure lasting 8 to 12 minutes. This device is made of silicone with inner and outer eyelid pads and temperature sensors that measure the eyelid temperature and heat the eyelids to 38 C to 42 C to melt meibum. Similar outcomes have been reported with LipiFlow treatment [50].

*MiBo Thermoflo.* The MiBo Thermoflo (MiBo Medical Group, Dallas, TX) is a treatment of DED that consists of a handheld probe with a double eye pad that transmits thermoelectric heat to the meibomian glands. The protocol consists of an initial 12-minute treatment per eyelid followed by a 10-minute session per eyelid one week later and a third session after another 2 weeks that is 8 to 10 minutes per lid [51].

*TearCare system.* The TearCare System (Sight Sciences, Menlo Park, CA) is a 12-minute in-office procedure for patients with DED. Four electrothermal iLid instruments are attached to the external surface of each eyelid and then regulated thermal energy is transmitted at a constant temperature (41 C –45 C) to melt the meibum using a TearCare controller. Patients can blink during the procedure, which increases meibum expression. Manual meibomian gland expression is performed using forceps to remove residual obstructions [52].

*Meibomian gland probing.* Intraductal meibomian gland probing, which is performed at the slit lamp, typically uses a 2-mm probe placed into each meibomian gland to mechanically remove its contents [28,53].

*BlephEx.* BlephEx (Scope Ophthalmics, London, UK) is a handheld device that contains an electromechanical unit and a disposable microsponge that is inserted and spins to debride and exfoliate the lash margin to treat blepharitis. BlephEx treatment combined with eyelid hygiene is associated with a reduction in quantity of *Demodex* [54].

*Devices*

*Nasal neurostimulation.* A variety of nasal neurostimulation devices have been shown to increase tear production by mechanical or chemical stimulation of the nasolacrimal reflex. These include:

1. The iTear 100 device (Olympic Ophthalmics, Isaquah, WA) stimulates the external branch of the anterior ethmoidal nerve on the side of the nose to activate the lacrimal functional unit [55].
2. TrueTear Intranasal Tear Neurostimulator (TrueTear Allergan Dublin, Ireland) [56] activates the nasal mucosal nerves. Although found to be safe and effective, it was discontinued.
3. Varenicline 0.03-mg solution (Tyrvaya Nasal Spray, Oyster Point Pharma) is a highly selective nicotinic acetylcholine receptor agonist that binds to the

trigeminal nerve when administered in the nose, activating the parasympathetic nervous system to stimulate tear production [57].

*Contact lenses.* Bandage contact lenses protect the surface of the eye and provide comfort by stabilizing the tear film, restoring epithelial cell turnover, and protecting cornea nerves. Extended-wear contact lens use has a risk of microbial keratitis [3,58].

Scleral lenses create a fluid-filled reservoir overlying the cornea in severe ocular surface diseases [33].

The BostonSight prosthetic replacement of the ocular surface ecosystem (PROSE; Boston Foundation for Sight, Needham, MA), approved by the FDA in 1994, is a rigid gas-permeable scleral lens filled with fluid to serve as a nociceptive barrier. Lenses are custom designed and can be used in severe ocular surface disease [58].

The EyePrintPro lens (Advanced Vision Technologies, Lakewood, CO) is also a customizable oxygen-transmissible scleral lens [59].

*Amniotic membrane.* Cryopreserved amniotic membrane grafts may be beneficial in moderate to severe DED that is refractory to medical treatments. Amniotic membranes can serve as a bandage to enable epithelialization and also have antiangiogenic, antiinflammatory, and antiscarring properties. Commercially available forms of amniotic membrane include AmbioDisk (Katena Products, Denville, NJ), which is sterilized, dehydrated, and stored at room temperature, and Prokera (Bio-Tissue, Miami, FL), which is cryopreserved at −80 C. Prokera products have a ring that holds the amniotic membrane [60,61].

## RECENT AND UPCOMING INNOVATIONS

### Diagnostic imaging

#### *Confocal microscopy*

In vivo confocal microscopy of the cornea is a newer application that has been developed to aid in the evaluation of DED.

Patients with DED have decreased epithelial cells [62]. A reported decrease in the density and altered morphology of the sub-basal and stromal nerve cells has been reported [63]. Reports also show increased epithelial Langerhans cells [64].

#### *Meibometry and meibography*

Meibometry can quantify the amount of lipid at the lid margin. Plastic tape is blotted onto the margin of the lid. A spot photometric reading using a Meibometer is taken from the lipid imprint can quantify the resting amount of lipid [65].

Using a transilluminator, examination of the everted eyelid with black-and-white photography or an infrared camera can allow more sophisticated visualization of the meibomian glands [66]. Laser confocal meibography allows better characterization of microscopic features such as glandular acinar unit density, acinar unit diameter, and periglandular inflammatory infiltrates and fibrosis [67]. OCT allows volumetric measurements of the meibomian glands [68].

*Interferometry*

Interferometry measures the interference between beams reflected by anterior and posterior surfaces to quantify the thickness of reflective materials, including the tear film. Patients with aqueous-deficient dry eye have a significantly thinner tear film by interferometry [69]. Interferometry also can identify the balance between the aqueous and lipid components of the tear film [70].

*Videokeratoscopy*

Corneal topography can aid in measuring changes in the tear film. The surface regularity index and surface asymmetry index can be used to evaluate the corneal surface and tear film [71].

*Fluorophotometry*

Fluorophotometry detects small changes in the corneal epithelium evaluating the barrier function of the cornea. Increased uptake of fluorescein can reveal subtle damage to the epithelium. Patients with DED have increased corneal permeability when measured by the fluorophotometer [72].

## Pipeline treatments

*Recombinant human nerve growth factor*

Nerve growth factor (NGF), which is naturally found in tears, may have a beneficial role in increasing tear production, enhancing corneal sensitivity, and causing nerve regeneration in DED. NGF (Oxervate) is authorized in the United States for treatment of neurotrophic keratitis, and studies have shown that recombinant human NGF (rhNGF) is safe and improves signs of DED. Tavilermide (MIM-D3), is a small-molecule NGF peptidomimetic that is a partial tropomyosin receptor kinase A(TrKA) agonist and has been studied in DED [73,74].

*Lacritin*

Lacritin is a glycoprotein secreted by the lacrimal gland's acinar cells that promotes basal tearing and has prosecretory and mitogenic properties that may have a beneficial role in treating DED [75].

*Lubricin*

Human lubricin supplementation also is being studied in DED. Lubricin (proteoglycan-4) is present in synovial fluid, on the ocular surface, and in meibomian glands, and is thought to reduce friction between the ocular surface and eyelid [76].

*Thymosin β4*

Thymosin β4 eye drops are being studied in DED and corneal neurotrophic defects because it is thought to play a role in corneal repair. Thymosin β4 is a naturally occurring G-actin–binding protein produced by most cells that decreases proinflammatory cytokine levels and promotes epithelial healing [77].

*Amniotic membrane extract eye drops*

Amniotic membrane extract and amniotic membrane extract drops are also being studied in acute corneal injury and ocular chemical burns and may promote reepithelialization of the cornea [78].

*Semifluorinated alkane eye drops*

Perfluorohexyloctane, a semifluorinated alkane, is a nonaqueous, nonblurring liquid that is commercialized in Europe, Australia, and New Zealand to treat evaporative DED. Perfluorohexyloctane has low surface tension enabling strong spreading properties, small drop sizes, and forms a film at the tear film-air interface to prevent evaporation. NOVO3 (100% perfluorohexyloctane) is an investigational drug in the United States that has shown improvement in DED and is currently undergoing phase 3 studies [79].

*Reproxalap ophthalmic solution*

Reproxalap (Aldeyra Therapeutics, Lexington, MA) is a small-molecule immune-modulating, covalent inhibitor of reactive aldehyde species (RASP). Increased levels of RASP are associated with several inflammatory ocular diseases, including DED. Phase 2 studies of reproxalap have shown improvement in signs and symptoms of DED [80].

*ALG-1007 (risuteganib) topical ophthalmic solution*

ALG-1007 (Allegro Ophthalmics, San Juan Capistrano, CA) is a topical application of risuteganib, a small peptide integrin regulator that regulates subunits involved in the complement 3 inflammatory pathway. Risuteganib blocks leukocyte adhesion and transendothelial migration, thereby decreasing ocular surface inflammation [81].

*Peptide melanocortin receptor agonist ophthalmic solution*

PL9643 (Palatin Technologies) is a peptide melanocortin receptor 1 and 5 agonist that is being studied in DED because of its antiinflammatory effects [82].

*Ophthalmic keratolytics*

Ophthalmic keratolytics (Azura Ophthalmics) is a topical eyelid ointment that prevents keratinization that is being studied to treat MGD [83].

## SUMMARY

DED is a multifactorial disorder caused by abnormalities of the tear film. DED may affect patients' vision, productivity, quality of life, and activities of daily living. Furthermore, DED has a large economic cost, including medical appointments, treatments, and procedures [84].

The diagnosis of DED requires taking a comprehensive history to assess for underlying medical conditions or environmental factors. Screening questionnaires are helpful in making the diagnosis and in determining the severity of disease. A thorough clinical evaluation includes a targeted grading of eyelids, conjunctiva, cornea, and tear function. There have been several advances that have occurred in ophthalmologic imaging that may be helpful in making an assessment at the cellular level, in evaluating the structure and function of the meibomian glands, and in grading the tear film.

There are various treatment options available to treat the different causes of DED. Clinicians should take a staged or stepwise approach in treating DED with consideration of the patients' symptoms and their underlying physiology. Treatments vary based on whether the patient's disease is caused by evaporative dry eye, aqueous deficiency, and/or inflammation. For patients with symptoms that have not significantly improved following implementation of conservative measures such as eyelid hygiene and lubricants, there are several prescription medications that can be used. Blood products have shown promise in improving symptoms and signs of DED. In-office procedures that target MGD can provide clinical improvement in evaporative DED. For patients with severe DED, contact lenses, amniotic membrane transplant, and neurostimulation can be used. Furthermore, surgical procedures can help ameliorate symptoms for certain patients, including those with conjunctivochalasis, exposure keratopathy, or eyelid malposition. Several investigational drugs that target various molecular pathways are currently in clinical trials.

Although DED affects millions of patients, several innovations have been implemented in order to more effectively treat the disease, ameliorate patients' symptoms, and reduce the impact on patients' lives.

## CLINICS CARE POINTS

- There are several questionnaires that can be useful tools to standardize symptomatic evaluation of dry eye and to monitor patients.
- Treatments vary for evaporative dry eye, aqueous deficiency, and/or inflammatory DED.
- In-office procedures that target meibomian gland dysfunction can improve evaporative DED.
- For patients with severe DED, prescription medications, blood products, contact lenses, amniotic membrane transplant, and neurostimulation can be used.

## Disclosure

The authors have nothing to disclose.

## References

[1] Stapleton F, Alves M, Bunya VY, et al. TFOS DEWS II epidemiology report. Ocul Surf 2017;15:334–65; https://doi.org/10.1016/j.jtos.2017.05.003.
[2] The definition and classification of dry eye disease: Report of the definition and classification subcommittee of the International Dry Eye Workshop (2007). Ocul Surf 2007;5(2):75–92.
[3] Jones L, Downie LE, Korb D, et al. TFOS DEWS II management and therapy report. Ocul Surf 2017;15:575–628; https://doi.org/10.1016/j.jtos.2017.05.006.
[4] Gomes JAP, Azar DT, Baudouin C, et al. TFOS DEWS II iatrogenic report. Ocul Surf 2017;15:511–38; https://doi.org/10.1016/j.jtos.2017.05.004.
[5] Fraunfelder FT, Sciubba JJ, Mathers WD. The role of medications in causing dry eye. J Ophthalmol 2012;2012:285851; https://doi.org/10.1155/2012/285851.
[6] Vitale S, Goodman LA, Reed GF, et al. Comparison of the NEI-VFQ and OSDI questionnaires in patients with Sjögren's syndrome-related dry eye. Health Qual Life Outcomes 2004;2:44; https://doi.org/10.1186/1477-7525-2-44.

[7] Schiffman RM, Christianson MD, Jacobsen G, et al. Reliability and validity of the ocular surface disease index. Arch Ophthalmol 2000;118:615–21; https://doi.org/10.1001/archopht.118.5.615.
[8] Chalmers RL, Begley CG, Caffery B. Validation of the 5-item dry eye questionnaire (DEQ-5): discrimination across self-assessed severity and aqueous tear deficient dry eye diagnoses. Cont Lens Anterior Eye 2010;33:55–60; https://doi.org/10.1016/j.clae.2009.12.010.
[9] Akowuah PK, Adjei-Anang J, Nkansah EK, et al. Comparison of the performance of the dry eye questionnaire (DEQ-5) to the ocular surface disease index in a non-clinical population. Cont Lens Anterior Eye 2021;101441; https://doi.org/10.1016/j.clae.2021.101441.
[10] Blackie C, Albou-Ganem C, Korb D. Questionnaire assists in dry eye disease diagnosis. Four-question survey helps evaluate patients' dry eye symptoms to improve screening. Ocul Surg News 2012.
[11] Ngo W, Situ P, Keir N, et al. Psychometric properties and validation of the standard patient evaluation of eye dryness questionnaire. Cornea 2013;32:1204–10; https://doi.org/10.1097/ICO.0b013e318294b0c0.
[12] Wolffsohn JS, Arita R, Chalmers R, et al. TFOS DEWS II diagnostic methodology report. Ocul Surf 2017;15(3):539–74; https://doi.org/10.1016/j.jtos.2017.05.001.
[13] Shimazaki J. Definition and diagnostic criteria of dry eye disease: historical overview and future directions. Invest Ophthalmol Vis Sci 2018;59:DES7-12; https://doi.org/10.1167/iovs.17-23475.
[14] Baudouin C, Aragona P, Van Setten G, et al. Diagnosing the severity of dry eye: a clear and practical algorithm. Br J Ophthalmol 2014;98:1168–76; https://doi.org/10.1136/bjophthalmol-2013-304619.
[15] Veres A, Tapasztó B, Kosina-Hagyó K, et al. Imaging lid-parallel conjunctival folds with OCT and comparing its grading with the slit lamp classification in dry eye patients and normal subjects. Invest Ophthalmol Vis Sci 2011;52:2945–51; https://doi.org/10.1167/iovs.10-5505.
[16] Lamberts DW, Foster CS, Perry HD. Schirmer test after topical anesthesia and the tear meniscus height in normal eyes. Arch Ophthalmol 1979;97:1082–5; https://doi.org/10.1001/archopht.1979.01020010536004.
[17] Vanley GT, Leopold IH, Gregg TH. Interpretation of tear film breakup. Arch Ophthalmol 1977;95:445–8; https://doi.org/10.1001/archopht.1977.04450030087010.
[18] Potvin R, Makari S, Rapuano CJ. Tear film osmolarity and dry eye disease: a review of the literature. Clin Ophthalmol 2015;9:2039–47; https://doi.org/10.2147/OPTH.S95242.
[19] Messmer EM, von Lindenfels V, Garbe A, et al. Matrix metalloproteinase 9 testing in dry eye disease using a commercially available point-of-care immunoassay. Ophthalmology 2016;123:2300–8; https://doi.org/10.1016/j.ophtha.2016.07.028.
[20] Ohashi Y, Ishida R, Kojima T, et al. Abnormal protein profiles in tears with dry eye syndrome. Am J Ophthalmol 2003;136:291–9; https://doi.org/10.1016/s0002-9394(03)00203-4.
[21] Latkany R, Lock BG, Speaker M. Tear film normalization test: a new diagnostic test for dry eyes. Cornea 2006;25:1153–7; https://doi.org/10.1097/01.ico.0000240085.21105.51.
[22] Begley C, Caffery B, Chalmers R, et al. Review and analysis of grading scales for ocular surface staining. Ocul Surf 2019;17:208–20; https://doi.org/10.1016/j.jtos.2019.01.004.
[23] Dogru M, Tsubota K. Pharmacotherapy of dry eye. Expert Opin Pharmacother 2011;12:325–34; https://doi.org/10.1517/14656566.2010.518612.
[24] Miljanović B, Trivedi KA, Dana MR, et al. Relation between dietary n-3 and n-6 fatty acids and clinically diagnosed dry eye syndrome in women. Am J Clin Nutr 2005;82:887–93; https://doi.org/10.1093/ajcn/82.4.887.

[25] Dry Eye Assessment and Management Study Research Group, Asbell PA, Maguire MG, Pistilli M, et al. n-3 Fatty acid supplementation for the treatment of dry eye disease. N Engl J Med 2018;378:1681–90; https://doi.org/10.1056/NEJMoa1709691.
[26] Liu J, Dong Y, Wang Y. Vitamin D deficiency is associated with dry eye syndrome: a systematic review and meta-analysis. Acta Ophthalmol 2020;98:749–54; https://doi.org/10.1111/aos.14470.
[27] Finis D, König C, Hayajneh J, et al. Six-month effects of a thermodynamic treatment for MGD and implications of meibomian gland atrophy. Cornea 2014;33:1265–70; https://doi.org/10.1097/ICO.0000000000000273.
[28] Thode AR, Latkany RA. Current and emerging therapeutic strategies for the treatment of meibomian gland dysfunction (MGD). Drugs 2015;75:1177–85; https://doi.org/10.1007/s40265-015-0432-8.
[29] Pucker AD, Ng SM, Nichols JJ. Over the counter (OTC) artificial tear drops for dry eye syndrome. Cochrane Database Syst Rev 2016;2:CD009729; https://doi.org/10.1002/14651858.CD009729.pub2.
[30] Berdy GJ, Abelson MB, Smith LM, et al. Preservative-free artificial tear preparations. Assessment of corneal epithelial toxic effects. Arch Ophthalmol 1992;110:528–32; https://doi.org/10.1001/archopht.1992.01080160106043.
[31] Ervin A-M, Law A, Pucker AD. Punctal occlusion for dry eye syndrome. Cochrane Database Syst Rev 2017;6:CD006775; https://doi.org/10.1002/14651858.CD006775.pub3.
[32] Sall K, Stevenson OD, Mundorf TK, et al. Two multicenter, randomized studies of the efficacy and safety of cyclosporine ophthalmic emulsion in moderate to severe dry eye disease. CsA Phase 3 Study Group. Ophthalmology 2000;107:631–9; https://doi.org/10.1016/s0161-6420(99)00176-1.
[33] O'Neil EC, Henderson M, Massaro-Giordano M, et al. Advances in dry eye disease treatment. Curr Opin Ophthalmol 2019;30:166–78; https://doi.org/10.1097/ICU.0000000000000569.
[34] Tauber J, Schechter BA, Bacharach J, et al. A Phase II/III, randomized, double-masked, vehicle-controlled, dose-ranging study of the safety and efficacy of OTX-101 in the treatment of dry eye disease. Clin Ophthalmol 2018;12:1921–9; https://doi.org/10.2147/OPTH.S175065.
[35] Matossian C, Trattler W, Loh J. Dry eye treatment with topical cyclosporine 0.1% in chondroitin sulfate ophthalmic emulsion. Clin Ophthalmol 2021;15:1979–84; https://doi.org/10.2147/OPTH.S308088.
[36] Sheppard JD, Donnenfeld ED, Holland EJ, et al. Effect of loteprednol etabonate 0.5% on initiation of dry eye treatment with topical cyclosporine 0.05. Eye Contact Lens 2014;40:289–96; https://doi.org/10.1097/ICL.0000000000000049.
[37] Haber SL, Benson V, Buckway CJ, et al. Lifitegrast: a novel drug for patients with dry eye disease. Ther Adv Ophthalmol 2019;11; https://doi.org/10.1177/2515841419870366.
[38] Marsh P, Pflugfelder SC. Topical nonpreserved methylprednisolone therapy for keratoconjunctivitis sicca in Sjögren syndrome. Ophthalmology 1999;106:811–6; https://doi.org/10.1016/S0161-6420(99)90171-9.
[39] Foulks GN, Borchman D, Yappert M, et al. Topical azithromycin therapy for meibomian gland dysfunction: clinical response and lipid alterations. Cornea 2010;29:781–8; https://doi.org/10.1097/ICO.0b013e3181cda38f.
[40] Yoo S-E, Lee D-C, Chang M-H. The effect of low-dose doxycycline therapy in chronic meibomian gland dysfunction. Korean J Ophthalmol 2005;19:258; https://doi.org/10.3341/kjo.2005.19.4.258.
[41] Foulks GN, Borchman D, Yappert M, et al. Topical azithromycin and oral doxycycline therapy of meibomian gland dysfunction: a comparative clinical and spectroscopic pilot study. Cornea 2013;32:44–53; https://doi.org/10.1097/ICO.0b013e318254205f.

[42] Drew VJ, Tseng C-L, Seghatchian J, et al. Reflections on dry eye syndrome treatment: therapeutic role of blood products. Front Med 2018;5:33; https://doi.org/10.3389/fmed.2018.00033.
[43] Anitua E, Muruzabal F, Tayebba A, et al. Autologous serum and plasma rich in growth factors in ophthalmology: preclinical and clinical studies. Acta Ophthalmol 2015;93:e605–14; https://doi.org/10.1111/aos.12710.
[44] Sanchez-Avila RM, Merayo-Lloves J, Muruzabal F, et al. Plasma rich in growth factors for the treatment of dry eye from patients with graft versus host diseases. Eur J Ophthalmol 2020;30:94–103; https://doi.org/10.1177/1120672118818943.
[45] Alio JL, Rodriguez AE, Ferreira-Oliveira R, et al. Treatment of dry eye disease with autologous platelet-rich plasma: a prospective, interventional, non-randomized study. Ophthalmol Ther 2017;6:285–93; https://doi.org/10.1007/s40123-017-0100-z.
[46] Wang Y, Carreno-Galeano JT, Singh RB, et al. Long-term outcomes of punctal cauterization in the management of ocular surface diseases. Cornea 2021;40:168–71; https://doi.org/10.1097/ICO.0000000000002384.
[47] Yokoi N, Inatomi T, Kinoshita S. Surgery of the conjunctiva. In: Geerling G, Brewitt H, editors. Dev Ophthalmol, vol. 41. Basel: KARGER; 2008. p. 138–58; https://doi.org/10.1159/000131086.
[48] Dell SJ, Gaster RN, Barbarino SC, et al. Prospective evaluation of intense pulsed light and meibomian gland expression efficacy on relieving signs and symptoms of dry eye disease due to meibomian gland dysfunction. Clin Ophthalmol 2017;11:817–27; https://doi.org/10.2147/OPTH.S130706.
[49] Finis D, Hayajneh J, König C, et al. Evaluation of an automated thermodynamic treatment (LipiFlow®) system for meibomian gland dysfunction: a prospective, randomized, observer-masked trial. Ocul Surf 2014;12:146–54; https://doi.org/10.1016/j.jtos.2013.12.001.
[50] Tauber J, Owen J, Bloomenstein M, et al. Comparison of the iLUX and the LipiFlow for the Treatment of Meibomian Gland dysfunction and symptoms: a randomized clinical trial. Clin Ophthalmol 2020;14:405–18; https://doi.org/10.2147/OPTH.S234008.
[51] Kislan T. New, targeted technology for treating the root cause of dry eye disease (DED) MiBo Medical n.d. Avilable at: https://mibomedicalgroup.com/articles/. Accessed February 28, 2021.
[52] Karpecki P, Wirta D, Osmanovic S, et al. A prospective, post-market, multicenter trial (CHEETAH) suggested TEARCARE® system as a safe and effective blink-assisted eyelid device for the treatment of dry eye disease. Clin Ophthalmol 2020;14:4551–9; https://doi.org/10.2147/OPTH.S285953.
[53] Maskin SL. Intraductal meibomian gland probing relieves symptoms of obstructive meibomian gland dysfunction. Cornea 2010;29:1145–52; https://doi.org/10.1097/ICO.0b013e3181d836f3.
[54] Epstein IJ, Rosenberg E, Stuber R, et al. Double-masked and unmasked prospective study of terpinen-4-ol lid scrubs with microblepharoexfoliation for the treatment of demodex blepharitis. Cornea 2020;39:408–16; https://doi.org/10.1097/ICO.0000000000002243.
[55] Ji MH, Moshfeghi DM, Periman L, et al. Novel extranasal tear stimulation: pivotal study results. Transl Vis Sci Technol 2020;9:23; https://doi.org/10.1167/tvst.9.12.23.
[56] Cohn GS, Corbett D, Tenen A, et al. Randomized, controlled, double-masked, multicenter, pilot study evaluating safety and efficacy of intranasal neurostimulation for dry eye disease. Invest Ophthalmol Vis Sci 2019;60:147; https://doi.org/10.1167/iovs.18-23984.
[57] Wirta D, Vollmer P, Paauw J, et al. Efficacy and safety of OC-01 (Varenicline) nasal spray on signs and symptoms of dry eye disease: the ONSET-2 phase 3, randomized trial. Ophthalmology 2021;S0161-6420(21):00836–8; https://doi.org/10.1016/j.ophtha.2021.11.004.

[58] Goyal S, Hamrah P. Understanding neuropathic corneal pain–gaps and current therapeutic approaches. Semin Ophthalmol 2016;31:59–70; https://doi.org/10.3109/08820538.2015.1114853.
[59] Nguyen MTB, Thakrar V, Chan CC. EyePrintPRO therapeutic scleral contact lens: indications and outcomes. Can J Ophthalmol 2018;53:66–70; https://doi.org/10.1016/j.jcjo.2017.07.026.
[60] Arya SK, Bhala S, Malik A, et al. Role of amniotic membrane transplantation in ocular surface disorders. Nepal J Ophthalmol 2010;2:145–53; https://doi.org/10.3126/nepjoph.v2i2.3722.
[61] McDonald MB, Sheha H, Tighe S, et al. Treatment outcomes in the DRy Eye amniotic membrane (DREAM) study. Clin Ophthalmol 2018;12:677–81; https://doi.org/10.2147/OPTH.S162203.
[62] Zhang X, Chen Q, Chen W, et al. Tear dynamics and corneal confocal microscopy of subjects with mild self-reported office dry eye. Ophthalmology 2011;118:902–7; https://doi.org/10.1016/j.ophtha.2010.08.033.
[63] Labbé A, Liang Q, Wang Z, et al. Corneal nerve structure and function in patients with non-sjogren dry eye: clinical correlations. Invest Ophthalmol Vis Sci 2013;54:5144–50; https://doi.org/10.1167/iovs.13-12370.
[64] Lin H, Li W, Dong N, et al. Changes in corneal epithelial layer inflammatory cells in aqueous tear-deficient dry eye. Invest Ophthalmol Vis Sci 2010;51:122–8; https://doi.org/10.1167/iovs.09-3629.
[65] Chew CK, Jansweijer C, Tiffany JM, et al. An instrument for quantifying meibomian lipid on the lid margin: the Meibometer. Curr Eye Res 1993;12:247–54; https://doi.org/10.3109/02713689308999470.
[66] Srinivasan S, Menzies K, Sorbara L, et al. Infrared imaging of meibomian gland structure using a novel keratograph. Optom Vis Sci 2012;89:788–94; https://doi.org/10.1097/OPX.0b013e318253de93.
[67] Wise RJ, Sobel RK, Allen RC. Meibography: a review of techniques and technologies. Saudi J Ophthalmol 2012;26:349–56; https://doi.org/10.1016/j.sjopt.2012.08.007.
[68] Kobayashi A, Yoshita T, Sugiyama K. In vivo findings of the bulbar/palpebral conjunctiva and presumed meibomian glands by laser scanning confocal microscopy. Cornea 2005;24:985–8; https://doi.org/10.1097/01.ico.0000160976.88824.2b.
[69] Hosaka E, Kawamorita T, Ogasawara Y, et al. Interferometry in the evaluation of precorneal tear film thickness in dry eye. Am J Ophthalmol 2011;151:18–23.e1; https://doi.org/10.1016/j.ajo.2010.07.019.
[70] Arita R, Morishige N, Fujii T, et al. Tear interferometric patterns reflect clinical tear dynamics in dry eye patients. Invest Ophthalmol Vis Sci 2016;57:3928–34; https://doi.org/10.1167/iovs.16-19788.
[71] Szczesna DH, Alonso-Caneiro D, Iskander DR, et al. Predicting dry eye using noninvasive techniques of tear film surface assessment. Invest Ophthalmol Vis Sci 2011;52:751–6; https://doi.org/10.1167/iovs.10-5173.
[72] Fahim MM, Haji S, Koonapareddy CV, et al. Fluorophotometry as a diagnostic tool for the evaluation of dry eye disease. BMC Ophthalmol 2006;6:20; https://doi.org/10.1186/1471-2415-6-20.
[73] Sacchetti M, Lambiase A, Schmidl D, et al. Effect of recombinant human nerve growth factor eye drops in patients with dry eye: a phase IIa, open label, multiple-dose study. Br J Ophthalmol 2020;104:127–35; https://doi.org/10.1136/bjophthalmol-2018-312470.
[74] Meerovitch K, Torkildsen G, Lonsdale J, et al. Safety and efficacy of MIM-D3 ophthalmic solutions in a randomized, placebo-controlled Phase 2 clinical trial in patients with dry eye. Clin Ophthalmol 2013;7:1275–85; https://doi.org/10.2147/OPTH.S44688.
[75] Vijmasi T, Chen FYT, Balasubbu S, et al. Topical administration of lacritin is a novel therapy for aqueous-deficient dry eye disease. Invest Ophthalmol Vis Sci 2014;55:5401–9; https://doi.org/10.1167/iovs.14-13924.

[76] Lambiase A, Sullivan BD, Schmidt TA, et al. A two-week, randomized, double-masked study to evaluate safety and efficacy of lubricin (150 μg/mL) eye drops versus sodium hyaluronate (HA) 0.18% eye drops (Vismed®) in patients with moderate dry eye disease. Ocul Surf 2017;15:77–87; https://doi.org/10.1016/j.jtos.2016.08.004.
[77] Sosne G, Dunn SP, Kim C. Thymosin β4 significantly improves signs and symptoms of severe dry eye in a phase 2 randomized trial. Cornea 2015;34:491–6; https://doi.org/10.1097/ICO.0000000000000379.
[78] Murri MS, Moshirfar M, Birdsong OC, et al. Amniotic membrane extract and eye drops: a review of literature and clinical application. Clin Ophthalmol 2018;12:1105–12; https://doi.org/10.2147/OPTH.S165553.
[79] Tauber J, Wirta DL, Sall K, et al. A randomized clinical study (SEECASE) to assess efficacy, safety, and tolerability of NOV03 for treatment of dry eye disease. Cornea 2021;40:1132–40; https://doi.org/10.1097/ICO.0000000000002622.
[80] Clark D, Tauber J, Sheppard J, et al. Early onset and broad activity of reproxalap in a randomized, double-masked, vehicle-controlled phase 2b trial in dry eye disease. Am J Ophthalmol 2021;226:22–31; https://doi.org/10.1016/j.ajo.2021.01.011.
[81] Lindstrom R, Donnenfeld E, Holland E, et al. Safety and efficacy of ALG-1007 topical ophthalmic solution – A synthetic peptide that regulates inflammation, in patients with dry eye disease: an exploratory phase I, open-label, single-center clinical study. AJOCT 2020;3:10; https://doi.org/10.25259/AJOCT_1_2020.
[82] Spana C, Taylor AW, Yee DG, et al. Probing the role of melanocortin type 1 receptor agonists in diverse immunological diseases. Front Pharmacol 2018;9:1535; https://doi.org/10.3389/fphar.2018.01535.
[83] Azura Ophthalmics Announces Primary Endpoints Met in Phase 2 Trial of Investigational Treatment for Contact Lens Discomfort. 2021. Available at: https://eyewire.news/articles/azura-ophthalmics-announces-primary-endpoints-met-in-phase-2-trial-of-investigational-treatment-for-contact-lens-discomfort/. Accessed February 28, 2021.
[84] Sarezky D, Massaro-Giordano M, Bunya VY. Novel diagnostics and therapeutics in dry eye disease. Adv Ophthalmol Optom 2016;1:1–20; https://doi.org/10.1016/j.yaoo.2016.03.016.

Advances in Ophthalmology and Optometry 7 (2022) 345–365

ADVANCES IN OPHTHALMOLOGY AND OPTOMETRY

# Update on the Classification and Management of Corneal Dystrophies

Vivian L. Qin, MD, Devin Cohen, MD,
Tomas Andersen, MD, MPH, Stephen E. Orlin, MD*

Scheie Eye Institute, Perelman School of Medicine, University of Pennsylvania, 51 North 39th Street, Philadelphia, PA 19104, USA

**Keywords**

• Corneal dystrophies • Corneal transplant • Genetics • Histopathology • Corneal epithelium • Corneal stroma • Corneal endothelium

**Key points**

- The most recent IC3D classification (2015) categorizes the corneal dystrophies based on genetic, clinical, and histologic characteristics.
- Most of the corneal dystrophies now have the causative gene identified.
- Treatment varies based on symptomatic severity and anatomic area of the cornea affected.
- Future directions include focusing on corneal regeneration without the use of donor grafts, including injection of cultured endothelial cells and gene therapy.

## INTRODUCTION

The corneal dystrophies are a group of inherited and predominantly bilateral and symmetric conditions often characterized by the accumulation of corneal deposits (Table 1).With the advancement of genetic and improved phenotypic analyses in more recent years, inconsistencies in the historical nomenclature and classification of these conditions have become increasingly apparent. In 2005, the International Committee for Classification of Corneal Dystrophies (IC3D) held its inaugural meeting to develop and maintain a revised nomenclature that was published in 2008 [1]. This classification system was organized anatomically based on the main layer affected: (1) epithelial and subepithelial,

*Corresponding author. *E-mail address:* Stephen.orlin@pennmedicine.upenn.edu

https://doi.org/10.1016/j.yaoo.2022.03.012

**Table 1**
Key clinical characteristics of the epithelial corneal dystrophies

| Dystrophy | Inheritance | Gene | IC3D Category | Key Signs | Key Symptoms |
|---|---|---|---|---|---|
| Epithelial Basement Membrane Dystrophy | Rarely inherited | When inherited: TGFBI on 5q31 | Majority degenerative. Rarely 1 | Maps, dots, fingerprint lines, or bleb patterns | Asymptomatic, mild irregular astigmatism, recurrent erosions |
| Meesmann Corneal Dystrophy | Autosomal dominant | KRT3 (12q13), KRT12 (17q12) | 1 | Intraepithelial microcysts | Asymptomatic, glare, photophobia, recurrent erosions, decreased vision |
| Lisch Epithelial Corneal Dystrophy | X-linked dominant | Unknown gene at Xp22.3 | 2 | Whorl-like, radial, band-shaped, flame-shaped, feathery, or club-shaped opacities | Asymptomatic, decreased vision |
| Gelatinous Droplike Corneal Dystrophy | Autosomal recessive | TACSTD2 on 1p32 | 1 | Subepithelial lesions, Mulberry configuration, superficial vascularization, Kumquat-like lesions | Photophobia, erosive episodes, decreased vision |
| Subepithelial Mucinous Corneal Dystrophy | Autosomal dominant or X-linked | Unknown | 4 | Subepithelial fibrillar deposits | Recurrent erosions, decreased vision |
| Epithelial Recurrent Erosion Dystrophies | Autosomal dominant | Unknown | 3 | Diffuse subepithelial fibrosis | Recurrent erosions, decreased vision |

(2) Bowman layer, (3) stromal, and (4) Descemet and endothelial dystrophies, and included standardized descriptive templates. In 2015, the IC3D published an update to the previous classification based on the most recent published literature at the time [2]. The anatomic classification of dystrophies was slightly modified to: (1) epithelial and subepithelial, (2) epithelial-stromal *TGFB1*, (3) stromal, and (4) endothelial. Key changes included the revised grouping of the *TGFB1* dystrophies, the removal of Grayson-Wilbrandt corneal dystrophy due to lack of substantial evidence, the elimination of congenital hereditary endothelial dystrophy 1 (CHED1), and the reclassification of CHED2 as CHED. Dystrophies continued to be categorized from 1 to 4 based on the level of evidence (ie, category 1: well-defined with identified gene and specific mutation, category 4: suspected dystrophy without convincing evidence) [2].

The corneal dystrophies vary in the severity of their associated symptoms, which can vary on a spectrum from asymptomatic, to mild discomfort due to epithelial erosions, to severely blurred vision due to corneal opacification or edema. Accordingly, management approaches vary based on the severity of symptoms and the layer of cornea affected.

Here we aim to provide an updated description of the corneal dystrophies based on the most recent 2015 IC3D classification. We also aim to provide an update on the medical and surgical management of these dystrophies, from medical to surgical treatment, including a preview of future innovations currently being explored.

## SIGNIFICANCE/IN-DEPTH ANALYSIS

### Epithelial and Subepithelial Dystrophies

#### *Epithelial basement membrane dystrophy*

Epithelial basement membrane dystrophy is the most common of the anterior corneal dystrophies. It is a bilateral, often asymmetric, condition, which develops between the ages of 20 and 50 years and is characterized by subepithelial microcysts, fingerprint lines, and geographic maplike lines [3,4] (Fig. 1).

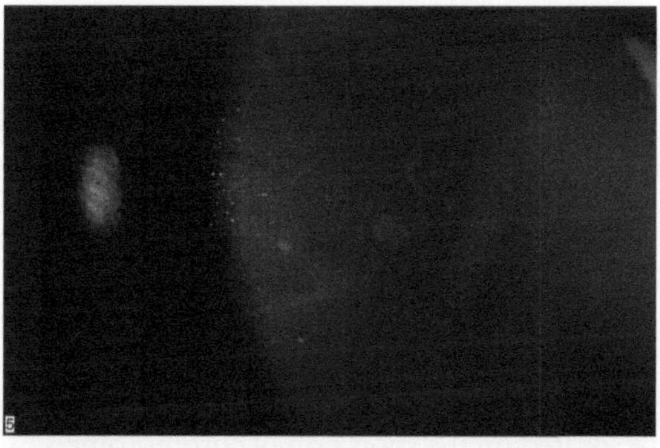

**Fig. 1.** Slit lamp photo showing the map, dot, fingerprint changes of EBMD.

Histologically, there is often an irregular, thickened epithelial basement membrane, which may invaginate into the overlying epithelium [5]. Although some cases seem to have autosomal dominant inheritance, most consider this condition to be an age-related degeneration of the cornea [6]. Although most patients remain asymptomatic, about 10% develop painful recurrent corneal erosions thought to be the result of poor hemidesmosomal attachments between the abnormal basement membrane and Bowman layer [4].

*Meesmann epithelial corneal dystrophy*

Meesmann epithelial corneal dystrophy (MECD) is a rare, bilateral dystrophy characterized by many intraepithelial vesicles in whorled or wedge-shaped patterns most numerous in the interpalpebral cornea. This condition typically occurs in late childhood or early adulthood and progresses slowly. Typical examination findings include diffuse gray opacities in varying patterns. The epithelial basement membrane may be irregular, thickened, multilayered, and insinuate into the overlying epithelium [2]. It is caused by heterozygous mutations in either the *KRT3* or *KRT12* genes, which encode corneal-specific keratins K3 and K12, respectively. K3 and K12 help to form cytoskeletal filaments that stabilize epithelial cells. Twenty-three mutations in *KRT12* and 3 in *KRT3* have been reported to cause MECD [7]. MECD is typically asymptomatic but cyst rupture can lead to lacrimation, photophobia, irritation, and decreased visual acuity.

*Lisch epithelial corneal dystrophy*

Lisch epithelial corneal dystrophy presents both unilaterally and bilaterally and is usually slowly progressive. It is characterized by gray, band-shaped, club-shaped, and feathery opacities, which may appear in whorled patterns [2]. It is inherited via an X-linked dominant inheritance pattern and has been mapped to the Xp22.3 gene [8]. Histopathology demonstrates sheets of cells with vacuolated cytoplasm. Patients typically do not experience recurrent corneal erosion, and only become visually symptomatic if opacities occur in the visual axis. Treatment usually only is indicated when visually symptomatic and disease recurrence is common [9].

*Gelatinous droplike corneal dystrophy*

Gelatinous droplike corneal dystrophy (GCD) is a bilateral and usually symmetric condition, which typically presents between ages 8 and 18 years. It is characterized by corneal subepithelial and stromal deposits of gelatinous amyloid material classically described as giving the corneal surface a mulberry-like appearance. Four distinct phenotypic varieties have been described: band keratopathy, stromal opacity, kumquat-like, and typical mulberry. The mulberry and the band keratopathy types tend to occur in the early to intermediate stage, whereas the kumquat-like type tends to occur in the very late stage [10]. GCD is caused by a homozygous biallelic loss-of-functional mutation of the tumor-associated calcium signal transducer 2 (TACSTD2) gene located on the short arm of chromosome 1. This gene encodes for TACSTD2 glycoprotein, which acts as a cell surface receptor and plays a role in cell adhesion. Thus, its loss of function can lead to an increase in epithelial permeability [11]. This dystrophy may be characterized by recurrent corneal epithelial erosions and/or progressively worsening vision.

*Subepithelial mucinous corneal dystrophy*
Subepithelial mucinous corneal dystrophy (SMCD) is the least well-characterized dystrophy among the epithelial and subepithelial dystrophies. Beyond its initial description in 1993 in just one family, there have been no further reports [2]. Based on the limited information available, it appears to be inherited in an autosomal dominant or possibly X-linked pattern [2,12]. Genetic locus and gene remain unknown [2]. Examination is notable for bilateral subepithelial opacities and haze that correspond to subepithelial deposits of fibrillar material. Clinically, patients present in childhood with recurrent corneal erosions and subsequently develop progressive vision loss [2,12].

*Epithelial recurrent erosion dystrophies*
The epithelial recurrent erosion dystrophies (EREDs) comprise 3 distinct variants: Franceschetti corneal dystrophy (FRCD), Dystrophia Smolandiensis (DS), and Dystrophia Helsinglandica (DH). They present with childhood-onset of recurrent epithelial erosions that diminish in severity by the fourth decade of life [2]. The erosions are complicated by diffuse subepithelial fibrosis that eventually leads to central corneal opacification and visual impairment in 50% of case [2]. In FRCD, light microscopy and transmission electron microscopy are notable for irregularly sized basal epithelial cells that by immunohistochemistry demonstrate reduced expression of desmosome proteins [2,13]. DS is notable for keloid formation by light microscopy and absence of the Bowman layer with abnormal subepithelial nerves by confocal microscopy [2,14]. Among the 3, DH may lead to less diminished visual acuity [15]. They all are inherited in an autosomal dominant pattern, but it remains unknown whether they are distinct entities or allelic variants with variable expressivity of the same genetic disorder [2].

## Epithelial-Stromal *TGFB1* dystrophies
The epithelial-stromal TGFBI dystrophies include Reis-Bücklers corneal dystrophy (RBCD), Thiel-Behnke corneal dystrophy (TBCD), lattice corneal dystrophy (LCD, classic and variant types), and granular corneal dystrophy (GCD, types 1 and 2) (Table 2). They all are autosomal dominant monogenic dystrophies involving the transforming growth factor beta-induced (TGFBI) gene at the 5q31 locus [2]. Their inclusion in the 2015 IC3D Classification within their own category based on the implicated gene reflects the overall goal of the IC3D to characterize corneal dystrophies more precisely through genetics rather than solely by anatomic layer [2]. Further diagnostic techniques help to distinguish among the sometimes phenotypically similar epithelial-stromal TGFBI dystrophies [16].

*Reis-Bücklers corneal dystrophy*
RBCD was formerly known as corneal dystrophy of Bowman layer, type I and GCD, type 3 [2]. This condition presents in children who develop painful

**Table 2**
Key clinical characteristics of the epithelial-stromal *TGFB1* corneal dystrophies

| Dystrophy | Inheritance | Gene | IC3D Category | Key Signs | Key Symptoms |
|---|---|---|---|---|---|
| Reis-Bücklers Corneal Dystrophy | Autosomal dominant | TGFBI on 5q31 | 1 | Diffuse opacities with clear interruptions. Rod-shaped bodies by E.M. | Recurrent erosions, decreased vision |
| Thiel-Behnke Corneal Dystrophy | Autosomal dominant | TGFBI on 5q31 | 1 | Multiple flecks with reticular formation. Curly fibers by E.M. | Similar but less aggressive course compared to Reis-Bücklers |
| Lattice Corneal Dystrophy, Type 1 and variants | Autosomal dominant | TGFBI on 5q31 | 1 | Branching refractile lattice lines | Recurrent erosions, decrease vision by 4th decade |
| Granular Corneal Dystrophy, Type 1 | Autosomal dominant | TGFBI on 5q31 | 1 | Granules superficial to Bowman's layer. Rod-shaped bodies by E.M. similar to RBCD | Glare and photophobia, recurrent erosions, decreased vision |
| Granular Corneal Dystrophy, Type 2 | Autosomal dominant | TGFBI on 5q31 | 1 | Short lines or dashes that typically do not cross | Recurrent erosions, decreased vision |

recurrent erosions complicated by progressive loss of vision due to irregular geographic opacifications at the level of the Bowman layer, extending posteriorly into the stroma (Fig. 2) [2,16]. Transmission electron microscopy reveals subepithelial electron-dense rod-shaped bodies that by immunohistochemistry are immunopositive for transforming growth factor beta-induced protein [2,16–18]. Erosions are managed conservatively, whereas advanced cases with vision loss often require phototherapeutic keratectomy (PTK), penetrating keratoplasty (PK), or anterior lamellar keratoplasty [16]. Disease recurrence remains common despite surgical intervention [16].

*Thiel-Behnke corneal dystrophy*

TBCD was formerly known as corneal dystrophy of Bowman layer, type II, honeycomb-shaped corneal dystrophy, curly fibers corneal dystrophy, and Waardenburg-Jonkers corneal dystrophy [2]. TBCD portends a similar but less aggressive course as compared with RBCD, with less frequent episodes of recurrent corneal erosions and later onset of deterioration of vision [2]. Compared with the irregular opacities with clear intervening stroma in early RBCD, the lesions in TBCD include reticular flecks that progress to symmetric

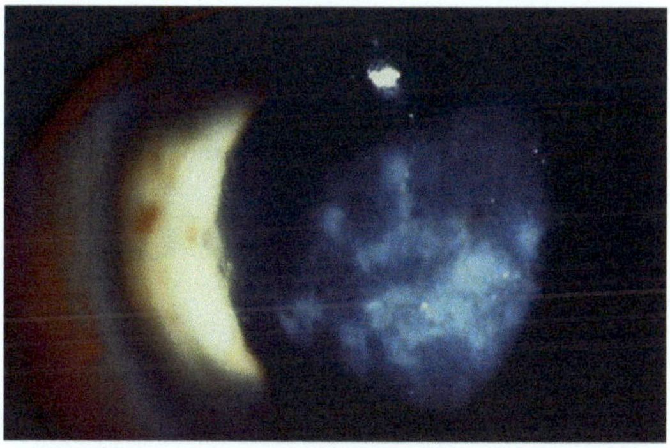

**Fig. 2.** Slit lamp photo showing the coarse geographic opacities of Reis-Bucklers.

subepithelial honeycomb opacities [2]. Transmission electron microscopy helps to differentiate TBCD from RBCD by revealing curly collagen fibers in the former as compared with the rod-shaped bodies in the latter [2,16–18]. A pathognomonic finding by light microscopy is replacement of the Bowman layer with a wavy, sawtooth pattern of fibrotic material [2,18]. Similar treatments exist for TBCD as for RBCD [16]. Disease recurrence in TBCD is slightly less common relative to RBCD [16].

*Lattice corneal dystrophy (type 1 and variants)*

LCD was formerly known as Biber-Haab-Dimmer corneal dystrophy [2]. LCD encompasses classic LCD (type 1) and LCD variants (types IIIA, I/IIIA, IV, and polymorphic amyloidosis) [2]. Classic LCD patients present with childhood erosive attacks and deterioration of vision by the fourth decade of life [2]. Characteristically lesions progress from initial flecks to lattice lines that start centrally and superficially and spread peripherally and posteriorly, sparing the far peripheral stroma, Descemet membrane, and endothelium [2]. Vision impairment is pronounced when diffuse central and paracentral subepithelial haze accompanies the lattice lines (Fig. 3) [2]. Light microscopy demonstrates epithelial atrophy, disruption of the Bowman layer, and distortion of corneal lamellae by amyloid deposition [2]. The LCD variants tend to have a later onset as compared with classic LCD type 1. Types IIIA and I/IIIA present with corneal erosions, whereas type IV and polymorphic amyloidosis typically do not cause erosion [2]. Lattice lines may be larger in type IIIA, thinner in type I/IIIA, smaller in type IV, and absent in polymorphic amyloidosis [2]. LCD type 2 (gelsolin type or Meretoja syndrome) is not considered a true corneal dystrophy, but rather systemic amyloidosis with corneal lattice lines [1].

*Granular corneal dystrophy (type 1)*

GCD type 1 (GCD1) was formerly known as corneal dystrophy Groenouw type 1 [2]. Symptoms progress from recurrent erosions during childhood to glare and photophobia and to diminished vision [2,16]. The lesions initially

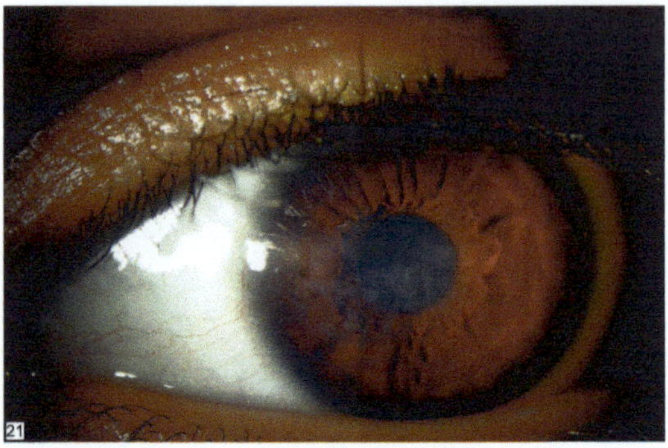


**Fig. 3.** Slit lamp photo showing the coarse linear opacities and haze of Lattice corneal dystrophy.

develop as brownish granules anterior to the Bowman layer [2]. With age they progress to snowflake and crushed bread crumb appearances [2]. Importantly, these opacities do not extend toward the limbus [2]. Although drop out of granules during erosive episodes may help clear the stroma, GCD nonetheless continues to progress and often requires interventions such as PTK [2,16].

*Granular corneal dystrophy (type 2)*

GCD type 2 (GCD2) is formerly known as Avellino dystrophy and combined granular-lattice dystrophy [2]. GCD2 presents most frequently during adolescence with painful epithelial erosions, although homozygotes may present as early as the first few years of life [2]. In most patients, superficial stromal white dots progress to being thornlike and eventually discoid (Fig. 4) [2]. Patients may additionally demonstrate dashlike lines that typically do not form the lattice configurations seen in LCD [2]. GCD2 is worsened by central corneal

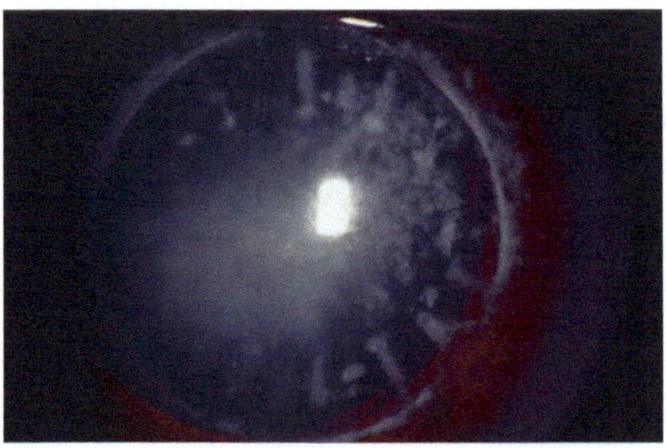

**Fig. 4.** Slit lamp photo showing the stellate opacities along suture tracks at graft host junction in patient following PK with granular corneal dystrophy type 2 (Avellino dystrophy).

injury and therefore care must be taken to avoid laser in situ keratomileusis, photorefractive keratectomy, and laser-assisted in situ epithelial keratomileusis [2,16]. Superficial PTK may help diminish anterior stromal haze as a temporizing measure before keratoplasty [2].

## Stromal Dystrophies

Seven corneal dystrophies have been classified as stromal corneal dystrophies (Table 3).

*Macular corneal dystrophy*

Macular corneal dystrophy, formerly Groenouw corneal dystrophy type II, is a slowly progressive condition that leads to severe decreased vision in the second to third decade of life. Gray-white flecklike opacities develop centrally and extend peripherally toward the limbus and deep toward Descemet membrane, accompanied by a diffuse stromal haze (Fig. 5) [2]. This condition is the only stromal dystrophy that is autosomal recessive, and more than 150 mutations have been mapped to chromosome 16q22 (*CHST6*), which is involved in the synthesis of keratan sulfate [19]. Glycosoaminoglycans (GAGs) accumulate throughout the stroma and will stain with Alcian blue and colloidal iron, and also can be seen as hyperreflective accumulations on optical coherence tomography [20].

*Schnyder corneal dystrophy*

Schnyder corneal dystrophy, formerly Schnyder crystalline corneal dystrophy, is a slowly progressive condition that causes moderately decreased vision (particularly in photopic conditions) and glare. Patients under 23 years present with a ringlike central corneal opacity and/or subepithelial crystals, those 23 to 38 years will develop arcus lipoides, and those over 38 years will develop diffuse stromal haze (Fig. 6) [2]. This condition is autosomal dominant and has been mapped to chromosome 1p36 (*UBIAD1*), likely involved in lipid and cholesterol transport and metabolism [21]. Cholesterol and phospholipids deposit intracellularly and extracellularly, stain with Oil-red-O and Sudan black.

*Congenital stromal corneal dystrophy*

Congenital stromal corneal dystrophy, formerly congenital hereditary stromal dystrophy, is a bilateral, nonprogressive condition that presents at or shortly after birth, causing strabismus, nystagmus, and amblyopia in afflicted children. Patients present with flaky, feathery stromal opacities throughout the stroma [2]. This condition is autosomal dominant and has been mapped to chromosome 12q21.33 (*DCN*). This decorin gene is responsible for maintaining regular spacing between collagen fibrils, and microscopy shows abnormal amorphous areas separating normal stromal lamellae [22].

*Fleck corneal dystrophy*

Fleck corneal dystrophy, formerly Francois-Neetens corneal dystrophy, often is asymptomatic, nonprogressive condition that begins at or shortly after birth.

**Table 3**
Key clinical characteristics of the stromal corneal dystrophies

| Dystrophy | Inheritance | Gene | IC3D Category | Key Signs | Key Symptoms |
|---|---|---|---|---|---|
| Macular Corneal Dystrophy | AR | 16q22 (*CHST6*) | 1 | Gray-white flecks and diffuse haze ("snowflakes and fog") | Severely decreased vision in 20s-30s |
| Schnyder Corneal Dystrophy | AD | 1p36 (*UBIAD1*) | 1 | <23: central corneal opacity<br>23–38: arcus lipoides<br>>38: diffuse stromal haze | Moderately decreased vision (esp photopic), glare |
| Congenital Stromal Corneal Dystrophy | AD | 12q21.33 (*DCN*) | 1 | Flaky feathery white opacities | Strabismus, nystagmus, amblyopia |
| Fleck Corneal Dystrophy | AD | 2q34 (*PIKFYVE*) | 1 | Discrete "dandruff" flecks in clear stroma | Mostly asymptomatic |
| Posterior Amorphous Corneal Dystrophy | AD | 12q21.22 (*KERA, LUM, DCN, EPYC*) | 1 | Diffuse gray-white sheets in posterior stroma | Mildly decreased vision |
| Central Cloudy Dystrophy of Francois | Unknown (AD?) | Unknown | 4 | Multiple polygonal opacities separated by cracklike clear areas | Asymptomatic |
| Pre-Descemet Corneal Dystrophy | X-linked (if associated with ichthyosis)<br>Unknown (if isolated) | Xp22.31 (*STS*)<br>Unknown (if isolated) | 1 (X-linked)<br>4 (Isolated) | Focal, fine polymorphic deep stromal opacities | Asymptomatic |

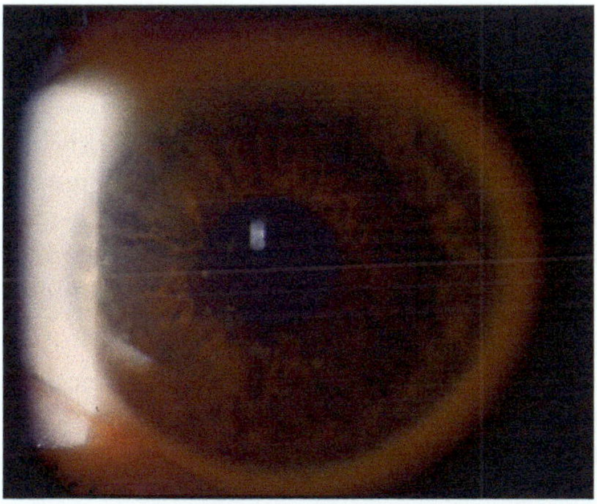

**Fig. 5.** Slit lamp photo showing the flecklike opacities and haze of macular corneal dystrophy.

Patients present with discrete dandruff-like speck- and ring-shaped opacities scattered throughout the otherwise clear stroma [2]. The condition is autosomal dominant, mapped to chromosome 2q34 (*PIKFYVE*, previously *PIP5CK3*). Microscopy shows deposits of both GAGs and lipids, due to mutations causing impaired endosomal sorting [23].

*Posterior amorphous corneal dystrophy*

Posterior amorphous corneal dystrophy causes mildly decreased visual acuity due to diffuse gray-white sheetlike opacities primarily in the posterior stroma, which may be centroperipheral or peripheral. The cornea may be thin and flat, and thus associated with hyperopia [2]. The condition is autosomal dominant,

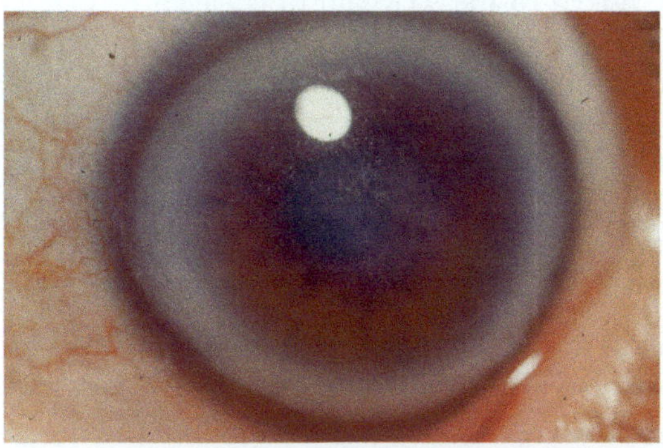

**Fig. 6.** Slit lamp photo showing the central crystalline deposits, panstromal opacity, and dense arcus of Schnyder corneal dystrophy.

and like CSCD, has been mapped to 12q21.33 (deletion of *KERA, LUM, DCN, EPYC*) [24].

*Central cloudy dystrophy of Francois*

Central cloudy dystrophy of Francois is the least well genetically characterized of the stromal dystrophies. This asymptomatic and nonprogressive condition presents with multiple polygonal gray opacities separated by lines of clear zones, indistinguishable from the appearance of the degenerative condition posterior crocodile shagreen [2,25]. The gene involved is unknown.

*Pre-Descemet corneal dystrophy*

Pre-Descemet corneal dystrophy is characterized by focal, fine, polymorphic gray opacities located in the deep stroma. Several subgroups exist–in particular, one type associated with X-linked ichthyosis has been mapped to chromosome Xp22.31 (*STS*), whereas the punctiform and polychromatic subtype is autosomal dominant, and the isolated form is not well-characterized genetically [2,26]. Microscopy shows posterior stromal keratocytes with lipofuscinlike lipid deposits [2].

## Endothelial Dystrophies

*Fuchs endothelial corneal dystrophy*

Fuchs endothelial corneal dystrophy (FECD) is the most common dystrophy of the corneal endothelium (Table 4). It is a bilateral disease characterized by loss of endothelial cells with accumulation of extracellular matrix and formation of posterior excrescences of Descemet membrane called guttae. The endothelial loss usually begins centrally and extends peripherally. Loss of endothelial cell pump function can lead to edema, formation of bullae, and eventually subepithelial fibrosis. Both early and late-onset forms have been described. The late-onset is the classic form typically inherited in an autosomal dominant fashion with initial signs presenting between the fourth and fifth decade of life. The rare early-onset form also is autosomal dominant and will present in the first decade of life [27]. Mutations causing early-onset FECD have been exclusively linked to the α2 chain of collagen 8 (*COL8A2*). *COL8* forms a short-chain ECM protein, secreted by endothelial cells, which comprises the main component of the Descemet membrane [28]. Many mutations have been linked to late-onset Fuchs, with variants in transcription factor 4 from CTG trinucleotide repeat expansion being the most common among them [29]. Rupture of bullae can occur in advanced disease, causing pain, epiphora, and anterior chamber reaction. Low-grade inflammation leads to fibrosis and eventually neurotrophic keratopathy and recurrent ulcers [27].

*Posterior polymorphous corneal dystrophy*

Posterior polymorphous corneal dystrophy (PPCD) is a rare bilateral condition, which can present with variable phenotypes and often is asymmetric between eyes. Poorly differentiated endothelial cells secrete abnormally thickened Descemet membrane, and endothelial dysfunction leads to focal or diffuse corneal edema. The endothelium becomes multilayered with degenerated

**Table 4**
Key clinical characteristics of endothelial corneal dystrophies

| Dystrophy | Inheritance | Gene | IC3D Category | Key Signs | Key Symptoms |
|---|---|---|---|---|---|
| Fuchs Endothelial Corneal Dystrophy | Sometimes autosomal dominant | Early-onset: Col8A2 on 1p34.3-p32<br>Later-onset: other associations | 1, 2, or 3 | Guttata, endothelial decompensation, stromal edema, bullous keratopathy, subepithelial fibrosis | Decreased vision, recurrent erosions |
| Posterior Polymorphous Corneal Dystrophy | Autosomal dominant. Sometimes not inherited | PPCD1: unknown gene on 20p11.2-q11.2<br>PPCD2<br>PPCD2: COL8A2 on 1p34.3-p32.3<br>PPCD3: ZEB1 on 10p11.22 | 1 or 2 | Opacities of Descemet membrane and endothelium (geographic, vesicular, railroad tracks, occasionally diffuse) | Asymptomatic, decreased vision |
| Congenital Hereditary Endothelial Dystrophy | Autosomal recessive | SLC4A11 on 20p13 | 1 | Diffuse haze, ground-glass milky appearance, corneal thickening. Rarely increased Intraocular pressure, band keratopathy. | Decreased vision with nystagmus. Minimal tearing or light sensitivity |
| X-Linked Endothelial Corneal Dystrophy | X-linked dominant | Unknown gene on Xq25 | 2 | Males: diffuse haze, ground-glass milky appearance, moon crater endothelial changes, band keratopathy<br>Females: moon crater endothelial changes | Males: blurred vision<br>Females: Asymptomatic |

endothelial cells, fibroblastlike cells, and epitheliallike cells with microvilli, keratin, and desmosomes. Groupings of vesicles and grayish deposits often are observed in vesicular, bandlike, or diffuse distributions. The epitheliallike cells can migrate across the anterior chamber angle onto the anterior iris surface where they can secrete basement membrane material leading to iridocorneal adhesions causing corectopia and ectropion uvea. Angle closure can occur leading to an increased risk of glaucoma. Corneal steepening may occur leading to significant astigmatism or even keratoconus. PPCD can be classified as 1 to 4 depending on the causative genetic mutations with PPCD1 associated with mutation in the promoter of OVOL2 gene (20p11.22), PPCD2 with mutation in COL8A2 gene (1p34.2-p32.3), PPCD3 with mutation in ZEB1 gene (10p11.22), and PPCD4 with mutation in GRHL2 gene (8q22 [30]).

*Congenital hereditary endothelial dystrophy*

Congenital hereditary endothelial dystrophy (CHED) is a bilateral nonprogressive condition, which typically presents as corneal opacification either at birth or in early infancy. It is the result of endothelial dysfunction leading to disruption of collagen fibrils, Descemet thickening, and stromal edema, which can result in 2 to 3 times the normal corneal thickness. It is inherited in an autosomal recessive fashion with the mutation occurring on the gene SLC4A11 on chromosome 20p13. This gene codes for a transmembrane protein, which codes for bicarbonate transporter-related-protein-1 (BTR1) helping to pump fluid from the corneal stroma into the aqueous humor [31].

*X-linked endothelial corneal dystrophy*

X-linked endothelial corneal dystrophy (XECD) is the least common of the corneal endothelial dystrophies and has only been reported in a single Austrian family where 35 trait carriers were identified among 4 generations. The carriers displayed variable pathology, spanning from asymptomatic changes to congenital corneal edema. In this lineage, some men presented with corneal opacification at birth, whereas women tended to present with milder endothelial irregularities resembling moon craters. The latter, described in other conditions as having a peau d'orange texture, were common to all individuals with XECD. Subepithelial band keratopathy was common among men and considered the most consistent hallmark of XECD in its later stages. XECD is inherited in an autosomal recessive fashion that has been linked to an 8 Mb region of Xq25; however, the exact gene responsible for this disease currently is unknown [32].

## RELEVANCE AND FUTURE AVENUES

Management of the different types of corneal dystrophies varies based on the severity of the dystrophy, the specific subjective complaints, and the depth of the cornea affected. Treatment is not indicated for symptoms with asymptomatic disease. For example, patients with fleck corneal dystrophy often have minimal symptoms and normal vision, so no specific management is indicated.

Several of the corneal dystrophies, particularly the epithelial dystrophies, can cause recurrent corneal erosions, which can be managed in a stepwise approach. Initial conservative management of recurrent corneal erosions consists of frequent lubrication of the ocular surface with drops and ointment. Medical options beyond lubrication include bandage contact lenses, serum eye drops, and amniotic membranes [33]. For refractory erosions, surgical options include anterior stromal puncture needle or with nd:YAG laser, alcohol deamination of epithelium, mechanical epithelial debridement with or without diamond burr polishing (DBD), and excimer laser PTK. In anterior stromal puncture, a needle tip is used to induce subepithelial fibrosis to cause the epithelium to adhere to the stroma [33]. In epithelial debridement, the central corneal area is mechanically removed to treat corneal erosions and visually significant epithelial irregularities. This treatment was found to be an effective method to improve visual acuity in EBMD [34].

A 2009 study explored the effect of epithelial debridement alone versus debridement in conjunction with DBD with results demonstrating a lower rate of recurrences when DBD is also performed. DBD is believed to decrease recurrence rate via its creation of a smooth substrate upon which the epithelium can regenerate as well as by stimulating fibrosis, which can improve epithelial adhesion [35].

PTK is a technique effective for dystrophies with lesions primarily localized to the Bowman layer and through the anterior one-third of the stroma. It has been used in the management of EBMD, Reis-Buckler, Thiel-Behnke, GCD, LCD, macular corneal dystrophy, and Schnyder corneal dystrophy [36]. In this technique, the epithelium is removed, and then an excimer laser ablates Bowman's layer and the anterior stroma, revealing a clear and smooth surface upon which the epithelium can regrow with strong adhesions. PTK for corneal dystrophies has been shown to result in improvements in visual acuity and symptoms of corneal erosions, and often is preferred as an initial surgical option over other more invasive procedures [36].

One retrospective study compared the efficacy and complication rate of PTK and DBD to find that although there was an increased rate of subepithelial haze and erosion in the PTK group compared with the DBD group, there was no significant difference between the 2 groups in subjective symptoms, recurrence, or visual acuity outcomes [37].

Recurrence of superficial dystrophies after epithelial debridement frequently is observed, often leading to consideration of corneal transplantation. In an attempt to try to prevent the need for corneal transplantation, the use of Mitomycin C has been explored to help prevent recurrence of anterior stromal dystrophies such as Meesmann and Lisch with encouraging results. Although the mechanism is not fully understood, it is thought to work by inhibiting stromal and epithelial proliferation through its DNA cross-linking effect [38]. Similarly, the use of amniotic membrane grafting has been attempted in Gelatinous droplike dystrophy with the thought that the graft's anti-inflammatory and antifibrotic effect would help to reduce fibrosis after PTK. One case report demonstrated that although it did not prevent or even delay recurrence, it did improve subjective discomfort [39]. This, therefore, could represent an effective treatment modality in cases where the main goal is pain management.

Corneal transplantation is used to replace dystrophic host cornea with healthy donor cornea, and techniques have advanced to target the transplantation of specific corneal layers. PK is a full-thickness corneal transplant and has historically been the dominant surgical procedure. It has been used to manage corneal dystrophies affecting any layer of the cornea. For stromal dystrophies not involving the Descemet membrane or the endothelium, deep anterior lamellar keratoplasty (DALK) has been shown to be safe and effective at improving visual acuity [40]. In this procedure, all layers are transplanted except the Descemet membrane and the endothelium, thus avoiding the complication of endothelial rejection that is seen in PK [41]. Endothelial keratoplasties (EKs) revolutionized the treatment of endothelial dysfunction and have become the preferred technique for the treatment of endothelial dystrophies, specifically Fuchs, which is the leading indication for EK in the United States [42]. Descemet stripping (automated) EK (DSEK or DSAEK) was introduced in 2003, whereas Descemet membrane EK (DMEK) was introduced in 2006, and both procedures have become increasingly adopted over time with early rapid improvement in vision [42]. A known risk for all of the transplant procedures for corneal dystrophies in particular is recurrence of the corneal dystrophy in the graft. The dystrophies that have been shown to most likely recur are RBCD, TBCD, GCD, LCD, and MCD.

Several techniques may be used to help prevent recurrence after corneal transplant or to address recurrence should it occur. A simple, but effective, strategy is the use of a BCL, which acts by reducing the rate of epithelial turnover. Allogenic limbal stem cell transplant is a more involved approach, which may help to prevent recurrence in certain conditions. Particularly, this has been studied in Gelatinous droplike dystrophy where it helped to prevent recurrence for 2 years after DALK [43]. Donor cells were detected on the graft years after transplantation suggesting that they contribute to epithelization in the long-term postoperative period [43]. Finally, the use of Boston keratoprosthesis can be considered in cases of graft failure, especially in diseases like GDLD that have well demonstrated high recurrence rates. Although the procedure can be highly successful, it must be performed with caution, given the possibility of devastating complications such as formation of retroprosthetic membrane, corneal stromal necrosis, and endophthalmitis [44].

Limitations to the use of keratoplasties include a worldwide shortage of human donor corneas and the inherent risk of graft failure or rejection, which has spurred investigation into alternatives that do not require donor tissue. For Fuchs, the most common reason for corneal transplantation in the United States, Descemet stripping only (DSO) has emerged as a promising surgical treatment option since its introduction in 2014 [45,46]. DSO involves creating a small 4-5 mm central descemetorrhexis without placement of any donor graft, and results thus far have shown promising rates of corneal clearing in patients with less severe disease and primarily central guttae, although the optimal patient characteristics for this procedure have yet to be clarified [46]. A related major advancement has been the use of Rho kinase inhibitors (ROCK inhibitors) as an adjuvant medical therapy to DSO. ROCK inhibitors have been shown to aid in the repopulation of corneal endothelial cells and promote wound healing [47]. Early studies have investigated topical ripasudil, a selective ROCK inhibitor, in the treatment of Fuchs as a supplement to DSO [48,49]. In a prospective study published in 2019, patients who underwent DSO with ripasudil were reported to have more rapid visual recovery as well as higher endothelial cell density than patients who underwent DSO alone [48]. Clinical trial results of DSO with ripasudil published in 2021 showed that the intervention was effective in achieving short-term corneal clearance, without any serious adverse events [49]. There remain many unanswered questions about the optimal use of DSO and ROCK inhibitors, and further studies are needed to investigate patient selection, long-term clinical outcomes, and potential applications in other endothelial corneal dystrophies.

Another exciting development in treating endothelial failure without requiring a donor graft may be the use of human corneal endothelial cells (hCECs). The first in-human clinical trial of hCEC injection therapy began in 2013, and 5-year outcomes were reported in 2021 [50]. Cultured hCECs supplemented with a ROCK inhibitor were injected into the anterior chamber of patients with endothelial failure of various etiologies. Five-year outcomes showed that 10 of 11 patients maintained complete corneal restoration with good best-corrected visual acuity, without any local or systemic adverse events [50]. This promising long-term data may represent the first steps toward using cultured cells to achieve clinical outcomes similar to DSAEK and DMEK without the drawbacks of using donor tissue.

The causative genes of many of the corneal dystrophies now have been identified and characterized with Mendelian inheritance, making them possible candidates for targeted treatment with gene therapy. However, gene therapy to treat corneal dystrophies remains in preliminary stages. For example, experimental studies have explored using the CRISPR/Cas9 system in a model of TGFbeta-1 diseases [51]. Another experimental study showed that a short-interfering RNA (siRNA) was able to knock down the mutant keratin 12 allele in cells cultured from corneal biopsies of patients with MECD [52]. Researchers have begun developing oligonucleotides to target the repeat trinucleotide expansion in the *TCF4* gene in Fuchs [53]. Targeted genetic manipulation to treat corneal dystrophies is an area that requires careful and extensive future investigation.

## SUMMARY

The major corneal dystrophies in the most recent IC3D classification represent an updated classification and nomenclature created in 2015, revised from the earlier 2008 published IC3D classification. Overall, the updated classifications incorporated the most up-to-date clinical, histopathologic, and genetic information to more precisely characterize dystrophies that were historically defined phenotypically. The disease templates describe inheritance patterns, genetic information, clinical signs and symptoms, and advanced imaging techniques that help distinguish among similar corneal dystrophies. Through careful evaluation of patients, focusing on identifying the layer of cornea affected, the morphology and distribution of lesions, and the presence of a family history and genetic basis helps to enable accurate diagnosis.

The premier advantage available today that was unavailable to those describing corneal dystrophies in the 19th and early 20th centuries is the ability to ascertain the genetic underpinning for corneal dystrophies. Many of the dystrophies listed in the 2015 IC3D classification are category C1, with a known identified gene and mutation. Exceptions to these genetically characterized corneal dystrophies include LECD, for which chromosomal loci but not the implicated gene have been identified; the EREDs, for which no chromosomal locus has been identified; XECD for which a region on the X chromosome but not the precise gene has been identified, and SMCD and CCDF, for which genetic evidence is lacking. With additional research, all valid dystrophies may eventually become categorized as C1, in which a specific mutation in a specific gene is identified. In cases where genetic information cannot be ascertained, some dystrophies may eventually be included in the removed dystrophies category, which currently includes Grayson-Wilbrandt corneal dystrophy. Factors that may continue to help the study of the diagnosis and management of corneal dystrophies include adhering to the recommendations of the IC3D to be consistent in the naming and characterization of dystrophies based on the specific templates and to be cautious in proposing new corneal dystrophies without defining both phenotype and genotype.

Some aspects of the management of corneal dystrophies have and will continue to remain constant. For instance, in cases of recurrent corneal erosions, conservative management begins with topical lubrication and prophylactic antibiotics. Subsequent management involves such interventions as anterior stromal puncture and PTK. Of course, for dystrophies causing severe vision changes, corneal transplantation often is performed. The paradigm has shifted toward transplanting smaller amounts of tissue, with procedures such as DSAEK and DMEK for dystrophies that are endothelial in origin. Even more recent advances have explored surgical treatment options away from those requiring donor tissue, such as DSO. Future innovations continue to focus on minimally invasive options focused on corneal regeneration, including the use of injected cultured endothelial cells. The preliminary experiments involving gene therapy also present an exciting future in the management of corneal dystrophies. As the genetic underpinnings of corneal dystrophies become more well understood, an increasing number of corneal dystrophies may be targeted with such techniques as CRISPR and siRNA, which have demonstrated preliminary success in some cases.

In conclusion, the study of corneal dystrophies has progressed since they were first described in the 1890s. The IC3D provided structure to the classification of corneal dystrophies in 2008 and again in 2015 based on ongoing advances in imaging, histopathologic, and genetic techniques. Looking toward the eventual next IC3D revision, the disease templates may include more C1 dystrophies, and specific gene therapy targets may be defined as part of the understanding of the pathophysiology and management of corneal dystrophies.

## CLINICS CARE POINTS

- When evaluating patients with a suspected corneal dystrophy, take a family history.
- Recurrent corneal erosions should be managed in a stepwise fashion from topical lubrication to surgical options including epithelial debridement, anterior stromal puncture, and phototherapeutic keratectomy.
- Corneal transplantation should be reserved for replacement of very visually significant dystrophic host cornea with anatomically targeted donor tissue.

## DISCLOSURE

The authors have nothing to disclose.

## References

[1] Weiss JS, Møller HU, Lisch W, et al. The IC3D classification of the corneal dystrophies. Cornea 2008;27(Suppl 2):S1.
[2] Weiss JS, Møller HU, Aldave AJ, et al. IC3D classification of corneal dystrophies-edition 2. Cornea 2015;34(2):117–59.
[3] Laibson PR, Krachmer JH. Familial occurrence of dot (microcystic), map, fingerprint dystrophy of the cornea. Invest Ophthalmol 1975;14(5):397–9.
[4] El Sanharawi M, Sandali O, Basli E, et al. Fourier-domain optical coherence tomography imaging in corneal epithelial basement membrane dystrophy: a structural analysis. Am J Ophthalmol 2015;159(4):755–63.e1.
[5] Characteristics of corneal dystrophies: a review from clinical, histological and genetic perspectives. Int J Ophthalmol 2016; https://doi.org/10.18240/ijo.2016.06.20.
[6] Werblin TP, Hirst LW, Stark WJ, et al. Prevalence of map-dot-fingerprint changes in the cornea. Br J Ophthalmol 1981;65(6):401–9.
[7] Allen EHA, Courtney DG, Atkinson SD, et al. Keratin 12 missense mutation induces the unfolded protein response and apoptosis in Meesmann epithelial corneal dystrophy. Hum Mol Genet 2016;25(6):1176–91.
[8] Lisch W, Büttner A, Oeffner F, et al. Lisch corneal dystrophy is genetically distinct from Meesmann corneal dystrophy and maps to Xp22.3. Am J Ophthalmol 2000;130(4):461–8.
[9] Kurbanyan K, Sejpal KD, Aldave AJ, et al. In Vivo Confocal microscopic findings in lisch corneal dystrophy. Cornea 2012;31(4):437–41.
[10] Kaza H, Barik MR, Reddy MM, et al. Gelatinous drop-like corneal dystrophy: a review. Br J Ophthalmol 2017;101(1):10–5.
[11] Paliwal P, Gupta J, Tandon R, et al. Identification and characterization of a novel TACSTD2 mutation in gelatinous drop-like corneal dystrophy. Mol Vis 2010;16:729–39.
[12] Feder RS, Jay M, Yue BYJT, et al. Subepithelial mucinous corneal dystrophy. Clinical and pathological correlations. Arch Ophthalmol (Chicago, Ill 1960) 1993;111(8):1106–14.
[13] Lisch W, Bron AJ, Munier FL, et al. Franceschetti hereditary recurrent corneal erosion. Am J Ophthalmol 2012;153(6):1073–81.e4.

[14] Hammar B, Lagali N, Ek S, et al. Dystrophia Smolandiensis: a novel morphological picture of recurrent corneal erosions. Acta Ophthalmol 2010;88(4):394–400.
[15] Hammar B, Björck E, Lind H, et al. Dystrophia Helsinglandica: a new type of hereditary corneal recurrent erosions with late subepithelial fibrosis. Acta Ophthalmol 2009;87(6): 659–65.
[16] Soh YQ, Kocaba V, Weiss JS, et al. Corneal dystrophies. Nat Rev Dis Prim 2020;6(1); https://doi.org/10.1038/S41572-020-0178-9.
[17] Kobayashi A, Sugiyama K. In vivo laser confocal microscopy findings for Bowman's layer dystrophies (Thiel-Behnke and Reis-Bücklers corneal dystrophies). Ophthalmology 2007;114(1):69–75.
[18] Kuchle M, Green WR, Volcker HE, et al. Reevaluation of corneal dystrophies of Bowman's layer and the anterior stroma (Reis-Bücklers and Thiel-Behnke types): a light and electron microscopic study of eight corneas and a review of the literature. Cornea 1995;14(4): 333–54.
[19] Klintworth GK, Smith CF, Bowling BL. CHST6 mutations in North American subjects with macular corneal dystrophy: A comprehensive molecular genetic review. Mol Vis 2006;12(March):159–76.
[20] Nowinska AK, Wylegala E, Teper S, et al. Phenotype and genotype analysis in patients with macular corneal dystrophy. Br J Ophthalmol 2014;98(11):1514–21.
[21] Weiss JS, Kruth HS, Kuivaniemi H, et al. Mutations in the UBIAD1 gene on chromosome short arm 1, region 36, cause Schnyder crystalline corneal dystrophy. Invest Ophthalmol Vis Sci 2007;48(11):5007–12.
[22] Bredrup C, Knappskog PM, Majewski J, et al. Congenital stromal dystrophy of the cornea caused by a mutation in the decorin gene. Invest Ophthalmol Vis Sci 2005;46(2):420–6.
[23] Li S, Tiab L, Jiao X, et al. Mutations in PIP5K3 are associated with François-Neetens mouchetée fleck corneal dystrophy. Am J Hum Genet 2005;77(1):54–63.
[24] Aldave AJ, Rosenwasser GOD, Yellore VS, et al. Linkage of Posterior Amorphous Corneal Dystrophy to Chromosome 12q21.33 and Exclusion of Coding Region Mutations in KERA, LUM, DCN, and EPYC. Invest Ophthalmol Vis Sci 2010;51(8):4006.
[25] Strachan IM. Cloudy central corneal dystrophy of François. Five cases in the same family. Br J Ophthalmol 1969;53(3):192–4.
[26] Hung C, Ayabe RI, Wang C, et al. Pre-descemet corneal dystrophy and x-linked ichthyosis associated with deletion of Xp22.31 containing the STS gene. Cornea 2013;32(9): 1283–7.
[27] Matthaei M, Hribek A, Clahsen T, et al. Fuchs endothelial corneal dystrophy: clinical, genetic, pathophysiologic, and therapeutic aspects. Annu Rev Vis Sci 2019;5(1):151–75.
[28] Mok J-W, Kim H-S, Joo C-K. Q455V mutation in COL8A2 is associated with Fuchs' corneal dystrophy in Korean patients. Eye 2009;23(4):895–903.
[29] Wieben ED, Aleff RA, Tang X, et al. Trinucleotide Repeat Expansion in the Transcription Factor 4 (TCF4) Gene Leads to Widespread mRNA Splicing Changes in Fuchs' Endothelial Corneal Dystrophy. Invest Ophthalmol Vis Sci 2017;58(1):343–52.
[30] Guier CP, Patel BC, Stokkermans TJ, Gulani AC. Posterior Polymorphous Corneal Dystrophy. 2021 Nov 2. In: StatPearls [Internet]. Treasure Island (FL): StatPearls Publishing; 2022 Jan-. PMID: 28613630.
[31] Patel SP, Parker MD. SLC4A11 and the pathophysiology of congenital hereditary endothelial dystrophy. Biomed Res Int 2015;2015:1–7.
[32] Schmid E, Lisch W, Philipp W, et al. A New, X-linked Endothelial Corneal Dystrophy. Am J Ophthalmol 2006;141(3):478–87.e3.
[33] Miller DD, Hasan SA, Simmons NL, et al. Recurrent corneal erosion: a comprehensive review. Clin Ophthalmol 2019;13:325.
[34] Itty S, Hamilton SS, Baratz KH, et al. Outcomes of epithelial debridement for anterior basement membrane dystrophy. Am J Ophthalmol 2007;144(2); https://doi.org/10.1016/j.ajo.2007.04.024.

[35] Wong VWY, Chi SCC, Lam DSC. Diamond burr polishing for recurrent corneal erosions: results from a prospective randomized controlled trial. Cornea 2009;28(2):152–6.
[36] Nagpal R, Maharana PK, Roop P, et al. Phototherapeutic keratectomy. Surv Ophthalmol 2020;65(1):79–108.
[37] Sridhar M, Rapuano CJ, Cosar CB, et al. Phototherapeutic keratectomy versus diamond burr polishing of Bowman's membrane in the treatment of recurrent corneal erosions associated with anterior basement membrane dystrophy. Ophthalmology 2002;109(4):674–9.
[38] Yeung JYT, Hodge WG. Recurrent Meesmann's corneal dystrophy: treatment with keratectomy and mitomycin C. Can J Ophthalmol 2009;44(1):103–4.
[39] Alex AF, Eter N, Uhlig CE. Combined excimer laser photoablation and amniotic membrane overlay for relief of symptomatic discomfort in gelatinous drop-like corneal dystrophy. Cornea 2015;34(10):1316–7.
[40] Unal M, Arslan OS, Atalay E, et al. Deep anterior lamellar keratoplasty for the treatment of stromal corneal dystrophies. Cornea 2013;32(8):301–5.
[41] Unal S, Argin A, Arslan E, et al. Bilateral complete avulsion of ocular globes in a Le Fort III maxillofacial fracture: a case report and review of the literature. Eur J Ophthalmol 2005;15(1):123–5.
[42] Price MO, Feng MT, Price FW. Endothelial keratoplasty update 2020. Cornea 2021;40(5): 541–7.
[43] Omoto M, Shimmura S, Hatou S, et al. Simultaneous deep anterior lamellar keratoplasty and limbal allograft in bilateral limbal stem cell deficiency. Jpn J Ophthalmol 2010;54(6):537–43.
[44] Fadlallah A, Jakobiec FA, Mendoza PR, et al. Boston Type I Keratoprosthesis for treatment of gelatinous drop-like corneal dystrophy after repeated graft failure. Semin Ophthalmol 2015;30(2):150–3.
[45] Borkar DS, Veldman P, Colby KA. Treatment of fuchs endothelial dystrophy by descemet stripping without endothelial keratoplasty. Cornea 2016;35(10):1267–73.
[46] Blitzer AL, Colby KA. Update on the surgical management of fuchs endothelial corneal dystrophy. Ophthalmol Ther 2020;9(4):757–65.
[47] Schlötzer-Schrehardt U, Zenkel M, Strunz M, et al. Potential Functional Restoration of Corneal Endothelial Cells in Fuchs Endothelial Corneal Dystrophy by ROCK Inhibitor (Ripasudil). Am J Ophthalmol 2021;224:185–99.
[48] Macsai MS, Shiloach M. Use of Topical Rho Kinase Inhibitors in the Treatment of fuchs dystrophy after descemet stripping only. Cornea 2019;38(5):529–34.
[49] Moloney G, Garcerant Congote D, Hirnschall N, et al. Descemet stripping only supplemented with topical ripasudil for fuchs endothelial dystrophy 12-Month Outcomes of the Sydney Eye Hospital Study. Cornea 2021;40(3):320–6.
[50] Numa K, Imai K, Ueno M, et al. Five-Year Follow-up of First 11 Patients Undergoing Injection of Cultured Corneal Endothelial Cells for Corneal Endothelial Failure. Ophthalmology 2021;128(4):504–14.
[51] Christie KA, Courtney DG, Dedionisio LA, et al. Towards personalised allele-specific CRISPR gene editing to treat autosomal dominant disorders. Sci Rep 2017;7(1):1–11.
[52] Courtney DG, Atkinson SD, Allen EHA, et al. SiRNA silencing of the mutant keratin 12 allele in corneal limbal epithelial cells grown from patients with Meesmann's epithelial corneal dystrophy. Invest Ophthalmol Vis Sci 2014;55(5):3352–60.
[53] Hu J, Rong Z, Gong X, et al. Oligonucleotides targeting TCF4 triplet repeat expansion inhibit RNA foci and mis-splicing in Fuchs' dystrophy. Hum Mol Genet 2018;27(6):1015–26.

Advances in Ophthalmology and Optometry 7 (2022) 367–382

ADVANCES IN OPHTHALMOLOGY AND OPTOMETRY

# Surgical Management of the Aphakic Eye

Tianyu Liu, MD*, Brian J. Nguyen, MD, Samantha L. Marek, MD, Stephen E. Orlin, MD

Scheie Eye Institute, University of Pennsylvania, 51 North 39th Street, Philadelphia, PA 19104, USA

**Keywords**

• Aphakia • ACIOL • Iris-fixated IOL • Sulcus IOL • Scleral-fixated IOL • Sutureless IOL • Yamane

**Key points**

- Current approaches to the surgical correction of aphakia include anterior chamber intraocular lenses (IOL), iris-fixated IOLs, sulcus IOLs, and scleral-fixated IOLs with or without sutures.
- Anterior chamber and iris-fixated IOLs technically are easier to place but are associated with risks including corneal decompensation, uveitis, and glaucoma, whereas scleral-fixated IOLs require longer operative times and specialized equipment and can be associated with suture breakage or erosion.
- Current techniques for secondary IOL implantation have comparable efficacy and safety outcomes, and patient and surgeon factors should be considered in choosing a surgical approach.

## INTRODUCTION

Aphakia refers to the absence of the lens of the eye. Optical aphakia implies that the natural or pseudophakic lens is still in the eye, but not within the visual axis. Causes of aphakia include congenital aphakia, trauma, surgical removal, or lens subluxation, which can occur in a variety of conditions including simple ectopia lentis, ectopia lentis et pupillae, microspherophakia, pseudoexfoliation, and various inherited metabolic disorders. Untreated aphakia results in several complications for the patient including high hyperopia, loss of accommodation,

*Corresponding author. *E-mail addresses:* Tianyu.Liu@pennmedicine.upenn.edu (T.L.); brian.nguyen@pennmedicine.upenn.edu (B.J.N.); samantha.marek@pennmedicine.upenn.edu (S.L.M.); stephen.orlin@pennmedicine.upenn.edu (S.E.O.)

https://doi.org/10.1016/j.yaoo.2022.03.016

aphakic bullous keratopathy, aphakic glaucoma, and risk of retinal tears and detachments [1].

Nonsurgical management of the aphakic eye is one option for patients who are deemed to be poor candidates for surgery. The high hyperopia resulting from aphakia can be corrected by spectacles or contact lenses, but both have their disadvantages. High-plus spectacles create several optical problems including excessive image magnification, pincushion effect, a ring scotoma in the temporal field, and cosmetic issues of thick lenses. Contact lenses mitigate some of these optical issues but are associated with risks including corneal hypoxia or edema, corneal abrasions, and microbial keratitis [2].

For patients who are good surgical candidates, implanting a secondary intraocular lens (IOL) can reduce some long-term risks of aphakia while achieving excellent visual and functional outcomes. A variety of approaches for secondary IOL placement exist, including anterior chamber IOLs (ACIOLs), iris-fixated IOLs, sulcus placement of IOLs with or without optic capture, and sutured and sutureless scleral-fixated IOLs. Each approach is associated with specific advantages and disadvantages, and the technique of choice should be tailored to the patient's history and risks. This article reviews each of the primary approaches for secondary IOL placement and concludes with a discussion of new developments in surgical techniques for the management of aphakia.

## SIGNIFICANCE AND IN-DEPTH ANALYSIS OF THE TOPIC

### Epikeratophakia

Epikeratophakia is a technique that was historically used for correction of aphakia but has since fallen out of favor. In this procedure, a lathed corneal lenticle from a human donor is placed on the deepithelialized surface of the recipient cornea and sutured into a prepared groove on the host cornea. This procedure was based on keratomileusis surgery performed initially by Jose Barraquer in 1949 and modified by Kaufman, Werlin, and Klyce in the 1980s. Although theoretically appealing because the lathed tissue could be prepared for correcting refractive errors up to 20 diopters (D), the procedure fell out of favor because of irregular astigmatism and improvement in IOL implant technology described later in the article [3].

### Anterior chamber intraocular lenses

ACIOLs are lenses that are placed in the anterior chamber and supported by the angle. ACIOLs represent one option for the correction of aphakia, particularly when poor capsular support exists, and sulcus placement is not possible.

Before the 1980s, ACIOLs were the most commonly used lenses for the correction of aphakia, but subsequently fell out of favor because the closed-loop design caused mechanical trauma to the corneal endothelium and angle, with resultant corneal decompensation and glaucoma [4,5]. Newer ACIOLs have an open loop design that has a better safety profile. A diagram of anterior chamber intraocular lens with open loop haptics can be found in this source [6].

The improvement in design leads to minimal vault of the lens, reducing corneal endothelial damage and iris chafing. Furthermore, this design minimizes contact area with the angle, reducing fibrosis and erosion of angle structures [4].

The most popular ACIOL lens options today are open loop ACIOLs and Artisan iris claw lenses [7]. Open loop ACIOLs are nonfoldable but flexible polymethyl methacrylate (PMMA) lenses placed into the anterior chamber supported by the angle. Artisan iris claw lenses are fixated directly to the iris and are described in detail in the following section. Both are safe and effective options. These lenses require large incisions, often scleral tunnels, for placement because the lenses are not foldable [8]. Several other ACIOL options exist, including foldable acrylic lenses, but these are not often used.

Open-loop ACIOLs have a more favorable risk profile than sutured posterior chamber IOLs (PCIOLs), avoiding complications such as suture erosion and suture-related endophthalmitis. ACIOLs also are technically easier to master and require shorter operating times, which is beneficial for patients who cannot tolerate longer or deeper sedation [9]. Complications of ACIOL placement include hyphema, pupil distortion, glaucoma, corneal decompensation, pupil block, and cystoid macular edema [8]. ACIOLs should be always combined with a peripheral iridectomy to prevent pupil-block glaucoma. Care also should be taken to avoid migration of the footplates through the iridectomy. When placed properly, ACIOLs are a safe and effective option for both primary and secondary IOL placement to correct aphakia.

### Iris-fixated intraocular lenses

Iris-fixated IOLs can be another option for lens placement in eyes with inadequate capsular support for either in-the-bag or sulcus placement. IOLs can be affixed to the iris in several ways. The Artisan iris claw lens (Ophtec B.V., Groningen, Netherlands) is a nonfoldable PMMA lens that is placed into the anterior chamber but is attached to the iris by enclaving the midperipheral iris through claws in the haptics [7]. The iris claw lenses can be placed in a retropupillary position also, which has similar visual outcomes to being placed in the anterior chamber, but is possibly associated with a higher complication rate, especially IOL dislocation [10].

Alternatively, a posterior chamber lens may be sutured to the iris using various techniques. Initially described in 1976, the McCannel iris suture is a popular method for fixating an IOL to the iris [11]. Using a 10-0 monofilament suture, the needle is introduced through the peripheral cornea and passed from anterior to posterior iris, under the haptic of the IOL, from posterior to anterior iris, and then out through the cornea (Fig. 1). The ends of the suture are brought out through a paracentesis and tied securely, thus docking the IOL to the posterior surface of the iris. This technique was modified by Chang [12] in 2004 by using Siepser slip knot with the McCannel technique to simplify the procedure. In this modification, the suture is initially placed using the McCannel technique and then tied with a slip knot. The slip knot is achieved by pulling a loop of suture out through the paracentesis, passing the free tip of

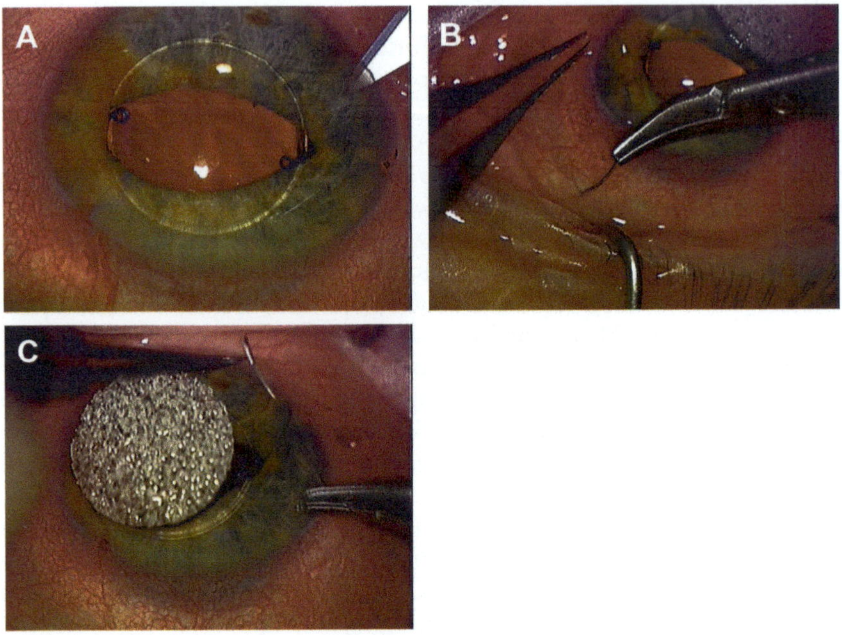


**Fig. 1.** Posterior iris intraocular lens fixation using McCannel iris suture technique. (*A*) Making the paracentesis. (*B*) Passing the needle through the peripheral cornea and iris. (*C*) Completing the needle pass through the peripheral cornea.

the other end through the loop, and pulling down to slide the knot onto the haptic. Long Vannas scissors are then used to cut the suture ends. If the lens is placed during a combination procedure, it can be sutured in alternative ways, such as in an open-sky manner during concurrent penetrating keratoplasty or placed posteriorly through a limbal approach after vitrectomy [13].

Benefits of this type of IOL placement over scleral-fixated PCIOLs include generally shorter surgical time and not requiring transscleral fixation sutures. However, this method is more technically challenging than placement of an open-loop ACIOL [4].

Drawbacks of iris-fixated lenses include pupil irregularities, iris chafing, pigment dispersion, chronic inflammation, glare, haloes, pupil block, and anterior synechiae formation [14]. This method also requires an intact anterior segment, because iris fixation will not work in cases of significant anterior chamber disruptions or iris irregularities [4].

## Sulcus placement of intraocular lenses

If adequate capsular support exists, lenses can be placed in the sulcus between the iris and ciliary processes, potentially avoiding some of the complications of ACIOLs or iris-fixated IOLs [15]. This method can be useful in cases of capsular rupture or zonular dehiscence, but adequate capsular support must exist to prevent the lens from falling posteriorly.

The entire lens can be placed into the sulcus, but is prone to decentering and tilt, which can lead to iris chafing, pigment dispersion, glaucoma, chronic inflammation, and macular edema [16]. A more stable approach is to place the haptics in the sulcus and capture the optic through a continuous curvilinear capsulorhexis (CCC) in the anterior capsule, the posterior capsule, or both. This way, the lens is stabilized and vaulted away from the iris, reducing the risks seen without optic capture. The optic capture technique was first published by Gimbel and DeBroff in 1994 [17] based on a technique described in a film from Neuhann and Neuhann in 1991 [18]. The capsulorhexis should be 1 to 2 mm smaller than the diameter of the optic. The haptics are placed into the sulcus, and then gentle pressure is placed on the optic 90° away from the haptics to capture the optic through the CCC [15].

Choosing the appropriate lens is important for sulcus placement. Options include 3-piece acrylic lenses, 3-piece silicone lenses, and 1-piece PMMA lenses [15]. Three-piece lenses tend to be favored over one-piece lenses because one-piece PMMA lenses require a large incision of about 6 to 7 mm. Three-piece silicone lenses have longer haptic lengths (13.5 mm) compared with three-piece acrylic lenses (13 mm). However, silicone lenses should be avoided if future vitrectomy with silicone oil placement may be needed, such as in eyes with a history of trauma, complicated cataract surgery, or other risk factors for retinal pathology.

One-piece acrylic lenses should not be placed in the sulcus because they are designed for in-the-bag placement only [19]. One-piece acrylic lenses are prone to iris chafing and subsequent complications, such as uveitis-glaucoma-hyphema syndrome (UGH syndrome, Fig. 2), due to their bulky haptics with a tacky textured finish and a flatter optic that is not vaulted away from the iris. These lenses are also too short for many eyes and can become displaced.

Apart from UGH syndrome, complications from sulcus-placed IOLs include chronic or recurrent inflammation, macular edema, and intraocular hemorrhage. Most often, these are due to single-piece acrylic IOLs placed in the sulcus or sulcus-placed lenses without optic capture, leading to iris-lens touch

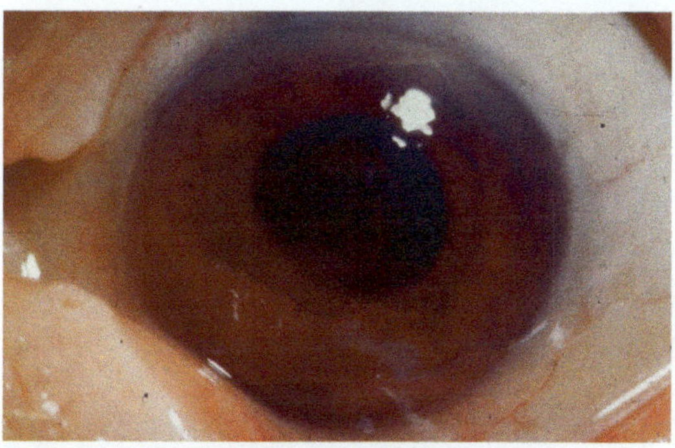

**Fig. 2.** Uveitis-glaucoma-hyphema (UGH) syndrome.

[15,19]. With proper lens choice and placement, sulcus IOL placement is a safe and effective approach to correcting aphakia when adequate capsular support exists.

## Sutured scleral-fixated intraocular lenses

If inadequate capsular support occurs for sulcus placement, lenses can be sutured directly to the sclera in the sulcus position. Techniques for scleral fixation vary in terms of ab interno versus ab externo approaches, fixation options, and suture and lens choices.

Ab interno scleral fixation was introduced by Smiddy and colleagues [20] in 1990. This approach involves passing a 10-0 Prolene suture on a curved needle through a corneoscleral incision under the level of the iris. The needle is then rotated to pass through a partial thickness scleral flap 90° away. The free ends of the suture are then tied to the haptics and repeated on the opposite side [20].

Ab externo scleral fixation was introduced by Lewis [20] in 1991. This approach involves docking a 10-0 Prolene suture on a straight needle at the level of the ciliary sulcus into a hollow 28-gauge needle through scleral flaps, allowing for 2-point fixation. The suture is cut in the middle through a corneal incision, and each new free end is tied to each haptic of the IOL. Entry is through a limbal-based 3-mm triangular partial thickness scleral flap [21,22] (Fig. 3).

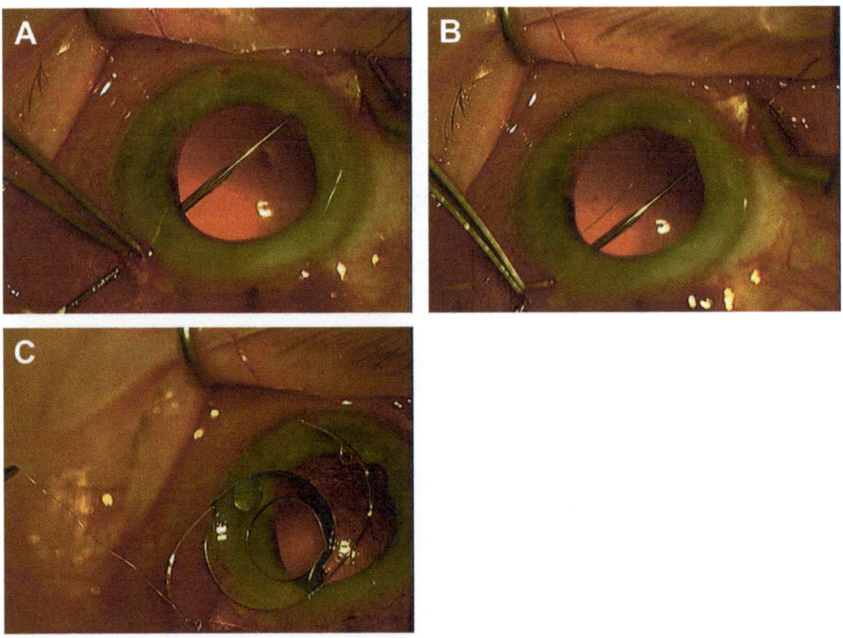


**Fig. 3.** Ab externo scleral fixation of a posterior chamber intraocular lens. (*A*) Docking the suture needle into a hollow 28-gauge needle. (*B*) Docking a second suture needle for 4-point fixation. (*C*) Tying the cut end of the suture to the eyelet of a CZ70BD lens.

Two studies using ultrasound biomicroscopy to compare the postoperative position of IOLs sutured via an ab interno versus ab externo method found comparable albeit low rates of sulcus positioning (approximately 30%) in both approaches [23,24].

Multiple advances have been made since the introduction of these techniques including 4-point fixation, endoscopy, and alternate suture choices. A 4-point fixation variation allows for a wider fixation of the haptics and more stability, decreasing the risk of postoperative tilt or astigmatism. A 10-0 Prolene suture is passed through the scleral flap and docked into a 26-gauge needle superiorly and externalized (see Fig. 4A). The externalized suture is then tied to the haptic. Another suture is passed in the same fashion 1 mm radially from the initial entrance and again tied to the haptic. It is repeated 180° away, thereby creating 4-point fixation [25] (see Fig. 4B).

Endoscopy is a technique introduced by Althaus and Sundmacher [26] in 1993 to directly visualize the sulcus. Endoscopy can be used in either ab interno or externo approaches to confirm correct placement of the suture tract [26].

In 2014, Khan and colleagues [27] introduced ab externo scleral fixation using an 8-0 Gore-Tex suture. The investigators reported no suture erosion or breakage at 1 year [28]. This finding is compared with a 28% breakage rate over 6 years for 10-0 Prolene suture reported by Vote and colleagues [29]. Because the exposed knots of the Gore-Tex sutures can cause scleral inflammation and necrosis, it is imperative to bury them.

Options for scleral fixation require IOLs with eyelets to accommodate the fixating sutures. The Akreos AO60 lens (Bausch + Lomb, Bridgewater, NJ, USA) is a hydrophilic acrylic lens with 4 haptics allowing for 4-point fixation. However, it is associated with a high rate of visually significant opacification when exposed to air or silicone oil during vitrectomy, and thus may not be a good option for patients at risk of subsequent retinal pathology [30]. The CZ70BD lens (Alcon, Geneva, Switzerland) is a PMMA single-piece IOL with eyelets in the middle of the haptic arms (Fig. 4). However, it is not foldable

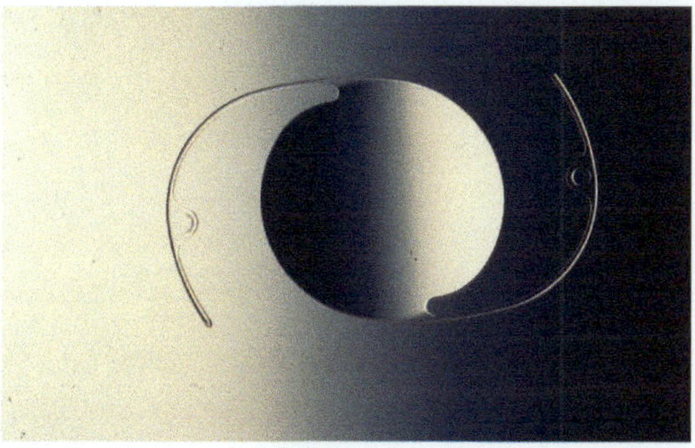

**Fig. 4.** CZ70BD lens with eyelets for suture fixation.

and requires a 7-mm incision for insertion. The enVista MX60 lens (Bausch + Lomb) is a 1-piece hydrophobic acrylic IOL that has eyelets at the haptic-optic junction and is foldable. In contrast to the Akreos hydrophilic acrylic lens, the PMMA and hydrophobic acrylic lenses may be better choices in patients with anticipated future vitreoretinal surgery given the lower risk of opacification.

### Sutureless scleral-fixated intraocular lenses

Sutured scleral-fixated IOLs are associated with unique risks including suture breakage or erosion through the conjunctiva (Fig. 5). These risks can be avoided by securing the IOL to the sclera without suturing.

Maggi and Maggi [31] were the first to describe sutureless IOL fixation using an IOL with 3 polytetrafluoroethylene loops serving as haptics, which were externalized through the sclera with a spring needle mechanism, and then cauterized to prevent slippage into the eye. The investigators presented 23 cases over 8 years with variable visual outcomes [31].

Scharioth and Pavlidis [32] described a sutureless IOL fixation technique using scleral tunnels. A 24-gauge cannula is used to create 2 straight sclerotomies with limbus-parallel tunnels at 50% scleral thickness, 180° from each other. The haptics of a 3-piece IOL are externalized through the sclerotomies and buried in the scleral tunnels [32]. A retrospective study of 63 patients across 4 European institutions undergoing this technique with a mean follow-up of 6.8 months found a significant increase in mean best corrected visual acuitylog (BCVA) from 1.25 logMAR (logarithm of the minimum angle of resolution [MAR]) to 0.40 logMAR, with 73% gaining 2 or more lines. Complications included temporary corneal edema (7.9%), persistent intraocular pressure (IOP) elevation (3.2%), spontaneous IOL dislocation (3.2%), vitreous hemorrhage (3.2%), macular edema (1.6%), persistent hypotony (1.6%), iris capture (1.6%), and traumatic IOL subluxation (1.6%), all of which occurred within 4 weeks of surgery [33].

In 2008, Agarwal and colleagues [34] described a sutureless IOL fixation technique in which the haptics are secured with fibrin glue under scleral flaps.

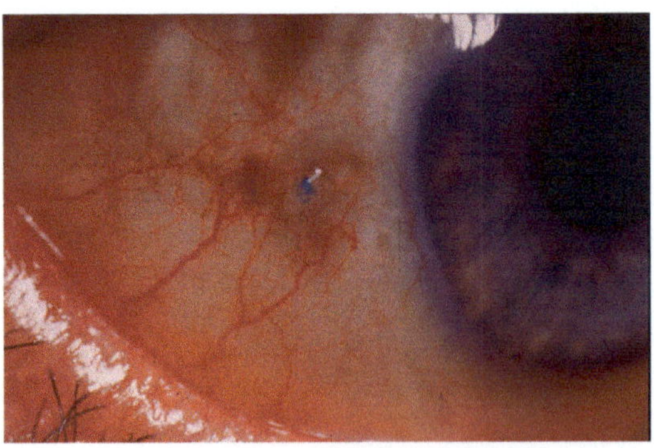

**Fig. 5.** Suture exposure in sutured scleral-fixated intraocular lens.

Two partial-thickness limbal-based scleral flaps are made 180° apart, and 2 straight sclerotomies are made under the scleral flaps. Each haptic is externalized through the sclerotomies, and the flaps are glued with reconstituted fibrinogen and thrombin [34]. Subsequent modifications included using a handshake technique to externalize the haptics and burying the haptic tips into scleral tunnels. The largest series to date included 735 eyes from a single Indian institution with a mean follow-up of 16.6 months. The mean postoperative decimal equivalent BCVA was 0.38 among eyes with rigid 1-piece IOLs and 0.39 among eyes with foldable 3-piece IOLs. Among eyes with rigid 1-piece IOLs, early complications included optic capture (3.4%), anterior uveitis (3%), corneal edema (0.8%), and transient elevated IOP (0.4%) and late complications included IOL decentration (4.3%), haptic displacement (4.1%), optic capture (3.4%), macular edema (1.4%), retinal detachment (1%), and chronic vitritis (0.4%). Complication rates were not reported for eyes with foldable 3-piece IOLs [35]. The same group reported long-term results (mean follow-up 8.2 years) from 91 eyes, most of which underwent implantation of 3-piece hydrophobic acrylic lenses with flexible PMMA haptics. The mean preoperative and postoperative BCVA was 0.61 and 0.5 logMAR, respectively, with no significant change. Haptic visibility was graded as none (50%), mild (33.5%), moderate (9.3%), and severe (7%), with no cases of haptic tip erosion or conjunctival rub. Long-term complications included glaucoma (7.7%), haptic luxation (4.4%), macular edema (3.2%), rhegmatogenous retinal detachment (3.2%), and corneal decompensation (3.2%) [36]. McKee and colleagues [37] reported outcomes of the glue technique in 50 eyes from a single US institution with 2 modifications: creation of the sclerotomies and scleral flaps with a diamond blade, lifting only 2 edges of each flap, and use of IOLs with haptic materials less prone to breakage or kinking (primarily STAAR CQ2015 lens with modified C-loop polyimide haptics). The investigators found an improvement in mean BCVA from 20/200 to 20/50 at 3 to 15 months follow-up, with complications including transient hypotony (22%), hyphema and vitreous hemorrhage (4%), macular edema (4%), and breakage of the haptic-optic junction in 1 eye 3 months postoperatively requiring IOL exchange [37].

Yamane and colleagues [38] described a sutureless IOL fixation technique using 27-gauge needles without the use of glue or scleral flaps. Two lamellar scleral dissections 1.5 mm in length and 50% scleral thickness are made 1.7 mm from the limbus, 180° apart; 27-gauge needles are used to make angled sclerotomies at the end of each scleral dissection and limbal parallel tunnels opposite the sclerotomies. The haptics are inserted into the 27-gauge needles and simultaneously externalized and then inserted into the scleral tunnels [38]. Yamane and colleagues [38] subsequently described a modification of this technique involving creation of angled sclerotomies with 30-gauge thin-walled needles without scleral dissection, as well as cauterization of the haptic ends after externalization to make 0.3-mm diameter flanges, which are pushed back into the scleral tunnels. In their series of 100 eyes with mean 20.6 months follow up, mean BCVA improved from 0.25 logMAR preoperatively to 0.04 to 0.12 logMAR at 6 to 36 months postoperatively, with mean IOL tilt of 3.4° and mean refractive difference from predicted value of −0.21 D. Complications included iris capture (8%), vitreous hemorrhage (5%), elevated IOP (3%), transient hypotony (2%), transient corneal edema (1%), and macular edema (1%), with no cases of IOL dislocation [39]. Of note, although the Yamane and other sutureless scleral fixation techniques avoid the risk of suture exposure seen with sutured scleral fixation, the haptics themselves can become exposed (Fig. 6).

The CT LUCIA 602 lens (Carl Zeiss AG, Oberkochen, Germany) is a 3-piece hydrophobic IOL that has been recommended by some for use with the Yamane technique due do its polyvinylidene fluoride haptics, which may be less susceptible to breakage. A biomechanical study comparing the CT LUCIA 602 lens with 3 three-piece IOLs with PMMA haptics found that significantly greater force was required to cause dislocation or optic-haptic disinsertion of the CT LUCIA 602 lens [40], although there have been no long-term clinical studies directly comparing rates of dislocation between these lenses when used with the Yamane technique.

## CURRENT RELEVANCE AND FUTURE AVENUES

### Minimizing suture erosion with scleral pockets and Z-sutures

One well-described complication of sutured scleral-fixated IOLs is suture erosion through the flap and conjunctiva, which may serve as a potential conduit for postoperative endophthalmitis. Since the original scleral flap method, multiple alternative techniques including scleral pockets and Z-sutures have been developed to minimize this risk of suture erosion.

In 2006, Hoffman and colleagues [41] described a scleral tunnel technique that uses a scleral pocket created through a clear corneal incision. With this technique, 2 clear corneal limbal incisions are made 180° from each other at the position of the anticipated haptics. Two corresponding scleral pockets are dissected posteriorly extending approximately 3.0 mm. A 1.0-mm paracentesis is made anterior to the clear corneal incision. Then a 27-gauge needle is advanced through the conjunctiva and scleral pocket 1.0 mm posterior to the

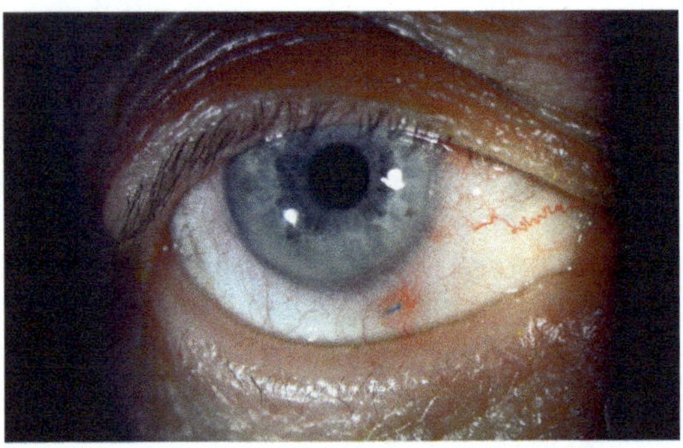

**Fig. 6.** Haptic exposure in intraocular lens fixated with Yamane technique.

surgical limbus, and the operation proceeds in ab externo fashion with 4-point fixation. Once the needles are removed, a Sinskey hook is used to pull the trailing sutures through the corneal incision so that they now pass through the incision, the scleral pocket, and through the ciliary sulcus into the eye. The sutures are then tied and slid under the roof of the scleral pocket. The same process is repeated on the opposite side for the other haptic. The scleral pockets do not require suturing [41].

Compared with the scleral flap approach, using scleral pockets avoids conjunctival dissection and scleral cauterization, which reduces patient discomfort. Furthermore, because the knot is covered by the partial thickness scleral pocket, this technique obviates knot coverage and rotation. No wound suturing is required, which reduces the risk of surgically induced astigmatism from radial sutures. The degree of flattening with the clear corneal incision in this technique is minimized through the small arc length and the ability to use superficial 300-μm incisions. Finally, this double-pass technique creates 4-point fixation, reducing the risk of lens tilt. Budoff and colleagues [42] reported a 1-year retrospective study of 17 patients who had posteriorly dislocated PCIOLs rescued with the Hoffman technique and reported excellent visual outcomes improving from an average BCVA of 20/500 preoperatively to 20/54 postoperatively; 3 eyes had decentration with 2 requiring additional surgical repair [42]. In a separate study of 31 aphakic eyes from iatrogenic or posttraumatic cause with secondary implantation using the Hoffman technique, the mean BCVA remained stable from 20/39 preoperatively to 20/40 at 1 year postoperatively, with no dislocations reported [43].

Another variation of sutured scleral fixation that reduces the risk of suture erosion involves the use of Z-sutures. Szurman and colleagues [44] first described the Z-suture knotless technique in 2010. With this technique, the IOL is implanted and fixated using an ab externo technique with a double-armed 10-0 Prolene suture resulting in 2 exit suture sites in the sclera. The external Z-suture begins with a partial-thickness scleral pass adjacent to the exit site and parallel to the limbus. The suture then is passed in the opposite direction close to the initial pass and is repeated 5 times. The suture is then cut flush with the sclera without any knot. When assessed ex vivo in the laboratory setting, 5 passes resisted a maximal tractional force of 0.41 N, exceeding the tensile strength of the Prolene suture. In their review of 45 cases of IOL fixation with Z-sutures over an average of 22.4 months, no cases of erosion, loosening, scleral atrophy, or chronic inflammation occurred. The prominent advantage of this technique is that it provides strong fixation without leaving a knot, thereby preventing the risk of erosion and resultant risk of endophthalmitis. Furthermore, the technique does not require extensive conjunctival dissection, is relatively straightforward to perform, and is applicable to any type of implant that requires transscleral suturing [44]. Dimopoulos and colleagues [45] reported longer-term retrospective data from 66 eyes over 64 months undergoing scleral fixation using the Z-suture technique, with traumatic aphakia as the leading indication. The mean preoperative visual acuity was 20/103 with no significant change at multiple time points up to 10 years. The investigators reported 11 failures due to breakage (16.7%) at 7.5 years with trauma as a predictive factor for postoperative dislocation, although there were no reports of suture erosion. It was concluded that the knotless Z-suture was a safe technique in patients with aphakia, although they believed longevity could be improved with more advanced suture material [45].

### Modifications of the Yamane sutureless fixation technique

The Yamane technique has become one of the most common approaches to sutureless scleral fixation, and numerous modifications have been proposed since its initial publication, including improvements in needle docking and flange creation, applying flanges to novel techniques, and using Yamane fixation in combination surgeries.

Since publishing their original technique, Yamane and colleagues have developed a needle stabilizer tool to help improve the positioning and angle of the sclerotomy needles.[45] Modifications have been made to the haptic needle docking technique due in part to the difficulty of docking the trailing haptic, including passing the trailing haptic to the other hand via a handshake technique, docking one or both haptics outside of the eye, and docking the haptics in the posterior chamber. Improvements in flange creation have also been described, including using a needle holder to flatten the flange for improved stability [46].

Yamane-style flanges have been applied to other techniques such as refixating glued IOLs, securing capsular tension segments, and establishing 4-point fixation. Gelman and Garg [47] described a technique of trimming and creating Yamane-style flanges to refixate glued IOLs that had extruded through the conjunctiva. Canabrava and colleagues [48] described a modification of the Yamane technique in which a 5-0 polypropylene haptic was removed from a 3-piece IOL and used to fixate a capsular tension segment to the sclera using flanged ends ("double-flanged technique"). The investigators subsequently described a method of fixating an IOL with 4 eyelets to the sclera using two 5-0 polypropylene sutures with flanged ends ("four-flanged technique") [48].

Finally, recent reports have established the feasibility of combining Yamane-fixated lenses with concurrent anterior or posterior segment surgeries. Cervantes [49] described a technique of concurrent Descemet-stripping endothelial keratoplasty and secondary IOL implantation by the Yamane method, which can be used in cases of pseudophakic or aphakic bullous keratopathy. The Yamane technique has been combined with concurrent pars plana vitrectomy for posteriorly dislocated crystalline or artificial lenses [50].

### Correction of pediatric aphakia

Although the focus of this article is to discuss surgical approaches to adult aphakia, these newer techniques are being used in pediatric patients as well. Owing to the risks of corneal decompensation, chronic inflammation, and glaucoma, ACIOLs and iris-fixated lenses are not typically recommended for children [51]. Because of suture-related risks with suture-fixated IOLs, including suture erosion with IOL decentration and suture-related endophthalmitis, nonsutured techniques are being explored; this is especially important for pediatric patients who have a much longer life expectancy of the lens in the eye. The Yamane technique has been shown to be safe and effective in children but is more technically challenging due to smaller orbits and less space to work with [52]. Other possible options include glued intrascleral fixation as well as a sutureless and glueless technique using scleral flaps [53,54]. Both these options have been shown to have minimal complications with no reports of IOL tilt or decentration. However, all these newer techniques are limited by short follow-up, and the long-term outcomes for pediatric patients undergoing these techniques are unclear.

## SUMMARY

A diverse and growing array of options exists for the surgical correction of aphakia. Current strategies for secondary IOL implantation include anterior chamber placement, iris fixation, sulcus placement, and scleral fixation with or without sutures. Each technique is associated with unique advantages and disadvantages and should be considered in light of the patient's anatomy, history, and risk factors.

Historically, ACIOLs were the most popular option for correcting aphakia due to the ease of implantation, short operative times, and lesser requirement for specialized instruments. Subsequent open-loop designs helped overcome some of the limitations of closed-loop designs, but ACIOLs still carry risks of lens decentration, iris tucking, UGH syndrome, and endothelial decompensation with subsequent corneal edema. Iris-fixated IOLs share some of the advantages and disadvantages of ACIOLs. This approach permits the lens to be placed further away from the corneal endothelium, but is somewhat more technically challenging to perform, and can inhibit mydriasis and thus interfere with subsequent posterior segment examinations.

In contrast to anterior chamber and iris-fixated IOLs, placing a lens in the sulcus achieves a more physiologic position with more predictable refractive outcomes. However, it can only be done when adequate capsular support exists. When insufficient capsular support exists, sutured or sutureless scleral-fixated IOLs can similarly achieve physiologic positioning, with decreased risk of endothelial decompensation and UGH syndrome. However, this approach is the most technically challenging, requiring increased operative time and vitrectomy equipment, with a heightened risk of uveal damage and retinal tears or detachments. Furthermore, sutured scleral-fixated IOLs carry a risk of suture breakage or erosion with subsequent endophthalmitis.

Although the benefits and disadvantages of each technique are different, a recent Ophthalmic Technology Assessment by the American Academy of Ophthalmology indicated no superiority of a particular IOL implantation technique in the absence of zonular report. Given comparable visual acuity and safety outcomes, surgeons should consider the patient's anatomy and history as well as their own experience in surgical planning and decision making [55].

## CLINICS CARE POINTS

- For aphakic patients with adequate capsular support, consider placement of a 3-piece IOL in the sulcus with optic capture through a CCC.
- For aphakic patients with inadequate capsular support and a formed anterior segment, consider placement of an anterior chamber IOL or iris-sutured IOL, but monitor for corneal decompensation, chronic inflammation, and glaucoma.
- For aphakic patients with inadequate capsular support at risk for anterior segment complications, consider placement of a sutured or sutureless PCIOL, but monitor for suture/haptic erosion or breakage.

## Disclosure

The authors have nothing to disclose.

## References

[1] Plager DA, Bothun ED, Freedman SF, et al. Complications at 10 years of follow-up in the Infant Aphakia Treatment Study. Ophthalmology 2020;127(11):1581–3.
[2] Shahid SM, Flores-Sanchez BC, Chan EW, et al. Scleral-fixated intraocular lens implants—evolution of surgical techniques and further developments. Eye 2021;35(11):2930–61.
[3] Morgan KS. Visual rehabilitation of aphakic children. IV. Epikeratophakia. Surv Ophthalmol 1990;34(5):379–84.
[4] Wagoner M, Cox TA, Ariyasu RG, et al. Intraocular lens implantation in the absence of capsular support: a report by the American Academy of Ophthalmology. Ophthalmology 2003;110(4):840–59.
[5] Mahapatra SK, Mannem N. Anterior chamber intraocular lens – an effective alternative in traumatic and surgical aphakia in the era of scleral-fixated intraocular lens. Indian J Ophthalmol 2021;69(6):1404–8.
[6] KELMAN®MULTIFLEX™1IIISTERILE UV-Absorbing PMMASingle-Piece Anterior Chamber Lenses. Product Information. Alcon Laboratories, Inc. Accessed January 14, 2022. Available at: http://embed.widencdn.net/pdf/plus/alcon/djcplhttyy/10-500-086_us_en.pdf?u=4rqn9d.
[7] Moschos MM, Nitoda E. The correction of aphakia using anterior chamber intraocular lens. vivo 2016;30:733–8.
[8] Bayramlar H, Hepsen IF, Ekic OC, et al. Comparison of the results of primary and secondary implantation of flexible open-loop anterior chamber intraocular lens. Eye 1998;12:826–8.
[9] Donaldson KE, Gorscak JJ, Budenz DL, et al. Anterior chamber and sutured posterior chamber intraocular lenses in eyes with poor capsular support. J Cataract Refract Surg 2005;31:903–9.
[10] Toro MD, Longo A, Avitabile T, et al. Five-year follow-up of secondary iris-claw intraocular lens implantation for the treatment of aphakia: Anterior chamber versus retropupillary implantation. PLoS ONE 2019;14(4):1–13.
[11] McCannel M. A retrievable suture idea for anterior uveal problems. Ophthalmic Surg 1976;7(2):98–103.
[12] Chang DF. Siepser slipknot for McCannel iris-suture fixation of subluxated intraocular lens. J Cataract Refract Surg 2004;30:1170–6.
[13] Zeh WG, Price FW. Iris fixation of posterior chamber intraocular lenses. J Cataract Refract Surg 2000;26:1028–34.
[14] Condon GP, Masket S, Krandemann C, et al. Small-incision iris fixation of foldable intraocular lenses in the absence of capsule support. Ophthalmology 2007;114(7):1311–8.

[15] Mehta R, Aref AA. Intraocular lens implantation in the ciliary sulcus: challenges and risks. Clin Ophthalmol 2019;13:2317–23.
[16] Gimbel HV, DeBroff BM. Intraocular lens optic capture. J Cataract Refract Surg 2004;30: 200–6.
[17] Gimbel HC, DeBroff BM. Posterior capsular rhexis with optic capture: maintaining a clear visual axis after pediatric cataract surgery. J Cataract Refract Surg 1994;20(6):658–64.
[18] Neuhann T, Neuhann Th. "The Rhexis-Fixated Lens," film presented at the Symposium on Cataract, IOL and Refractive Surgery," Boston, April 1991.
[19] Chang DF, Masket S, Miller KM, et al. Complications of sulcus placement of single-piece acrylic intraocular lenses. J Cataract Refract Surg 2009;35:1445–58.
[20] Smiddy WE, Sawusch MR, O'Brien TP, et al. Implantation of scleral-fixated posterior chamber intraocular lenses. J Cataract Refract Surg 1990;16(6):691–6.
[21] Lewis JS. Ab externo sulcus fixation. Ophthalmic Surg 1991;22(11):692–5.
[22] Solomon K, Gussler JR, Gussler C, et al. Incidence and management of complications of transsclerally sutured posterior chamber lenses. J Cataract Refract Surg 1993;19(4): 488–93.
[23] Kamal AM, Hanafy M, Ehsan A, et al. Ultrasound biomicroscopy comparison of ab interno and ab externo scleral fixation of posterior chamber intraocular lenses. J Cataract Refract Surg 2009;35(5):881–4.
[24] Horiguchi L, Garcia PN, Malavazzi GR, et al. Ultrasound biomicroscopy comparison of ab interno and ab externo intraocular lens scleral fixation. J Ophthalmol 2016;2016: 9375091.
[25] Rao SK, Gopal L, Fogla R, et al. Ab externo 4-point scleral fixation. J Cataract Refract Surg 2000;26(1):9–10.
[26] Althaus C, Sundmacher R. Intraoperative intraocular endoscopy in transscleral suture fixation of posterior chamber lenses: consequences for suture technique, implantation procedure, and choice of PCL design. Refract Corneal Surg 1993;9(5):333–9.
[27] Khan MA, Gerstenblith AT, Dollin ML, et al. Scleral fixation of posterior chamber intraocular lenses using gore-tex suture with concurrent 23-gauge pars plana vitrectomy. Retina 2014;34(7):1477–80.
[28] Khan MA, Gupta OP, Smith RG, et al. Scleral fixation of intraocular lenses using Gore-Tex suture: clinical outcomes and safety profile. Br J Ophthalmol 2016;100(5):638–43.
[29] Vote BJ, Tranos P, Bunce C, et al. Long-term outcome of combined pars plana vitrectomy and scleral fixated sutured posterior chamber intraocular lens implantation. Am J Ophthalmol 2006;141(2):308–12.
[30] Patel NA, Fan KC, Yannuzzi NA, et al. Akreos AO60 intraocular lens opacification after retinal detachment repair. Ophthalmol Retina 2020;4(8):854–6.
[31] Maggi R, Maggi C. Sutureless scleral fixation of intraocular lenses. J Cataract Refract Surg 1997;23(9):1289–94.
[32] Scharioth GB, Pavlidis MM. Sutureless intrascleral posterior chamber intraocular lens fixation. J Cataract Refract Surg 2007;33:1851–4.
[33] Scharioth GB, Prasad S, Georgalas I, et al. Intermediate results of sutureless intrascleral posterior chamber intraocular lens fixation. J Cataract Refract Surg 2010;36:254–9.
[34] Agarwal A, Kumar DA, Jacob S, et al. Fibrin glue-assisted sutureless posterior chamber intraocular lens implantation in eyes with deficient posterior capsules. J Cataract Refract Surg 2008;34:1433–8.
[35] Kumar DA, Agarwal A. Glued intraocular lens: a major review on surgical technique and results. Curr Opin Ophthalmol 2013;24:21–9.
[36] Kumar DA, Agarwal A, Dhawan A, et al. Glued intraocular lens in eyes with deficient capsules: retrospective analysis of long-term effects. J Cataract Refract Surg 2021;47: 496–503.

[37] McKee Y, Price FW, Feng MT, et al. Implementation of the posterior chamber intraocular lens intrascleral haptic fixation technique (glued intraocular lens) in a United States practice: outcomes and insights. J Cataract Refract Surg 2014;40:2099–105.
[38] Yamane S, Inoue M, Arakawa A, et al. Sutureless 27-gauge needle-guided intrascleral intraocular lens implantation with lamellar scleral dissection. Ophthalmology 2014;121(1): 61–6.
[39] Yamane S, Sato S, Maruyama-Inoue M, et al. Flanged intrascleral intraocular lens fixation with double-needle technique. Ophthalmology 2017;124:1136–42.
[40] Ma KK, Yuan A, Sharifi S, et al. A biomechanical study of flanged intrascleral haptic fixation of three-piece intraocular lenses. Am J Ophthalmol 2021;227:45–52.
[41] Hoffman RS, Fine IH, Packer M. Scleral fixation without conjunctival dissection. J Cataract Refract Surg 2006;32(11):1907–12.
[42] Budoff G, Miller CG, Halperin SJ, et al. One-year outcomes of a novel technique for rescuing and scleral fixating a posterior dislocated intraocular lens–bag complex without conjunctival opening (Hoffman pockets). Retina 2016;36(10):1935–40.
[43] Haszcz D, Nowomiejska K, Oleszczuk A, et al. Visual outcomes of posterior chamber intraocular lens intrascleral fixation in the setting of postoperative and posttraumatic aphakia. BMC Ophthalmol 2016;16(1):1–6.
[44] Szurman P, Petermeier K, Aisenbrey S, et al. Z-suture: a new knotless technique for transscleral suture fixation of intraocular implants. Br J Ophthalmol 2010;94(2):167–9.
[45] Dimopoulos S, Dimopoulos V, Blumenstock G, et al. Long-term outcome of scleral-fixated posterior chamber intraocular lens implantation with the knotless Z-suture technique. J Cataract Refract Surg 2018;44(2):182–5.
[46] Yamane S, Maruyama-Inoue M, Kadonosono K. Needle stabilizer for flanged intraocular lens fixation. Retina 2019;39:801.
[47] Gelman RA, Garg S. Novel Yamane technique modification for haptic exposure after glued intrascleral haptic fixation. Am J Ophthalmol Case Rep 2019;14:101–4.
[48] Canabrava S, Canedo Domingos Lima AC, Ribeiro G. Four-flanged intrascleral intraocular lens fixation technique: no flaps, no knots, no glue. Cornea 2020;39:527–8.
[49] Cervantes LJ. Combined double-needle flanged-haptic intrascleral fixation of an intraocular lens and Descemet-stripping endothelial keratoplasty. J Cataract Refract Surg 2017;43: 593–6.
[50] Najafi M, Yamane S, Johnston RH. Modified flanged intrascleral fixation of intraocular lens for vitreoretinal surgeons. Ophthalmic Surg Lasers Imaging Retina 2020;51(2):125–7.
[51] Epley KD, Shainberg MJ, Leuder GT, et al. Pediatric secondary lens implantation in the absence of capsular support. J AAPOS 2001;5(5):301–6.
[52] Sternfeld M, Basith SST, Kurup SP, et al. Secondary intraocular lens implantation using the flanged intrascleral fixation technique in pediatric aphakia: case series and review of literature. J AAPOS 2020;24(5):286.e1–6.
[53] Kumar DA, Agarwal A, Prakash D, et al. Glued intrascleral fixation of posterior chamber intraocular lens in children. Am J Ophthalmol 2012;153(4):594–601.
[54] Kannan NB, Kohli P, Pangtey BPS, et al. Evaluation of sutureless, glueless, flapless, intrascleral fixated posterior chamber intraocular lens in children with ectopia lentis. J Ophthalmol 2018;2018:1–6.
[55] Shen JF, Deng S, Hammersmith KM, et al. Intraocular lens implantation in the absence of zonular support: an outcomes and safety update: a report by the American Academy of Ophthalmology. Ophthalmology 2020;127(9):1234–58.

# Oculoplastics

Advances in Ophthalmology and Optometry 7 (2022) 383–400

ADVANCES IN OPHTHALMOLOGY AND OPTOMETRY

# Teprotumumab

## A Major Advance in the Treatment of Thyroid Eye Disease Management

Caroline Y. Yu, MD, Jamie A. Keen, MD, Erin M. Shriver, MD*

Department of Ophthalmology and Visual Sciences, University of Iowa, 200 Hawkins Drive, Iowa City, IA 52242, USA

**Keywords**

• Thyroid eye disease • Graves' ophthalmopathy • Teprotumumab
• Orbital inflammation • Dysthyroid optic neuropathy • Strabismus • Oculoplastics

**Key points**

- Thyroid eye disease can lead to permanent visual impairment as well as several other debilitating ocular and orbital conditions with significant morbidity.
- Teprotumumab is a recent FDA-approved treatment for thyroid eye disease that can improve proptosis, diplopia, and quality of life.
- Before initiating teprotumumab, it is important to counsel patients on the associated side effects and perform regular screening examinations to monitor for changes during treatment.

## INTRODUCTION

Thyroid eye disease (TED), also known as Graves' ophthalmopathy, is a chronic inflammatory disease that can cause permanent disfigurement and visual disability. It is relatively uncommon in the general population, with studies estimating an overall prevalence of 155/100,000 population to 250/100,000 population [1,2]. Among patients with Graves' disease, the incidence of TED becomes as high as 25% to 40%, with women being affected nearly 3 to 5 times more frequently than men [3,4]. Manifestations of TED within the ocular adnexa and orbit include eyelid retraction, proptosis, extraocular muscle dysfunction, and periorbital edema. TED patients also can suffer from exposure keratopathy and dysthyroid optic neuropathy (DON), which both can

*Corresponding author. *E-mail address:* erin-shriver@uiowa.edu

https://doi.org/10.1016/j.yaoo.2022.03.008

lead to permanently decreased visual acuity. Studies have shown that patients with TED are more likely to report difficulty with activities of daily living such as driving and reading, experience emotional distress, and have an increased risk of suicide [5–7].

Early studies on the natural history of TED suggest that it follows a biphasic pattern, classically titled "Rundle's curve." The initial active state is thought to last 1 to 3 years before transitioning to a more static, fibrotic state [8]. Traditionally, most medical treatments were targeted at the active phase of TED as this phase was thought to have the most inflammatory activity. The severity of disease varies greatly between patients, with only about 5% to 6% of TED patients having moderate to severe disease [9]. Vision loss due to DON and exposure keratopathy occurs in about 3% to 7% of TED patients [10–12]. Because of the variability in disease presentation, it is helpful to grade TED activity and symptom severity to guide treatment. Rubrics for assessing TED activity and severity include the Clinical Activity Score (CAS) [13]; N-no signs of symptoms, O-only signs no symptoms, S-soft tissue involvement, P-proptosis, E-extraocular muscle involvement, C-corneal involvement, S-sight loss (NO-SPECS) [14]; the vision, inflammation, strabismus, and appearance (VISA) system [15]; and the European Group of Graves' Orbitopathy (EUGOGO) classification [16].

Based on disease activity and severity, patients may be treated with conservative localized therapies aimed at mild symptom management or treatment may escalate to systemic corticosteroid therapy, orbital radiation (ORT), immunomodulatory agents, or surgery [17]. For mild, active TED, conservative management typically includes artificial tears, collaboration with the endocrinologist to maintain a euthyroid status, encouragement of smoking cessation, and consideration of selenium supplementation [18,19]. One long-standing treatment option for active TED is ORT, which can be used alone or in conjunction with corticosteroids [20] and has been shown to have variable results [21–24]. Other frequent treatment options for active TED patients are oral or intravenous corticosteroid therapy, but these have been shown to have little to no impact on long-term strabismus and proptosis outcomes and can be associated with significant side effects [25–27]. The use of immunomodulatory agents including rituximab and tocilizumab has been studied in TED and have shown limited success in improving diplopia and proptosis in patients being treated with these medications, and the risk of severe adverse effects such as infections and neutropenia exists [28,29]. Finally, surgical options such as decompression, strabismus surgery, and eyelid procedures are available but generally reserved for patients that are clinically stable. The one exception to this is in patients with DON, who may require surgical treatment to save their vision even if they are not clinically stable. Not only are there significant cost, morbidity, and a degree of unpredictability associated with surgical treatment but also a significant delay can occur before patients are stable enough to undergo surgical treatment [30–33].

In January 2020, teprotumumab (Horizon Therapeutics, Dublin, Ireland) became the first Food and Drug Administration-approved treatment for TED. Teprotumumab is a human monoclonal antibody that binds to insulin-like growth factor 1 receptor (IGF-1R) delivered via a series of intravenous infusions. The initial phase II and III randomized controlled trials showed promising results in terms of proptosis, diplopia, CAS, and quality of life as well as a relatively favorable side effect profile [34,35]. Since its approval, many publications have expounded on the role of teprotumumab in various clinical settings, as well as its safety profile and clinical effect. Teprotumumab expands treatment options for TED patients and has the potential to change the course of the disease. Therefore, it is important for clinicians to familiarize themselves with the pathophysiology, safety profile, and clinical efficacy of teprotumumab in TED.

## PATHOPHYSIOLOGY OF THYROID EYE DISEASE: THE ROLE OF INSULIN-LIKE GROWTH FACTOR 1 RECEPTOR

While the pathophysiology of TED is not yet completely understood, it is thought that TED is an autoimmune orbital inflammatory condition associated with abnormal orbital fibroblast activity that leads to the characteristic soft-tissue remodeling seen in the disease [36,37]. It is unclear what initially triggers the loss of immune tolerance, but autoimmunity against the thyrotropin receptor (TSHR) and overexpression of IGF-1R are hypothesized to play a central role [38–40]. Studies have shown that patients with TED have a higher expression of IGF-1R in their T cell, orbital fat, extraocular muscle, and fibroblast cell populations than healthy controls [39,40]. Evidence shows a shared pathway between TSHR and IGF-1R, specifically that IGF-1R may play a role in potentiating the effect of TSHR and can lead to a more robust stimulation of hyaluronan secretion [41–43]. IGF-1R also may be elevated in chronic, clinically inactive TED compared with controls [44].

## TREATMENT LANDSCAPE FOR THYROID EYE DISEASE—ANTI-INFLAMMATORY THERAPIES

Before the development of teprotumumab, no targeted treatments specifically for TED existed, and the available treatment options primarily aimed at decreasing the inflammation and mitigating patient symptoms.

For mild, active, treatment-naive TED, selenium supplementation was demonstrated to decrease eyelid retraction and improve CAS [13] by 1.9 points at 6 months and 2.2 points at 12 months in one European trial [19]. Selenium is found in a high concentration in the thyroid gland in control populations, has antioxidant properties when incorporated into selenoprotein, and has been shown to reduce thyroid peroxidase-antibody (TPO) titers [45,46]. However, unlike in Europe, selenium deficiency is uncommon in the United States [47], and no published data are available for its efficacy in non–selenium-deficient populations.

For moderate to severe active TED, corticosteroids have been a first-line option and can be administered orally, intravenously, and locally. Not only has it been shown to be effective in the setting of DON but it also decreases the risk of TED exacerbation following radioactive iodine therapy [48]. Corticosteroids can improve soft-tissue changes including eyelid retraction [49] and subjective diplopia [50], but multiple studies have shown that there is no significant effect on proptosis [26,51,52]. The optimal route of delivery is debated, with some data showing higher efficacy of intravenous corticosteroids than oral steroids in terms of optic neuropathy and CAS [50,51,53]. The dosing schedule also varies, with the 2021 EUGOGO guidelines recommending up to a cumulative dose of 4.5 g as well as possibly using mycophenolate in conjunction with corticosteroids to improve treatment response rates [18,51]. However, corticosteroids have some important limitations. Even with intravenous corticosteroids, the positive response rate is only around 60% to 70% [51,54,55], and recurrence of active disease is common with both tapering and cessation of corticosteroid therapy [56]. Additionally, both oral and intravenous corticosteroids are associated with several serious and potentially life-threatening systemic side effects such as hepatotoxicity, hypertension, mood disruption, and diabetes [57].

ORT is another option, often used as an adjunctive therapy to corticosteroids. When used as a monotherapy, ORT may improve diplopia, eyelid retraction, and soft-tissue changes, as well as decrease the need for surgical intervention [20,23,58]. When used in conjunction with corticosteroids, a greater decrease occurs in mean ophthalmopathy index value, which is a numerical score based on NOSPECS [59], and a decrease in the cumulative dose of steroids needed [60]. However, studies have found that there is no significant improvement in rectus muscle hypertrophy or proptosis with radiation [23,61,62].

More recently, biological therapies have been used to treat TED patients with mixed results. These include tocilizumab, rituximab, adalimumab, and infliximab. Published data for the efficacy of these treatments are limited at this time, with tocilizumab, an interleukin-6 (IL-6) inhibitor, and rituximab, a CD20 inhibitor, being the best studied. Tocilizumab, is an anti-IL-6 receptor monoclonal antibody and has been shown in one study to be effective in treating patients with steroid-resistant TED. Specifically, the study found that 86.7% of the treatment group experienced at least a 2-point improvement in CAS score. On the other hand, no significant difference occurred in proptosis between placebo and control by week 40 of treatment [29]. There also have been several case reports in the United States that described improvements in CAS in patients treated with tocilizumab [63,64].

Rituximab is another biological therapy that has been investigated in TED patients. The antibody targets the CD20 antigen, causing depletion of B lymphocytes. To date, less than 50 TED patients have been reported to have received rituximab for TED, and these reports have shown variable results [65–67]. Of the 2 randomized studies published, one report found no additional benefit of rituximab treatment compared with placebo [66], while another study found lower CAS scores in the rituximab group at 16, 20, and 24 weeks compared with methylprednisolone [65]. Salvi and colleagues additionally reported that all patients who received rituximab had at least some improvement in their CAS score by 24 weeks, exhibited improved extraocular motility by 52 weeks, and did not display evidence of disease reactivation by 52 weeks [65].

Adalimumab, a tumor necrosis factor-α (TNF- α) antagonist, was studied in one prospective nonrandomized trial and showed mixed results with a statistically significant improvement in inflammatory score in patients with a higher baseline inflammatory index only [68]. Finally, infliximab, another TNF-α inhibitor, has been reported in one case report to successfully treat a patient with TED [69]. While these treatments do show promise as alternative options for the traditional treatment modalities for TED, limited data exist on the efficacy of these medications. They also are associated with a high cost and significant side effect profile including drug-induced lupus, transaminitis, and infections.

## TEPROTUMUMAB: MECHANISM OF ACTION

Teprotumumab is a human monoclonal antibody with high affinity and specificity for the extracellular cysteine-rich alpha-subunit domain of IGF-1R. It was initially studied in solid tumors and sarcomas, with a phase I clinical trial showing a mild side effect profile [70]. Based on data showing the pivotal role of IGF-1R in the pathophysiology of TED, a multicenter phase II clinical trial was conducted studying its use in TED in 2013 [34]. Teprotumumab's pharmacokinetic profile includes a relatively long half-life of 19.9 days, slow clearance via the reticuloendothelial system, and limited volume of distribution [71]. In the randomized clinical trials, an initial dose of 10 mg/kg followed by 7 doses of 20 mg/kg every 3 weeks was administered [34,35]. Although there have not been clinical studies to establish optimal dosing for teprotumumab to date, this dosing regimen was chosen to maintain teprotumumab through concentrations above 20 μg/mL, a concentration that theoretically achieves more than 90% IGF-1R saturation [72].

## SAFETY PROFILE OF TEPROTUMUMAB

Teprotumumab is associated with a relatively mild side effect profile, but there are some important risks to discuss with patients. It has not been studied in pregnant patients, so pregnancy is considered an absolute contraindication to treatment, and contraception is required for men and women if applicable during treatment and up to 6 months after treatment. The most common side effects include risk of exacerbation or initiation of inflammatory bowel disease (IBD), hearing-related impairment, hyperglycemia, nausea, alopecia, fatigue, and muscle spasms [34,35]. Several cases of IBD associated with teprotumumab treatment have been reported in the literature, thus it generally is considered a contraindication to treatment [34,73,74]. The Treatment of Graves'

Orbitopathy (Thyroid Eye Disease) to Reduce Proptosis with Teprotumumab Infusions in a Randomized, Placebo-Controlled, Clinical Study (OPTIC) phase III trial excluded patients with a preexisting history of IBD [35], so limited data exist on this patient subpopulation. One publication showed development of ulcerative colitis after initiation of teprotumumab in a patient without any prior history of IBD, but this patient had a family history of IBD [73]. Therefore, before initiation of teprotumumab, a thorough personal and family history of autoimmune disease should be obtained, and patients should be counseled to seek care if they develop new gastrointestinal symptoms.

Another important side effect that patients should be educated about is potential hearing-related impairment. Between 10% and 46% of TED patients receiving teprotumumab have been reported to experience subjective hearing symptoms including hypoacusis, autophony, and tinnitus, and cases of teprotumumab-associated audiology testing changes have been reported [74–77]. IGF-1R is known to play an important role in inner ear regulation [78,79], and current studies suggest that teprotumumab may potentiate sensorineural hearing loss in patients with underlying hearing impairment [75–77]. At this time, it is recommended that patients receive a baseline audiology screening to evaluate for possible underlying hearing impairment and to monitor patients closely for hearing changes [75–77,79].

In addition, patients should be counseled on the risk of hyperglycemia. Because IGF-1R and the insulin receptor are structurally similar, IGF-1R inhibitors are known to be associated with hyperglycemia [80]. In the phase II study, 12% of teprotumumab patients developed hyperglycemia [34]. Of these patients, the hyperglycemia was grade 1 (<160 mg/dL fasting glucose) in those without a history of diabetes and grade 2 to 3 in those with a history of diabetes (grade 2: >160–250 mg/dL fasting glucose, grade 3: >250–500 mg/dL fasting glucose) [34]. When hyperglycemia occurred, it was well controlled with medication adjustment in all patients [34]. No universal guideline exists, but some recommend checking a baseline hemoglobin A1C (HbA1C) within 1 month of teprotumumab initiation, close management and titration of diabetes therapy as needed for patients with a known history of diabetes, and frequent fasting glucose testing for patients with a history of glucose intolerance or no known history of diabetes [81].

Finally, other rare adverse events that have been reported are encephalopathy [82] and intracerebral hemorrhage [83], but whether there is a causal relationship to teprotumumab is unclear.

## CLINICAL EFFECT OF TEPROTUMUMAB

Although teprotumumab is still a relatively new therapeutic option for TED patients, initial studies have shown promising results in terms of CAS, proptosis, and diplopia.

The initial phase II and III multicenter, randomized, double-masked clinical trials showed a statistically significant response rate compared with placebo in CAS, proptosis reduction in the more proptotic eye by $\geq$2 mm, Gorman diplopia score, and Graves' ophthalmopathy-specific quality-of-life questionnaire 24 weeks after treatment [34,35]. Interestingly, in the pooled data from the 2 trials, 71.4% of teprotumumab-treated patients achieved a clinically significant proptosis response (defined as ≥2 mm), which was apparent as early as week 6 after teprotumumab initiation and was maintained up to 28 weeks after treatment initiation [35,36,84]. Orbital volumetric analysis of a subgroup of patients showed a reduction in extraocular muscle and orbital fat volume by 33% and 29% on average, suggesting that teprotumumab may be able to reverse the changes that lead to proptosis in TED [85]. Furthermore, extraocular muscle diameter as measured by orbital echography in a separate case series demonstrated an average of 14.6% reduction in total extraocular muscle diameter [86].

Longer-term, follow-up data were published in the OPTIC-X study, which showed that 56% of patients maintained their proptosis response by week 72 after treatment initiation and that 40% of the nonresponders did experience a clinically significant proptosis response following an additional 8 teprotumumab infusions [83]. While the patients enrolled in the initial trials were predominantly Caucasian, subgroup analysis from pooled data from both trials showed no significant difference in proptosis or diplopia response rate based on patient gender, age, tobacco use status, time to diagnosis of Graves' disease, baseline CAS, and TSH-binding inhibitor immunoglobulin (TBII) with the exception of decreased diplopia response in tobacco users and those with a TBII less than 10 IU/L at baseline [87].

Two TED patients treated with teprotumumab are depicted in Figs. 1 and 2.

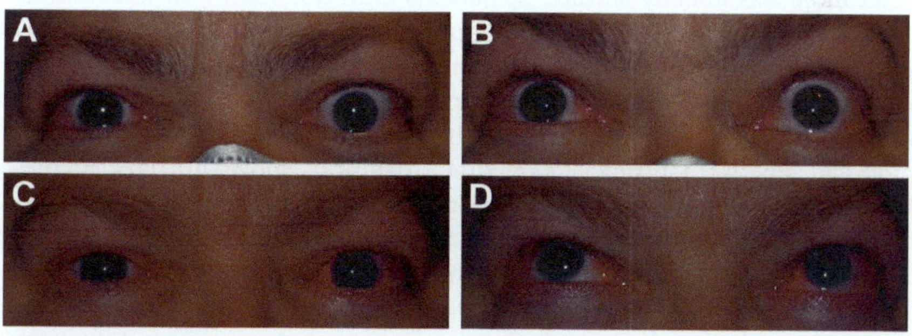


**Fig. 1.** A 55-year-old woman with a history of choroidal melanoma of the right eye treated with plaque brachytherapy and a 10-month history of thyroid eye disease treated with teprotumumab. External photographs in (*A*) primary gaze and (*B*) upgaze before teprotumumab initiation demonstrated bilateral proptosis, upper and lower eyelid retraction, restricted upgaze, and a Clinical Activity Score (CAS) of 6. External photographs in (*C*) primary gaze and (*D*) upgaze 4 weeks after completion of 8 doses of teprotumumab demonstrated improvement in proptosis (right eye 4 mm, left eye 3 mm), decreased bilateral eyelid retraction, improved extraocular motility, and a CAS of 5 (increased from 3 mid treatment because of the onset of scleritis in the left eye).

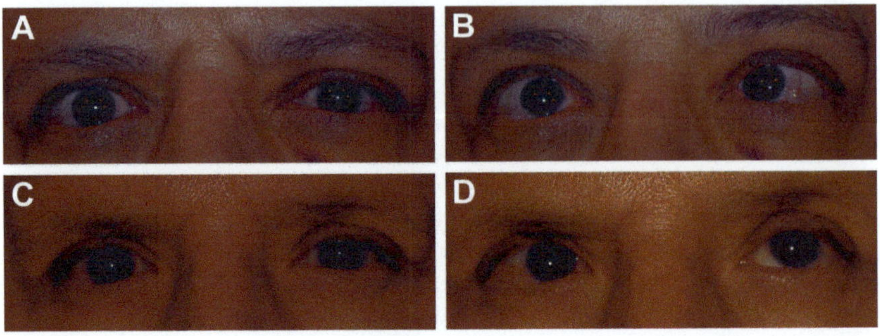

**Fig. 2.** A 59-year-old man with a history of dysthyroid optic neuropathy status after bilateral medial orbital wall and floor decompression 5 months before teprotumumab treatment. External photographs in (*A*) primary and (*B*) upgaze before teprotumumab initiation showed bilateral proptosis, upper and lower eyelid retraction, restricted upgaze, and a Clinical Activity Score (CAS) of 6. External photographs in (*C*) primary gaze and (*D*) upgaze immediately after completion of 8 doses of teprotumumab demonstrated improved proptosis (right eye 4.5 mm, left eye 6 mm), improved extraocular motility, and a CAS reduced to 0.

## CLINICAL APPLICATIONS OF TEPROTUMUMAB: FUTURE AVENUES

Currently teprotumumab is the only FDA-approved treatment for TED with promising initial data not only in patients with acute, active TED but also in those with other stages of TED. To date, several hundred cases of TED treated with teprotumumab have been reported in the literature, including for the treatment of DON [88–94] and chronic TED [83,95–98] (Table 1). Although the medication was initially studied in patients with less than 9 months duration and a CAS of 4 or greater [34,35], teprotumumab may be beneficial in patients with DON and chronic (active and inactive) TED. Several case series have demonstrated improvement in best-corrected visual acuity, afferent pupillary defect, and color vision in patients with DON following treatment with teprotumumab [88–94]. Chronic TED, which has been shown to have increased IGF-1R expression even in inactive patients, also may respond to teprotumumab treatment. Several case series have demonstrated a decrease in proptosis, CAS, and lid retraction following teprotumumab treatment in chronic active and inactive TED [83,95–101]. While initial data on teprotumumab are promising with evidence of reversal of orbital changes, longer term follow-up is needed to ascertain whether teprotumumab treatment can decrease the need for future surgical management and if the clinical improvement can be sustained over the long term. Further studies directly comparing the efficacy of teprotumumab to that of other treatments such as corticosteroids and other immunomodulatory agents are needed to determine the best treatment algorithm for patients with TED.

From a socioeconomic standpoint, it is important to note that the medication can be costly to the patient. Currently, teprotumumab is estimated to cost

**Table 1**
Summary of publications regarding patients treated with teprotumumab

| Study | Study type | Population | n | Outcome timepoint | Mean Δ proptosis (mm) | Mean Δ in clinical activity score (CAS) | Diplopia response[b] |
|---|---|---|---|---|---|---|---|
| Smith et al, [34] 2017 | Phase II randomized double masked, placebo-controlled multicentre trial | Acute (duration <9 mo), CAS >4 | 42 | 24 wk | −2.46 ± 0.20 | −3.43 (SD 0.18) | 68% Diplopia response vs 20% in placebo group |
| Douglas et al, [35] 2020 | Phase III randomized double masked, placebo-controlled multicentre trial | Acute (duration <9 mo), CAS >4 | 41 | 24 wk | −2.79 (95% CI: −3.40, 2.17) | CAS response rate (58.5%)[a] | 68% Diplopia response vs 29% in placebo group |
| Douglas et al, OPTIC-X [83], 2021 | Randomized, Placebo controlled clinical extension study | Placebo treated from phase III trial | 37 | 24 wk | −3.5 ± 1.7 | CAS response rate (65.6%)[a] | 60.9% Diplopia response |

(*continued on next page*)

**Table 1**
**(*continued*)**

| Study | Study type | Population | n | Outcome timepoint | Mean Δ proptosis (mm) | Mean Δ in clinical activity score (CAS) | Diplopia response[b] |
|---|---|---|---|---|---|---|---|
| Douglas et al, OPTIC-X [83], 2021 | Randomized, placebo controlled clinical extension study | Nonresponders or clinical flare from phase III trial | Nonresponders (3), flare (9) | 24 wk | Nonresponders: $-1.5 \pm 0.9$<br>Flare: $-1.9 \pm 1.2$ | N/A | Nonresponders: N/A<br>Flare: 3/3 with complete diplopia resolution |
| Ugradar et al, [97] 2021 | Retrospective review | Chronic (>2 y) with CAS $\leq 3$ | 31 | After 3 or more infusions | −3.5 (SD 0.40) and −3.0 (SD 0.30) | −1.8 (SD 1) | 67% Diplopia response rate |
| Ozzello et al, [96] 2021 | Retrospective review | Chronic with CAS $\leq 1$ | 9 | After 8 infusions | $-4.0 \pm 2.4$ | N/A | N/A |
| Diniz et al, [94] 2021 | Cross-sectional cohort study | Heterogeneous | 21 | Varying treatment timepoints ($5.6 \pm 2.0$ infusions) and length of follow-up (30 wk $\pm$ 11 wk) | $-2.5 \pm 1.8$ | $-2.2 \pm 1.4$ | Mean Δ GDS: $-0.75 \pm 1.1$ |
| Sears et al, [90] 2021 | Case series | DON | 10 | 0–33 wk After completion of 8 infusions | $-4.8 \pm 2.7$ | $-5.25 \pm 1.2$ | N/A |

| | | | | | | | |
|---|---|---|---|---|---|---|---|
| Yu et al, [98] 2021 | Case series | Chronic | 6 | After 8th infusions for 5/6 patients. 1/6 Patients after 6th infusion | −3.8 ± 2.1 | −1.5 (SD 3) | No GDS reported. Patient 1 improved in all directions. Patient 2 improved in all directions, except in supraduction |
| Chiou et al, [93] 2021 | Case report | Chronic with DON (11 y and 7 y) | 2 | Following 3rd infusion | Patient 1: −45 OD, −3 OS<br>Patient 2: −3 OD, 4 OS | Patient 1: −6<br>Patient 2: −1 | N/A |
| Ozzello et al, [95] 2020 | Case report | Chronic (≥3 y) | 1 | Following 3rd infusion | −5 OD, −6 OS | −1 | N/A |
| Sears et al, [89] 2021 | Case report | Chronic (17 mo) with DON | 1 | 21 wk | −2 OD, −4 OS | −3 | N/A |
| Slentz et al, [91] 2021 | Case report | Acute (6 mo) with DON | 1 | 25 wk | −5 OD, −5 OS | −5 | No GDS reported. Improved abduction, no change to supraduction and infraduction |

(*continued on next page*)

**Table 1 (*continued*)**

| Study | Study type | Population | n | Outcome timepoint | Mean Δ proptosis (mm) | Mean Δ in clinical activity score (CAS) | Diplopia response[b] |
|---|---|---|---|---|---|---|---|
| Hwang et al, [88] 2021 | Case report | Acute (8 mo) with DON | 1 | Following 8th infusion, except for CAS, which was reported after 4th infusion | −5 OD, −45 OS | −6 | |
| Lopez et al, [92] 2021 | Case report | Acute with DON | 1 | 24 wk | −3 OD, −5 OS | N/A | No GDS reported subjectively improved diplopia with residual 25 prism diopters of comitant esotropia 1 mo after treatment completion |

*Abbreviations:* CAS, clinical activity score; DON, dysthyroid optic neuropathy; GDS, Gorman diplopia score; OD, right eye; OS, left eye

[a]CAS response rate was defined as achieving a CAS of 0 to 1.

[b]Diplopia response was defined as improvement by one or more grades in GDS.

$14,900 per vial, or an estimated total of $342,700 for a 70-kg patient [83]. In addition, there is a cost associated with the infusions and associated testing, as well as the indirect costs incurred from travel to and from the infusion location and time off from work to receive these infusions. However, this should be weighed against the overall typical economic burden of TED, which includes both direct costs, such as surgical treatment and immunosuppressive agents, and indirect costs, such as disability and work impairment. One German study estimated a total cost of between $4662 and $8964 per TED patient per year for both direct health care-related and indirect costs associated with TED [99], while Singh and colleagues found over $135.5 million was spent in the emergency and inpatient setting alone for TED in 2017 in the United States [100].

In addition to teprotumumab, there are ongoing trials for other targeted medications for TED. These include secukinumab, a human monoclonal anti-interleukin-17-A antibody, a medication currently approved for the treatment of psoriatic arthritis, moderate to severe plaque psoriasis, and axial spondyloarthritis (ClinicalTrials.gov Identifier: NCT04737330). Other preclinical studies are examining the possibility of small molecular TSHR antagonists for the treatment of TED, as these may have the additional benefit of targeting IGF-1R-independent signaling pathways in TED as well as treating underlying Graves' disease [101,102].

This review is aimed to summarize the current state of understanding about TED management including teprotumumab. As the first FDA-approved medication for treatment of TED, teprotumumab has shown promising initial findings, especially with regard to reversal of orbital changes. Before initiating teprotumumab, it is important to carefully screen and counsel patients on possible side effects of the medication. At this time, clinical experience with this medication is limited, and additional studies and long-term follow-up data are needed to better understand the full clinical utility of teprotumumab. Future management of TED will likely build on lessons learned from this novel targeted therapy.

## CLINICS CARE POINTS

- Thyroid eye disease (TED) is a disfiguring and potentially vision-threatening orbital inflammatory disease that can drastically reduce patients' quality of life.
- Traditional therapies for TED include glucocorticoids and orbital radiation, which primarily function by addressing the inflammation in the active phase of TED.
- Teprotumumab is a targeted insulin-like growth factor (IGF-1R) antagonist and is the first FDA-approved treatment for TED.
- Randomized controlled trials have showed that teprotumumab is effective at decreasing proptosis, Clinical Activity Score (CAS), and diplopia in patients with acute, active TED. Multiple case series have suggested that teprotumumab also may be effective in patients with dysthyroid optic neuropathy (DON), chronic active TED, and chronic inactive TED, but more studies are needed to

determine which patients are most likely to benefit from teprotumumab, optimal dosage, and duration of treatment, as well as if clinical improvement can be sustained long term.

- Clinicians and patients should be aware about the potential side effects of teprotumumab treatment including initiation or exacerbation of inflammatory bowel disease, hearing-related impairment, hyperglycemia, nausea, alopecia, fatigue, and muscle spasms. It has not been studied in pregnant patients, so pregnancy is considered an absolute contraindication to treatment, and contraception is required for men and women if applicable during treatment and up to 6 months after treatment.

## DISCLOSURE

E.M. Shriver is a consultant/advisor for Horizon Therapeutics. The other authors have no financial or other conflicts of interests to disclose.

## References

[1] Abraham-Nordling M, Bystrom K, Torring O, et al. Incidence of hyperthyroidism in Sweden. Eur J Endocrinol 2011;165(6):899–905.
[2] Bartley GB. The epidemiologic characteristics and clinical course of ophthalmopathy associated with autoimmune thyroid disease in Olmsted County, Minnesota. Trans Am Ophthalmol Soc 1994;92:477–588.
[3] Chin YH, Ng CH, Lee MH, et al. Prevalence of thyroid eye disease in Graves' disease: A meta-analysis and systematic review. Clin Endocrinol 2020;93(4):363–74.
[4] Bartalena L, Piantanida E, Gallo D, et al. Epidemiology, natural history, risk factors, and prevention of Graves' orbitopathy. Front Endocrinol 2020;11:615993.
[5] Kahaly GJ, Petrak F, Hardt J, et al. Psychosocial morbidity of Graves' orbitopathy. Clin Endocrinol 2005;63(4):395–402.
[6] Park JJ, Sullivan TJ, Mortimer RH, et al. Assessing quality of life in Australian patients with Graves' ophthalmopathy. Br J Ophthalmol 2004;88(1):75–8.
[7] Ferløv-Schwensen C, Brix TH, Hegedüs L. Death by Suicide in Graves' Disease and Graves' Orbitopathy: A Nationwide Danish Register Study. Thyroid 2017;27(12):1475–80.
[8] Rundle FF. Management of exophthalmos and related ocular changes in Graves' disease. Metabolism 1957;6(1):36–48.
[9] Tanda ML, Piantanida E, Liparulo L, et al. Prevalence and natural history of Graves' orbitopathy in a large series of patients with newly diagnosed Graves' hyperthyroidism seen at a single center. J Clin Endocrinol Metab 2013;98:1443–9.
[10] Bahn RS. Graves' ophthalmopathy. N Engl J Med 2010;362(8):726–38.
[11] Barrio-Barrio J, Sabater AL, Bonet-Farriol E, et al. Graves' Ophthalmopathy: VISA versus EUGOGO Classification, Assessment, and Management. J Ophthalmol 2015;2015:249125.
[12] Biondi B, Bartalena L, Cooper DS, et al. The 2015 European Thyroid Association Guidelines on Diagnosis and Treatment of Endogenous Subclinical Hyperthyroidism. Eur Thyroid J 2015;4(3):149–63.
[13] Mourits MP, Prummel MF, Wiersinga WM, et al. Clinical activity score as a guide in the management of patients with Graves' ophthalmopathy. Clin Endocrinol 1997;47(1):9–14.
[14] Werner SC. Modification of the classification of the eye changes of Graves' disease. Am J Ophthalmol 1977;83(5):725–7.
[15] Dolman PJ, Rootman J. VISA classification for Graves orbitopathy. Ophthal Plast Reconstr Surg 2006;22(5):319–24.
[16] Bartalena L, Baldeschi L, Dickinson A, et al. Consensus statement of the European Group on Graves' orbitopathy (EUGOGO) on management of GO. Eur J Endocrinol 2008;158(3):273–85.

[17] Bartley GB, Fatourechi V, Kadrmas EF, et al. The treatment of Graves' ophthalmopathy in an incidence cohort. Am J Ophthalmol 1996;121(2):200–6.
[18] Bartalena L, Kahaly GJ, Baldeschi L, et al. The 2021 European Group on Graves' orbitopathy (EUGOGO) clinical practice guidelines for the medical management of Graves' orbitopathy. Eur J Endocrinol 2021;185(4):G43–67.
[19] Marcocci C, Kahaly GJ, Krassas GE, et al. Selenium and the course of mild Graves' orbitopathy. N Engl J Med 2011;364(20):1920–31.
[20] Bradley EA, Gower EW, Bradley DJ, et al. Orbital radiation for graves ophthalmopathy: a report by the American Academy of Ophthalmology. Ophthalmology 2008;115(2):398–409.
[21] Rajendram R, Bunce C, Lee RWJ, et al. Orbital radiotherapy for adult thyroid eye disease. Cochrane Database Syst Rev 2012;7:CD007114.
[22] Shams PN, Ma R, Pickles T, et al. Reduced risk of compressive optic neuropathy using orbital radiotherapy in patients with active thyroid eye disease. Am J Ophthalmol 2014;157(6):1299–305.
[23] Kazim M, Trokel S, Moore S. Treatment of acute Graves orbitopathy. Ophthalmology 1991;98(9):1443–8.
[24] Wakelkamp IM, Tan H, Saeed P, et al. Orbital irradiation for Graves' ophthalmopathy: Is it safe? A long-term follow-up study. Ophthalmology 2004;111(8):1557–62.
[25] Zang S, Ponto KA, Kahaly GJ. Clinical review: intravenous glucocorticoids for Graves' orbitopathy: efficacy and morbidity. J Clin Endocrinol Metab 2011;96(2):320–32.
[26] Tu X, Dong Y, Zhang H, et al. Corticosteroids for Graves' ophthalmopathy: systematic review and meta-analysis. Biomed Res Int 2018;2018:4845894.
[27] van Geest RJ, Sasim IV, Koppeschaar HP, et al. Methylprednisolone pulse therapy for patients with moderately severe Graves' orbitopathy: a prospective, randomized, placebo-controlled study. Eur J Endocrinol 2008;158(2):229–37.
[28] Stan MN, Garrity JA, Carranza Leon BG, et al. Randomized controlled trial of rituximab in patients with Graves' orbitopathy. J Clin Endocrinol Metab 2015;100(2):432–41.
[29] Perez-Moreiras JV, Gomez-Reino JJ, Maneiro JR, et al. Efficacy of tocilizumab in patients with moderate-to-severe corticosteroid-resistant graves orbitopathy: a randomized clinical trial. Am J Ophthalmol 2018;195:181–90.
[30] Borumandi F, Hammer B, Kamer L, et al. How predictable is exophthalmos reduction in Graves' orbitopathy? A review of the literature. Br J Ophthalmol 2011;95(12):1625–30.
[31] Jefferis JM, Jones RK, Currie ZI, et al. Orbital decompression for thyroid eye disease: methods, outcomes, and complications. Eye 2018;32(3):626–36.
[32] Ben Simon GJ, Wang LL, McCann JD, et al. Primary-gaze diplopia in patients with thyroid-related orbitopathy undergoing deep lateral orbital decompression with intraconal fat debulking: A retrospective analysis of treatment outcome. Thyroid 2004;14:379–83.
[33] Barker L, Mackenzie K, Adams GG, et al. Long-term surgical outcomes for vertical deviations in thyroid eye disease. Strabismus 2017;25(2):67–72.
[34] Smith TJ, Kahaly GJ, Ezra DG, et al. Teprotumumab for thyroid-associated ophthalmopathy. N Engl J Med 2017;376(18):1748–61.
[35] Douglas RS, Kahaly GJ, Patel A, et al. Teprotumumab for the treatment of active thyroid eye disease. N Engl J Med 2020;382(4):341–52.
[36] Shan SJ, Douglas RS. The pathophysiology of thyroid eye disease. J Neuroophthalmol 2014;34(2):177–85.
[37] Khong JJ, McNab AA, Ebeling PR, et al. Pathogenesis of thyroid eye disease: review and update on molecular mechanisms. Br J Ophthalmol 2016;100(1):142–50.
[38] Bahn RS, Dutton CM, Natt N, et al. Thyrotropin receptor expression in Graves' orbital adipose/connective tissues: potential autoantigen in Graves' ophthalmopathy. J Clin Endocrinol Metab 1998;83:998–1002.
[39] Smith TJ, Hegedüs L, Douglas RS. Role of insulin-like growth factor-1 (IGF-1) pathway in the pathogenesis of Graves' orbitopathy. Best Pract Res Clin Endocrinol Metab 2012;26(3):291–302.

[40] Janssen JAMJL, Smith TJ. Lessons learned from targeting IGF-I receptor in thyroid-associated ophthalmopathy. Cells 2021;10(2):383.
[41] Tsui S, Naik V, Hoa N, et al. Evidence for an association between thyroid-stimulating hormone and insulin-like growth factor 1 receptors: a tale of two antigens implicated in Graves' disease. J Immunol 2008;181(6):4397–405.
[42] Krieger CC, Place RF, Bevilacqua C, et al. TSH/IGF-1 Receptor Cross Talk in Graves' ophthalmopathy pathogenesis. J Clin Endocrinol Metab 2016;101(6):2340–7.
[43] Krieger CC, Neumann S, Gershengorn MC. TSH/IGF1 receptor crosstalk: mechanism and clinical implications. Pharmacol Ther 2020;209:107502.
[44] Ugradar S, Shi L, Wang Y, et al. Teprotumumab for non-inflammatory thyroid eye disease (TED): evidence for increased IGF-1R expression. Eye 2021;35(9):2607–12.
[45] Ventura M, Melo M, Carrilho F. Selenium and thyroid disease: from pathophysiology to treatment. Int J Endocrinol 2017;2017:1297658.
[46] Hu Y, Feng W, Chen H, et al. Effect of selenium on thyroid autoimmunity and regulatory T cells in patients with Hashimoto's thyroiditis: a prospective randomized-controlled trial. Clin Transl Sci 2021;14(4):1390–402.
[47] Sadaka A, Nguyen K, Malik A, et al. Vitamin D and selenium in a thyroid eye disease population in Texas. Neuroophthalmology 2019;43(5):291–4.
[48] Acharya SH, Avenell A, Philip S, et al. Radioiodine therapy (RAI) for Graves' disease (GD) and the effect on ophthalmopathy: a systematic review. Clin Endocrinol 2008;69(6):943–50.
[49] Lee SJ, Rim TH, Jang SY, et al. Treatment of upper eyelid retraction related to thyroid-associated ophthalmopathy using subconjunctival triamcinolone injections. Graefes Arch Clin Exp Ophthalmol 2013;251(1):261–70.
[50] Currò N, Covelli D, Vannucchi G, et al. Therapeutic outcomes of high-dose intravenous steroids in the treatment of dysthyroid optic neuropathy. Thyroid 2014;24(5):897–905.
[51] Marcocci C, Bartalena L, Tanda ML, et al. Comparison of the effectiveness and tolerability of intravenous or oral glucocorticoids associated with orbital radiotherapy in the management of severe Graves' ophthalmopathy: results of a prospective, single-blind, randomized study. J Clin Endocrinol Metab 2001;86(8):3562–7.
[52] Kahaly GJ, Pitz S, Hommel G, et al. Randomized, single blind trial of intravenous versus oral steroid monotherapy in Graves' orbitopathy. J Clin Endocrinol Metab 2005;90(9):5234–40.
[53] Bartalena L, Pinchera A, Marcocci C. Management of Graves' ophthalmopathy: reality and perspectives. Endocr Rev 2000;21(2):168–99.
[54] Sisti E, Menconi F, Leo M, et al. Long-term outcome of Graves' orbitopathy following high-dose intravenous glucocorticoids and orbital radiotherapy. J Endocrinol Invest 2015;38(6):661–8.
[55] Bartalena L, Marcocci C, Pinchera A. Treating severe Graves' ophthalmopathy. Baillieres Clin Endocrinol Metab 1997;11(3):521–36.
[56] Marino M. Acute and severe liver damage associated with intravenous glucocorticoid pulse therapy in patients with Graves' ophthalmopathy. Thyroid 2004;14(5):403–6.
[57] Bartalena L, Krassas GE, Wiersinga W, et al. Efficacy and safety of three different cumulative doses of intravenous methylprednisolone for moderate to severe and active Graves' orbitopathy. J Clin Endocrinol Metab 2012;97(12):4454–63.
[58] Mourits MP, van Kempen-Harteveld ML, García MB, et al. Radiotherapy for Graves' orbitopathy: randomised placebo-controlled study. Lancet 2000;355(9214):1505–9.
[59] Marcocci C, Bartalena L, Bogazzi F, et al. Role of orbital radiotherapy in the treatment of Graves' ophthalmopathy. Exp Clin Endocrinol 1991;97(2–3):332–7.
[60] Limone PP, Bianco L, Mellano M, et al. Is concomitant treatment with steroids and radiotherapy more favorable than sequential treatment in moderate-to-severe graves orbitopathy? Radiol Med 2021;126(2):334–42.

[61] Ohtsuka K, Sato A, Kawaguchi S, et al. Effect of steroid pulse therapy with and without orbital radiotherapy on Graves' ophthalmopathy. Am J Ophthalmol 2003;135(3): 285–90.
[62] Gorman CA, Garrity JA, Fatourechi V, et al. A prospective, randomized, double-blind, placebo-controlled study of orbital radiotherapy for Graves' ophthalmopathy. Ophthalmology 2001;108(9):1523–34.
[63] Russell DJ, Wagner LH, Seiff SR. Tocilizumab as a steroid sparing agent for the treatment of Graves' orbitopathy. Am J Ophthalmol Case Rep 2017;7:146–8.
[64] Copperman T, Idowu OO, Kersten RC, et al. Subcutaneous tocilizumab for thyroid eye disease: simplified dosing and delivery. Ophthalmic Plast Reconstr Surg 2019;35(3):e64–6.
[65] Salvi M, Vannucchi G, Currò N, et al. Efficacy of B-cell targeted therapy with rituximab in patients with active moderate to severe Graves' orbitopathy: a randomized controlled study. J Clin Endocrinol Metab 2015;100(2):422–31.
[66] Stan MN, Garrity JA, Carranza Leon BG, et al. Randomized controlled trial of rituximab in patients with Graves' orbitopathy. J Clin Endocrinol Metab 2015;100(2):432–41.
[67] Vannucchi G, Campi I, Covelli D, et al. Efficacy profile and safety of very low-dose rituximab in patients with Graves' orbitopathy. Thyroid 2021;31(5):821–8.
[68] Ayabe R, Rootman DB, Hwang CJ, et al. Adalimumab as steroid-sparing treatment of inflammatory-stage thyroid eye disease. Ophthalmic Plast Reconstr Surg 2014;30(5): 415–9.
[69] Durrani OM, Reuser TQ, Murray PI. Infliximab: a novel treatment for sight-threatening thyroid associated ophthalmopathy. Orbit 2005;24(2):117–9.
[70] Winn BJ, Kersten RC. Teprotumumab: interpreting the clinical trials in the context of thyroid eye disease pathogenesis and current therapies. Ophthalmology 2021;128(11): 1627–51.
[71] Xin Y, Xu F, Gao Y, et al. Pharmacokinetics and Exposure-Response Relationship of Teprotumumab, an Insulin-Like Growth Factor-1 Receptor-Blocking Antibody, in Thyroid Eye Disease. Clin Pharmacokinet 2021;60(8):1029–40.
[72] Smith TJ, Kahaly GJ, Ezra DG, et al. Teprotumumab for thyroid-associated ophthalmopathy. Supplementary Material: Protocol. N Engl J Med 2017;376:1748–61.
[73] Ashraf DC, Jankovic I, El-Nachef N, et al. New-onset of inflammatory bowel disease in a patient treated with teprotumumab for thyroid associated ophthalmopathy. Ophthalmic Plast Reconstr Surg 2021;37(5):e160–4.
[74] Safo MB, Silkiss RZ. A case of ulcerative colitis associated with teprotumumab treatment for thyroid eye disease. Am J Ophthalmol Case Rep 2021;22:101069.
[75] Belinsky I, Creighton FX Jr, Mahoney N, et al. Teprotumumab and hearing loss: case series and proposal for audiologic monitoring. Ophthalmic Plast Reconstr Surg 2021;38(1): 73–8.
[76] Kossler A, Sears CM, Dosiou C. Hearing Loss and Teprotumumab. J Endocr Soc 2021;5(Suppl 1):A839.
[77] Yu CY, Correa T, Simmons BA, et al. Audiology findings in patients with teprotumumab associated otologic symptoms. Am J Ophthalmol Case Rep 2021;24:101202.
[78] Chern A, Gudis DA, Dagi Glass LR. Teprotumumab and hearing loss: hear the warnings. Orbit 2021;40(4):355–6.
[79] Rodríguez-de la Rosa L, Lassaletta L, Calvino M, et al. The role of insulin-like growth factor 1 in the progression of age-related hearing loss. Front Aging Neurosci 2017;9:411.
[80] Goldman JW, Mendenhall MA, Rettinger SR. Hyperglycemia associated with targeted oncologic treatment: mechanisms and management. Oncologist 2016;21(11):1326–36.
[81] Lee HBH, Mariash CN, Yoon MK, et al. Teprotumumab and hyperglycemia guidelines to monitor for hyperglycemia in teprotumumab. Ophthalmic Plast Reconstr Surg 2021;37(4):393.
[82] Hoang TD, Nguyen NT, Chou E, et al. Rapidly progressive cognitive decline associated with teprotumumab in thyroid eye disease. BMJ Case Rep 2021;14(5):e242153.

[83] Douglas RS, Kahaly GJ, Ugradar S, et al. Teprotumumab efficacy, safety, and durability in longer-duration thyroid eye disease and re-treatment: OPTIC-X Study. Ophthalmology 2021;S0161-6420(21):00818–826.
[84] Douglas RS. Teprotumumab, an insulin-like growth factor-1 receptor antagonist antibody, in the treatment of active thyroid eye disease: a focus on proptosis. Eye 2019;33(2): 183–90.
[85] Jain AP, Gellada N, Ugradar S, et al. Teprotumumab reduces extraocular muscle and orbital fat volume in thyroid eye disease. Br J Ophthalmol 2020;106(2):165–71.
[86] Tran C, Pham CM, Simmons BA, et al. Echographic assessment of extraocular muscle response to teprotumumab. Ophthalmic Plast Reconstr Surg 2021.
[87] Kahaly GJ, Douglas RS, Holt RJ, et al. Teprotumumab for patients with active thyroid eye disease: a pooled data analysis, subgroup analyses, and off-treatment follow-up results from two randomised, double-masked, placebo-controlled, multicentre trials. Lancet Diabetes Endocrinol 2021;9(6):360–3724.
[88] Hwang CJ, Nichols EE, Chon BH, et al. Bilateral dysthyroid compressive optic neuropathy responsive to teprotumumab. Eur J Ophthalmol 2021 120672121991042.
[89] Sears CM, Azad AD, Dosiou C, et al. Teprotumumab for dysthyroid optic neuropathy: early response to therapy. Ophthalmic Plast Reconstr Surg 2021;37(3S):S157–60.
[90] Sears CM, Wang Y, Bailey LA, et al. Early efficacy of teprotumumab for the treatment of dysthyroid optic neuropathy: a multicenter study. Am J Ophthalmol Case Rep 2021;23: 101111.
[91] Slentz DH, Smith TJ, Kim DS, et al. Teprotumumab for optic neuropathy in thyroid eye disease. JAMA Ophthalmol 2021;139(2):244–7.
[92] Lopez MJ, Herring JL, Thomas C, et al. Visual recovery of dysthyroid optic neuropathy with teprotumumab. J Neuroophthalmol 2021.
[93] Chiou CA, Reshef ER, Freitag SK. Teprotumumab for the treatment of mild compressive optic neuropathy in thyroid eye disease: a report of two cases. Am J Ophthalmol Case Rep 2021;22:101075.
[94] Diniz SB, Cohen LM, Roelofs KA, et al. Early experience with the clinical use of teprotumumab in a heterogenous thyroid eye disease population. Ophthalmic Plast Reconstr Surg 2021;37(6):583–91.
[95] Ozzello DJ, Kikkawa DO, Korn BS. Early experience with teprotumumab for chronic thyroid eye disease. Am J Ophthalmol Case Rep 2020;19:100744.
[96] Ozzello DJ, Dallalzadeh LO, Liu CY. Teprotumumab for chronic thyroid eye disease. Orbit 2021;1–8.
[97] Ugradar S, Kang J, Kossler AL, et al. Teprotumumab for the treatment of chronic thyroid eye disease. Eye (Lond) 2021.
[98] Yu CY, Simmons BA, Pham CM, et al. The role of teprotumumab in chronic, clinically active thyroid eye disease. Eye (Lond) 2021.
[99] Ponto KA, Merkesdal S, Hommel G, et al. Public health relevance of Graves' orbitopathy. J Clin Endocrinol Metab 2013;98(1):145–52.
[100] Singh G, Sehgal M, Mithal A, et al. Thyroid eye disease in the United States: data from emergency department visits and hospitalizations. Presented at: 2021 AACE Virtual Annual Meeting, May 26–29, 2021.
[101] Neumann S, Krieger CC, Gershengorn MC. Targeting TSH and IGF-1 Receptors to Treat Thyroid Eye Disease. Eur Thyroid J 2020;9(Suppl 1):59–65.
[102] Marcinkowski P, Hoyer I, Specker E, et al. A new highly thyrotropin receptor-selective small-molecule antagonist with potential for the treatment of Graves' orbitopathy. Thyroid 2019;29(1):111–23.

Advances in Ophthalmology and Optometry 7 (2022) 401–432

ADVANCES IN OPHTHALMOLOGY AND OPTOMETRY

# Diagnosis and Management of Irritated Eyelids

Christine Ryu, MD, Rao V. Chundury, MD*

Truhlsen Eye Institute, University of Nebraska Medical Center, 3902 Leavenworth Street, Omaha, NE 68105, USA

**Keywords**

• Periorbital dermatitis • Eyelid irritation • Blepharitis
• Meibomian gland dysfunction

**Key points**

- Irritated, erythematous eyelids can be caused by a wide variety of conditions that can be categorized into blepharitis, immunologic, inflammatory, infectious, and neoplastic.
- Conditions such as anterior blepharitis, posterior blepharitis, and rosacea do not have a cure and require maintenance therapy for symptom control. The chronicity and maintenance regimen should be discussed with patients.
- Steroids are the first-line treatment of most immunologic and inflammatory conditions but should be used at the lowest dose and shortest course possible to minimize side effects.
- Malignancy should be considered on the differential for eyelid irritation, especially in a unilateral presentation of a typically bilateral process or refractory to treatment.
- Involvement beyond the eyelid, such as ocular surface, posterior segment, optic nerve, or systemic, should be treated or referred to an appropriate specialist.

## INTRODUCTION

Eyelid irritation is one of the most frequent complaints encountered by the eyecare provider. Several factors make eyelid irritation common and bothersome enough for patients to seek evaluation. The eyelids are a high-risk area for irritation, as they usually are exposed to the environment. The eyelid skin is the thinnest skin in the body at 0.55 mm, compared with 2 mm for the remainder

*Corresponding author. *E-mail address:* rao.chundury@unmc.edu

https://doi.org/10.1016/j.yaoo.2022.03.017

of the face [1]. Exposure to allergens and irritants, therefore, is more likely to affect this thin skin. Irritating agents can become trapped by the orbicularis muscle and lead to prolonged exposure [2]. The risk of nonmelanoma skin cancers increases with ultraviolet radiation, and 80% of the cases manifest on the head and neck; the eyelids alone account for 5% of nonmelanoma skin cancers [3]. Aside from physical discomfort, eyelid changes such as discoloration and edema can lead patients to avoid work and socializing, as the eyelids cannot be easily covered up. This psychosocial morbidity should not be underestimated. The eyelids are especially important due to their specialized structure and function. Loss of lid integrity can lead to ocular sequelae such as decreased vision and poor quality of life.

Despite how common it is, eyelid irritation can be frustrating to diagnose. The correct diagnosis can elude the provider for numerous reasons. First, overlapping signs and symptoms exist between conditions, such as pruritis or scaling overlying lesions. As the disease progresses from acute to chronic phases, the presentation can change. Conditions can masquerade as others, such as sebaceous cell carcinoma mimicking meibomian gland dysfunction. In addition, patients frequently present with more than one distinct condition.

Even with the correct diagnosis, treatment can prove unsatisfactory for both patients and clinicians, as many causes of eyelid irritation are chronic, lifelong conditions without a cure. Patients with these conditions should be counseled on the chronicity and given realistic expectations that they will need maintenance management including warm compresses and lid hygiene for symptom control.

This article discusses the diagnosis and management of eyelid irritation. More space has been dedicated to the subtypes of blepharitis and dermatitis, as they are the most frequent culprits and the most frustrating to treat. Several other important conditions on the differential diagnosis of erythematous, irritated eyelids will be covered in less detail. Some of these conditions can have associated ocular presentations such as keratopathy, which will not be discussed in depth here. Clinicians should keep in mind that this article is not an exhaustive list.

## SIGNIFICANCE

### Blepharitis

Blepharitis is inflammation of the eyelid margins and is one of the most common causes of irritated eyelids, seen in 37% and 47% of patients by ophthalmologists and optometrists, respectively [4]. Patients present with pruritis, irritation, burning, and erythema. Often these symptoms are worse in the morning, in contrast to dry eyes from aqueous deficiency, which worsen as the day progresses.

Anterior blepharitis is inflammation of the eyelid margin anterior to the gray line, including the eyelid skin and lash follicles. Anterior blepharitis is further categorized into seborrheic and staphylococcal.

Many of these conditions commonly are found with others, such as staphylococcal blepharitis with rosacea and atopic dermatitis [5]. Some of these associations are believed to be causal. Background information, presenting signs and symptoms, and management have been summarized in Table 1

*Staphylococcal blepharitis*

The pathogenesis has been linked to bacteria. One proposition is the direct infection by *Staphylococcus spp.* Several studies have found a higher prevalence of *Staphylococcus aureus* in patients with staphylococcal blepharitis compared with controls; however, *S aureus* is culture positive in only about 50% of patients with staphylococcal blepharitis, whereas coagulase-negative *Staphylococci* (CoNS) is culture positive in greater than 90% [6,7]. Another study found higher quantitative burden of normal commensal bacteria found in nonblepharitis patients [8]. Others have proposed hypersensitivity to *S aureus* [9,10] or its exotoxins [11]. In addition, the bacterial lipases produced by blepharitis bacterial strains are more likely to hydrolyze meibum components into free fatty acids, which causes ocular irritation [12] and has been demonstrated to promote S aureus growth in vitro [22].

*Posterior blepharitis*

Similar to staphylococcal blepharitis, bacteria are involved in pathogenesis. Patients have a greater quantity of normal lid flora [7,12,25,[7,12,25], and CoNS strains are more likely to produce lipases that hydrolyze meibum components into irritating free fatty acids [12]. The free fatty acids can directly irritate the ocular surface and promote hyperkeratinization, worsening MGD [51].

*Rosacea*

Severe ocular rosacea can be seen with minimal cutaneous involvement [36]. Up to 58% of patients with cutaneous rosacea develop ocular rosacea, and 20% of patients can present with ocular rosacea before cutaneous manifestations [52,53]. About 2% to 4.5% of periorbital dermatitis cases are caused by rosacea [54].

Demodex *blepharitis*

*Demodex* is a commensal mite of the eyelashes, nose, forehead, and cheeks [43]. It is a part of normal skin fauna especially with increasing age. Demodex has been found in about 30% of symptomatic patients with seborrheic blepharitis but also in about 30% of nonblepharitis patients [55], confirming that their presence alone is not pathogenic. Increased burden is a potential cause for symptomatic pathogenesis, but no minimum mite concentration triggering pathogenic demodicosis has been determined [45]. *Demodex* can carry *Staphylococcus spp.*, *Streptococcus spp.*, and other bacteria. Bacterial superantigens and *Demodex* waste may trigger blepharitis or rosacea through delayed hypersensitivity or innate immune response [44].

## Immunologic

The eyelids are involved in about 8.6% to 12.9% of all dermatitis presentations, and dermatitis confined to only the eyelids is about 4.44% to 4.7% of cases [56–59]. All 3 subtypes of dermatitis have some pruritis, edema, and erythema of

**Table 1**
Blepharitis

| Condition | Background | Signs and Symptoms | Management |
|---|---|---|---|
| Staphylococcal blepharitis (Fig. 1) | • Subtype of anterior blepharitis<br>• Pathogenesis linked to bacteria. Proposed mechanisms include<br>o Direct infection by *Staphylococcus spp.* [6,7]<br>o Higher quantitative burden of normal commensal bacteria [8]<br>o Hypersensitivity to *Staphylococcus aureus* or exotoxins [9,10,11]<br>o Bacterial lipases hydrolyzing meibum into irritating components [12]<br>• Frequently found with rosacea and atopic dermatitis | • Hard, brittle, crusty scales (collarettes) surrounding lash bases [5]<br>• Lid margin erythema<br>• Chronic changes: trichiasis, madarosis, poliosis, lid margin notching, thickening, and scarring [5,13]<br>• More severe signs and symptoms (eg, severe pruritis and irritation, eyelids stuck together on waking up) than seborrheic or posterior blepharitis | • First line: erythromycin or bacitracin ointment [7,14] (fusidic acid is an appropriate alternative [15])<br>• Topical azithromycin [14]<br>• Gentamicin, neomycin, and tetracyclines also effective [7]<br>• MRSA coverage: trimethoprim, besifloxacin [14]<br>• Methicillin-resistant CoNS: vancomycin [16]<br>• Severe or refractory cases: systemic tetracyclines or systemic azithromycin [14,17–19] |
| Seborrheic blepharitis (Fig. 2) | • Subtype of anterior blepharitis<br>• Pathogenesis linked to *malassezia* yeasts [20]<br>• Frequently found with posterior blepharitis [5]<br>• 95% of patients have seborrheic dermatitis [6,21] | • Soft, greasy scales on anterior lid margin<br>• Mild lid erythema and inflammation<br>• Lash changes rare (eg, madarosis, trichiasis) [22]<br>• Most common symptom: burning | • Often improves with lid hygiene alone<br>• Concurrent seborrheic dermatitis must be treated to prevent relapses of seborrheic blepharitis [21,23]<br>• Tea tree oil wipes may offer longer symptom relief compared with baby shampoo [24]<br>• Topical antibiotics do not improve seborrheic blepharitis [21] |

| | | | |
|---|---|---|---|
| Posterior blepharitis (Fig. 3) | • Also called meibomian gland dysfunction (MGD)<br>• Pathogenesis linked to bacteria. Proposed mechanisms include:<br>o Higher quantitative burden of normal commensal bacteria [7,12,25]<br>o Bacterial lipases hydrolyzing meibum into irritating components [12]<br>• Obstructive form<br>o Hyperkeratinization and narrowing of meibomian gland ducts with upstream acinar enlargement [5]<br>• Meibum has a higher melting point of >40°C, making it less expressible at physiologic eyelid temperatures of 33–37°C [18,26]<br>• Hypersecretory form<br>o Hyperproduction of normal consistency meibum<br>• Predisposed to chalazia<br>• Frequently found with rosacea | • Burning sensation<br>• Mattering at eyelid margins<br>• Obstructive form [9]<br>o Clogged meibomian gland openings<br>o Thick or absent meibum on manual expression<br>o Foamy or oily tear film<br>• Hypersecretory form [6]<br>o Patent meibomian gland openings<br>o Dilated ducts<br>• Chronic changes: lid margin thickening scalloping, erythema, telangiectasias, trichiasis, meibomian gland atrophy, and fibrosis | • Topical azithromycin [14]<br>• Topical cyclosporine A [14,27]<br>• Topical tacrolimus: shown to improve meibomian gland secretion, telangiectasias, and some symptoms in MGD that had been refractory to lid hygiene, topical antibiotics, and systemic antibiotics [28]<br>• Intraductal meibomian gland probing: mechanically dilates obstructed meibomian glands. Allows immediate release of built-up meibum, easier penetration of topical therapies into the glands, longer-term patency of gland opening, and even regrowth of atrophied glands [29].<br>• LipiFlow: applies heat and pulsatile pressure to melt and express thickened meibum [18].<br>• Intense pulsed light (IPL): nonlaser light to the skin causing local heating, melting of meibum, and thrombosis of telangiectatic vessels, thereby improving lid redness and decreasing delivery of inflammatory cytokines [18,30]. IPL may additionally decrease bacteria and *demodex* [30,31]<br>• Severe or refractory cases: systemic tetracyclines or azithromycin [14,17,18,19] |

(*continued on next page*)

**Table 1**
**(*continued*)**

| Condition | Background | Signs and Symptoms | Management |
|---|---|---|---|
| Angular blepharitis (Fig. 4) | • Inflammation primarily affecting lateral and/or medial canthi<br>• Classically associated with *Moraxella spp.*, less commonly with *Staphylococcus spp* | • *M spp.*: wet, macerated canthal skin with gray mucous exudate<br>• *Staphylococcus spp.*: similar to staphylococcal blepharitis but limited to canthal angles, may have combined anterior and angular blepharitis [32]<br>• Possible conjunctival injection [33] | • Erythromycin or bacitracin ointment<br>• Vitamin B6 supplementation alone helped in a case series [34] |
| Rosacea (Fig. 5) | • Chronic inflammatory disease with increased inflammation, angiogenesis, mast cell dysfunction, and neurovascular dysregulation<br>• Pathogenesis multifactorial, may involve *Demodex* [35]<br>• Environmental triggers: spicy food, alcohol, UV exposure, emotional stress, vigorous exercise<br>• Frequently found with staphylococcal blepharitis, posterior blepharitis, and demodicosis | • Ocular rosacea: lid margin inflammation, telangiectasias, anterior and posterior blepharitis, frequent chalazia<br>• Other signs include facial erythema, flushing, telangiectasias, pustules, papules, and hypertrophic sebaceous glands<br>• Chronic changes: plague, hypertrophic skin changes, rhinophyma | • Conservative measures avoidance of triggers, use of mild and lipid free soaps, use of sunscreen [36,37]<br>• Topical cyclosporine A [14,27]<br>• Topical tacrolimus [38]<br>• Topical metronidazole (antimicrobial, antiinflammatory, and immunosuppressive) [39]<br>• Topical ivermectin (antiinflammatory, anti-Demodex) [40,41]<br>• Topical brimonidine (reduce erythema and mast cell activity) [42]<br>• Newer therapies targeting molecules specific to the pathogenesis of rosacea such as interleukin-17 and Toll-like receptors are under investigation [37,38]<br>• Management of anterior blepharitis, posterior blepharitis, and symptomatic demodicosis |

| | | | |
|---|---|---|---|
| *Demodex* blepharitis Fig. 6 | • Normal commensal mite of face [43]<br>• Trigger for pathogenic demodicosis unclear but proposed mechanism include<br>  ○ Increased quantity and burden<br>  ○ Introduction of bacteria carried by *Demodex*<br>  ○ Delayed hypersensitivity or innate immune response to *Demodex* waste or bacterial superantigens [44] | • Cylindrical sleeves at lash bases [45]<br>• *Demodex folliculorum*<br>  ○ Consume follicular epithelial cells and lay eggs within follicle, leading to mechanical abrasions<br>  ○ Anterior blepharitis, reactive hyperkeratinization, follicular distension trichiasis [44,46]<br>• *Demodex brevis*<br>  ○ Mechanically block meibomian glands and shed exoskeleton within glands<br>  ○ Posterior blepharitis, granulomatous inflammation, frequent chalazia [44,46] | • If asymptomatic, does not require treatment<br>• First line: tea tree oil or its active ingredient terpinene-4-ol (anti-Demodex, antibacterial, antifungal, and antiinflammatory) [14,43,45,47,48]<br>  ○ Weekly lid scrubs with 50% tea tree oil solution<br>  ○ Daily lids scrub with 5% tea tree oil solution<br>  ○ Tea tree oil shampoo<br>• Topical 4% pilocarpine gel [49]<br>• Topical ivermectin [14,40]<br>• IPL [31]<br>• Permethrin cream [50]<br>• Refractory cases: oral ivermectin or oral metronidazole [14,47] |

*Abbreviations:* CoNS, coagulase-negative Staphylococci; UV, ultraviolet.

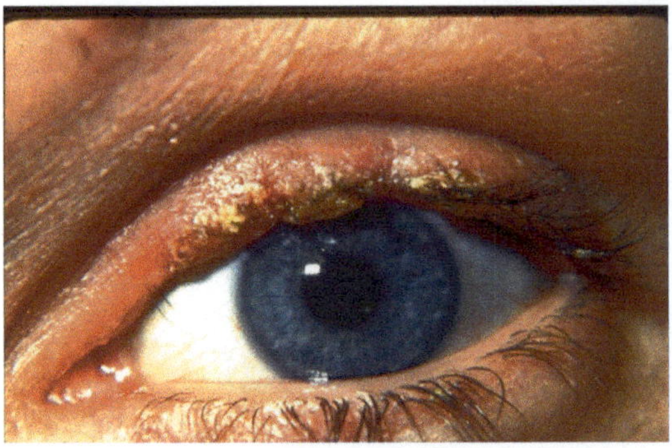

**Fig. 1.** Staphylococcal blepharitis. Erythematous upper lid margin with ulceration and prominent yellow crusting. (Reproduced, with permission, from Coleman AL, *Eye Care Skills*, Managing the Red Eye, American Academy of Ophthalmology, Copyright 1996.)

eyelids. Pruritis is worse in allergic contact dermatitis, and burning is classic for irritant contact dermatitis [23]. If chronic, skin lesions can progress to lichenification, fissuring, hyperpigmentation, ectropion, ptosis, and worsening of dermatochalasis [60,61]. More information can be found in Table 2

*Allergic contact dermatitis*

Allergic contact dermatitis (ACD) is a delayed-type hypersensitivity reaction triggered by an allergen-specific activation of the acquired immune system. Because this sensitization process depends on each individual, only some people exposed to the same chemical will develop hypersensitivity [38]. Once sensitized, patients will usually manifest signs 24 to 48 hours after exposure to the allergen, although presentation can be delayed up to 96 hours [36,38]. Some of

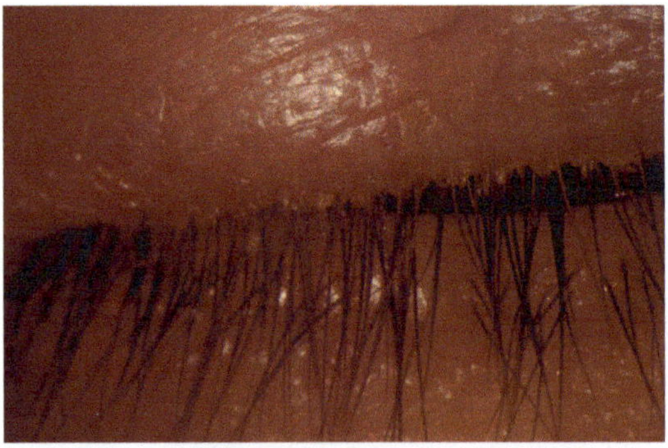

**Fig. 2.** Seborrheic blepharitis. Soft, greasy scales at the base of upper lid lashes. Lower lid margin also seems to have greasy scales. No erythema or telangiectasias are observed. (Reproduced, with permission, from Waring GO, *2021-2022 Basic and Clinical Science Course*, Section 13, Refractive Surgery, American Academy of Ophthalmology, Copyright 2011.)

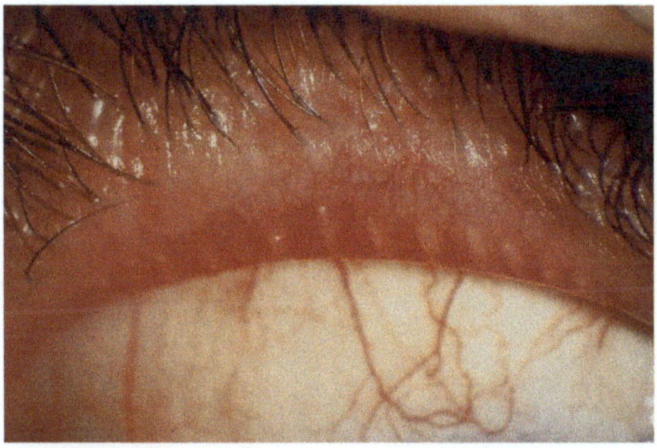

**Fig. 3.** Posterior blepharitis of an upper eyelid. The meibomian glands are capped with thickened meibum, and telangiectasias are present on the thickened lid margin. (Reproduced, with permission, from Weisenthal RW, *2017-2018 Basic and Clinical Science Course*, Section 8, Cornea and External Disease, American Academy of Ophthalmology, Copyright 2017.)

the most common allergens are listed in Table 3. ACD is the most common cause of periorbital dermatitis, accounting for 30% to 50% of eyelid dermatitis, although some have reported up to 75% [54,56–59,62,78].

*Irritant contact dermatitis*

Irritant contact dermatitis (ICD) is a nonspecific inflammation involving the innate immune response. The irritant disrupts epidermal integrity, and its direct toxicity triggers the innate immune system [61]. Unlike ACD, no inflammation specific to the offending agent exists. Patients present with an acute, immediate reaction after exposure. Common irritants include detergents, acids, and solvents. Many ACD allergens are weak irritants, and at higher

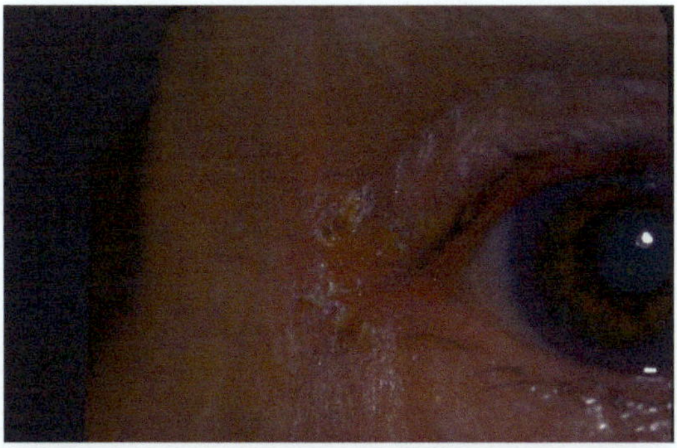

**Fig. 4.** Angular blepharitis. Wet, cracked lateral canthal angle surrounded by dried, crusty scales. Remainder of upper and lower eyelids shown do not seem thickened or erythematous. (Reproduced, with permission, and developed by the BCSC Committee, *External Disease and Cornea*, Part I: External Disease, American Academy of Ophthalmology, Copyright 1994.)

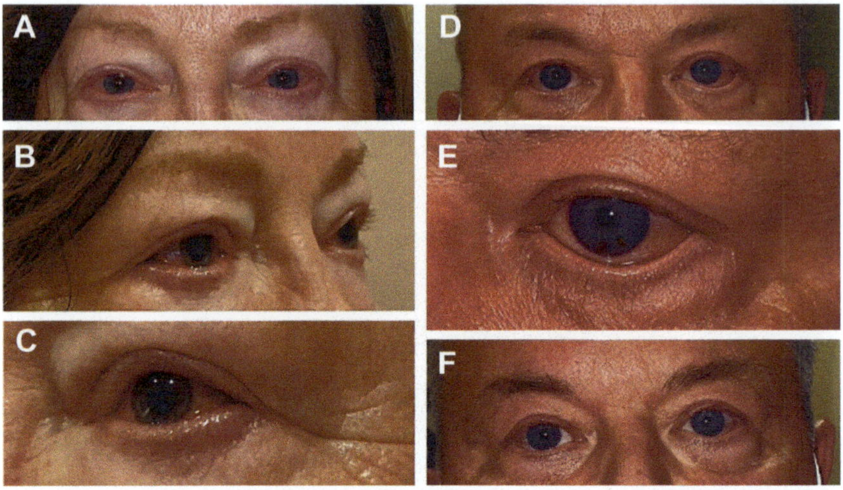


**Fig. 5.** Rosacea blepharitis. (*A–C*) A 76-year-old woman with long-standing rosacea blepharitis not improved on artificial tears, Lotemax ointment, and warm compresses. Erythema and edema of bilateral upper and lower eyelids (*A*) and thickening of eyelid margins (*B, C*). (*D–F*) A 64-year-old man with moderate facial erythema, eyelid erythema, and left lower lid ectropion (*E*). After treatment with minocycline and topical metronidazole, facial and eyelid erythema and left lower lid ectropion are much improved (*F*).

concentrations, they can lead to ICD. Because of its inherent toxicity, an irritant will trigger an ICD response in most people [61]. ICD accounts for 7% to 20% of periocular dermatitis [1,54,57–59,61].

*Atopic dermatitis*

Atopic dermatitis (AD) is a chronic skin condition associated with asthma and allergic rhinitis. AD is a multifactorial condition with genetic and

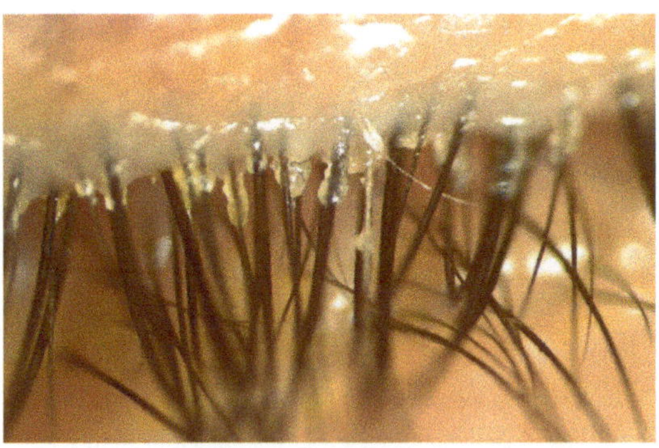

**Fig. 6.** Demodex blepharitis. Cylindrical sleeves surrounding lash bases. (Reproduced, with permission, from Feder RS, *2021-2022 Basic and Clinical Science Course*, Section 8, Cornea and External Disease, American Academy of Ophthalmology, Copyright 2021.)

**Table 2**
Immunologic causes of eyelid irritation

| Condition | Background | Signs and Symptoms | Condition-Specific Management |
|---|---|---|---|
| Allergic contact dermatitis (ACD) (Fig. 7) | • Allergens-specific delayed-type hypersensitivity reaction<br>• Direct exposure: direct contact of allergen to eyelids (eg, eye makeup, eye drops) [54,60]<br>• Ectopic exposure: application of allergen not primarily on eyelids<br>o Hair products<br>o Nail polish and artificial nails leaving ACD streaks on face [62]. Periungual ACD rare as this skin is less sensitive [2,58]<br>o Gold jewelry or gold lid weight [60,63,64]<br>• Airborne exposure: aerosolized or volatile allergen (eg, pollen, dust mites, air fresheners, paint fumes), accounts for 20% of ACD [65]<br>• Steroid hypersensitivity: sensitization to topical steroid or its vehicle [66,67]<br>o Paradoxic worsening or lack of improvement on topical steroids<br>o Incidence of 0.2%–5% | • Erythema, edema, papules, and vesicles within 24–48 h after exposure to allergen (can be delayed up to 96 h) [23,61]<br>• Each exposure leads to another fresh crop of vesicles [61] | • Topical cyclosporine A (less effective than tacrolimus and pimecrolimus) [68]<br>• Ultraviolet B (UVB) phototherapy and psoralen plus ultraviolet A (PUVA)<br>Photochemotherapy: especially helpful if patients are unable to avoid allergens<br>• "Consort dermatitis": others who frequently interact with the patient may need to avoid patient's allergens (eg, for patient with gold hypersensitivity, patient's spouse avoids wearing gold jewelry) [63]<br>• Hypersensitivity to steroids<br>o Refer for patch testing with standardized steroid tray and patient's own products<br>o Use class C and D1 topical steroids (dexamethasone, clobetasol, rimexolone) [69] |

(*continued on next page*)

**Table 2**
**(*continued*)**

| Condition | Background | Signs and Symptoms | Condition-Specific Management |
|---|---|---|---|
| Irritant contact dermatitis (ICD) | • Innate immune system response to direct toxicity or irritant (eg, detergents, acids, solvents)<br>• Immediate reaction after exposure | • Burning > pruritis<br>• Erythema, edema, macules, papules, blisters | • No additional ICD-specific management |
| Atopic dermatitis (AD) (Fig. 8) | • Chronic skin condition from dysregulation of innate immunity with hyperactivation of Th2 response and IgE [70]<br>• More frequent colonization by bacteria [70–72]<br>• Rubbing and scratching triggers additional Th-2 response• | • Pruritis<br>• Bilateral medial upper eyelids most frequently affected<br>• Erythema, scaling, fissuring, oozing [59]<br>• Loss of eyelashes and eyebrow hairs form rubbing [23,72]<br>• Dennie-Morgan lines: symmetric infraorbital skin folds<br>• Allergic shiners: symmetric purple-gray infraorbital discoloration from venous stasis [23,73] | • Acute AD: medium-potency topical steroids [23]<br>• Chronic AD: low-potency topical steroids |
| *General Management of Dermatitis*<br>• Avoidance of offending allergens or irritants<br>• Emollients to restore skin barrier [73]<br>  ○ Ointments have better moisture retention than lotions and creams<br>  ○ Select products with fewest additives possible<br>• Avoidance of touching affected areas to decrease introduction of allergens/irritants and minimize mechanical trauma<br>• Avoidance of cosmetics or other topical agents until skin barrier is restored<br>• Topical tacrolimus and pimecrolimus [65,74,75] | | • Steroids for ACD and ICD [23,68]<br>  ○ Low-potency topical steroids for most cases<br>  ○ Moderate or severe dermatitis: medium-potency topical steroids<br>  ○ Extensive facial involvement or greater than 20% of body surface area: systemic steroids<br>• Pruritis control<br>  ○ Cool compresses<br>  ○ Avoidance of topical anesthetics and topical antihistamines—risk of developing sensitization [23,76]<br>  ○ Systemic steroids [23] or topical steroids with oral antihistamines [77] | |

*Abbreviation:* IgE, immunoglobulin E.

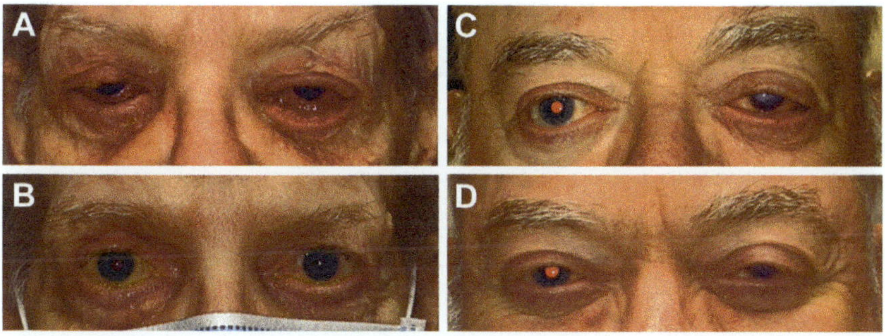


**Fig. 7.** Allergic contact dermatitis. (*A–B*) A 92-year-old man on latanoprost and Cosopt presenting with severe bilateral eyelid redness, swelling, irritation, ptosis, and ectropion (*A*). Patient was managed by switching to preservative free glaucoma medications, prednisolone eye drops, tacrolimus ointment, and left temporary tarsorrhaphy with significant improvement (*B*). (*C–D*) A 73-year-old man using Combigan in left eye only presenting with left lower lid ectropion along with swelling, mild erythema, and irritation of the left upper and lower lids (*C*). Signs and symptoms resolved after discontinuing Combigan and using Lotemax ointment (*D*).

environmental factors that leads to dysregulation of innate immunity and hyperactivation of Th-2 response and immunoglobulin E [70]. Patients have an increased susceptibility to skin infections and are more frequently colonized by a greater number of bacteria [70]. The eyelids specifically are colonized by *S aureus* in 67% of patients with AD compared with 6% of non-AD patients [71]. About 20% to 42% of patients with AD develop eyelid involvement [72]. Eyelid AD accounts for 11.3% to 25% of periorbital dermatitis [1,54,58,59,62].

### Inflammatory

*Psoriasis, discoid lupus erythematosus, and dermatomyositis*

Psoriasis, discoid lupus erythematosus (DLE), and dermatomyositis are all inflammatory conditions with skin manifestations. Psoriasis has typical lesions

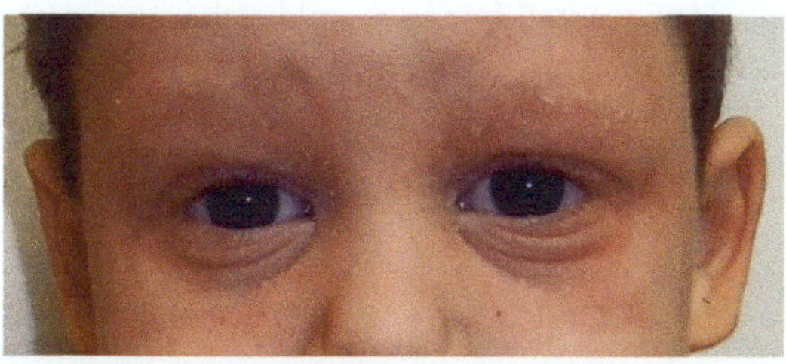

**Fig. 8.** Atopic dermatitis. Bilateral upper and lower eyelid erythema, edema, and flaking. Note the prominent Dennie-Morgan folds and allergic shiners of lower eyelids. Patient also has loss of eyebrow hairs from vigorous itching. (Reproduced, with permission, from Wallace BS, *Focal Points*: Dermatologic Disorders of the Periocular Region, American Academy of Ophthalmology, Copyright 2020.)

**Table 3**
Common contact allergens

| | |
|---|---|
| • Ophthalmic drops<br>o Brimonidine<br>o Benzalkonium chloride<br>• Topical anesthetics<br>o Benzocaine<br>• Topical antibiotics<br>o Neomycin<br>o Bacitracin<br>• Topical steroids<br>• Adhesives<br>• Gold<br>o Jewelry<br>o Lid weights<br>• Occupational exposures<br>o Resins<br>o Construction materials<br>• New clothing (fabric dyes and resins) | • Hair products<br>o Dyes<br>o Shampoo<br>o Conditioner<br>• Cosmetics<br>• Eyelash curlers<br>• Nail polish<br>• Artificial nails<br>• Facial & body skin care products<br>o Body wash<br>o Lotions<br>o Lip care<br>o Perfumes<br>• Household products<br>o Laundry detergent and fabric softeners<br>o Cleaning solutions<br>o Paint |

often found throughout the body, but chronic eyelid inflammation can lead to evolving and variable presentations. DLE can have variable presentations and masquerade as other conditions such as blepharitis, which can delay diagnosis for years when the patient lacks other signs of DLE and systemic lupus erythematosus. The symmetric and violaceous heliotrope rash is pathognomonic for dermatomyositis. More information is summarized in Table 4.

### Infectious

*Hordeola, chalazia, preseptal cellulitis, herpes zoster ophthalmicus, erysipelas, and necrotizing fasciitis*

Presentation is summarized in Table 5 and some examples are shown in Figs. 9–13. Preseptal cellulitis, erysipelas, and early necrotizing fasciitis present similarly with eyelid pain, erythema, edema, and fever. Erysipelas can be distinguished by sharply demarcated borders, unlike the poorly defined borders of preseptal cellulitis. Some signs that differentiate necrotizing fasciitis are a dusky violaceous hue, pain extending beyond erythema, pain out of proportion, bullae, and rapid progression [27,77].

### Neoplastic

*Actinic keratosis, squamous cell carcinoma, sebaceous cell carcinoma, cutaneous T-cell lymphoma*

Presentation is summarized in Table 6 and examples are shown in Figs. 14–17. All of these conditions can involve the margin and masquerade as blepharitis and chalazia [95–100]. Histopathological confirmation is essential. Some clues hinting at malignancy include significantly asymmetric blepharitis and worsening or persistent symptoms despite treatment.

**Table 4**
Inflammatory causes of eyelid irritation

| Condition | Background | Signs and Symptoms | Management |
|---|---|---|---|
| Psoriasis | • Chronic inflammatory disease that most commonly affects skin<br>• Scalp, hairline, and eyebrow involvement common. Remainder of face less commonly involved and seen in only 17%–46% of psoriasis cases [49]<br>• Eyelid psoriasis accounts for 2.3%–3.8% of eyelid dermatitis [1,54,56,62]<br>• Eyelid involvement often coincide with systemic flares of psoriasis [79]<br>• Higher prevalence of staphylococcal and posterior blepharitis [80,79] | • Sharply demarcated, irregular, salmon or red plaques covered by silvery scale<br>• Chronic inflammation leads to trichiasis, ectropion, symblepharon, ptosis, madarosis, punctal stenosis [49] | • Eyelid hygiene<br>• Emollients<br>• Low-potency topical steroids such as 1% hydrocortisone<br>• Low-dose retinoids [81]<br>• Ultraviolet B (UVB) phototherapy [81]<br>• Tacrolimus ointment [82] |
| Discoid lupus erythematosus (DLE) | • Most common cutaneous manifestation of systemic lupus erythematosus (SLE), a chronic autoimmune disease<br>• Rarely can present with isolated eyelid DLE without any other DLE or SLE manifestations [83,84] | • Most commonly erythematous, coin-shaped, raised plaque with overlying scale<br>• Alternatively, can present with atrophy, edema, pigmentary changes, or telangiectasias [83–85]<br>• Chronic, untreated changes can lead to permanent lid scarring, | • First line: hydroxychloroquine [83,84]<br>• Other immunosuppressants (methotrexate, azathioprine, cyclophosphamide) [83,86]<br>• Smoking cessation [83,85]<br>• Sun protection<br>• Pimecrolimus and tacrolimus ointment [84,86] |

(*continued on next page*)

**Table 4**
***(continued)***

| Condition | Background | Signs and Symptoms | Management |
|---|---|---|---|
| | | entropion, ectropion, symblepharon, madarosis, trichiasis<br>• Can mimic blepharoconjunctivitis [9,83,85]<br>• Typically bilateral and asymmetric [85] | • Other tried treatments with few numbers: topical steroids, intralesional steroids, systemic steroids [83,86] |
| Dermatomyositis | • Rare inflammatory microangiopathy affecting skin and muscles | • Heliotrope rash: symmetric violaceous discoloration of the upper eyelids, may extend to malar region [87]<br>  ○ Pathognomonic for dermatomyositis<br>  ○ May worsen after sun exposure | • Refer to primary care or rheumatology for work-up and management<br>• Systemic steroids, immunosuppressants, intravenous immunoglobulin depending on severity and disease response [87] |

**Table 5**
Infectious causes of eyelid irritation

| Condition | Background | Signs and Symptoms | Management |
|---|---|---|---|
| Hordeolum (Fig. 9) | • Acute bacterial infection of eyelid margin<br>Internal: meibomian gland<br>External: gland of Zeis | • Painful, erythematous papule along eyelid margin | • Antibiotics are not required<br>• Warm compresses help with hordeolum drainage and prevent progression to a chalazion |
| Chalazion (Fig. 10) | • Lipogranulomatous inflammation of meibomian glands or glands of Zeis caused by spillover of meibum [88]<br>• Noninfectious but can be due to chronic hordeola<br>• Noninfectious causes include obstructive MGD, rosacea, and demodicosis | • Painless eyelid papule | • Antibiotics are not required<br>• Many chalazia improve with time and warm compresses<br>• If chronic, intralesional triamcinolone or incision and curettage can be done |
| Preseptal Cellulitis(Fig. 11) | • Acute infection superficial to orbital septum | • Unilateral eyelid erythema, edema, and tenderness<br>• Systemic signs such as fever, malaise, elevated white blood cell counts | • Oral or intravenous broad-spectrum antibiotics covering gram-positive and gram-negative bacteria to start, then narrowed down as cultures result |
| Herpes zoster opthalmicus(Fig. 12) | • Reactivation of varicella zoster virus in cranial nerve V1 distribution<br>• Frontal nerve most commonly affected<br>• Nasociliary nerve as Hutchinson sign (lesions on the tip, side, or root of nose) is a strong predictor | • Prodromal signs and symptoms such as fever, malaise, pain along V1 dermatome<br>• Acute onset erythematous rash of painful macules, papules, and vesicles on unilateral forehead and eyelid | • Oral acyclovir or valacyclovir<br>• Intravenous acyclovir for sever ophthalmic disease or systemic illness<br>• Bacitracin or erythromycin ointment for skin lesions |

(continued on next page)

**Table 5**
**(*continued*)**

| Condition | Background | Signs and Symptoms | Management |
|---|---|---|---|
| | of ocular inflammation and loss of corneal sensation [89] | • New vesicles form for 3–7 d, followed by crusting and healing over 2–6 wk<br>• Occasionally presents in zoster sine herpete form without vesicles [89] | |
| Erysipelas | • Superficial skin infection by *Streptococcus pyogenes*<br>• Underlying lymphatic involvement [90] | • Acute onset of sharply demarcated, erythematous lesion that progressively enlarges<br>• May develop overlying vesicles and pustules<br>• Usually bilateral but asymmetric [90]<br>• Systemic signs such as fever | • Penicillin<br>• Although erysipelas often resolves on its own, it can also progress to more severe skin infection [89]<br>• Untreated *Streptococcus pyogenes* infections can lead to rheumatic fever |
| Necrotizing Fasciitis(Fig. 13) | • Acute infection of subcutaneous soft tissue and fascia<br>• Rapid progression along fascial planes<br>• Most common causative agent: beta-hemolytic *Streptococcus* | • Edema, dusky violaceous hue, pain extending beyond erythema, pain out of proportion, bullae, rapid progression [73,91]<br>• Orbital involvement is rare but can include decreased vision, APD, proptosis, ophthalmoplegia [92]<br>• Systemic signs such as fever, hypotension | • Intravenous broad-spectrum antibiotics<br>• Aggressive surgical debridement<br>• Hyperbaric oxygen can inhibit bacterial exotoxin production, kill anaerobes, and improve tissue viability [90]<br>• Intravenous immunoglobulin: adjunctive therapy to neutralize bacterial exotoxins [93]<br>• Conservative surgical management with close observation suggested if necrosis is limited to eyelids [94] |

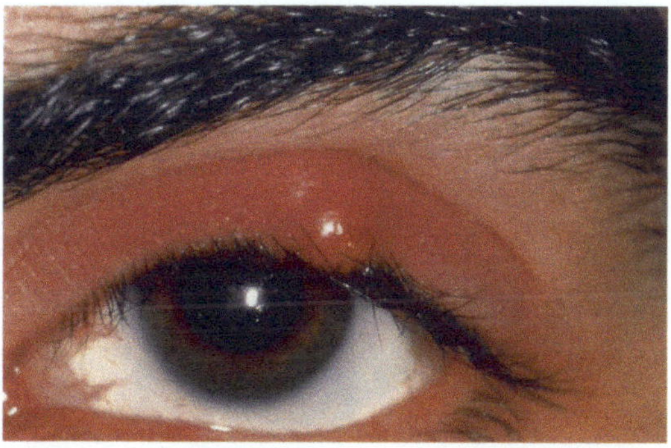

**Fig. 9.** Hordeolum. Upper lid hordeolum with surrounding erythema of upper lid. Area of purulent-appearing material from 4 to 6 o'clock of hordeolum. (Reproduced, with permission, from Feder RS, *2021-2022 Basic and Clinical Science Course*, Section 8, Cornea and External Disease, American Academy of Ophthalmology, Copyright 2021.)

## PRESENT RELEVANCE AND FUTURE AVENUES

### Blepharitis

All patients with blepharitis should practice lid hygiene. The process begins with warm compresses, where a clean washcloth soaked in hot water or heating pack is placed over the eyelids for 5 to 10 minutes; this softens any debris and melts solidified meibum. In patients with posterior blepharitis, gentle massaging helps express the now liquefied meibum. Next, the lid margins and lash bases are scrubbed gently with diluted baby shampoo, commercially available lid scrubs (eg, OCuSOFT, SteriLid), or 0.01% hypochlorous acid (Avenova). A washcloth, finger, cotton pad, or Q-tip can be used; this mechanically removes loosened debris and decreases bacterial burden. After the lids have been cleaned, antibiotic ointment can be applied to the lid margin.

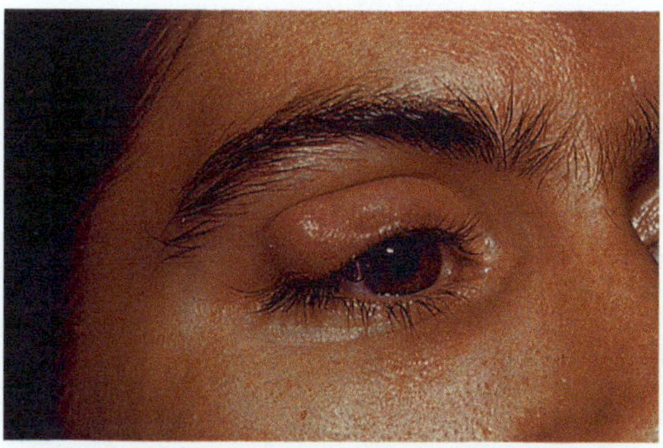

**Fig. 10.** Chalazion. Large upper lid chalazion. (Reproduced, with permission, from Johns KJ, *Eye Care Skills*, Managing the Red Eye, American Academy of Ophthalmology, Copyright 2009.)

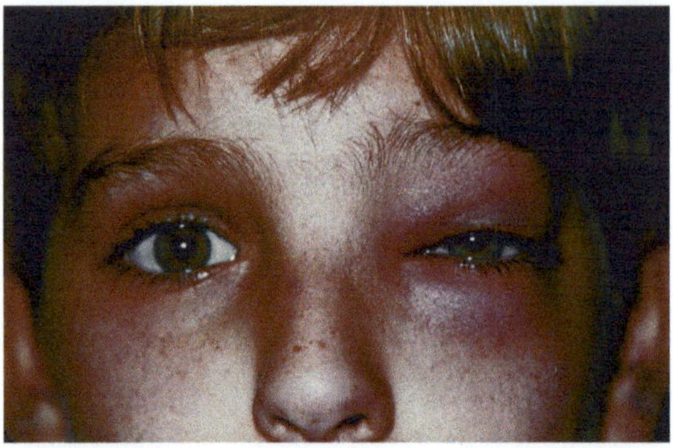

**Fig. 11.** Preseptal cellulitis. Edema and poorly demarcated erythema of left upper and lower eyelids. (Reproduced, with permission, from Blomquist PH, *Practical Ophthlamology*, 8th Edition, American Academy of Ophthalmology, 2021.)

Topical azithromycin suppresses bacterial lipase production; has antiinflammatory effects; and improves lid erythema, meibomian gland secretions, and subjective symptoms in both anterior and posterior blepharitis [15]. Topical azithromycin also decreases the quantity of lid CoNS and *Corynebacteria* [115].

Systemic antibiotics are added when the blepharitis is severe or refractory. Tetracyclines and azithromycin are most used, as they suppress bacterial lipase production and have antiinflammatory effects [14,17–19]. Doxycycline and minocycline are more lipophilic and achieve higher concentrations in tears and eyelids [18]. Once symptoms are under control, patients frequently require chronic low-dose maintenance to inhibit bacterial lipase production [17].

Topical steroids can be used in short courses for acute inflammation or corneal involvement such as phlyctenular or marginal keratitis [5,18]. Long-term use is not recommended given side effects including cataracts and

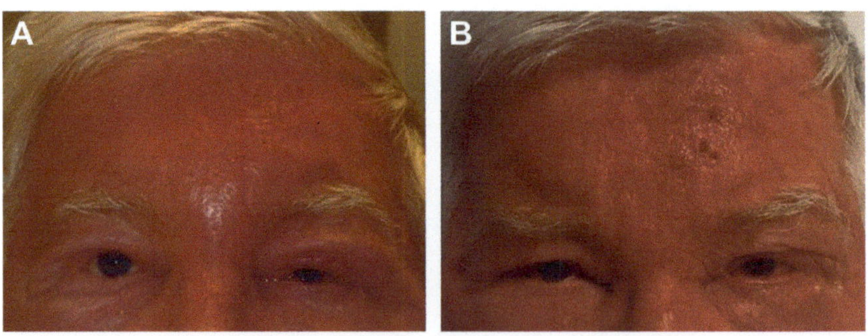


**Fig. 12.** Herpes zoster ophthalmicus. A 81-year-old man presenting with acute edema and erythema of left eyelids and face (*A*). Presentation was preceded with 3 weeks of left eye pain. Vesicles appeared 1 day later in cranial nerve V1 distribution (*B*).

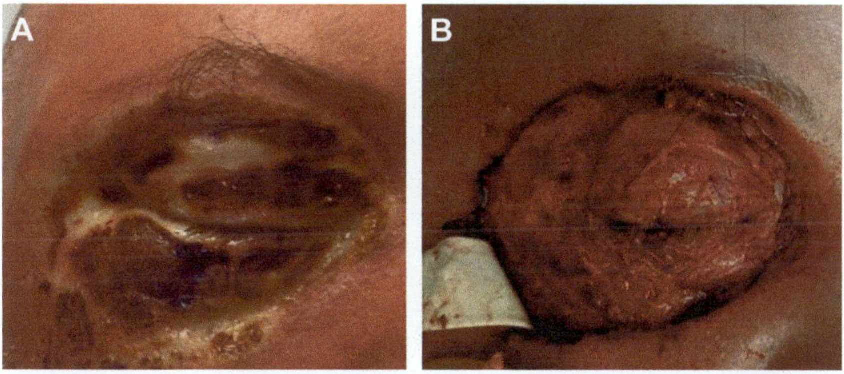


**Fig. 13.** Necrotizing fasciitis. A 50-year-old man presenting with severe right upper and lower eyelid edema, blanched skin, overlying eschars, and brown drainage (*A*). After initial debridement of necrotic tissues (*B*).

increased IOP. Combination topical ointments with antibiotic and steroid are effective as acute treatment [14]. Tobramycin-loteprednol combination offers the most favorable risk-benefit ratio [14].

Topical nonsteroidal antiinflammatory medications such as cyclosporine A and lifitegrast can decrease eyelid inflammation and dry eye symptoms, which frequently are found along with blepharitis. Cyclosporine A has been shown to improve meibomian gland secretions [14,27]. Topical omega-3 fatty acid can decrease inflammation and improve dry eye symptoms, but oral omega-3 fatty acid supplementation has conflicting results [18].

Additional management more specific to each condition is discussed in greater detail in Table 1.

## Immunologic

Management is summarized in Table 2. For ACD, ICD, and AD, patients should avoid any offending allergens or irritants; repeated contact will lead to recurrent exacerbations of symptoms. Topical steroids have long been the mainstay of treatment, but tacrolimus and pimecrolimus are becoming more common. Although first approved for AD, they are increasingly shown to effectively and rapidly improve ACD and ICD as well while avoiding steroid side effects such as skin atrophy, telangiectasias, and hyperpigmentation [65,74,75]. Mild transient burning and pruritis were the only adverse effects [75].

## Inflammatory

Management is summarized in Table 4. Many patients have involvement of extraorbital skin and other organ systems, which should be managed with other appropriate specialists such as primary care physicians, dermatologists, and rheumatologists.

**Table 6**
Neoplastic causes of eyelid irritation

| Condition | Background | Signs and Symptoms | Management |
|---|---|---|---|
| Actinic keratosis (AK) (Fig. 14) | • Premalignant, dysplastic lesion of epidermal keratocytes | • Most typical presentation: hyperkeratotic, scaly, "sandpaper" textured papule or macule<br>• Alternative presentation [95]:<br>○ Cutaneous horns<br>○ Pigmented lesions<br>○ Margin-involvement masquerading as blepharitis<br>• May have pruritis | • Surgical resection with permanent pathology, Mohs, frozen section<br>• Less common [101–107]<br>○ Cryotherapy, photodynamic therapy (PDT)<br>○ Topical such as 5-fluorouracil, imiquimod, diclofenac, ingenol mebutate |
| Squamous cell carcinoma (SqCC) (Fig. 15) | • Malignant lesion of squamous epithelium<br>• Most common on medial canthus and lower lids<br>• Frequent involvement of lid margins [96]<br>• SqCC in situ (Bowen disease) is confined within epidermis | • Firm plaque or nodule with overlying scaly keratinization<br>• Erosions, fissures, ulcer, spontaneous bleeding with lesion progression<br>• Alternative presentations [96,97]:<br>○ Cutaneous horn<br>○ Papilloma<br>○ Masquerading as chronic blepharitis or chalazion<br>• Bowen disease: erythematous plaque | • Most common [108,102]<br>○ Surgical resection with Mohs, frozen section control, permanent pathology<br>○ Radiation<br>• Less common<br>○ Cryotherapy<br>○ Electrodesiccation with curettage<br>○ PDT<br>• Tropical such as 5-fluorouracil and imiquimod as pretreatment before surgery or for poor surgical candidates<br>• Immunotherapy such as pembrolizumab, erlotinib [109,110] |

| | | | |
|---|---|---|---|
| Sebaceous cell carcinoma (SbCC) (Fig. 16) | • Rare, aggressive malignant lesion of sebaceous glands<br>o Meibomian glands<br>o Glands of Zeis<br>o Caruncle<br>• Eyelid margin and tarsal conjunctiva frequently involved [67] | • Painless, yellowish nodule or thickening of eyelid margin<br>• Frequently mimics: [98,99]<br>o Blepharitis, chalazia, and blepharoconjunctivitis<br>o SqCC, basal cell carcinoma | • Surgical resection with Mohs, frozen section control, or wide local excision [111]<br>• For diffuse lesions, conjunctival map biopsies [111]<br>• For local invasion confined to orbit, exenteration<br>• Adjuvant cryotherapy and topical mitomycin C [99]<br>• Radiation can be adjuvant or primary treatment in poor surgical candidates [67,111] |
| Cutaneous T-cell lymphoma (CTCL) (Fig. 17) | • Epidermal infiltration of malignant T-cells | • Progression through 3 stages<br>o Patches<br>o Infiltrative plaques<br>o Nodular tumors<br>• Common presentations include cicatricial ectropion, diffuse lid thickening, blepharitis, erythematous patches, ulceration [100,112]<br>• Symptoms include pruritis and burning [113] | • All stages: lid hygiene, electron beam therapy [94]<br>• Early patch stage: topical corticosteroids, ultraviolet B (UVB) phototherapy [94,114]<br>• Plaque stage: topical nitrogen mustard, psoralen plus ultraviolet A (PUVA) photochemotherapy [100]<br>• Less common: topical imiquimod, methotrexate, interferon-alpha, retinoids [100,113] |

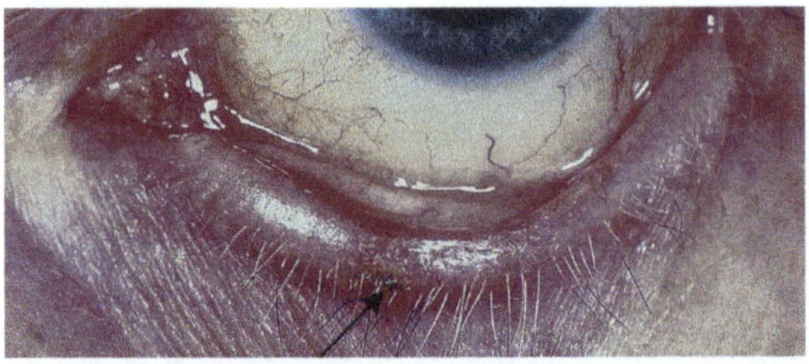

**Fig. 14.** Actinic keratosis. Left lower eyelid margin actinic keratosis (*arrow*) that appears as focal area of anterior blepharitis crusting at lash bases and overlying dark lesions. (Reproduced, with permission, from Foster JA, *2017-2018 Basic and Clinical Science Course*, Section 07, Orbit, Eyelids, and Lacrimal System American Academy of Ophthalmology, Copyright 2017.)

## Infectious

Management is summarized in Table 5. Of note, early recognition is essential for necrotizing fasciitis.

## Neoplastic

Management is summarized in Table 6. Most actinic keratosis, squamous cell carcinoma, and sebaceous cell carcinoma (SbCC) are primarily managed surgically. Various topical therapies are under investigation but require more data and careful use as they can cause ocular surface irritation.

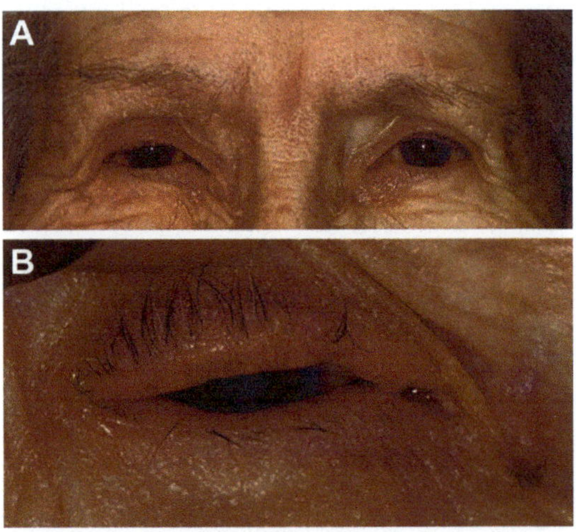


**Fig. 15.** Squamous cell carcinoma.(*A*) A 91-year-old woman presenting with pain, erythematous, crusting of right eyelids. Signs and symptoms were more prominent on the right upper eyelid. (*B*) Limited improvement on conservative measures such as preservative free artificial tears and medicated drops lead to biopsy.

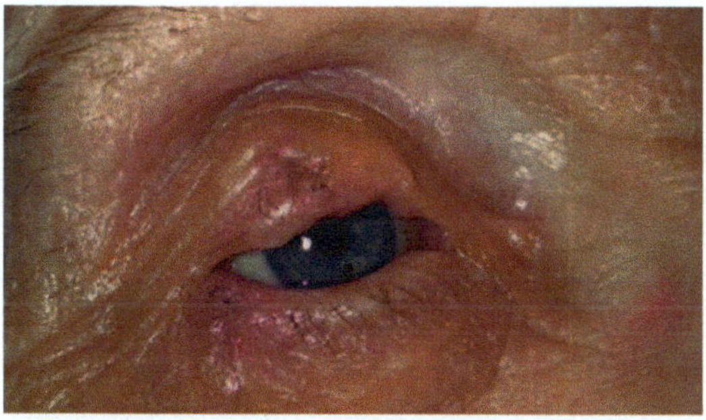

**Fig. 16.** Sebaceous cell carcinoma. Distortion of upper eyelid along with erythema, swelling, and lash loss of upper and lower eyelids. (Reproduced, with permission, from Purdy EP, *Focal Points*, Malignant Eyelid Tumors and Their Management, AmericanAcademy of Ophthalmology, Copyright 2018.)

## SUMMARY

All eye care providers will encounter patients with eyelid irritation. Thorough history taking can lead to the diagnosis. If the patient presents in a chronic phase, asking about the initial signs and symptoms might provide clues. When allergic or irritant contact dermatitis is suspected, patients should be asked about contact with a thorough list of possible offending agents, some of which are listed in Table 3. Many patients do not require formal patch testing if an offending agent is identified and successfully avoided. When an offending agent is not easily identified or symptoms persist even with avoidance, patients should be referred for patch testing to identify the specific allergen.

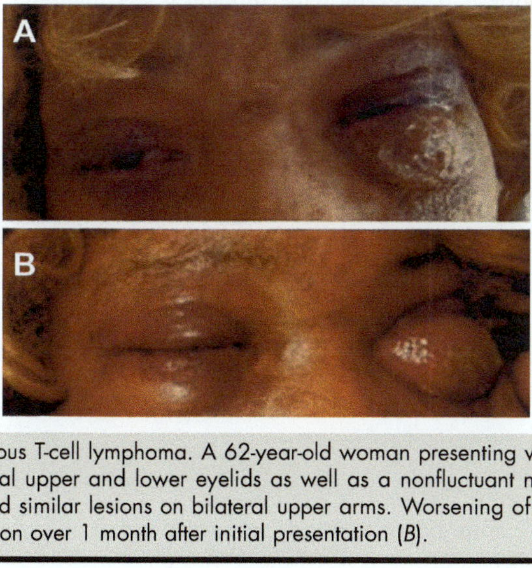


**Fig. 17.** Cutaneous T-cell lymphoma. A 62-year-old woman presenting with thickening and crusting of bilateral upper and lower eyelids as well as a nonfluctuant nodule of left lower lid (*A*). Patient had similar lesions on bilateral upper arms. Worsening of erythema, edema, and left lower lesion over 1 month after initial presentation (*B*).

When examining, attention should be paid to the laterality and location of the lesions, the appearance of the lash bases, and loss of lashes. Some findings are pathognomonic, such as cylindrical sleeves of lash bases for demodicosis. Assessing the face, head, and neck for skin involvement and systemic signs such as a rash on the rest of the body, weakness, joint pain, and fever can point toward the correct diagnosis.

Some findings signal more ominous conditions and should expedite workup and management. When patients present with eyelid erythema and edema along with fever and chills, patients should be assessed for infectious causes. Other warning signs include hypotension or shock. Patients with afferent pupillary defect, ophthalmoplegia, or other cranial nerve deficits should be worked up for orbital cellulitis, necrotizing fasciitis, mucormycosis, and cavernous sinus thrombosis.

When patients present with concerning signs such as lash loss or unilateral blepharitis, the clinician should revisit a wider differential diagnosis. The potential for malignancies should not be forgotten. In a study of 60 cases of SbCC, the diagnosis was suspected in only one-third of cases at initial presentation [99]. Suspicious lesions should be biopsied without delay to decrease morbidity and mortality.

Even with all the information, some conditions will be difficult to correctly diagnose immediately. Patients should be followed to monitor improvement. Patch testing should be considered for refractory dermatitis, as ACD may be present with other conditions such as AD and seborrheic blepharitis. Patients also may benefit from getting patch tested with their own products, as the allergen will not be found in standard trays in up to 12.5% of patch-tested patients [54].

The authors propose a diagnostic flowchart to aid with diagnosis in Fig. 18. Several caveats exist to this flowchart. First, there are always exceptions to the rule, and patients can and will present with unusual manifestations. Typically, bilateral conditions can present with unilateral involvement and vice versa.

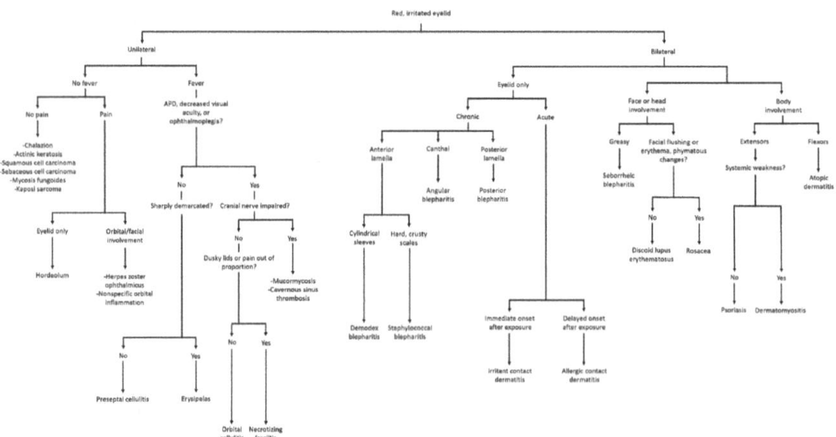


**Fig. 18.** Diagnostic flowchart for erythematous, irritated eyelids.

Some conditions that are associated with other systemic or facial findings may present with isolated eyelid findings. For example, atopic dermatitis, psoriasis, and discoid lupus erythematosus may present with eyelid changes exclusively without rashes and plaques elsewhere. Malignancies such as SbCC and cutaneous T-cell lymphoma are known to have variable presentations and masquerade as more benign conditions. Patients also can present with more than one of these conditions simultaneously.

For chronic conditions such as anterior and posterior blepharitis, rosacea, and AD, patients should be counseled on this chronicity and the almost guaranteed risk of relapse without maintenance therapy. With the proper expectations, patients are less likely to be frustrated with symptom flares and more adherent with long-term use of warm compresses, lid scrubs, and ocular surface lubrication.

Topical steroids are the first-line treatment of several of the conditions discussed, including ACD, ICD, and AD. They also are used for acute inflammatory episodes of phlyctenular or marginal keratitis that may present with blepharitis. Although steroids work well, multiple side effects occur such as skin atrophy, telangiectasias, increased intraocular pressure, and cataract formation. As such, the general rule is to use the lowest potency and shortest duration necessary.

Newer steroid-sparing agents tacrolimus and pimecrolimus have allowed decreased dependency on steroids. These agents have been approved for AD first and have been used with success. More recently, they have been applied for ACD, ICD, rosacea, and posterior blepharitis. Although not officially approved, tacrolimus and pimecrolimus are promising additions to therapeutic regimens.

Multispecialty ophthalmic care may be indicated in patients who have persistent or worsening eyelid irritation if it leads to ocular pathology such as aqueous tear deficiency, keratitis, and corneal ulcers. In addition, patients requiring systemic treatment and co-management of extraorbital manifestations should be referred to appropriate specialties such as dermatology and rheumatology.

## CLINICS CARE POINTS

- When patients with irritated eyelids present with fever, rule out infectious causes such as preseptal or orbital cellulitis, erysipelas, necrotizing fasciitis, and herpes zoster ophthalmicus. Avoid starting steroids until infection is ruled out.
- When presumed preseptal cellulitis is accompanied by pain out of proportion, dusky hue, or rapid progression, consider necrotizing fasciitis.
- Unilateral or very asymmetric blepharitis is suspicious for malignancy and should be biopsied promptly if minimal improvement with conservative management.
- When patients present with pruritis and cylindrical sleeves at eyelash bases, treat with tea tree oil products for demodicosis.
- When patients worsen with topical steroids, consider patch testing for steroid hypersensitivity

## Disclosure

The authors have nothing to disclose.

## References

[1] Ayala F, Fabbrocini G, Bacchilega R, et al. Eyelid dermatitis: an evaluation of 447 patients. Am J Contact Dermat 2003;14(2):69–74.
[2] Rozas-Muñoz E, Gamé D, Serra-Baldrich E. Allergic contact dermatitis by anatomical regions: diagnostic clues. dermatitis de contacto alérgica por regiones anatómicas. Claves Diagnósticas *Actas Dermosifiliogr (Engl Ed* 2018;109(6):485–507.
[3] Scotto J, Fears TR, Fraumeni JF. Incidence of non-melanoma skin cancer in the United States. US National Cancer Institute; 1981. Available at. http://www.ciesin.columbia.edu/docs/001-526/001-526.html NIH Pub. No. 82-2433.
[4] Lemp MA, Nichols KK. Blepharitis in the United States 2009: a survey-based perspective on prevalence and treatment. Ocul Surf 2009;7(2 Suppl):S1–14.
[5] Smith RE, Flowers CW Jr. Chronic blepharitis: a review. CLAO J 1995;21(3):200–7.
[6] McCulley JP, Dougherty JM, Deneau DG. Classification of chronic blepharitis. Ophthalmology 1982;89(10):1173–80.
[7] Dougherty JM, McCulley JP. Comparative bacteriology of chronic blepharitis. Br J Ophthalmol 1984;68(8):524–8.
[8] Groden LR, Murphy B, Rodnite J, et al. Lid flora in blepharitis. Cornea 1991;10(1):50–3.
[9] Bernardes TF, Bonfioli AA. Blepharitis. Semin Ophthalmol 2010;25(3):79–83.
[10] Seal D, Ficker L, Ramakrishnan M, et al. Role of staphylococcal toxin production in blepharitis. Ophthalmology 1990;97(12):1684–8.
[11] O'Brien TP. The role of bacteria in blepharitis. Ocul Surf 2009;7(2 Suppl):S21–2.
[12] Dougherty JM, McCulley JP. Bacterial lipases and chronic blepharitis. Invest Ophthalmol Vis Sci 1986;27(4):486–91.
[13] Amescua G, Akpek EK, Farid M, et al. Blepharitis preferred practice pattern. Ophthalmology 2019;126(1):P56–93.
[14] Pflugfelder SC, Karpecki PM, Perez VL. Treatment of blepharitis: recent clinical trials. Ocul Surf 2014;12(4):273–84.
[15] Jackson WB. Blepharitis: current strategies for diagnosis and management. Can J Ophthalmol 2008;43(2):170–9.
[16] Khan JA, Hoover D, Ide CH. Methicillin-resistant Staphylococcus epidermidis blepharitis. Am J Ophthalmol 1984;98(5):562–5.
[17] Dougherty JM, McCulley JP, Silvany RE, et al. The role of tetracycline in chronic blepharitis. Inhibition of lipase production in staphylococci. Invest Ophthalmol Vis Sci 1991;32(11):2970–5.
[18] Sabeti S, Kheirkhah A, Yin J, et al. Management of meibomian gland dysfunction: a review. Surv Ophthalmol 2020;65(2):205–17.
[19] Igami TZ, Holzchuh R, Osaki TH, et al. Oral azithromycin for treatment of posterior blepharitis. Cornea 2011;30(10):1145–9.
[20] Gupta AK, Bluhm R, Cooper EA, et al. Seborrheic dermatitis. Dermatol Clin 2003;21(3):401–12.
[21] Thygeson P, Vaughan DG Jr. Seborrheic blepharitis. Trans Am Ophthalmol Soc 1954;52:173–88.
[22] Shine WE, Silvany R, McCulley JP. Relation of cholesterol-stimulated Staphylococcus aureus growth to chronic blepharitis. Invest Ophthalmol Vis Sci 1993;34(7):2291–6.
[23] Beltrani VS. Eyelid dermatitis. Curr Allergy Asthma Rep 2001;1(4):380–8.
[24] Arici C, Mergen B, Yildiz-Tas A, et al. Randomized double-blind trial of wipes containing terpinen-4-ol and hyaluronate versus baby shampoo in seborrheic blepharitis patients [published online ahead of print, 2021 Jun 28]. *Eye (Lond)*.
[25] McCulley JP, Dougherty JM. Bacterial aspects of chronic blepharitis. Trans Ophthalmol Soc U K 1986;105(Pt 3):314–8.

[26] Borchman D, Foulks GN, Yappert MC, et al. Human meibum lipid conformation and thermodynamic changes with meibomian-gland dysfunction. Invest Ophthalmol Vis Sci 2011;52(6):3805–17.
[27] Prabhasawat P, Tesavibul N, Mahawong W. A randomized double-masked study of 0.05% cyclosporine ophthalmic emulsion in the treatment of meibomian gland dysfunction. Cornea 2012;31(12):1386–93.
[28] Sakassegawa-Naves FE, Ricci HMM, Moscovici BK, et al. Tacrolimus ointment for refractory posterior blepharitis. Curr Eye Res 2017;42(11):1440–4.
[29] Maskin SL, Testa WR. Growth of meibomian gland tissue after intraductal meibomian gland probing in patients with obstructive meibomian gland dysfunction. Br J Ophthalmol 2018;102(1):59–68.
[30] Goldberg DJ. Current trends in intense pulsed light. J Clin Aesthet Dermatol 2012;5(6): 45–53.
[31] Prieto VG, Sadick NS, Lloreta J, et al. Effects of intense pulsed light on sun-damaged human skin, routine, and ultrastructural analysis. Lasers Surg Med 2002;30(2):82–5.
[32] Thygeson P, Kimura SJ. Chronic conjunctivitis. Trans Am Acad Ophthalmol Otolaryngol 1963;67:494–517.
[33] van Bijsterveld OP. Bacterial proteases in Moraxella angular conjunctivitis. Am J Ophthalmol 1971;72(1):181–4.
[34] Mitsui Y, Hinokuma S, Tanaka C. Etiology of angular conjunctivitis. Am J Ophthalmol 1951;34(11):1579–86.
[35] Chang YS, Huang YC. Role of Demodex mite infestation in rosacea: a systematic review and meta-analysis. J Am Acad Dermatol 2017;77(3):441–7, e6.
[36] Tavassoli S, Wong N, Chan E. Ocular manifestations of rosacea: a clinical review. Clin Exp Ophthalmol 2021;49(2):104–17.
[37] Wladis EJ, Adam AP. Treatment of ocular rosacea. Surv Ophthalmol 2018;63(3):340–6.
[38] Akhyani M, Ehsani AH, Ghiasi M, et al. Comparison of efficacy of azithromycin vs. doxycycline in the treatment of rosacea: a randomized open clinical trial. Int J Dermatol 2008;47(3):284–8.
[39] Barnhorst DA Jr, Foster JA, Chern KC, et al. The efficacy of topical metronidazole in the treatment of ocular rosacea. Ophthalmology 1996;103(11):1880–3.
[40] Amir Ali A, Vender R, Vender R. The role of IL-17 in papulopustular rosacea and future directions. J Cutan Med Surg 2019;23(6):635–41.
[41] Shah PP, Stein RL, Perry HD. Update on the management and treatment of Demodex blepharitis [published online ahead of print, 2021 Nov 4]. Cornea.
[42] Kim M, Kim J, Jeong SW, et al. Inhibition of mast cell infiltration in an LL-37-induced rosacea mouse model using topical brimonidine tartrate 0.33% gel. Exp Dermatol 2017;26(11): 1143–5.
[43] Kheirkhah A, Casas V, Li W, et al. Corneal manifestations of ocular demodex infestation. Am J Ophthalmol 2007;143(5):743–9.
[44] Liu J, Sheha H, Tseng SC. Pathogenic role of Demodex mites in blepharitis. Curr Opin Allergy Clin Immunol 2010;10(5):505–10.
[45] Gao YY, Di Pascuale MA, Li W, et al. High prevalence of Demodex in eyelashes with cylindrical dandruff. Invest Ophthalmol Vis Sci 2005;46(9):3089–94.
[46] English FP, Nutting WB. Demodicosis of ophthalmic concern. Am J Ophthalmol 1981;91(3):362–72.
[47] Navel V, Mulliez A, Benoist d'Azy C, et al. Efficacy of treatments for Demodex blepharitis: a systematic review and meta-analysis. Ocul Surf 2019;17(4):655–69.
[48] Cheng AM, Sheha H, Tseng SC. Recent advances on ocular Demodex infestation. Curr Opin Ophthalmol 2015;26(4):295–300.
[49] Fulk GW, Murphy B, Robins MD. Pilocarpine gel for the treatment of demodicosis–a case series. Optom Vis Sci 1996;73(12):742–5.

[50] Hecht I, Melzer-Golik A, Sadi Szyper N, et al. Permethrin cream for the treatment of demodex blepharitis. Cornea 2019;38(12):1513–8.
[51] Shine WE, McCulley JP. Role of wax ester fatty alcohols in chronic blepharitis. Invest Ophthalmol Vis Sci 1993;34(13):3515–21.
[52] Starr PA, Macdonald A. Oculocutaneous aspects of rosacea. Proc R Soc Med 1969;62(1): 9–11.
[53] Ghanem VC, Mehra N, Wong S, et al. The prevalence of ocular signs in acne rosacea: comparing patients from ophthalmology and dermatology clinics. Cornea 2003;22(3): 230–3.
[54] Feser A, Plaza T, Vogelgsang L, et al. Periorbital dermatitis–a recalcitrant disease: causes and differential diagnoses. Br J Dermatol 2008;159(4):858–63.
[55] Kemal M, Sümer Z, Toker MI, et al. The prevalence of demodex folliculorum in blepharitis patients and the normal population. Ophthalmic Epidemiol 2005;12(4):287–90.
[56] Amin KA, Belsito DV. The aetiology of eyelid dermatitis: a 10-year retrospective analysis. Contact Dermatitis 2006;55(5):280–5.
[57] Landeck L, John SM, Geier J. Topical ophthalmic agents as allergens in periorbital dermatitis. Br J Ophthalmol 2014;98(2):259–62.
[58] Valsecchi R, Imberti G, Martino D, et al. Eyelid dermatitis: an evaluation of 150 patients. Contact Dermatitis 1992;27(3):143–7.
[59] Warshaw EM, Voller LM, Maibach HI, et al. Eyelid dermatitis in patients referred for patch testing: retrospective analysis of North American contact dermatitis group data, 1994-2016. J Am Acad Dermatol 2021;84(4):953–64.
[60] Chisholm SAM, Couch SM, Custer PL. Etiology and management of allergic eyelid dermatitis. Ophthalmic Plast Reconstr Surg 2017;33(4):248–50.
[61] Nosbaum A, Vocanson M, Rozieres A, et al. Allergic and irritant contact dermatitis. Eur J Dermatol 2009;19(4):325–32.
[62] Guin JD. Eyelid dermatitis: experience in 203 cases. J Am Acad Dermatol 2002;47(5): 755–65.
[63] McDaniel LM, Couch SM. Allergic eyelid dermatitis as the sole manifestation of gold hypersensitivity. Ophthalmic Plast Reconstr Surg 2017;33(4):e80–2.
[64] Björkner B, Bruze M, Möller H, et al. Allergic contact dermatitis as a complication of lid loading with gold implants. Dermatitis 2008;19(3):148–53.
[65] Feser A, Mahler V. Periorbital dermatitis: causes, differential diagnoses and therapy. J Dtsch Dermatol Ges 2010;8(3):159–66.
[66] Gönül M, Gül U. Detection of contact hypersensitivity to corticosteroids in allergic contact dermatitis patients who do not respond to topical corticosteroids. Contact Dermatitis 2005;53(2):67–70.
[67] Song X, Jia R, Fan X. An update on eyelid sebaceous cell carcinoma. Int Ophthalmol Clin 2019;59(2):1–11.
[68] Morris S, Barlow R, Selva D, et al. Allergic contact dermatitis: a case series and review for the ophthalmologist. Br J Ophthalmol 2011;95(7):903–8.
[69] Huang CX, Yiannias JA, Killian JM, et al. Seven common allergen groups causing eyelid dermatitis: education and avoidance strategies. Clin Ophthalmol 2021;15:1477–90.
[70] Baker BS. The role of microorganisms in atopic dermatitis. Clin Exp Immunol 2006;144(1): 1–9.
[71] Nakata K, Inoue Y, Harada J, et al. A high incidence of Staphylococcus aureus colonization in the external eyes of patients with atopic dermatitis. Ophthalmology 2000;107(12): 2167–71.
[72] Beck KM, Seitzman GD, Yang EJ, et al. Ocular co-morbidities of atopic dermatitis. part i: associated ocular diseases. Am J Clin Dermatol 2019;20(6):797–805.
[73] Wolf R, Orion E, Tüzün Y. Periorbital (eyelid) dermatides. Clin Dermatol 2014;32(1): 131–40.

[74] Mensing CO, Mensing CH, Mensing H. Treatment with pimecrolimus cream 1% clears irritant dermatitis of the periocular region, face and neck. Int J Dermatol 2008;47(9):960–4.
[75] Freeman AK, Serle J, VanVeldhuisen P, et al. Tacrolimus ointment in the treatment of eyelid dermatitis. Cutis 2004;73(4):267–71.
[76] Belsito DV, Fransway AF, Fowler JF Jr, et al. Allergic contact dermatitis to detergents: a multicenter study to assess prevalence. J Am Acad Dermatol 2002;46(2):200–6.
[77] Pandit SA, Glass LRD. Non-glaucoma periocular allergic, atopic, and irritant dermatitis at an academic institution: a retrospective review. Orbit 2019;38(2):112–8.
[78] Cooper SM, Shaw S. Eyelid dermatitis: an evaluation of 232 patch test patients over 5 years. *Contact Dermatitis* 2000;42(5):291–3.
[79] Eustace P, Pierse D. Ocular psoriasis. Br J Ophthalmol 1970;54(12):810–3.
[80] Cruz NFSD, Brandão LS, Cruz SFSD, et al. Ocular manifestations of psoriasis. Arq Bras Oftalmol 2018;81(3):219–25.
[81] Wolf R. How to manage psoriasis of the eyelids. a glance at opinions of other dermatologists. Dermatologica 1986;173(3):105–8.
[82] Lebwohl M, Freeman AK, Chapman MS, et al. Tacrolimus ointment is effective for facial and intertriginous psoriasis. J Am Acad Dermatol 2004;51(5):723–30.
[83] Acharya N, Pineda R 2nd, Uy HS, et al. Discoid lupus erythematosus masquerading as chronic blepharoconjunctivitis. Ophthalmology 2005;112(5):e19–23.
[84] Wang X, Wang P, Wang M, et al. Discoid lupus erythematosus solely involving the eyelids: case report and literature review. Int J Dermatol 2021;60(10):1190–8.
[85] Ghauri AJ, Valenzuela AA, O'Donnell B, et al. Periorbital discoid lupus erythematosus. Ophthalmology 2012;119(10):2193–4, e11.
[86] Knott HM, Martínez JD. Innovative management of lupus erythematosus. Dermatol Clin 2010;28(3):489–99.
[87] Dalakas MC, Hohlfeld R. Polymyositis and dermatomyositis. Lancet 2003;362(9388): 971–82.
[88] Driver PJ, Lemp MA. Meibomian gland dysfunction. Surv Ophthalmol 1996;40(5): 343–67.
[89] Liesegang TJ. Herpes zoster ophthalmicus natural history, risk factors, clinical presentation, and morbidity. Ophthalmology 2008;115(2 Suppl):S3–12.
[90] Grosshans EM. The red face: erysipelas. Clin Dermatol 1993;11(2):307–13.
[91] Lazzeri D, Lazzeri S, Figus M, et al. Periorbital necrotising fasciitis. Br J Ophthalmol 2010;94(12):1577–85.
[92] Shield DR, Servat J, Paul S, et al. Periocular necrotizing fasciitis causing blindness. JAMA Ophthalmol 2013;131(9):1225–7.
[93] Aakalu VK, Sajja K, Cook JL, et al. Group A streptococcal necrotizing fasciitis of the eyelids and face managed with debridement and adjunctive intravenous immunoglobulin. Ophthalmic Plast Reconstr Surg 2009;25(4):332–4.
[94] Luksich JA, Holds JB, Hartstein ME. Conservative management of necrotizing fasciitis of the eyelids. Ophthalmology 2002;109(11):2118–22.
[95] López-Tizón E, Mencía-Gutiérrez E, Garrido-Ruíz M, et al. Clinicopathological study of 21 cases of eyelid actinic keratosis. Int Ophthalmol 2009;29(5):379–84.
[96] Reifler DM, Hornblass A. Squamous cell carcinoma of the eyelid [published correction appears in Surv Ophthalmol 1986 Jul-Aug;31(1):77]. Surv Ophthalmol 1986;30(6): 349–65.
[97] Sullivan TJ. Squamous cell carcinoma of eyelid, periocular, and periorbital skin. Int Ophthalmol Clin 2009;49(4):17–24.
[98] Bernardini FP. Management of malignant and benign eyelid lesions. Curr Opin Ophthalmol 2006;17(5):480–4.
[99] Shields JA, Demirci H, Marr BP, et al. Sebaceous carcinoma of the eyelids: personal experience with 60 cases. Ophthalmology 2004;111(12):2151–7.

[100] Cook BE Jr, Bartley GB, Pittelkow MR. Ophthalmic abnormalities in patients with cutaneous T-cell lymphoma. Ophthalmology 1999;106(7):1339–44.
[101] Lagler CN, Freitag SK. Management of periocular actinic keratosis: a review of practice patterns among ophthalmic plastic surgeons. Ophthalmic Plast Reconstr Surg 2012;28(4): 277–81.
[102] Moran JM, Phelps PO. Periocular skin cancer: diagnosis and management. Dis Mon 2020;66(10):101046.
[103] Stockfleth E, Sibbring GC, Alarcon I. New topical treatment options for actinic keratosis: a systematic review. Acta Derm Venereol 2016;96(1):17–22 [published correction appears in acta derm venereol. 2016 mar;96(3):431].
[104] Couch SM, Custer PL. Topical 5-fluorouracil for the treatment of periocular actinic keratosis and low-grade squamous malignancy. Ophthalmic Plast Reconstr Surg 2012;28(3): 181–3.
[105] Batra R, Sundararajan S, Sandramouli S. Topical diclofenac gel for the management of periocular actinic keratosis. Ophthalmic Plast Reconstr Surg 2012;28(1):1–3.
[106] Toledo-Alberola F, Belinchón-Romero I, Guijarro-Llorca J, et al. Photodynamic therapy as a response to the challenge of treating actinic keratosis in the eyelid area. Actas Dermosifiliogr 2012;103(10):938–9.
[107] Ross AH, Kennedy CT, Collins C, et al. The use of imiquimod in the treatment of periocular tumours. Orbit 2010;29(2):83–7.
[108] Thosani MK, Schneck G, Jones EC. Periocular squamous cell carcinoma. Dermatol Surg 2008;34(5):585–99.
[109] Yin VT, Pfeiffer ML, Esmaeli B. Targeted therapy for orbital and periocular basal cell carcinoma and squamous cell carcinoma. Ophthalmic Plast Reconstr Surg 2013;29(2):87–92.
[110] Habib LA, Wolkow N, Freitag SK, et al. Advances in immunotherapy and periocular malignancy. Semin Ophthalmol 2019;34(4):327–33.
[111] Owen JL, Kibbi N, Worley B, et al. Sebaceous carcinoma: evidence-based clinical practice guidelines. Lancet Oncol 2019;20(12):e699–714.
[112] Game JA, Davies R. Mycosis fungoides causing severe lower eyelid ulceration. Clin Exp Ophthalmol 2002;30(5):369–71.
[113] Colossi CG, Mondadori J, Barreto PKM, et al. Mycosis fungoides: analysis of ophthalmologic findings in a series of cases. Case Rep Dermatol Med 2019;2019:2380598, Published 2019 Jan 20.
[114] Hodak E, Pavlovsky L. Phototherapy of mycosis fungoides. Dermatol Clin 2015;33(4): 697–702.
[115] Haque RM, Torkildsen GL, Brubaker K, et al. Multicenter open-label study evaluating the efficacy of azithromycin ophthalmic solution 1% on the signs and symptoms of subjects with blepharitis. Cornea 2010;29(8):871–7.

# Uveitis

Advances in Ophthalmology and Optometry 7 (2022) 433–448

ADVANCES IN OPHTHALMOLOGY AND OPTOMETRY

# Uveitic Glaucoma

Erick Rivera-Grana, MD[a,1], Stephanie M. Llop, MD[b,*]

[a]Department of Ophthalmology, University of Puerto Rico Medical Sciences Campus, PO Box 365067, San Juan, PR 00936, USA; [b]Bascom Palmer Eye Institute, University of Miami Miller School of Medicine, 900 Northwest 17th Street, Miami, FL 33136, USA

**Keywords**

• Uveitis • Glaucoma • Uveitic glaucoma • Inflammatory glaucoma

**Key points**

- Uveitic glaucoma treatment differs greatly from other glaucoma syndromes, and, therefore, it should not be treated equally. Concomitant treatment of inflammation and elevated intraocular pressure must be achieved in a timely fashion to minimize chronic complications.
- No clear treatment algorithm exists, and there is limited data studying glaucoma treatment modalities for uveitic glaucoma.
- Further studies are needed to establish best treatment approaches for uveitic glaucoma depending on the etiology.

## INTRODUCTION

Uveitis is defined as an inflammation involving uveal tissue, which consists of 3 main components: iris, ciliary body, and choroid. Raised intraocular pressure (IOP) is a frequent complication of chronic and recurrent uveitis. In some conditions, such as Posner-Schlossman and herpetic uveitis, the IOP may be elevated at presentation [1,2]. Uveitic glaucoma (UG) is defined as increased IOP with associated optic nerve damage, causing characteristic glaucomatous vision loss in patients with uveitis [3]. In the United States, it is estimated that approximately 20% of patients with uveitis develop glaucoma [1,4]. IOP spikes in patients with uveitis tend to be higher, and progression of glaucomatous optic neuropathy is faster [5]. The first-line treatment for most noninfectious uveitis is corticosteroid medications, which predispose patients to ocular hypertension and may eventually lead to glaucomatous damage causing

[1]Present address: 2878 El Monte Street. Urb El Monte. Ponce. PR 00716.

*Corresponding author: *E-mail address:* sxl1789@med.miami.edu

https://doi.org/10.1016/j.yaoo.2022.03.014

steroid-induced glaucoma (SIG). The pathophysiology of UG may differ depending on the underlying inflammatory etiology of uveitis. For example, acute uveitis (eg, herpetic uveitis and Posner-Schlossman syndrome [PSS]) are characterized by acute IOP elevation at presentation of inflammation. In contrast, chronic anterior uveitis (eg, sarcoid-associated uveitis) may develop a gradual increase in IOP [3]. Elevation of IOP can be due to open-angle, closed-angle, or mixed mechanisms and steroid-induced processes coexisting [6]. Owing to these variances of etiologies and the addition of possible steroid-induced IOP spikes, the management of UG differs from the standard management of patients with open-angle or closed-angle glaucoma without uveitis. It is essential to be aware of the differences in etiology and management of UG for better IOP and inflammatory control of these patients, which eventually will result in better visual acuity and reduce long-term complications. This article describes the epidemiology, different pathogenesis, and most current medical and surgical treatment modalities for UG.

## SIGNIFICANCE

Approximately 20% of patients with uveitis may develop UG. It is more common in chronic uveitis with an incidence of 11% after 5 years [5]. In other studies, the prevalence of UG has been reported to be as high as 46% in patients with chronic uveitis [7]. No sex predilection seems to exist. Any form of ocular inflammation may be associated with an increased IOP. UG commonly is correlated with increased IOP, although the elevation may occur intermittently, as opposed to primary glaucoma, where pressure-independent mechanisms may be related [3]. The rise of IOP in patients with active inflammation can be a diagnostic challenge due to the uncertainty if the IOP imbalance is due to acute inflammatory changes, anatomic changes of aqueous pathway, or concurrent steroid-induced response. It is thought that UG occurs because of a myriad of events. UG can be caused by open- or closed-angle mechanisms as well as mixed mechanisms.

### Pathogenesis

#### *Open-angle*

An open-angle mechanism is the more common form of UG [5]. Acute anterior uveitis commonly causes hypotonic states because of ciliary body hyposecretion of aqueous humor. In chronic or recurrent inflammation, associated morphologic changes occur in the trabecular meshwork (TM), resulting in increased outflow resistance leading to increased IOP. In intraocular inflammation, the blood-aqueous barrier is disrupted, leading to increased deposition of proteins, inflammatory cells, and debris on the TM, causing an obstruction. The TM endothelium has the ability of phagocytosis; the increase in debris deposition causes increased phagocytosis, leading to cell migration out of the TM. With decreased endothelial cells, reduced trabecular function occurs, resulting in increased IOP [1]. Another factor contributing to high IOP when disruption of the blood-aqueous barrier exists is direct protein deposition in the TM and increased aqueous viscosity causing a sludge effect [1]. Physicians should be aware that patients with no apparent cellularity but with chronic flare have an increased risk of raised IOP. A study by Holland showed that increased flare is a predictor of complications in children with chronic anterior uveitis, including raised IOP [8].

Chronic inflammation may lead to permanent TM morphologic changes, and these changes have been observed to improve with anti-inflammatory treatment.

Herpetic uveitis and PSS are different from other subtypes of infectious and noninfectious uveitis. They present with acute increased IOP since the initial onset of inflammation. Several studies have shown that this initial IOP spike is due to TM inflammation called "trabeculitis." Hogan and colleagues [9] showed that patients with herpetic keratouveitis presented with a thickened trabecular band infiltrated with fibrin and inflammatory cells on histologic studies. Townsend and Kauffman demonstrated that rabbit models with herpetic keratouveitis developed severe infiltration of inflammatory cells in the TM [10]. These findings are examples in the literature that suggest how direct inflammation plays a role in the acute elevation of IOP in herpetic uveitis.

The most common first-line treatment for noninfectious uveitis involves corticosteroid use. Topical corticosteroids have been associated with a rise of 6 to 15 mm Hg from baseline in about one-third of the general population [11]. The exact mechanism by which corticosteroids induce elevation of IOP is not clearly understood, but the most regarded cause is decreased TM outflow [12].

*Closed-angle*

A closed-angle UG mechanism can result because of multiple reasons. The most common cause being posterior synechiae formation. Owing to the aqueous humor's physiologic posterior to anterior outflow, the presence of extensive posterior synechiae can lead to iris bombé, causing a pupillary block. Chronic anterior chamber inflammation may lead to peripheral anterior synechiae (PAS), which could block the TM. This can be avoided with good inflammatory control. A pupil will rarely completely seclude if adequate anti-inflammatory therapy is being given, even if there are nearly 360° of posterior synechiae [13]. Another form of closed angle can be from uveal effusions, which cause forward rotation of the ciliary body and iris root obstructing the TM; this is mainly observed in posterior uveitides such as Vogt-Koyanagi-Harada syndrome (VKH) [5].

## Signs and symptoms

Patients can present with nonspecific symptoms usually associated with increased IOP, such as blurred or decreased visual acuity, eye redness, eye pain, and corneal edema. Periodic monitoring with ancillary testing with optical coherence tomography and visual fields is recommended to assess and monitor optic neuropathy involvement and progression. Understanding the underlying etiology of uveitis can provide helpful information on the pathophysiology of IOP elevation and appropriate treatment of both IOP and inflammation.

## Uveitis etiologies associated with uveitic glaucoma

### *Herpetic uveitis*

Herpes simplex (HSV) and varicella zoster (VZV) viruses are the 2 most common herpes viruses associated with uveitis and increased IOP. An estimated 28% to 45% of patients with HSV keratouveitis develop transient elevated IOP [14]. Secondary glaucoma is the most common complication in patients with herpetic uveitis [5]. Acute increase in IOP in the presence of active iridocyclitis is the hallmark of a herpetic etiology associated with both HSV and VZV. Previous studies of HSV and associated ocular hypertension have shown cellular changes in the TM suggestive of trabeculitis as a cause of elevated IOP [15]. The IOP spikes can be secondary to obstruction of the TM by inflammatory cells and debris and can be as high as 50 to 60 mm Hg. Clinically it is characterized by acute onset, unilateral anterior uveitis, which can be associated with keratitis. Diffuse or sectoral iris atrophy demonstrated by retro illumination at the slit lamp is characteristic of herpetic uveitis but no longer considered pathognomonic of VZV, as it can also be seen with HSV and CMV [5].

Treatment of viral anterior uveitis includes topical corticosteroids and cycloplegic agents. Systemic antiviral drugs such as acyclovir (400–800 mg 5 times/d) or valacyclovir (500 mg–1 g, 3 times/d) can be used for HSV and VZV; low dose for HSV and higher dose for VZV. Prolonged corticosteroid treatment might be required with gradual taper. Management of herpetic secondary glaucoma can be complex, and it depends on several factors: inflammation and elevated IOP. One should never undertreat the inflammation due to fear of steroid response. For IOP management, medical treatment is considered the first line. Historically, there has been a hesitance to use prostaglandins analogs in patients with herpetic uveitis. Several recent reports have shown adequate efficacy and safety [16,17]. If the IOP cannot be adequately controlled with medical management, surgical intervention may be necessary. Inflammation should be suppressed before surgery for better outcomes. Surgical treatments may include glaucoma drainage devices (GDDs) and trabeculectomies.

### *Posner-Schlossman syndrome*

It is also known as glaucomatocyclitic crisis and usually manifests as a recurrent unilateral, mild, acute, nongranulomatous anterior uveitis. Episodes can last from several hours to several days. Clinical signs include markedly elevated IOP, corneal edema, low-grade cell, and flare. IOP elevation in PSS differs from other herpetic etiologies in that it is of greater magnitude ranging from 40 to 70 mm Hg, and usually resolves spontaneously [5,7]. Recent studies suggest cytomegalovirus (CMV) as a possible cause of PSS. An anterior chamber tap is recommended for PCR testing. There is some evidence of a potential role of antiviral therapy in CMV-positive cases. Topical ganciclovir 0.15% with a loading dose of 1 drop 6 times/d and then tapering over 3 months depending on anterior chamber inflammation can be given, while remaining on a minimum maintenance therapy of 3 to 4 times daily [18]. Oral valgancyclovir 900 mg BID for 2 weeks, then 450 mg BID as a maintenance dose can be used [19]. Even though it is generally considered a benign self-limited condition, prompt diagnosis and treatment are paramount since approximately 25% of patients may develop UG [5]. The exact etiology of glaucoma development in PSS is not known. A vascular etiology triggering endothelial dysfunction leading to unstable oxygen supply and disturbance of small vessel autoregulation is the most likely cause [5,20,21].

First-line treatment consists of topical corticosteroids along with antiglaucoma medications. In recurrent cases where surgical management is necessary, limited data exist on comparative procedures to accurately assess the best first-line approach. Artini and Bani published a retrospective case series of 5 patients with PSS-associated glaucoma who underwent trabeculectomy with mitomycin C and found successful results in IOP control [20]. Their study certainly has limitations but shows that trabeculectomy can be an option in these patients.

*Juvenile idiopathic arthritis uveitis*

Juvenile idiopathic arthritis (JIA) is the most common systemic disorder associated with anterior segment inflammation in the pediatric population. It is characterized by arthritis that starts before 16 years of age and episodes that last a minimum of 6 weeks. Clinically, JIA uveitis is associated with bilateral nongranulomatous, asymptomatic anterior segment uveitis. The prevalence of glaucoma ranges from 14% to 42% [5,22,23]. Owing to the natural course of asymptomatic inflammation, pediatric patients with arthritis are to be constantly monitored. Apart from monitoring anterior chamber cell activity, a study by Holland demonstrated the importance of chronic flare in developing long-term complications in patients with JIA [8]. The etiology of glaucoma in these patients can be open angle or closed angle because of posterior synechiae and PAS formation.

The treatment of glaucoma in these patients has particular challenges because of the chronicity and the different mechanisms of glaucoma, but it is crucial to achieve adequate control of inflammation early in the disease to avoid chronic inflammatory complications. The management of glaucoma in JIA uveitis patients consists of IOP-lowering medications as first-line treatment. If severe, glaucoma surgery, which can be either trabeculectomy or GDD, must be considered. Surgery should be performed after good inflammation control has been achieved. Kafkala and colleagues [24] published a retrospective chart review evaluating the safety and efficacy of Ahmed valves and found that Ahmed valve implantation can be an effective and safe procedure for treating pediatric UG. Surgery targeting the drainage angle has been a more recent development in pediatric UG. There have been reports of success with gonioscopy-assisted transluminal trabeculectomy (GATT). This technique targets the pathophysiology of JIA-associated glaucoma [25].

*Vogt-Koyanagi-Harada syndrome*

VKH is a chronic, bilateral, granulomatous panuveitis. Secondary angle-closure glaucoma may occur when choroidal inflammation results in the forward rotation of the ciliary body [5]. This type of glaucoma can be the presenting sign of VKH. Ultrasound biomicroscopy can be used to observe the choroidal thickening and anterior rotation of the ciliary body. Inflammatory insults may produce elevated IOP due to trabeculitis, progressive synechiae angle closure, or iris bombé [26]. Veerappan and colleagues studied the incidence of glaucoma in VKH and found that approximately two-thirds of the eyes that developed glaucoma had PAS and/or posterior synechiae, primarily in iris bombé configuration. These observations suggest that secondary angle closure from VKH-associated inflammation is a major cause of glaucoma in eyes with VKH [26]. Other studies showed that the incidence of glaucoma in VKH could range from 10% to 45% [3,26].

The mainstay treatment for VKH is high-dose corticosteroids, which also can contribute to UG development in these patients. Glaucoma treatment consists of adequate inflammation control to decrease choroidal thickening in patients with ciliary body rotation. As the inflammation dissipates, the thickening reduces, and the anterior chamber deepens, relieving the secondary angle closure. In patients with PAS, synechiolysis can be performed. All other cases can be managed with glaucoma medications and GDD placement if inadequate control with medications.

*Sarcoid uveitis*

Sarcoidosis is a multisystem disease that can produce any form of intraocular inflammation. The most common ocular manifestations include panuveitis, snowballs, periphlebitis, mutton fat keratic precipitates, and iris nodules [3]. Sarcoidosis primarily affects people aged between 20 and 40 years and has a female and African American predominance. Sarcoidosis can have TM precipitates known as Berlin nodules, leading to obstruction of the TM and subsequent rise of the IOP. Owing to anterior segment inflammation, PAS can develop and cellular and inflammatory debris can precipitate in the TM, obstructing aqueous outflow. Mainstay treatment consists of topical and systemic steroids, which also can lead to SIG.

*Steroid-induced glaucoma*

Most cases of noninfectious intraocular inflammatory diseases are treated with some formulation of corticosteroid as first-line treatment. Approximately one-third of patients without a known diagnosis of glaucoma can develop increased IOP of 6 mm Hg to 15 mm Hg with the use of steroids [27]. The term corticosteroid responder is used when patients using corticosteroids medications develop increased IOP. Increased IOP can occur with any type and form of corticosteroids (local or systemic). Table 1 shows different topical anti-inflammatory agents and their IOP-elevating potencies. Table 2 shows different IVT steroid treatments and their risk of developing increased IOP.

The IOP rise commonly occurs 3 to 6 weeks after corticosteroid use and can occur at any point after this, even years later. The IOP spike response is dose and frequency-dependent [11]. The IOP generally can return to baseline within

**Table 1**
Different corticosteroid formulations with their IOP-elevating potencies

| | Relative Potency | Rise in IOP, mm Hg |
|---|---|---|
| *Dexamethasone, 0.1%* (equivalent to betamethasone 0.1%) | 24.0 | 22 |
| *Fluorometholone, 0.1%* | 21.0 | 6 |
| *Prednisolone acetate, 1%* | 2.3 | 10 |
| *Medrysone, 1%* | 1.7 | 1 |
| *Tetrahydrotriamcinolone, 0.25%* | 1.4 | 2 |
| *Hydrocortisone, 0.5%* | 1.0 | 3 |

*From* 2020-2021 Basic and Clinical Science Course (BCSC). Section 2 - Fundamentals and Principles of Ophthalmology. American Academy of Opthalmology; 2020:402.

2 weeks of corticosteroid cessation if there are no irreversible changes to the TM [11,27].

In corticosteroid responders, it is called steroid-induced ocular hypertension (SIOH) when there is increased IOP without optic nerve damage. If this pressure is elevated to a high enough magnitude and prolonged period, it can cause glaucomatous optic neuropathy. When this happens, it is termed SIG, which is considered a type of secondary open-angle glaucoma.

The pathogenesis of SIOH/SIG is attributed to increased resistance to aqueous outflow in the TM. The TM has glucocorticoid receptors. Steroids act on the receptors and alter cell migration and phagocytosis, causing decreased cellularity and increased extracellular matrix deposition, increasing outflow resistance [28]. Risk factors associated with developing SIG include older age, known history of primary open-angle glaucoma (POAG), connective tissue disease, high myopia, and type 1 diabetes mellitus [27,29,30]. It is

**Table 2**
Intravitreal steroid formulations and risk of developing ocular hypertension

| Medication | Dose | Percent (%) risk of developing ocular hypertension |
|---|---|---|
| Triamcinolone acetonide | 4 mg/0.1 mL | 32.1[a] |
| | 8 mg/0.2 mL | 31.8[a] |
| | 10 mg/0.2 mL | 30.0[a] |
| | 20 mg/0.2 mL | 39.8[a] |
| | 25 mg/0.2 mL | 45.9[a] |
| Fluocinolone acetonide implant | 0.59 mg | 65.9[a] |
| | 2.1 mg | 79.0[a] |
| Dexamethasone implant | 0.35 mg | 10.9[b] |
| | 0.7 mg | 15.3[b] |

[a]Ocular hypertension defined as IOP greater than 21 mm Hg or greater than 10 mm Hg from baseline.
[b]Ocular hypertension defined as IOP greater than 25 mm Hg or greater than 10 mm Hg from baseline.

*Adapted from* Kiddee W, Trope GE, Sheng L, Beltran-Agullo L, Smith M, Strungaru MH, Baath J, Buys YM. Intraocular pressure monitoring post intravitreal steroids: a systematic review. Surv Ophthalmol. 2013 Jul-Aug;58(4):291-310.

important to be aware that in children, the IOP elevation and optic nerve damage can be more severe at presentation and progress faster compared with adults [27]. Active monitoring of high-risk SIG patients is of utmost importance. IOP measurement should be planned at 2 weeks and then every 4 to 6 weeks for 2 to 3 months [27]. Treatment is to discontinue corticosteroid use, but this choice is not always an option in a patient with active uveitis. Medical management is similar to POAG, and all current commercial IOP-lowering medications can be used for IOP management. Approximately 1% to 5% of SIG patients develop unresponsive IOP elevation, which ultimately needs surgical management [27]. Of the available GDDs, valved devices, such as the Ahmed valve, provide less postoperative hypotony complications compared with trabeculectomy. A study by Papadaki and colleagues [31] showed Ahmed valve implantation in UG, with 77% and 50% success rates at 1 and 4 years, respectively. With the development and increased utilization of periocular and intraocular steroids, SIG is an increasing phenomenon that ophthalmologists should be highly aware of. Diligent follow-up schedules and prompt treatment are essential, specifically in high-risk SIG patients and the pediatric population.

## PRESENT RELEVANCE AND FUTURE DIRECTIONS TO CONSIDER OR INVESTIGATE

### Standard treatment approaches

*Traditional topical intraocular pressure-lowering medications*

IOP management with topical medications is different in patients with UG than in patients with noninflammatory glaucoma. Traditionally topical beta-blockers and carbonic-anhydrase inhibitors were used as first-line treatment, but recently a shift has occurred to using prostaglandin analogs (PGAs). In the past, resistance existed to using PGAs in patients with UG due to data demonstrating they could exacerbate inflammation. Some studies have shown their effective use in patients with well-controlled uveitis, including herpetic uveitis [5,17,32]. Siddique and colleagues [5] recommend that PGAs be used as first-line treatment in UG patients with quiescent uveitis. PGAs also provide the benefit of decreasing medication burden because of their once-a-day dosing, an important factor to consider in UG patients who probably are using other concurrent topical treatments for their inflammation. In patients with active inflammation, topical beta-blockers seem to be a more appropriate first-line treatment. Topical beta-blockers have a good safety and efficacy profile and are unlikely to worsen inflammation. Alpha-adrenergic agonists (eg, Brimonidine) are known to be vasoactive, which promote more access of proinflammatory mediators into eye tissue and have been associated with inducing granulomatous uveitis in several studies [33,34]. For these reasons, they should be used as third-line treatment. Fig. 1 demonstrates a step-wise approach for topical treatment in patients with UG.

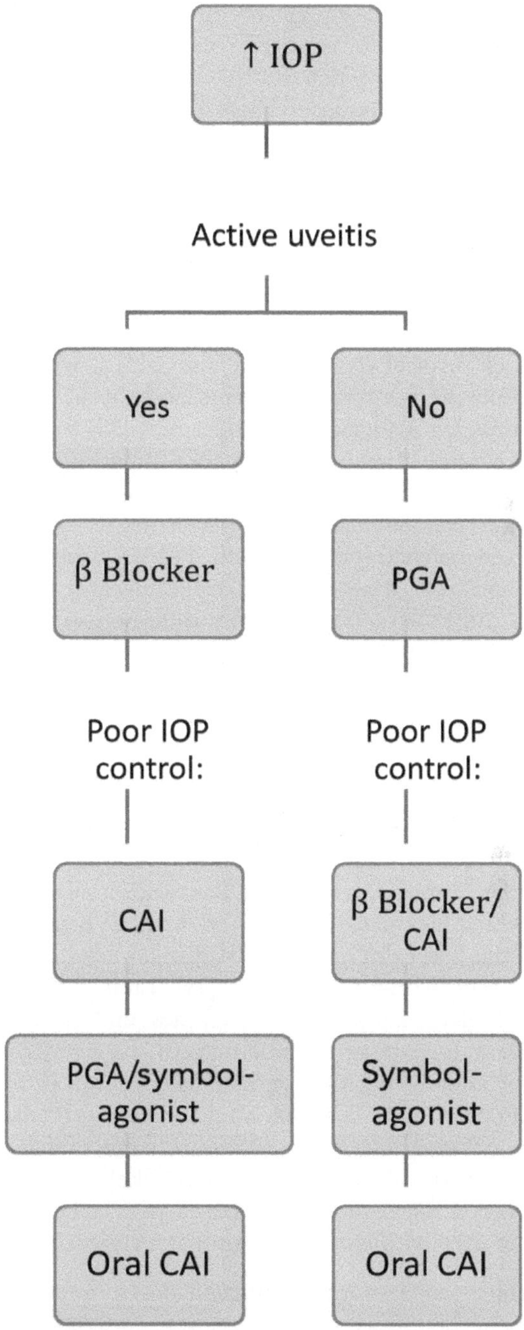


**Fig. 1.** A step-wise approach to using IOP-lowering medications in patients with UG. CAI, carbonic anhydrase inhibitor.

*Trabeculectomy*

Trabeculectomy is indicated for patients with closed-angle, open-angle, or combined mechanism glaucoma when IOP remains elevated despite maximum tolerated medical therapy. Associated risk factors for trabeculectomy failure include young age, black race, history of uveitis, previous ocular surgeries, or combined surgery [35]. The reason why uveitis is associated with trabeculectomy failure can be due to an increase in the number of inflammatory cells, which may alter wound healing, leading to increased scarring [35].

Previous studies have shown that trabeculectomy without the use of antimetabolites can be performed in patients with UG [36,37]. The use of adjuvant antifibrotic agents such as mitomycin C (MMC) has been shown to improve the success rate of surgical treatment of UG with a wide range of 50% to 90%, depending on the number of patients and the length of the follow-up period [38]. A study by Kaburaki and colleagues [39] found no difference in the rate of IOP control after 5 years when comparing trabeculectomy with MMC as initial surgical treatment for patients with UG and primary open-angle patients. Kanaya and colleagues performed a study comparing UG with age- and sex-matched patients with POAG who underwent MMC-trabeculectomy and also showed MMC-trabeculectomy effectively reduced IOP in both UG and POAG. No significant difference occurred in the success rate between UG and POAG [40]. These studies demonstrate that trabeculectomy is a viable surgical procedure in patients with controlled inflammation. Further prospective studies with long-term monitoring and inclusion of patients with uveitis can provide a better assessment of risk and benefits of trabeculectomy in this population.

*Glaucoma drainage devices*

GDD often are used for refractory UG cases. A meta-analysis published in 2016 compared the Ahmed valve and the Baerveldt implant in refractory glaucoma patients, which included UG and showed that both devices lower IOP comparably, but the Baerveldt had better surgical outcomes and was more successful in reducing glaucoma medications [41]. Limited data exist comparing different types of glaucoma-surgical techniques and most of them do not include UG patients. Iverson and colleagues retrospectively compared whether initial GDD implantation in UG eyes had better surgical outcomes and less complications compared with initial filtering surgery with adjuvant antifibrotic therapy. They concluded that both techniques were similar in IOP-lowering achievement, but the nonvalved GDD was more likely to maintain IOP control and avoid reoperation for glaucoma compared with trabeculectomy with antifibrotic therapy in eyes with chronic inflammatory glaucoma [42].

## Treatments apart from well-known intraocular pressure medications and filtering surgery

*Laser treatment*

*Laser trabeculoplasty.* Laser trabeculoplasty is the application of laser energy to the TM. Two types of lasers trabeculoplasties procedures exist, argon laser trabeculoplasty (ALT) and selective laser trabeculoplasty (SLT). These differ in the laser spot size and amount of energy applied to the TM.

In ALT, thermal damage applied to the TM causes shrinkage of collagen fibers, resulting in widening of TM, improving aqueous outflow. There is scarce literature available on the use of ALT in UG. The few available literature reports show that ALT is not a sufficient treatment and usually fails to control the IOP in uveitic eyes because of angle alterations [5,43].

SLT involves the application of laser energy to the TM, which is specifically absorbed by the pigmented trabecular cells, sparing thermal damage to adjacent tissue. A meta-analysis published in 2015 on the efficacy of SLT in open-angle glaucoma showed that one of the most common adverse effects of treatment was anterior chamber inflammation ranging from 0% to 89% of patients [44]. In patients with a history of intraocular inflammations, SLT is considered a relative contraindication [45]. Therefore, SLT has been used sparsely for cases of UG. Maleki and colleagues retrospectively evaluated the efficacy of SLT in 15 patients with uveitis who had received intravitreal steroids. They found that none of the eyes developed new or increased intraocular inflammation, and in 46.7% of eyes IOP was successfully reduced [46]. Zhou and colleagues retrospectively compared the efficacy of primary SLT in UG and SIG, comparing them to POAG. The study showed that UG patients had similar IOP decrease responses compared to POAG, but an increase in the use of hypotensive medications occurred after SLT. With this, they concluded that judicious SLT could be performed in select cases of UG [47]. SLT appears to be an appropriate treatment in some cases of UG. Further large-scale and controlled studies are needed to accurately assess the efficacy of these new treatment modalities in UG patients.

*Peripheral laser iridectomy versus surgical iridectomy.* Laser iridectomy applies laser energy, most commonly using the photo disruptive Q-switched Nd: YAG laser (Nd: YAG) or the photo-thermal Nd: YAG-KTP 532 nm, to the iris to create a hole and allow the aqueous humor to flow into the anterior chamber. It is commonly used in angle-closure glaucoma or as prophylaxis for narrow angles. In UG, patients with chronic anterior inflammation may develop posterior synechiae, and if these synechiae extend 360°, they can obstruct the normal aqueous outflow causing a phenomenon known as seclusion pupillae resulting in acute IOP elevation. One should consider whether an iris procedure is required at all for any given patient with uveitis, even if the person presents with a nearly secluded pupil. Laser peripheral iridectomies (PIs) are not without risks. Iris pigment dispersion associated with the procedure increases intraocular inflammation. A risk of hyphema exists, which can complicate IOP management. Betts and colleagues studied the risk factors for failure of both laser and surgical PIs in patients with uveitis. Young age, the use of ND: YAG laser, iris bombe, and postprocedure inflammation were significant risk factors for iridectomy failure. The median survival time for a YAG PI was 70 days versus 11 years for a surgical PI. For these reasons and complications associated with laser PI, they advocated for the use of early surgical PI rather than laser PI in patients with UG [48].

Patients with UG tend to have increased proteins, fibrin, and inflammatory debris in the aqueous humor, making it a "sticky aqueous." An outpouring of fibrin occurs at the PI site, which may close the small opening created with laser PI. Holland and Barton published an article in which they recommend not to perform prophylactic laser or surgical iridectomies in patients with UG who have well-controlled inflammation [13]. In patients who need iridectomies, such as patients with poorly controlled inflammation or iris bombé, they recommend surgical iridectomy over laser PI. Surgical iridectomy is less inflammatory, reducing pigment deposition into the anterior chamber; it also has the advantage that during the same procedure, one can perform synechialysis, creating a better contiguous space in the posterior chamber [13]. For these reasons, Holland and Barton also advocate for the use of surgical iridectomy over laser PI in patients with uveitis and angle-closure glaucoma [13].

*Minimally invasive glaucoma surgery*

Minimally invasive glaucoma surgery (MIGS) comprises a group of procedures that use microscopic-sized equipment and incisions to improve IOP in glaucoma. These procedures can be categorized into miniaturized versions of trabeculectomy, trabecular bypass operations, and suprachoroidal shunts. These include XEN gel stent, iStent, and Hydrus Microstent. Scarce evidence exists of the use of MIGS for UG. The idea behind the use of these procedures is to reduce the incidence of complications of the traditional glaucoma surgeries such as trabeculectomy and GDD, which are associated with an increased incidence of postoperative complications in uveitic eyes undergoing glaucoma surgery, including ocular hypotony, cystoid macular edema, and choroidal effusions.

The XEN hydrogel stent is a hydrophilic collagen implant, which drains aqueous from the anterior chamber to the subconjunctival space alleviating IOP [49]. Sng and colleagues prospectively treated with a XEN implant 24 eyes with UG, which had uncontrolled IOP despite maximal tolerated medical treatment. Eighty-three percent of studied patients had good control of glaucoma without requiring further surgical management and 62.5% of the eyes were medication-free for at least 12 months. The most common postoperative complication was transient (>30 mm Hg) rise in IOP in 15 eyes (62.5%) of patients, of which only 4 eyes required glaucoma medications at 12 months. Some sight-threatening complications occurred such as bleb-related infection (4.2%) and persistent hypotony (4.2%), although uncommon. To the authors' knowledge, this was the first reported sight-threatening complication associated with a XEN implant, which reinforces that patients with UG have different outcomes compared with POAG patients. XEN implantation may be more appropriate in uveitic eyes with mild to moderate visual field loss, as such IOP spikes may result in complete loss of remaining visual field in eyes with advanced visual field loss [50].

GATT is a procedure performed using a fiberoptic microcatheter. Sachdev and colleagues studied GATT in a series of 3 pediatric patients with JIA-associated UG. The illuminated fiberoptic catheter allows accurate cannulation of the Schlemm canal, avoiding false passage and reducing the risk of complications associated with traditional goniotomy. All 3 patients were treated intraoperatively with orbital floor triamcinolone 4%/bupivacaine 0.25% and were described as maintaining good inflammation control. In their series, GATT was effective in reducing IOP by 40% to 66% [25].

To the authors' knowledge, there are no additional studies evaluating other types of MIGS for use in UG. Further studies are needed to provide evidence-based results and risks of complications.

*New topical treatments*

A new treatment currently available is Rho-kinase inhibitor eye drops. This is the newest glaucoma drop medication in approximately 20 years. The mechanism of action is by lowering the resistance to outflow through the TM, which also decreases the production of fluid and episcleral venous pressure. It works at a cellular level within the TM decreasing actin-myosin contraction and reducing actin stress fibers and focal adhesions in the TM improving aqueous outflow. Ripasudil, a Rho-kinase inhibitor, has shown to have anti-inflammatory properties by inhibiting several proinflammatory mediators, which can provide further benefits in patients with UG [51,52]. Futakuchi and colleagues [51] and the ROCK-S study group collaborators published a study evaluating the efficacy and safety of a Rho-kinase inhibitor medication in secondary glaucoma, such as UG and SIG. They reported good IOP-lowering effects as well as a significant concomitant decrease in anterior segment inflammation. These all are promising new treatment modalities that still require further studies but provide a positive outlook into the future.

## SUMMARY

UG is a complex disease in which understanding the pathogenesis related to increased IOP will lead to improved treatment. New treatment modalities may help to halt the progression of the disease. In today's era of increased use of periocular and intraocular steroids and other medications, it is of utmost importance to better understand UG to improve the visual outcomes of patients with this disease. Increased IOP in UG can be due to a combination of open, closed, and mixed mechanisms that can be complicated by steroid-induced elevation of IOP and that treatment should not be the same as for primary glaucoma. As previous studies have shown us, the IOP spikes tend to be more severe, and optic neuropathy progression is more accelerated in UG than in patients with primary open- or chronic angle-closure glaucoma. Achieving successful results is directly correlated with prompt and aggressive treatment of both inflammation and IOP elevation. Further studies are needed to better assess different treatment modalities and improve the diagnosis of underlying etiologies.

## CLINICS CARE POINTS

- When assessing the treatment plan for uveitic glaucoma, never undertreat inflammation or intraocular pressure (IOP). IOP and inflammation should be both managed concomitantly.
- Uveitic glaucoma differs from other types of glaucoma and should be treated more aggressively to avoid irreversible damage.
- Inflammation should be controlled as much as possible before surgical management for better postoperative results.
- Surgical iridectomy is preferred over laser iridotomy in patients with acute IOP elevation due to iris bombe.

### Disclosure

The authors have nothing to disclose.

### References

[1] Sng CCA, Ang M, Barton K. 1st edition. Uveitis and glaucoma: new insights in the pathogenesis and treatment, vol. 221. Elsevier B.V.; 2015; https://doi.org/10.1016/bs.pbr.2015.06.008.
[2] Herbert HM, Viswanathan A, Jackson H, et al. Risk factors for elevated intraocular pressure in uveitis. J Glaucoma 2004;13(2):96–9.
[3] Kalogeropoulos D, Sung VCT. Pathogenesis of uveitic glaucoma. J Curr Glaucoma Pract 2018;12(3):125–38.
[4] Gregory AC, Zhang MM, Rapoport Y, et al. Racial influences of uveitic glaucoma: consolidation of current knowledge of diagnosis and treatment. Semin Ophthalmol 2016;31(4):400–4.
[5] Siddique SS, Suelves AM, Baheti U, et al. Glaucoma and uveitis. Surv Ophthalmol 2013;58(1):1–10.
[6] Muñoz-Negrete FJ, Moreno-Montañés J, Hernández-Martínez P, et al. Current approach in the diagnosis and management of uveitic glaucoma. Biomed Res Int 2015;2015; https://doi.org/10.1155/2015/742792.
[7] Bodh S, Kumar V, Raina U, et al. Inflammatory glaucoma. Oman J Ophthalmol 2011;4(1):3; https://doi.org/10.4103/0974-620x.77655.
[8] Holland GN. A reconsideration of anterior chamber flare and its clinical relevance for children with chronic anterior uveitis (an American Ophthalmological Society thesis). Trans Am Ophthalmol Soc 2007;105:344–64.
[9] Hogan MJ, Kimura SJ, Thygeson P. Pathology of herpes simplex kerato-iritis. Am J Ophthalmol 1964;57(4):551–64.
[10] Townsend WM, Kaufman HE. Pathogenesis of glaucoma and endothelial changes in herpetic kerato-uveitis in rabbits. Am J Ophthalmol 1971;71(4):904–10.
[11] Armaly MF, Becker B. Intraocular pressure response to topical corticosteroids. Fed Proc. 24(6):1274–8. Available at: http://www.ncbi.nlm.nih.gov/pubmed/5853148.
[12] Razeghinejad MR, Katz LJ. Steroid-induced iatrogenic glaucoma. Ophthalmic Res 2012;47(2):66–80.
[13] Holland GN, Barton K. Iridotomies on eyes with uveitis: Indications and technique. Br J Ophthalmol 2019;314221; https://doi.org/10.1136/bjophthalmol-2019-315221.
[14] Karbassi M, Raizman MB, Schuman JS. Herpes zoster ophthalmicus. Surv Ophthalmol 1992;36(6):395–410.

[15] Sungur GK, Hazirolan D, Yalvac IS, et al. Incidence and prognosis of ocular hypertension secondary to viral uveitis. Int Ophthalmol 2010;30(2):191–4.
[16] Horsley MB, Chen TC. The use of prostaglandin analogs in the uveitic patient. Semin Ophthalmol 2011;26(4–5):285–9.
[17] Markomichelakis NN, Kostakou A, Halkiadakis I, et al. Efficacy and safety of latanoprost in eyes with uveitic glaucoma. Graefes Arch Clin Exp Ophthalmol 2009;247(6):775–80.
[18] Wong JXH, Agrawal R, Wong EPY, et al. Efficacy and safety of topical ganciclovir in the management of cytomegalovirus (CMV)-related anterior uveitis. J Ophthalmic Inflamm Infect 2016;6(1):0–4.
[19] Bhoopat T, Takhar JS, Oldenburg CE, et al. Treatment of cytomegalovirus anterior uveitis at a north american tertiary center with oral valganciclovir. Cornea 2020;39(5):584–9.
[20] Artini W, Bani AP. The effectiveness of trabeculectomy with mitomycin C and releasable suture in posner-schlossman syndrome with secondary glaucoma: A case series. Niger J Clin Pract 2019;22(1):138–43.
[21] Su W-W, Cheng S-T, Ho W-J, et al. Glaucoma is associated with peripheral vascular endothelial dysfunction. Ophthalmology 2008;115(7):1173–8.e1.
[22] Kanski JJ, Shun-Shin GA. Systemic uveitis syndromes in childhood: an analysis of 340 cases. Ophthalmology 1984;91(10):1247–52.
[23] Wolf MD, Lichter PR, Ragsdale CG. Prognostic factors in the uveitis of juvenile rheumatoid arthritis. Ophthalmology 1987;94(10):1242–8.
[24] Kafkala C, Hynes A, Choi J, et al. Ahmed valve implantation for uncontrolled pediatric uveitic glaucoma. J AAPOS 2005;9(4):336–40.
[25] Sachdev A, Khalili A, Choi J, et al. Gonioscopy-assisted transluminal trabeculotomy in uveitic glaucoma secondary to juvenile idiopathic arthritis. J Glaucoma 2020;29(10):116–9.
[26] Veerappan M, Fleischman D, Ulrich JN, et al. The relationship of vogt–koyanagi–harada syndrome to ocular hypertension and glaucoma. Ocul Immunol Inflamm 2017;25(6):748–52.
[27] Roberti G, Oddone F, Agnifili L, et al. Steroid-induced glaucoma: epidemiology, pathophysiology, and clinical management. Surv Ophthalmol 2020;65(4):458–72.
[28] Feroze KB, Khazaeni L. Steroid induced glaucoma. 2021. Available at: https://www.ncbi.nlm.nih.gov/books/NBK430903/.
[29] Gaston H, Absolon MJ, Thurtle OA, et al. Steroid responsiveness in connective tissue diseases. Br J Ophthalmol 1983;67(7):487–90.
[30] Becker B, Bresnick G, Chevrette L, et al. Intraocular pressure and its response to topical corticosteroids in diabetes. Arch Ophthalmol 1966;76(4):477–83.
[31] Papadaki TG, Zacharopoulos IP, Pasquale LR, et al. Long-term results of Ahmed glaucoma valve implantation for uveitic glaucoma. Am J Ophthalmol 2007;144(1):62–9.
[32] Sallam A, Sheth HG, Habot-Wilner Z, et al. Outcome of raised intraocular pressure in uveitic eyes with and without a corticosteroid-induced hypertensive response. Am J Ophthalmol 2009;148(2):207–13.e1.
[33] Beltz J, Zamir E. Brimonidine induced anterior uveitis. Ocul Immunol Inflamm 2016;24(2):128–33.
[34] Cates CA, Jeffrey MN. Granulomatous anterior uveitis associated with 0.2% topical brimonidine. Eye (Lond) 2003;17(5):670–1.
[35] Broadway DC, Chang LP. Trabeculectomy, risk factors for failure and the preoperative state of the conjunctiva. J Glaucoma 2001;10(3):237–49.
[36] Stavrou P, Misson GP, Rowson NJ, et al. Trabeculectomy in uveitis Are antimetabolites necessary at the first procedure? Ocul Immunol Inflamm 1995;3(3):209–16.
[37] Stavrou P, Murray PI. Long-term follow-up of trabeculectomy without antimetabolites in patients with uveitis. Am J Ophthalmol 1999;128(4):434–9.

[38] Almobarak FA, Alharbi AH, Morales J, et al. Intermediate and long-term outcomes of mitomycin c-enhanced trabeculectomy as a first glaucoma procedure in uveitic glaucoma. J Glaucoma 2017;26(5):478–85.
[39] Kaburaki T, Koshino T, Kawashima H, et al. Initial trabeculectomy with mitomycin C in eyes with uveitic glaucoma with inactive uveitis. Eye 2009;23(7):1509–17.
[40] Kanaya R, Kijima R, Shinmei Y, et al. Surgical outcomes of trabeculectomy in uveitic glaucoma: a long-term, single-center, retrospective case-control study. J Ophthalmol 2021;2021; https://doi.org/10.1155/2021/5550776.
[41] Wang S, Gao X, Qian N. The Ahmed shunt versus the Baerveldt shunt for refractory glaucoma: a meta-analysis. BMC Ophthalmol 2016;16(1):1–7.
[42] Iverson SM, Bhardwaj N, Shi W, et al. Surgical outcomes of inflammatory glaucoma: a comparison of trabeculectomy and glaucoma-drainage-device implantation. Jpn J Ophthalmol 2015;59(3):179–86.
[43] Goldmann DB, Mellin KB. Argon laser trabeculoplasty in special forms of open-angle glaucoma. Klin Monbl Augenheilkd 1987;191(1):13–5.
[44] Wong MOM, Lee JWY, Choy BNK, et al. Systematic review and meta-analysis on the efficacy of selective laser trabeculoplasty in open-angle glaucoma. Surv Ophthalmol 2015;60(1):36–50; https://doi.org/10.1016/j.survophthal.2014.06.006.
[45] Koktekir BE, Gedik S, Bakbak B. Bilateral severe anterior uveitis after unilateral selective laser trabeculoplasty. Clin Exp Ophthalmol 2013;41(3):305–7.
[46] Maleki A, Swan RT, Lasave AF, et al. Selective laser trabeculoplasty in controlled uveitis with steroid-induced glaucoma. Ophthalmology 2016;123(12):2630–2.
[47] Zhou Y, Pruet CM, Fang C, et al. Selective laser trabeculoplasty in steroid-induced and uveitic glaucoma. Can J Ophthalmol 2021; https://doi.org/10.1016/j.jcjo.2021.05.006.
[48] Betts TD, Sims JL, Bennett SL, et al. Outcome of peripheral iridotomy in subjects with uveitis. Br J Ophthalmol 2020;104(1):8–10.
[49] Lewis RA. Ab interno approach to the subconjunctival space using a collagen glaucoma stent. J Cataract Refract Surg 2014;40(8):1301–6.
[50] Sng CCA, Wang J, Hau S, et al. XEN-45 collagen implant for the treatment of uveitic glaucoma. Clin Exp Ophthalmol 2018;46(4):339–45.
[51] Futakuchi A, Morimoto T, Ikeda Y, et al. Intraocular pressure-lowering effects of ripasudil in uveitic glaucoma, exfoliation glaucoma, and steroid-induced glaucoma patients: ROCK-S, a multicentre historical cohort study. Sci Rep 2020;10(1):2–12.
[52] Uchida T, Honjo M, Yamagishi R, et al. The Anti-Inflammatory Effect of Ripasudil (K-115), a Rho Kinase (ROCK) Inhibitor, on Endotoxin-Induced Uveitis in Rats. Invest Ophthalmol Vis Sci 2017;58(12):5584–93.

Advances in Ophthalmology and Optometry 7 (2022) i–iv

ADVANCES IN OPHTHALMOLOGY AND OPTOMETRY

# Solo Private Practice Journey

Priya Kalyam, MD

Legacy Eyelids & Cosmetic Surgery, 6835 Communications Parkway, Suite 520 Plano, TX 75024, USA

**Keywords**

• Oculofacial plastic surgery • Private practice • Business of medicine

**Key points**

- Solo practice offers control over the structure of your medical practice.
- The financial challenges of opening a solo practice can be overcome by strategic borrowing and budgeting.
- Business of medicine should be included in academic training to allow exposure to young physicians.

## INTRODUCTION

Starting a private practice immediately after fellowship or training is the least recommended path, and many new physicians often choose academics or join large group practices with administrators. Unfortunately, business in medicine is not emphasized in clinical training and without knowledge of operating a business, starting out on your own can seem very daunting. I would like to share my positive and negative experiences to help motivate other graduates that starting a private practice is doable and should be considered.

I had excellent training with great mentors in both academics and private practice with adequate exposure to business, but I was still very nervous and scared to start on my own. I joined a large private practice ophthalmology group with several locations, but I knew I wanted to eventually have an equity stake. Within a few months I learned that I did not have independence to be the doctor that I always dreamed to be. Often in large groups, layers of administrative burden exist, and I decided to confront the odds and start my own practice.

### A step forward

I joined many physician groups, forums, and spoke to mentors and other colleagues who traveled a similar path to seek guidance on how to start a private

*E-mail address:* priyakalyam@gmail.com

https://doi.org/10.1016/j.yaoo.2022.03.015

practice and prepared all the steps needed to start on my own. The first lesson I learned was that everything takes a lot of time to accomplish in the beginning no matter how well you are organized. A range of tasks emerged from my research: establishing a legal business entity, securing a business loan, finding an office space, choosing equipment, negotiating with representatives, and credentialing with insurance companies. None of these steps worked out on my expected timeline. It took me 3 months before I could open my doors (Table 1).

Choosing the location is the first step, as a business address is needed for setting up the remaining processes. I chose to sublease an office space to keep costs low in the beginning, and it allowed me to secure a place faster. If you are living in a large city, commercial rents can be very high and burdensome for a small practice. I also immediately applied for Medicare privileges that are needed before I could be credentialed with other commercial payers. Many physicians join organizations or use a third-party company to help with credentialing, but I chose to credential on my own, which took the same time (~30–60 days); this allowed me to keep expenses to zero, and no one is more responsible about your business as you are. Insurance companies often request many forms, and responding in a given timeline is essential. Also, credentialing on my own allowed me to negotiate with several insurance companies.

## Opening the practice

Although I subleased a few days per week, I was able to generate some revenue, and I started marketing. I strongly recommended tracking referral sources and sending thank you notes after patient visits. Taking time to meet local eye doctors and general physicians one-on-one helped establish rapport. I even provided offices with my cell phone number to reach me after hours. Creating a good first impression is very important in earning referrals to your practice.

**Table 1**
Starting a business

| Steps | Duration | Cost | Other tips |
|---|---|---|---|
| Setting up LLC | 1 h | \$0–\$500 | Can use CPA but doable on your own |
| Choosing business name/LOGO | 5 h | \$0–\$250 | Keep it short if possible—you will use it on all forms<br>Use local place name for easy search engine optimization |
| Credentialing | 90 d | \$0–\$3000 | Can use companies but can be doable on your own if you have time and are organized |
| Finding an office space | 30 d | \$0–\$1000 | Word of mouth, local society groups, realtors |
| Securing loan | 90 d | \$0 | Important to meet with local bankers and set good rapport. I found local banks to be more helpful than larger banks |

Subleasing allowed me time to secure bank loans and find a more permanent location. My family members helped me create a proforma for business and create financial projections to secure funding. Small business administration (SBA) also has great online resources to learn how to start and manage business. They provided me information for licenses, permits, and state regulations. Although numerous ways to secure loans exist, I found that SBA loans had the best interest rate, but they had many regulations and it takes a long time if you are in a hurry.

Once I secured finances, I was able to start the build out process for my permanent space, which took me about 7 months. I experienced construction delays due to the COVID pandemic. It was recommended to build extra rooms for future expansion and to have a large procedure room, which I now am glad to have followed that advice from my colleagues.

I strongly recommend furnishing office rooms as the practice expands. I only equipped 2 rooms and bought used equipments that were in good condition. All the representatives will tempt you to buy more by offering financing. Make sure to budget–budget ahead of time and stay on budget! Controlling expenses was most important to being financially successful. Always negotiate on everything (equipment, furniture, electronic medical records) and never accept the first price that marketing representatives offer. If they cannot decrease the price, you can ask them to add a freebie such as stools or other small equipment. Reaching out to local ophthalmology/optometry groups also helped me identify local eye doctors who were retiring. Every penny I saved allowed room for something else while staying within budget (Table 2).

## Day-to-day life

I also learned how to perform all tasks of my business from answering phone calls, scheduling patients for surgery, billing, and claims management; this

**Table 2**
Equipment costs

| Basic equipment | Cost | Tips |
|---|---|---|
| Slit lamp | $1500–$10000 | Start with local vendors, Facebook groups for used equipment |
| Exam chair | $3000–$8000 | I purchased from local vendor; also look at government auctions |
| Visual field machine | $6000–$8000 | Used machine; make sure it works before purchase. EBay is a good source too but read reviews |
| Office supplies: computers, printer, and so forth | $5000 | Thanksgiving sale. Costco, Amazon |
| Office medical supplies/ small instruments | $1000–$2000 | Eye Care and Cure; Henry Schein Ask them to add you to a group purchasing organization (GPO) for lower costs |

allowed me to train staff the way I want them to perform and also allowed me to trouble shoot any difficulties. I did not hire any employees until a few months into my practice, as I was subleasing. I used word of mouth to find interested candidates for my front desk and made them responsible for many tasks including answering telephone, scheduling, processing payments, and scanning charts. It is important to make your assistants understand the goals of your practice and make them feel part of the team. With a well-chosen and motivated staff, their performance goes beyond what is required.

### Things I wish I focused on during residency

I strongly encourage all residents and fellows to learn ICD 10 codes and CPT codes for the most common diseases in their specialties and learn how to fill out a superbill at the end of each patient visit during their training years; this is a great early step to learn billing no matter which avenue you choose to practice. In addition, pay attention to postoperative periods and modifiers needed. Ask questions!! Ask your mentors/front desk staff/billers and learn from their experience. Request your program directors to include a few billing lectures if that is not part of your curriculum already. In addition, American Academy of Ophthalmology has coding courses that you can take online or in-person courses in your home towns that focus on ophthalmology coding. Once you are on your own you learn a lot from your rejected claims and improve with time.

## SUMMARY

After a few years into solo private practice, I feel like we have finally established a routine. There were several ups and downs in the beginning, and administrative tasks can be very annoying, but I truly enjoy going to work every day. Although you may feel you are not generating enough revenue in the beginning, with perseverance you can easily surpass what you might make working for a large group practice. I find that providing the type of care I want for my patients, having the independence to make changes immediately to improve practice, and performing other duties as a business owner are fulfilling for my career. I am not saying solo private practice is for everyone, but if you have the ambition, work ethic, and motivation, it is definitely achievable. I also hope this article will help motivate those who are in residency or desiring a change in their current employment status. It is completely possible to succeed and well worth the investment in yourself.

### Disclosure

The author has nothing to disclose.

# EUTROPHICATION

**Ivica Angelovski**

Delve PUBLISHING

www.delvepublishing.com

# Eutrophication

*Ivica Angelovski*

**Delve Publishing**
4164 Lakeshore Road
Burlington, ON L7L 1A4
Canada
www.delvepublishing.com
Email: orders@arclereducation.com



ISBN: 978-1-77956-468-9 (Hardcover)

# ABOUT THE AUTHOR

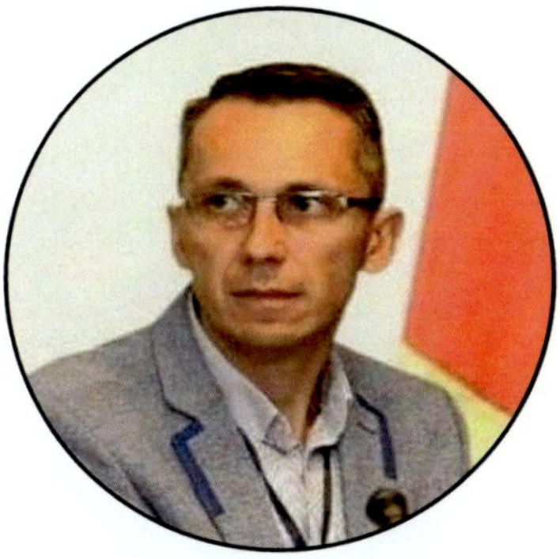

**Ivica Angelovski** was born in 1978 in North Macedonia, where he completed primary and secondary education, as well as the Faculty of Agricultural Sciences and Food. Ivica is a dedicated professional agronomist with over a wealth of experience in the field of agriculture production. He is currently engaged as Advisor Officer for Plant Health in the Ministry of Agriculture, Forestry and Water Economy in the Republic of North Macedonia. An expert on organic farming, plant nutrition, integrated pest management, vegetable production, seed technology and soil management his full list of qualifications run as tall as his experience. Ivica is a member of the Global panel for phytosanitary issues within the European Plant Protection Organization (EPPO), where he contributes to the work of this body. Also, he has a lifelong passion for agriculture, based on the many training sessions he visited during his career.

# TABLE OF CONTENTS

# LIST OF FIGURES

# PREFACE

The natural and artificial process that drives the biological succession of estuarine, freshwater, and other aquatic ecosystems  is called eutrophication. Larger scale studies of the land use change and biogeochemical cycles that control the gross productivity of human-impacted aquatic ecosystems have been involved in many studies, even though eutrophication involves the integration of biological and geological processes that are studied as individual entities. The process of natural eutrophication is very unpredictable and dependent on important site-specific components like biodiversity, climate-related variables, element balance and geomorphology. The functions of many major aquatic processes that influence eutrophication are by human influences. In the fields of aquatic research and management, such as impact assessment and the discussion of remedial actions, the ecosystem size is crucial.

The majority of scientists and aquatic ecologists  are more interested in knowing the cause of eutrophication. There is no conflict between observation at larger ecosystem scales and sampling and observation at smaller sizes. The migration of people into large cities, or urbanization, occurs after favorable economic developments. Concentrations of urban population can be found all over the world, usually in large cities. The flat plains become ideal locations for urban growth and draw people by offering employment possibilities. The man-made concrete walls dividing land from the sea have replaced beaches (natural). The installation of a pollution load management system for fertilizers is primarily responsible for the maintenance and improvement of the water quality. Analyses of issues of the coastal water environment, human activity management, regulatory structures that include laws and community activities, the development of water-related technologies, and other relevant topics are heavily influenced by the unique features (natural) of the site. All estuaries may be preserved as healthy environments that sustainably offer resources, as well as other benefits to nearby residents and tourists.

The primary focus of this book is the effect of human activity on the rate of eutrophication in various aquatic ecosystems worldwide. We can anticipate that this book will be helpful to students, engineers, aquatic ecologists, scientists, and managers concerned with water quality.

# INTRODUCTION

More effective management of anthropogenic processes to the watershed or water bodies by lowering loadings from agricultural, urban, or atmospheric sources can effectively reduce the physical, chemical, and biological problems. The accumulation of excess nutrients in coastal sites is closely associated with human activities both upstream and within estuaries, which are connected to decisions about their management and policy framing. One of the burning problems with nutrient control is runoff; control of agricultural sources receives attention, followed by control of atmospheric sources, regulation of urban sources, and control through other appropriate mechanisms. It is possible to decrease the amount of phosphorus (P) that is transported from agricultural land that is bonded to sediment by regulating erosion. There are techniques to regulate the amount of phosphorus (P) that is dissolved in runoff and the amount of nitrogen (N) that leaches into groundwater. The management of nutrients has received less attention because it involves a substantial amount of effort. Because the majority of the nitrogen (N) absorbed during grazing is redeposited as urine and dung, nitrogen surpluses within grazing systems frequently account for a sizable (large) fraction of the total fertilizer input (s). Since some of this nitrogen is unevenly available across the field and is not immediately available, it is not recycled effectively as expected. The subsurface deposition of inorganic fertilizer away from the zone of removal in surface runoff and the periodic plowing of soils to redistribute surface phosphorus throughout the root zone are effective management strategies for phosphorus adjustments to soils susceptible to phosphorus loss. It is currently advised by farm advisers and resource planners to evaluate soils for phosphate and nitrogen before applying manure to the farm land. However, plans for managing manure based on nitrogen are still dependent on crop requirements. Farmers and their consultants may underestimate the usefulness of manure as fertilizer if these evaluations are not made. The causes of eutrophication are explained in this book.

Chapter 1

# INTRODUCTION TO EUTROPHICATION

## Contents

## 1.1. INTRODUCTION

Anthropogenic eutrophication still is a major threat to inland waters, even though re-oligotrophication has advanced in a few areas (Ansari et al., 2011). Inland waters are now seriously threatened by a new risk brought about by climate change. The majority of direct effects come from temperature variations and related physico-chemical changes. Increased nutrient loading is one of the indirect consequences that are mediated by catchment processes like extreme weather occurrences or events.

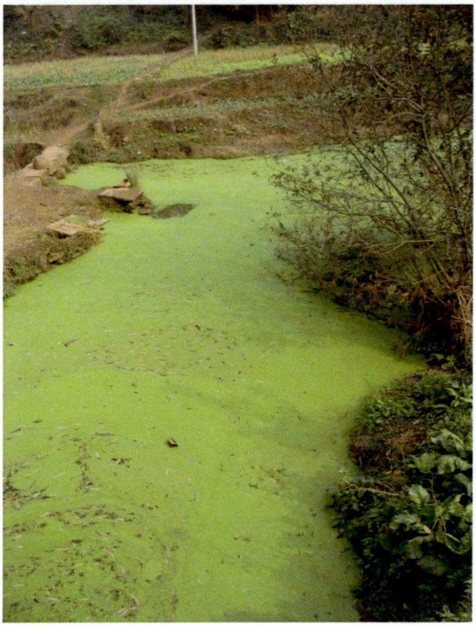

**Figure 1.1.** *Eutrophication.*

Source: https://upload.wikimedia.org/wikipedia/commons/7/74/River_algae_Sichuan.jpg,, Creative Commons License.

These effects will cause severe alterations to the physical and biological composition of the seas, based on future climate projections. An oligotrophic lake absorbs nutrient-poor wastewater from its drainage basin. The amount of organic matter produced in the exposed epilimnion is minimal. As a result, during the summer months, not much organic material sinks into the hypolimnion and less oxygen is used there. On the other hand, a eutrophic lake tends to be shallow. Rivers and groundwater that empty into its epilimnion carry more nutrients. The level of primary production is higher than in an oligotrophic environment. As a result, more organic matter accumulates in the hypolimnion, which is more susceptible to oxygen depletion. In the summer, the deep-water layer of a eutrophic lake turns anoxic.

Eutrophication (Figure 1.1) in freshwater systems is characterized as a syndrome of ecosystem reactions that happen when the concentration of chemical elements (nutrients) rises to a point where the ecosystem's primary production increases. Natural or artificial nutrient enrichment is possible, and it is typically brought about by human activity. Many detrimental consequences on the environment could arise, depending on the level of nutrient enrichment. The development of phytoplankton biomass in lakes is generally stimulated by nutrient augmentation because micro-algae and cyanobacteria typically grow more quickly than algae or plants (Mironiuk and Chojnacka, 2018).

## 1.2. EUTROPHICATION

Eutrophication lost its prominence in the late 1980s and was replaced with a focus on freshwater concerns other than nutrient enrichment (Wurtsbaugh et al., 2019). The effectiveness of the restoration efforts (Figure 1.2) contributed significantly to the reduction of public awareness of the eutrophication issue. The extensive installation of wastewater and sewage treatment plants enhanced the quality of the water by primarily reducing the organic load, especially phosphorus, which was designated as the primary target. In many industrialized countries, eutrophication was effectively controlled and reversed as a result of additional measures and a reduction in the anthropogenic nutrient load. Re-oligotrophication, which may be explained by empirical models, was eventually caused by the falling in-lake concentrations of chemical components, especially phosphorus. The treatment of point sources and their removal from the catchment, as a result, led to the majority of these significant advancements in lakes. Simultaneously, rivers started to appear increasingly eutrophic due to the significant decrease in organic matter, which was once more brought about by extensive sewage treatment. Early research on the organic load in running water systems, particularly the carbon enrichment from untreated sewage, was the main topic of many research studies. In many developing countries, rivers have become fully anoxic due to excessive emissions of organic waste. Subsequently, it became clear that nitrogen enrichment may also happen in rivers and streams as a direct result of anthropogenic modification of land use, as sewage treatment advanced and streams became less contaminated. Different regions are predicted to have different baseline levels of nutrients based on factors such as terrain, geology, and land use (Djodjic et al., 2021). Because it is more difficult to control nutrients in runoff water from urban and agricultural areas, diffuse sources are significantly more difficult to manage than point sources. However, when it comes to annual loads, runoff and erosion during winter storm events often account for the majority of P transfer from land to water. As a result, this phosphorus from dispersed sources may contribute very little to river eutrophication because the transfers typically occur outside of the peak biological demand window. Alternatively, determining and measuring P sources during times of low flow may be crucial to knowing eutrophication. The spring and summer months, when plants are growing, are when undesirable signs of river eutrophication mostly appear. This is because high water temperatures, long water residence periods, low flow, and an abundance of light all encourage rapid algal development. River eutrophication during the growth season is mostly caused by point discharges, which are an important source of dissolved, bioavailable phosphorus components at high concentrations. River water P concentrations from point sources can occasionally rise even further while diffuse agricultural runoff contributions are generally quite low due to less effluent dilution.

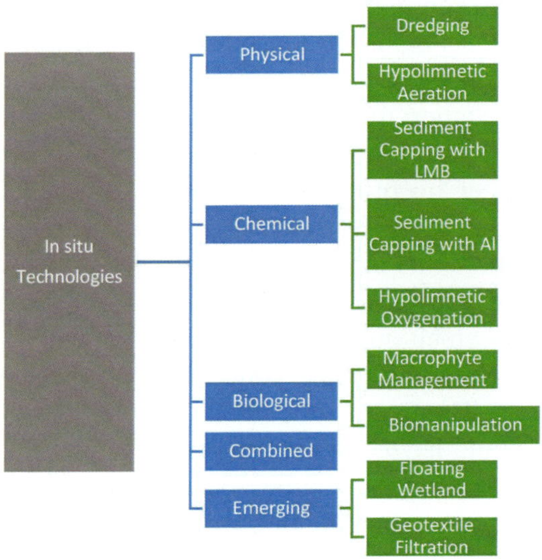


**Figure 1.2.** *Restoration.*

Source: Pereira AC, Mulligan CN. Practices for Eutrophic Shallow Lake Water Remediation and Restoration: A Critical Literature Review. Water. 2023; 15(12):2270. https://doi.org/10.3390/w15122270, Creative Commons License.

## 1.3. INTERACTIONS IN WATER

The intricate interactions among hydraulic nutrient flushing, light restriction or limitation, and water velocity are significant in regulating the growth of algae (Summers and Ryder, 2023). This implies that the effects of rivers with short retention times (less than three days) will differ from those of rivers with long retention times (more than three days) or riverine lakes. Some conceptual models explaining the development of eutrophic conditions in rivers were presented by many researchers based on a comparison with lake systems (>30 days retention period) and taking into account some of the essential elements. Phosphorus (P) and nitrogen (N) concentrations are the primary determinants of the autotrophic condition in flowing streams. In rivers and streams, there is a positive correlation between algal biomass and gross primary output or yield. Some researchers have determined the trophic level limits based on the nutritional reference concept/model. Rivers, lakes, and wetlands are under strain from diverse uses globally, especially eutrophication and pollution. As a result, the benefits that aquatic ecosystems can offer society have decreased and will continue to diminish.

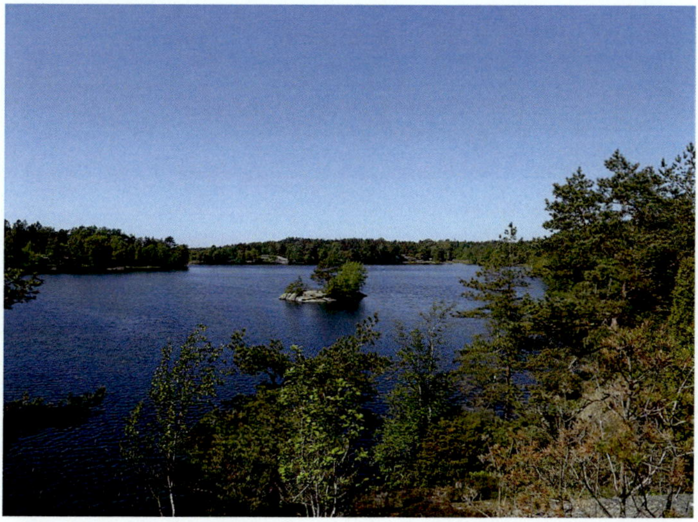

**Figure 1.3.** *Freshwater ecosystems.*

Source: https://en.wikipedia.org/wiki/Freshwater_biology#/media/File:Oxsjon_Vastergotland_Sweden_from_E_looking_N_May_29_2021.jpg, Creative Commons License.

The physical and chemical features of freshwater ecosystems (Figure 1.3) from various geological settings or ecoregions mean that many effects of climate change will be unpredictable and may have diverse effects on these systems. Furthermore, a region's climate and other environmental factors may differ from the average conditions in the area. The main environmental risks, especially to small lakes and ponds, will be the effects of population growth and economic development in a warmer climate. In arid regions, salinization will worsen and, in the worst situations, cause water bodies to disappear. Analysis of the combined or integrated effects of climate change (global warming) (Figure 1.4) and socio-economic driving forces on the future distribution of freshwater resources worldwide, using existing climate scenarios, clearly demonstrates increasing water stress due to growing water demands.

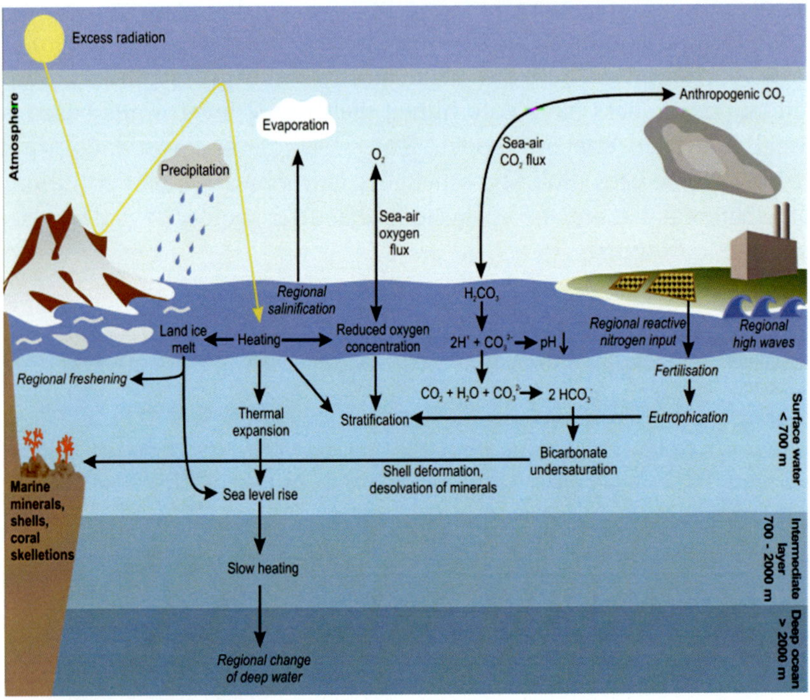


**Figure 1.4.** *Overview of climatic change.*

Source: https://en.wikipedia.org/wiki/File:Overview_of_climatic_changes_and_their_effects_on_the_ocean.png, Creative Commons License.

## 1.4. CLIMATE CHANGE IMPACTS

Certain areas may benefit from climate change due to reduced water stress and better water supply. Significant effects of climate change on freshwater systems include altered precipitation patterns, rising air temperatures, and increased concentrations of greenhouse gases, especially $CO_2$. A collection of lakes and streams, collectively referred to as an effect filter, might have multiple properties that modify changes in these environmental variables. Diverse limnological variables are influenced differently by these effect filters. Biological reactions have the maximum diversity, whereas physical variables exhibit the highest degree of similarity (Whittaker et al., 2001). Through point and especially nonpoint sources, the topography, geology, land use, and anthropogenic pressure impact the catchment dynamics. The concentration of nutrients in streams and rivers, which in turn feed and load standing water surfaces with nutrients and other materials, is mostly determined by erosion, timing, and runoff volume. Depending on the catchment geology, $CO_2$ can have an impact on freshwaters by lowering pH levels, which causes both running and stagnant water to become acidic. Lake morphometry, history, and geographic location all influence how it responds to climate fluctuation. Latitude and altitude will determine anticipated future changes in the length and timing of the ice/snow season. The size and depth of the lake have a significant impact on hydrodynamic patterns. These factors also affect the annual heat budget, temperature stratification during the summer, and the oxygen concentration in the hypolimnion, which can lead to internal nutritional loading. The retention time, which is a function of through-flow and morphometry, establishes whether internal or external processes predominate. Pelagic (Figure 1.5) and biological components of the food web are influenced by different important determinants, both directly (like temperature) and indirectly (like nutrients). Furthermore, a lake's past history can have a substantial impact on how it responds to climate change, with increased eutrophication through the release of nutrients. However, depending on what stage they are in, lakes with various histories will respond to the effects of climate change in different ways.

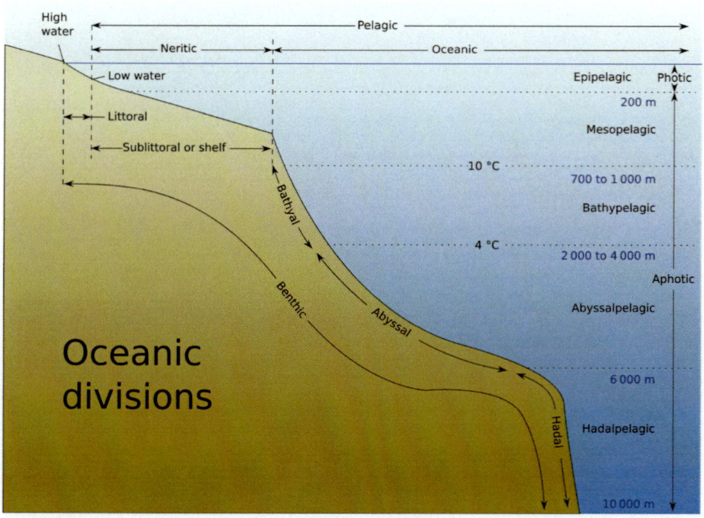


**Figure 1.5.** *Pelagic zones.*

Source: By Chris huh(Original text: K. Aainsqatsi) / K. Aainsqatsi – self-made(Original text: self-made), Public Domain, https://commons.wikimedia.org/w/index.php?curid=3251432, Creative Commons License.

## 1.5. HYDROLOGY

Changes in the hydrological runoff regime will happen if northern hemisphere winters become warmer and wetter and summers become hotter and drier as predicted (Hayhoe et al., 2007). Winter and spring-time are predicted to see higher discharges since more precipitation will fall as rain rather than snow. River and stream peaks are probably going to shift. Maximum runoff and intense rainfalls can cause erosion, floods, and nutrient leaching, all of which can contribute to the eutrophication of rivers. Discharge in areas covered by glaciers will first rise as a result of increased melting, then fall as the glaciers retreat. Increased rainfall during the rainy season may cause storms and flooding in tropical and subtropical areas. In temperate and high-latitude regions, rising summer temperatures will bring harsh/rough weather, decreased stream and river flow, and intense and extended thermal stratification. Since solubility decreases with rising temperature, there will be less oxygen accessible in these warmer lakes. Furthermore, if decomposition rates rise, they will require increased concentration of oxygen, which could cause deoxygenation in lakes' deeper regions. Eutrophication in rivers receiving point sources of nutrients will intensify due to decreasing inflows and rising water residence/retention time.

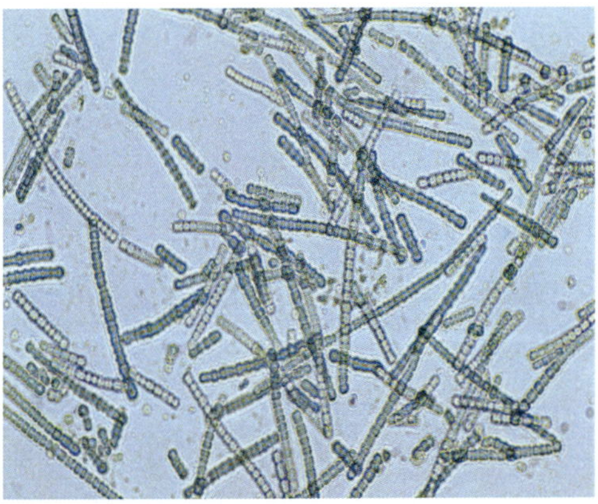

**Figure 1.6.** *Cyanobacteria.*

Source: https://en.wikipedia.org/wiki/Cyanobacteria#/media/File:CSIRO_ScienceImage_4203_A_bluegreen_algae_species_Cylindrospermum_sp_under_magnification.jpg, Creative Commons License.

This process will replace diatoms with cyanobacteria, (Figure 1.6) some of which are poisonous, fix nitrogen, or both. This will influence the quality of drinking water, biodiversity, and the environment. Hence, there will be a huge rise in the demand for water, especially in the developing countries. Since most developing nations are present in subtropical and tropical climates, where surface water is a primary source of drinking water, the situation is even worse there. Because of their low flushing rates and shallow annual mixing, deep tropical lakes are ideal climate monitors, because they let heat accumulate throughout global warming. The oldest lake in the East African Rift Valley and the second-deepest lake in the world, Lake Tanganyika, (Figure 1.7) has seen slower vertical mixing and lower primary production due to a steep density gradient brought on by warming.

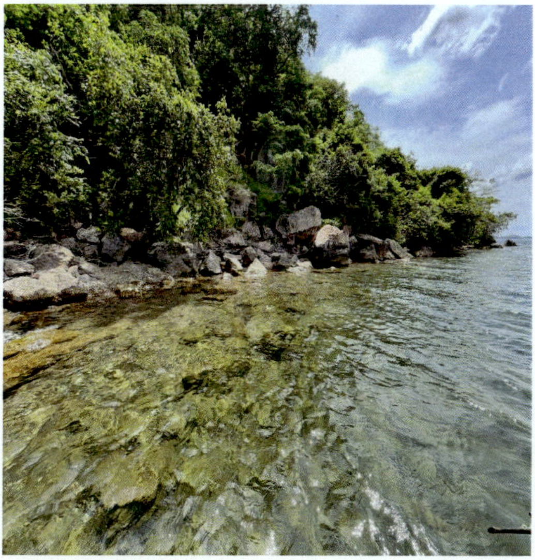

**Figure 1.7.** *Lake Tanganyika.*

Source: https://upload.wikimedia.org/wikipedia/commons/3/34/Clear_lake_Kagongo_Ward.jpg, Creative Commons License.

## 1.6. LAKES

The largest lake called Lake Baikal (Figure 1.8) is aggressively responding to climate change, according to analysis of water temperature and ice cover (Gorbarenko et al., 2014). By the end of the century, the Baikal region's climate, especially during the winter, will be wetter and warmer. The length of the ice-free season has grown while the average thickness of the lake's ice has decreased. The principal primary producers in the lake, the native diatoms, are impacted by the length of the ice cover. Unlike most other diatoms, these diatoms bloom under the ice in the spring and are heavily dependent on it for growth and reproduction. The primary food source for the crustaceans in this lake is these diatoms, which are then consumed by the fish in the lake.

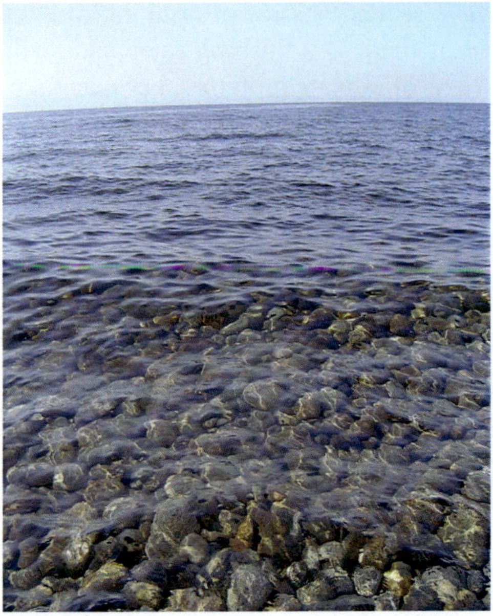

**Figure 1.8.** *Lake Baikal.*

Source: https://en.wikipedia.org/wiki/Lake_Baikal#/media/File:Baikal_1739.jpg, Creative Commons License.

Because freshwater seals reproduce/breed on the ice, shorter ice cover periods will eventually also affect the top predator in Baikal, the only freshwater seal in the world.

The melting of permafrost will have a secondary impact on ecosystem function due to climate change, aggravating anthropogenic stresses like industrial pollution and cultural eutrophication. Climate-related eutrophication will most likely result from increased erosion brought on by high winter runoff, higher water temperatures, and extended summer stratification. Increased runoff and soil erosion will increase the amount of nutrients that rivers and lakes receive, especially nitrogen.

Higher nitrogen concentrations are unlikely to have much impact, while higher phosphorus loads will mostly damage lakes. However, more nitrogen intake into rivers will result in more nitrogen being transported and accumulating downstream, which will eventually have an impact on estuaries, coastal zones, and even entire seas like the Baltic Sea (Figure 1.9).

Calcareous geological zones are mostly unaffected by greenhouse gases, especially carbon dioxide. Elevated $CO_2$ concentrations in crystalline and bed-rock regions will cause freshwaters to become acidic, much like the oceans.

However, a variety of factors, including adaptation mechanisms to some extent, particularly in cyanobacteria, which have evolved an efficient mechanism for concentrating $CO_2$, will determine the effects of higher concentrations of $CO_2$ on algal species.

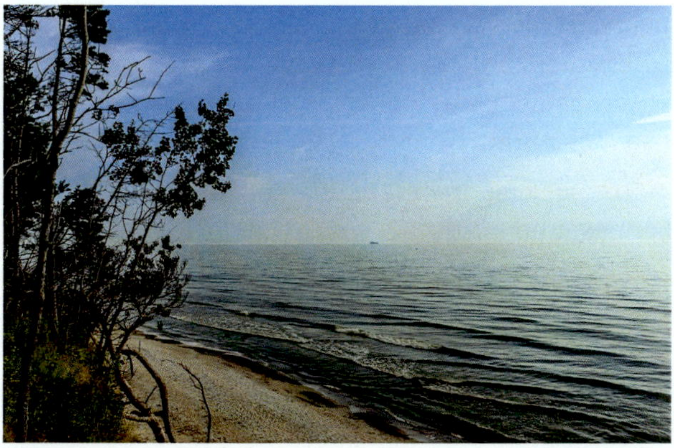

**Figure 1.9.** *Baltic Sea.*

Source: https://en.wikipedia.org/wiki/Baltic_Sea#/media/File:Sunny_day_on_the_coast_on_Baltic_sea.jpg, Creative Commons License.

The warm season is expected to see an increase in air temperature if atmospheric $CO_2$ doubles in the future (Schlesinger and Mitchell, 1987). If stream shading stays unchanged, this increase will result in an average rise in stream temperature due to the correlation between the annual average air and water temperatures. Research on how climate change affects inland waters needs to combine more and more data from properly planned experiments and findings from field-based studies. Moreover, ecological models must be used and relied upon for future change forecasts. Global trends in population expansion, energy consumption, and agricultural yield will exacerbate the effects of pollution and eutrophication on freshwater and coastal systems, particularly in developing countries. Eutrophication has to be understood as the result of numerous, cumulative exploitations of water ecosystems that have deteriorated and impaired the functions that these ecosystems typically supply. All of these effects are amplified by climate change. Simultaneously, we have to acknowledge that almost all systems globally react to eutrophication in various ways, resulting in issues unique to individual sites. The transformation and retention of nutrients, as well as physical boundary conditions, play a major role in the ensuing effects of local eutrophication. Eutrophication must be decreased to levels that are acceptable to natural ecosystems and human population. Adaptation efforts at all levels are required to foster the problems provided by climatic variability, particularly in developing nations.

## 1.7. COMPLICATIONS IN WATER ADAPTATION

Adaptation connected to water is complicated. Ecological, political, social, economic, and cultural variables must all be taken into account during adaptation. Variations in the quantity and quality of water require water managers as well as individual users of the water environment, such as industries, farmers, consumers and other stakeholders to respond and prepare practically. However, there are very few instances of concrete steps taken by the water sector to explicitly adapt to a changing climate.

This is partially because there are still uncertainties in forecasts of future hydrological changes, and partly because strategies may be impacted by other factors in addition to climate change. It is now well acknowledged that P inputs must be reduced in order to reduce the eutrophication of lakes, reservoirs, streams, and rivers.. Reactive nitrogen is frequently believed to be the primary regulating element for the eutrophication of coastal waters or estuaries (Howarth and Marino, 2006). However, reducing nitrogen input will have severe effects by favoring nitrogen-fixing cyanobacteria as a response of the phytoplankton community to high seasonal nitrogen constraint, therefore controlling reactive nitrogen alone will not be adequate to diminish eutrophication. Programs for managing freshwaters and coastal areas that aim to reduce eutrophication must include phosphorus control as a critical component. There are several theories, approaches, and strategies for reducing eutrophication, including biological control. The use of surface water for residential purposes in semi-arid areas appears to be affected by two major issues. The creation of chlorinated hydrocarbons during the water treatment process and the eutrophication of surface water bodies are these issues. Anthropogenic activities cause both issues to arise, either directly or indirectly. Certain nutrients found in lakes, reservoirs, streams, rivers, and near-shore marine water, such as silicate, phosphorus, and nitrogen are necessary for life and do not pose a threat to the ecosystem. Nutrients are life-supporting substances, not contaminants. When excessive inputs alter the ecosystem's initial characteristics, attributes, or functions, they become problematic. This phenomenon is known as the eutrophication of water bodies when it occurs. The presence of abundant plankton, algae, and water weeds is known as eutrophication. This condition affects the taste and odor of domestic water supplies and causes the development of trihalomethanes or THM precursors. Water eutrophication is the common factor that connects algal blooms, fish mortalities, edible shellfish, blue algae, and public health (Turner et al., 2021). The process of a water body becoming more abundant in aquatic plant life, such as algae and aquatic macrophytes (water weeds), is known as eutrophication. It is caused by an increase in the amount of nutrients that aquatic plants receive from both natural and man-made sources, particularly compounds that contain phosphorus and nitrogen. These nutrients disturb the natural balance of the organisms in the water and degrade the water quality.

The silt (Figure 1.10) that is rich in organic nutrients and minerals is carried into the freshly formed lakes by the runoff water. Wind-borne spores of bacteria, protozoa, and algae quickly establish a population and serve as the foundation of a food pyramid that gradually expands to accommodate populations of plants and animals. The remains of dead plants and animals at lake bottoms are broken down (degraded) by microorganisms. When plants die, they become food for decomposers like bacteria, fungi and earthworms. In addition, the lake ecology continues to get organic fertilizers and minerals from the sediments of surface water runoff from the nearby land. Bacteria and algae flourish in the nutrient-rich water. As long as the water contains a sufficient amount of dissolved oxygen, the breakdown process is predominantly aerobic. But when silt keeps coming in and organic matter accumulates, the aerobic bacteria use up the oxygen and start to allow other types of bacteria that take over the decay process. These are the anaerobic microorganisms that produce hydrogen sulfide and methane as byproducts of their decomposition. The process of adding nutrients to an environment that causes the amount of accessible oxygen in the water to drop is known as natural eutrophication. The succession from lake to marsh to meadow to forest is driven by this. Depending on the original state of the land, this natural succession process could occur anywhere over a period of 500–10.000 years or more (Webb, 1987). Ecosystems can receive nutrients more quickly when human activity speeds up this process. The flow of inorganic nutrients and organic substances into terrestrial, aquatic, and coastal marine environments is increased by runoff from agriculture, urbanization, and industrial development, particularly from septic systems and sewers as well as other human-related activities. Lakes are frequently categorized based on the amount of organic matter and nutrients they contain. They are divided into four primary types based on their trophic state: oligotrophic, mesotrophic, eutrophic, and dystrophic. Oligotrophic lakes (Figure 1.11) have limited plant growth and inadequate plant nutrition supplies. The waters of oligotrophic lakes are of high-drinking quality. Moreover, biological productivity is therefore typically poor.

Lakes that are mesotrophic have intermediate features. They sustain minimal plant development and have medium-level nutrients. The waters of these lakes are usually clear with submerged aquatic plants. Heavy plant growths can be found in eutrophic lakes due to their abundant supply of plant nutrients. Consequently, biological productivity is typically quite high. Deep waters show lower quantities of dissolved oxygen during times of limited circulation; the waters are turbid due to dense growths of phytoplankton or because they are rich in rooted aquatic plants. An increase in plant-available nutrients in the water suggests a growth in algal primary production. Chlorophyll, sunlight, carbon dioxide, nutrients, and other relevant elements are required by green plants for the process of photosynthesis to produce biomass and oxygen. While potassium, sulfur, iron, and molybdenum are micronutrients that are also necessary, the three most critical nutrients are silicate, phosphorus, and nitrogen.

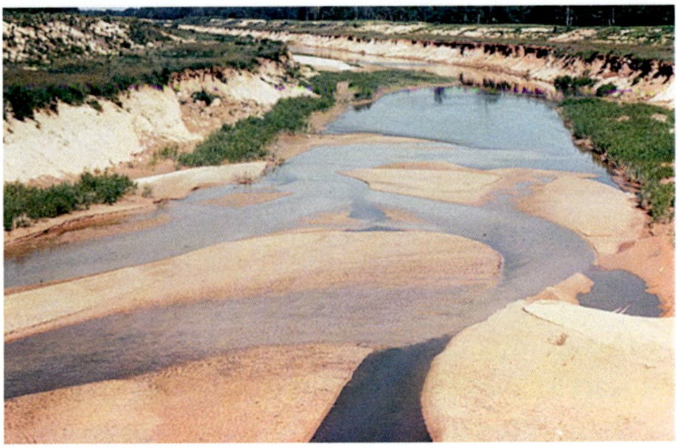

**Figure 1.10.** *Siltation of a waterway.*

Source: https://en.wikipedia.org/wiki/Siltation#/media/File:Siltation_or_Sedimentation.jpg, Creative Commons License.

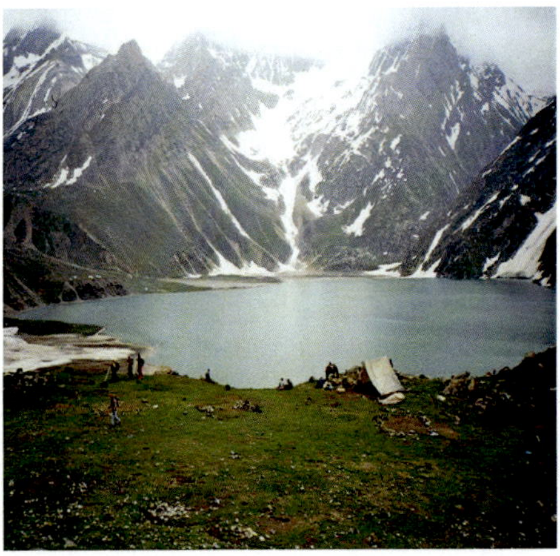

**Figure 1.11.** *Oligotrophic lakes.*

Source: https://en.wikipedia.org/wiki/Sheshnag_Lake#/media/File:Sheshnag4.jpg, Creative Commons License.

Algae (Figure 1.12) can grow to a greater depth in the water when sunlight can reach it. Chlorophyll is required by green plants to store solar energy. The amount of microscopic algae present in the water during the winter, before the spring bloom, can be ascertained by measuring the chlorophyll concentration in the water. High levels of phytoplankton microalgae, with a silicon skeleton (diatom) biomass in stratified water bodies that can result in algal blooms, are the primary source of eutrophication, which is primarily caused by an imbalance in the food web. In addition to the carbon, oxygen, and hydrogen that plants can directly get in the water and the carbon dioxide in the atmosphere, nitrogen (N) and phosphorus (P) are two essential nutrients for the growth of aquatic life. The development of diatoms requires silicate. The concentrations of nutrients in the water alter during eutrophication. One of the three nutrients may occasionally be completely incorporated into the aquatic life and hence unavailable for additional algal growth. The limiting factor is then used to describe this nutrient. In freshwater environments, P is typically the limiting nutrient for phytoplankton, but N is frequently the limiting nutrient in marine water, particularly during the summer.

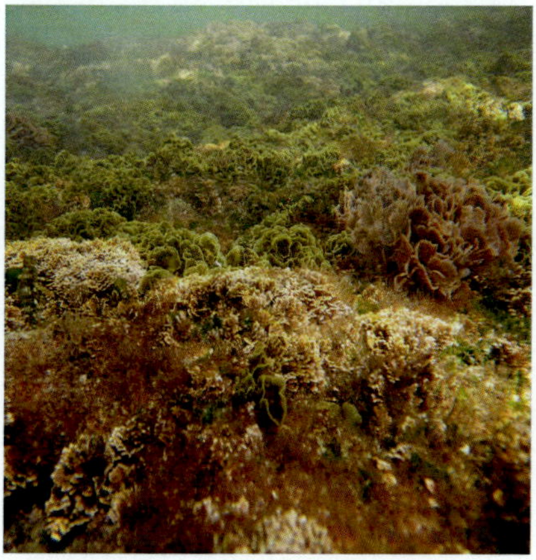

**Figure 1.12.** *Algae.*

Source: https://en.wikipedia.org/wiki/Algae#/media/File:NSW_seabed_1.JPG, Creative Commons License.

## 1.8. POLLUTION

In addition to fertilizer inputs, several environmental factors promote the development of eutrophication (Huang et al., 2017). The growth of aquatic algae is influenced by the thermal stratification of water bodies (lakes and reservoirs), temperature, and light. Eutrophication is a phenomenon that mostly occurs during the spring and summer periods (months) due to increased light and temperature conditions. Because of the shadow effect by algae and other living things, eutrophication itself influences how much light enters the water body and decreases photosynthesis in deep water layers. Drinking water disinfection is the process of treating water to eliminate or inactivate human pathogens, up to a certain safety threshold that needs to be maintained during water distribution, storage and usage. The process is dependent on the type and quantity of microorganisms, as well as the chemical and physical characteristics of the source water. Chemical substances known as chlorination disinfection by-products (DBPs) are produced when chlorine combines with water that contains natural organic matter (NOM) during the water treatment process. Water is treated using a wide range of disinfection techniques all over the world. All naturally occurring surface waters contain a complex matrix of organic material made up of fulvic and humic acids. The breakdown of organic materials from the watershed surroundings, such as leaves, aquatic plants, and human and animal waste, produces NOM. Total organic carbon (TOC) and watercolor are two measures of water quality that are thought to be reliable indications of the existence of NOM in natural water. Particulate organic carbon or POC and dissolved organic carbon or DOC make up TOC, with DOC accounting for over 99% of the total organic carbon or TOC. It has been established that elevated water color and TOC or DOC values indicate a substantial concentration of NOM(Golea et al., 2017). The type and quantity of disinfectant used to disinfect the water directly correlates with the possibility for the creation of DBPs. However, other factors that affect the formation of DBPs include the disinfectant and NOM in addition to pH, water temperature, water turbidity, disinfectant dose, chlorine demand, sunlight, and contact time i.e., the duration of time that the organisms are in contact with the disinfectant.

It is possible that a large number of these components are operating concurrently and antagonistically. DBPs come in a range of forms, including trihalomethanes (THMs), haloacetic acids (HAAs), and haloacetonitriles, which are produced by halogen substitution and/or oxidation reactions in all disinfection techniques (Mayer and Ryan, 2019). The popular disinfection techniques, including ozonation, chlorination, chloramination, and disinfection with chlorine gas, produce the DBPs. Trihalomethane has been the most problematic DBP of all of these, with a substantial quantity of data available. THMs are a family of chlorination DBPs that are created when chlorine reacts with dissolved organic molecules in water. It is possible to categorize the byproducts produced when natural waters are chlorinated into two groups. THM chemicals are derivatives of methane that have been chlorinated and brominated. They make up the first class of compounds. Chloroform ($CHCl_3$), dichlorobromomethane ($CHCl_2Br$), chlorodibromomethane ($CHClBr_2$), and bromoform ($CHBr_3$) are the four chemicals that are frequently included in this class. Chloroform is the most prevalent and frequently found among the four THMs. A complex mixture of comparatively nonvolatile chemicals with larger molecular weights than THM substances makes up the second class. The combination contains a huge number of distinct chemicals at minute concentrations, making it challenging to identify and quantify each individual molecule. As a result, the non-purgeable total organic halide (NPTOX) concentration is used to calculate the concentration of these compounds. The most prevalent DBPs in chlorinated drinking water are trihalomethanes. THMs are thought to be a sign that additional DBPs may be present. They are most likely harmful to people, as well as known to be carcinogenic in lab animals. THMs have been linked to low birth weight, miscarriage, colon and bladder cancer, as well as other unfavorable pregnancy outcomes.

## 1.9. FRESHWATER

The majority of freshwater areas on Earth are polymictic and shallow, usually no deeper than three meters (Herdendorf, 1990). Freshwaters have a wide range of uses and are very valuable for conservation and economy. Since the water depth is typically shallow enough to permit the establishment of submerged macrophytes, they can and often are dominated by littoral communities. The species richness of invertebrate, fish, and water-fowl communities is more diverse than in deep lakes.

Through modifications to the trophic structure, biodiversity, biogeochemical cycles, and seasonal dynamics, eutrophication, also known as nutrient enrichment, has an impact on the entire aquatic system. Many physico-chemical buffer mechanisms help submerged plants in these lakes maintain the clear or pure water state. Once a lake's nutritional threshold is exceeded, there could be a sudden change to a turbid state. Compared to cold temperate lakes, internal nitrogen cycling is comparatively more significant while external loading is comparatively less significant in warm lakes. When it comes to the same concentration of nutrients, warm lakes are typically more productive than cold ones. A community of omnivorous fish that is diversified puts strong predation pressure on zooplankton, making top-down control less significant. As a result, nutrient control becomes the determining factor for water purity. Restoration techniques for cold lakes include both top-down and bottom-up controls; for warm lakes, nutrient or bottom-up control techniques seem to be more important for eutrophication management. Regarding climate change, in both cold and warm climates, warming is probably going to make some eutrophication problems worse. It is anticipated that the structure and operations of cold temperate shallow lakes will resemble those of sub-tropical shallow lakes more because of the temperature increase, which will improve nutrient cycling and the top-down controls of omnivore and benthivorous fish.

## 1.10. IMPORTANCE OF WATER BODIES

Every civilization was established near a steady source of freshwater, typically found in large lakes or rivers utilized for irrigation, boating, swimming, and fishing, as well as for harvesting fish and other food supplies. However, most of the Earth's freshwater is shallow and primarily found in lowlands, with sources ranging from glaciers and geological disturbances to landslides and artificial or natural damming of rivers. Although shallow lakes have been used for various purposes, they are highly valuable both economically and environmentally. The natural resources and services provided by shallow lake wetlands have substantial monetary worth. Globally, natural systems contribute over 30 trillion US dollars annually—three times the gross domestic product (GDP) of all global economies combined (Costanza et al., 2014). Shallow lakes and wetlands are valued at trillions of dollars annually, more than forests and grasslands combined. Freshwater wetlands contribute over 10%, and wetlands overall contribute more than 25% of this total. Shallow lakes are generally less than 3 meters deep and polymictic, meaning thermal stratification is not stable and the water column mixes continuously. The shallow depth allows sufficient underwater light to support the growth of submerged macrophytes, leading to the predominance of littoral communities. Unlike deep lakes, where opportunities for submerged plant growth are restricted to near-shore regions, submerged macrophytes can cover a substantial portion of a shallow lake. These submerged plants play a vital role in shallow lakes and wetlands by providing food and habitat for various consumers. Additionally, they play an essential structural role in the ecosystem as a whole.

The littoral zone and shallow depth together lead to higher benthic–pelagic interaction and a stronger impact of sediment activities on the dynamics of the water column (Griffiths et al., 2017). Due to increased nutrient recycling that makes nutrients directly available to primary producers, particularly phytoplankton and periphyton, shallow lakes are more productive per unit area of water than deep lakes. Because of the significant influence of the littoral zone and the related macrophytes, shallow lakes have a higher species richness than deep lakes. Compared to turbid lakes, shallow lakes play a major role in biodiversity and serve as vital feeding grounds for land animals and waterfowl. Shallow lakes react non-linearly, rather than linearly, to external stimuli. According to the 'alternative stable states' hypothesis, under similar conditions and with a certain amount of stability against external forces, shallow lake ecosystems can exhibit at least two alternative states: a turbid state with phytoplankton and a clear state with dominance of submerged plants. There is greater biodiversity in shallow lakes with submerged vegetation, including fish, ducks, and invertebrates. Stability against agitations may be provided by several physical, chemical, and biological stabilizing feedback processes, many of which are based on interactions with submerged plants. The external influence that has been studied the most is enhanced nutrient availability, or eutrophication, particularly in temperate shallow lakes. The growth of submerged plants causes enhanced nutrient fixation in macrophytes and associated epiphytes, leaving less nutrients available for the phytoplankton, especially in summer; the increase in plant biomass greatly aids in reducing turbidity induced by sediment resuspension, which otherwise entails increased nutrient release to the water column. These are just a few of the physicochemical buffer mechanisms in north temperate shallow lakes that submerge plants used to stabilize the clear water state. Roots and plant surface areas, open to colonization by nitrifying and denitrifying bacteria, boost denitrification and, in turn, induce nitrogen-limited conditions; and submerged macrophytes may diminish phytoplankton by shading. Reduced sediment resuspension significantly promotes the clear water state, with the dominance of submerged plants. It is not totally understood why submerged plants encourage clear water conditions at identical P concentrations from their effects on light and nutrients.

## 1.11. FISH

During feeding, common fish species in Northern Europe, like the carp (*Cyprinus carpio*) (Figure 1.13) and freshwater bream (*Abramis brama*), (Figure 1.14) stir up sediment, which can significantly increase the amount of suspended matter and related nutrients in the water (Dobsikova and Velisek, 2015). In eutrophic lakes (without plants), these fish are frequently in high numbers. Some studies conducted in laboratories have demonstrated that submerged plants including Ceratophyllum, Myriophyllum, and *Chara* spp. chemically restrict the growth of phytoplankton. In temperate shallow lakes, cascading effects of submerged plants on phytoplankton indirectly affect fish and invertebrates, especially zooplankton. In vegetation, strong predator fishlike pike (*Esox lucius*) also survive. Lower predatory control of zooplankton, especially large-bodied species (*Daphnia*), is the result of several predatory fish exerting a strong top-down control on benthic-planktivorous fish, predominantly cyprinids. Large pelagic zooplankton species (Daphnia and other cladocerans) may use submerged plants as a daytime shelter to evade fish predation. Since many predators hunt by night, the risk of predation decreases, and the zooplankton goes to open water to feed on algae. Therefore, plant refuges aid in the regulation of phytoplankton biomass by zooplankton, preserving the quality (clearness) of the water. Large mussel grazers like Anodonta and Dreissena may be essential in removing phytoplankton from the water.

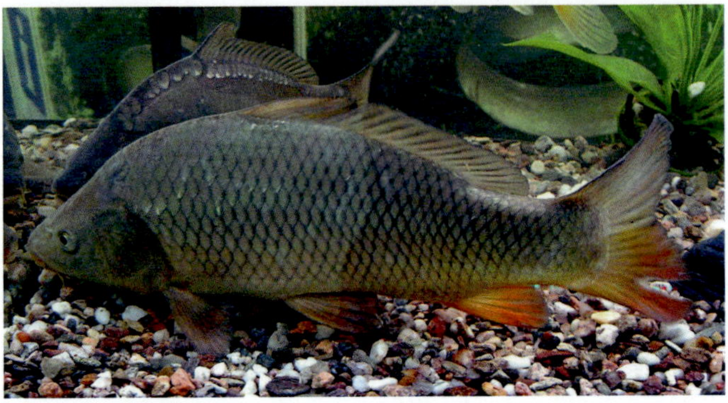

**Figure 1.13.** *Cyprinus carpio.*

Source: https://en.wiktionary.org/wiki/Cyprinus_carpio#/media/File:Carp_(Cyprinus_carpio)_in_aquarium.JPG, Creative Commons License.

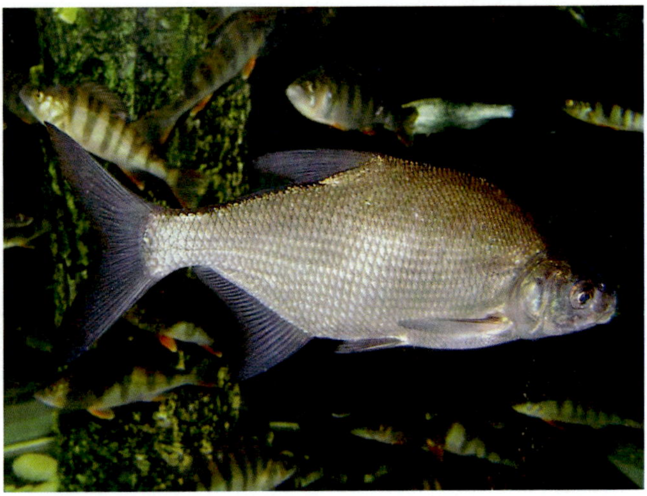

**Figure 1.14.** *Freshwater bream (Abramis brama).*

Source: https://en.wikipedia.org/wiki/Common_bream#/media/File:Carp_bream1.jpg, Creative Commons License.

Eutrophication is the product of excessive nutrient loading to the receiving lakes, which primarily reflects impacts caused by humans (Smith et al., 1999). Since most lowlands are being converted to agricultural or urban land, shallow lakes, which are primarily found in lowland areas, are extremely prone to nutrient enrichment, which can have a significant impact on nutrient flows. While all agricultural systems lack these conservation mechanisms and release nutrients into streams and other bodies of water, natural, pristine systems typically store organic matter and store nutrients. Domestic sewage, intensive agriculture, and industry are the main sources of external nutrient inputs that cause eutrophication, which disrupts the delicate nutrient cycles of the catchment terrestrial ecosystems. A multitude of biological alterations brought about by eutrophication have a detrimental impact on lake ecological conditions. Practical difficulties of eutrophication include decreased value for both commercial and recreational fisheries, harmful algal blooms, and more issues (problems) with using water for irrigation and domestic supply. Rapid economic growth and unsustainable exploitation practices are causing eutrophication in many developing nations to worsen. Significant efforts have been made in the western countries to address eutrophication. Intensive farming and other dispersed sources in the watershed are the main sources of nutrient loading to lakes in developed countries, whereas sewage water and fish farm waste are the main contributors in developing countries. It is anticipated that the eutrophication issue will worsen due to rising water demands brought on by an expanding human population and the consequences of global warming. But eutrophication is caused by important alterations in the food chain as well as by algal immediate response to rising nitrogen levels.

Fish at the top of the food chain react quite differently to higher nutrition levels. At low nutrient concentrations, predatory fishlike perch and pike become dominant; at high nutrient concentrations, cyprinids, particularly roach, carp, and bream, take over; at intermediate levels, the predatory fish survives. As a result, grazers of macroinvertebrates, such as snails, and zooplankton are heavily under threat from cyprinid predation. Benthivorous, bottom-feeding fish are more prevalent, which encourages sediment resuspension and raises turbidity (Adámek and Maršálek, 2013). When phosphorus concentrations rise over 0.15 mg TP $L^{-1}$, the level of zooplankton decreases because of the strong pressure from predators, resulting in a decrease in the ratio of zooplankton to phytoplankton biomass in northern temperate lakes. This ratio typically ranges from 0.5 to 0.8 in mesotrophic lakes to less than 0.2. This indicates that in lakes rich in nutrients, the phytoplankton is not under the control of the zooplankton. Reduced zooplankton grazing pressure coupled with an enhanced nutrient supply suggests a significant increase in phytoplankton biomass, which lowers water transparency. Small grazers (rotifers) take over the zooplankton community as a result of the increasing pressure from predators. Large phytoplankton taxa, such as filamentous cyanobacteria, may therefore flourish in eutrophic lakes. A drop in the number of snails, which are effective grazers of epiphytes on plants and are mediated by fish predation, will further degrade the underwater light environment for submerged plants. Turbid lakes with few major cyprinid fish species, mostly composed of cyanobacteria and green algae, little to no submerged vegetation, and a significantly diminished diversity of waterfowl have degraded conservation and biodiversity significance. For cold temperate shallow lakes, many crucial macrophyte feedback processes for maintaining clear water conditions have been extensively documented.

## 1.12. IMPACTS

The impacts of plants on trophic interactions appear to be more intricate in subtropical and Mediterranean lakes (Moi et al., 2021). While macrophytes can be significant in all forms i.e., emergent, submerged, floating leaved, and free-floating, their effects on trophic interactions and water quality might vary. Since the aquatic plants in these systems are not restricted by temperature, unlike those in cold temperate lakes, they can exist year-round. Particularly, compared to submerged plants, the effects of free-floating plants (*Salvinia* spp., and *Eichhornia crassipes*) (Figure 1.15) on water transparency appear to be much weaker. Plants marginally improve water clarity, and turbidity is common in nutrient-rich lakes with high plant biomass. One of the primary indirect stabilizing buffer mechanisms of submerged plants in shallow temperate lakes is to provide a shelter for large grazers against fish predation. Since denitrification is known to increase with increasing temperatures, it is expected to be a highly important stabilizing buffer mechanism of submerged plants in warm lakes for reducing the N availability for phytoplankton. Thus, it has frequently been proposed that N may be more limiting in warm lakes than in temperate lakes. Submerged macrophyte growth, however, does not lead to a decrease in inorganic N concentrations in shallow lakes in the Mediterranean and subtropic areas. Inefficient denitrification in the warmer lakes was also discovered in some studies on shallow lakes in South America, ranging from the subtropical to the tundra. This could be because of low-quality organic matter.

Large blooms may directly injure humans and other aquatic organisms because the majority of these genera like *Microcystis aeruginosa*, *M. panniformis*, *Planktothrix rubescents* (Figure 1.16), and *Aphanizomenon ovalisporum* have been observed to establish toxic strains in some reservoirs. Each bloom-forming species has a unique set of characteristics, to ensure their survival in environments that are frequently harsh for other phytoplankton. Certain cyanobacteria that generate blooms (*P. rubescens* and *Cylindrospermopsis raciborskii*) have the lowest light saturation values for growth and photosynthesis, and they generally require far less light than eukaryotic algae. Especially in calm conditions and/or during stratification, their gas vesicle regulation favors their location in the light gradient along the water column. Compared to other algae, bloom-forming cyanobacteria are effective at tapping into nutrient reserves that are not easily accessible.

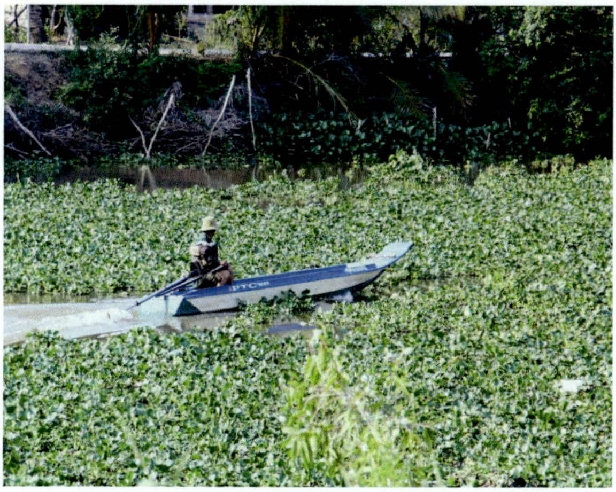

**Figure 1.15.** *Water hyacinth (Eichhornia crassipes).*

Source: https://upload.wikimedia.org/wikipedia/commons/7/77/LucbinhTien-Giang.jpg, Creative Commons License.

They can make use of vertical nutritional gradients, their quick maximal rate of P absorption, and their strong affinity for $NH_4$ due to buoyancy regulation. Both $CO_2$ and $HCO_3$ have effective carbon concentration processes, which enable them to compete over a broad pH range. Because of their large size, they can retain surplus C, N, and P, which helps to buffer environmental variations in the nutrient supply. Even in calm conditions, healthy cyanobacteria prevent sinking loss by regulating their buoyancy. Cyanobacteria exhibit a high degree of phenotypic variability in terms of the length of trichomes, and shape of the colony, although their forms are restricted to relatively simple shapes(Marquardt and Palinska, 2007).

This allows them to endure a variety of environmental conditions once their dominance has been established. *Microcystis morphotypes* have the ability to utilize and retain nutrients extremely well. They also benefit from the ability to regulate their buoyancy and the variety of their colony size and form, which is especially useful in an underwater environment with variable light levels. One of the most notable effects of nutrient buildup in the sediments due to certain hydrological patterns in reservoirs was the emergence of extremely heavy cyanobacterial blooms. Extended growing seasons are possible due to the characteristics of a Mediterranean environment, and Microcystis often begins its growing season at the end of February and continues until October or November.

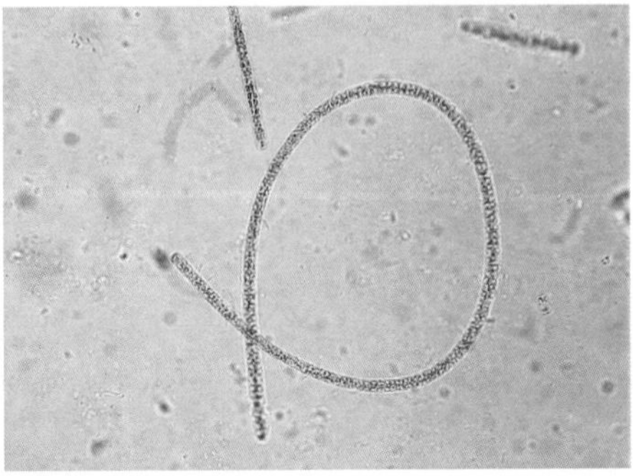

**Figure 1.16.** *Planktothrix rubescens.*

Source: https://en.wikipedia.org/wiki/Planktothrix#/media/File:Planktothrix_rube-scens.jpeg, Creative Commons License.

Chapter 2

# EUTROPHICATION AND BENTHIC VEGETATION

## Contents

## 2.1. INTRODUCTION

As a direct result of increased human activities, there is a tendency for marine coastal systems to be damaged more and more (Burkett and Davidson, 2012). This tendency started at the end of the previous century but became particularly evident throughout the past three to four decades. A growing number of different wastes and contaminants, such as fertilizers, enter the coastal areas through rivers. These wastes and contaminants come from several intensive land and marine uses, including industry, urbanization, agriculture, and mariculture. This led to rising levels of pollutants and nutrients in many shallow coastal areas, which are the main recipients of land runoff. In enclosed or semi-enclosed water bodies like fjords, bays, harbors, or estuaries, the release of wastes that transport nutrients has resulted in eutrophication, and in severe cases, hypertrophication. The process of naturally occurring or artificially induced enrichment with inorganic nutrient elements, primarily nitrogen, and phosphorus, beyond the maximum critical level of a system's ability to regulate itself for a balanced flow and cycling of nutrients is known as eutrophication. Naturally, there might be substantial differences in the critical values between oligotrophic and eutrophic environments.

A system and the way matter and energy move through it may alter as a result of eutrophication, although these modifications may not always be damaging to the system. Actually, it has long been believed that increasing the amount of nutrients available, where they frequently limit primary production, will improve benthic and pelagic productivity.

## 2.2. HYPERTROPHICATION

Hypertrophication, also known as nutrient pollution, refers to an excess of nutrients that exceed the maximum critical self-regulatory level to the point where, if nutrient loadings are not decreased, detrimental processes result in permanent changes in the aquatic communities. Many observations on structural and functional changes resulting in a general degradation of the coastal environment have documented the effects of air, marine, and terrestrial pollution on coastal ecosystems.

Numerous instances of correlative or causal ecological reactions to pollution include increased plankton production, which increases sedimentation and benthic yield. This could therefore result in mortality and oxygen deprivation episodes, as well as a die-back of the benthic and diseases that affect benthic and pelagic species. Some of the obvious effects are changes in the marine benthic vegetation, which is made up of seagrasses, macroalgae, and microalgae. These changes are likely related to both eutrophication and hypertrophication in specific as well as pollution in general (Battarbee, 2010). Even though eutrophication has been linked to all of the abovementioned phenomena, the data are highly varied, making it seem difficult to establish a causal relationship between increasing nutrient loadings and biological responses. The consequences of coastal eutrophication on marine macrophytes were primarily considered localized issues. These issues have been dominated by plankton blooms in the open sea, that are caused by eutrophication.

## 2.3. EFFECTS ON BENTHIC ORGANISMS

Changes in the microphytobenthos have been observed and documented along the European coasts in some locations ranging from the northernmost shores of the Atlantic and Baltic to the eastern parts of the Mediterranean and into the Black Sea (Kautsky et al., 2017). Many additional locations/sites would likely yield similar observations. The fact that changes in marine vegetation appear to be concentrated around the coasts of northern Europe must undoubtedly be related to increased industrialization and population density, but it may also be partially explained by the fact that more research has been done in the northern states than in any other region of Europe. There has been no attempt to tackle the marine eutrophication-macrophyte problem on a European level. The long-term impacts of nutrient pollution and coastal eutrophication have received minute attention.

These issues have occasionally been acknowledged and taken into account in regional, national, or international programs or agreements. There have been successful attempts to reduce pollution in several European countries, as evidenced by the recent signs/indications of de-eutrophication, or a decline in the amount of inorganic nutrients in coastal waters. Recently, research has been conducted in Europe on the mechanisms underlying the effects of pollution and eutrophication on benthic macro-vegetation. One such project is EUMAC (Eutrophication and Macrophytes), a cooperative EC-ENVIRONMENT project involving several European research centers and universities (Taylor, 1999). The fundamental reason EUMAC was the realization that eutrophication has complicated effects on coastal systems, especially on phytobenthic populations, which cannot be well described by a single factor or variable. Elevated nitrogen levels typically do not automatically result in the extensive growth of algae or other distinguished alterations to biological populations. Combined physical, chemical, and biological elements are effective in the transition from the input of extra nutrients to a coastal system to the actual manifestation of typical eutrophication effects. To effectively mitigate and regulate these interactions and safeguard and potentially rebuild coastal ecosystems, a deeper understanding of their mechanisms is necessary.

## 2.4. THE DISRUPTIVE EFFECTS OF NUTRIENTS

The nutrient enrichment, or eutrophication, of coastal waters due to human activity is currently seen as a serious global pollution problem. The natural nutrient cycles are essentially disrupted by the increased anthropogenic source of inorganic plant nutrients, which can also artificially boost primary production during periods of low activity. This may have significant ecological complications for species that are benthic and pelagic. For instance, there will be an increase in phytoplankton activity. While this can generally be advantageous by increasing fisheries, there is evidence that it has also led to the occurrence of some toxic and non-toxic phytoplankton blooms, (Figure 2.1) which have harmed recreational and fisheries activities.

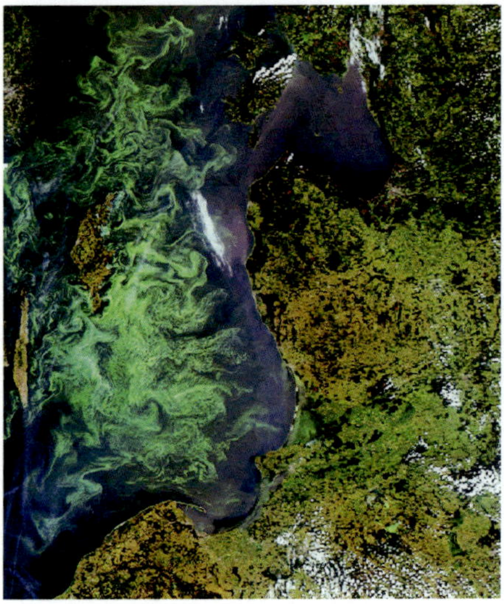

**Figure 2.1.** *Phytoplankton blooms.*

Source: https://upload.wikimedia.org/wikipedia/commons/6/6b/Envisat_image_of_a_phytoplankton_bloom_in_the_Baltic_Sea_ESA226711.jpg, Creative Commons License.

Many international reports are now emphasizing how benthic algal communities react to nitrogen effects. These usually relate to the occurrence of macroalgal growths that are excessive and the negative ecological and environmental effects that follow. The effect of other possible pollutants present in the carrying waters must be taken into account when analyzing the ecological impact of nutrients obtained from these anthropogenic sources, especially those that are released with sewage effluent. Both agricultural runoff and sewer effluent will include suspended particles, biological waste, and freshwater. Moreover, sewage contains a variety of surfactants and dispersants, as well as occasionally trace amounts of heavy metals, whereas agricultural runoff may contain herbicides, pesticides, and hydrocarbons. Several of these pollutants have an impact on marine benthic communities, especially on marine benthic algae. Thus, under conditions of heavy sediment loading, benthic algal photosynthetic yield would be lowered, and this could create problems for some benthic algae, especially those in the sublittoral zone.

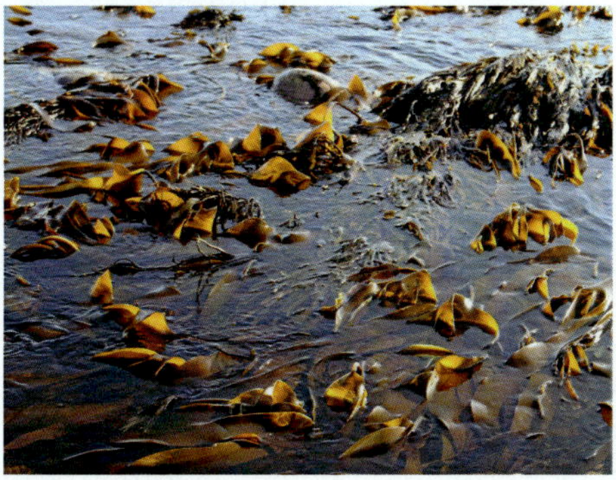

**Figure 2.2.** *Laminaria saccharina.*

Source: https://upload.wikimedia.org/wikipedia/commons/f/f8/Laminaria_saccharina_IMG_1029_listafyr.JPG, Creative Commons License.

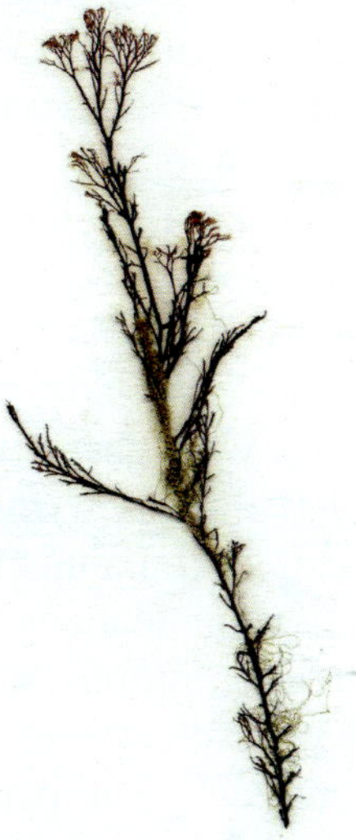

**Figure 2.3.** *Red algae (Polysiphonia nigrescens).*

Source: https://upload.wikimedia.org/wikipedia/commons/d/df/Polysiphonia_nigrescens_Helgoland.JPG, Creative Commons License.

*Laminaria saccharina* (Figure 2.2) gametophyte fertilization requires sufficient light (Cuijuan et al., 2005). The decrease of Fucus biomass in Kiel Bight, Western Baltic and the reduction of Macrocystis beds near sewage outfalls in California are among the reported effects of decreased light penetration caused by pollutants. Algae (adapted to low light) would also have a competitive advantage, as demonstrated by the populations of *Phyllophora truncata*, *Phycodrys rubens*, and *Polysiphonia nigrescens* (Figure 2.3) that are allegedly mostly displaced Fucus spp. below 2 m depths in Kiel Bight.

## 2.5. ALGAL ZONATION PATTERNS

Increased sediment loading has also been shown to alter algal zonation patterns and depth distributions (Eriksson and Johansson, 2005). The area of sewage outfalls, for instance, has been shown to have a reduced kelp depth range, with plants often limited to shallow water and very few young kelps existing beneath the old ones. Reduced water transparency has also been linked to changes in the South Kattegat (Baltic Sea) eelgrass depth penetration, which went from 10-12 m to 5-6 m between 1900 and 1989. There was more silt deposition close to sewage outfalls, which can negatively impact marine benthic algal ecosystems in many ways. The sediments can cover every substratum, interfering with the spore (larvae) attachment and recruitment processes. Sediments can also disturb spore surfaces when combined with water flow. In addition to lowering photosynthetic activity, deposits on algal thalli will also destroy algae species. The decline of kelp beds off the coast of southern California has been attributed to all of the mentioned detrimental effects of increased sedimentation on benthic communities. These effects have been well-recognized. The sediments impede the development of Macrocystis gametophytes. Silt had a similar negative effect on the growth of zoospores in Laminaria saccharina. Many sediments formed from effluents, especially those from sewage treatment plants, have a high organic loading, which has several effects on marine benthic ecosystems. Some researchers have reported that mussels are becoming more common and producing biomass in contaminated waters, particularly those near sewage outfalls. *Mytilus edulis* populations have decreased in conjunction with reductions in organic loading (pollution), such as when sewage effluent is redirected into deeper water or when treatment methods are improved (Beyer et al., 2017). There are important ecological consequences of the competitive advantage that mussels have when they are near sewage outfalls, particularly for marine benthic algae. Mussels compete with other algae for available space, cover the surfaces of other algae, and serve as highly effective filters for possibly settling spores. These observations suggest that mussels are not ideal substrata for many algae.

Likewise, numerous observations have indicated that there is an increase in grazing activity close to sewage outfalls; sea urchins, in particular, are known to feed on the organic material in the sewage. The decline of Macrocystis kelp beds in California has been attributed to an increase in grazers; these grazers put older kelp plants under high grazing pressure, attack holdfasts, and chew the stipe, resulting in the loss of the upper blade sections. Reports of relatively few young kelps being present near the outfalls support the idea that young plants are likewise mostly sensitive. Reports of increased numbers of detritivorous snails, such as Hydrobia, and increased grazing pressure on *Fucus vesiculosus* by the isopod *Idotea baltica* are among the other changes resulting from increased pollution-related grazer activity. The latter was attributed to the rise in Idothea abundance, most likely as a result of nutrient-related modifications in the Fucus phenolic content, which made the latter more susceptible to grazing activity. In addition to the secondary impacts of organic enrichment, several researchers have noted a significantly diminished and specialized flora in situations of extreme pollution with high organic loading. In particular, species of Lyngbya and Phormidium appear to predominate. This is an important observation. The low pH levels and anaerobic conditions likely contributed to the abundance of blue-green algae. It is also important to note that sediments formed from sewage may include hazardous materials. The experiments utilizing gametophytes of the kelp Macrocystis revealed this for deeper sediments; re-exposure of these contaminated sediments by disturbance would therefore have unfavorable ecological effects. Some researchers observed that silt had inhibitory effects on algae. The sewage effluent has shown to be inhibitory to marine species given the potential existence of conservative materials in it, including heavy metals, different organic chemicals, pesticides, surfactants, detergents, chlorine, etc. Three Sargassum spp. were inhibited by municipal wastewater. The toxic chemicals are associated with sewage spills, some researchers also considered the possibility that the observed decreases in the numbers of brown and red algal species near outfalls could be caused by the toxic effects of detergents or surfactants present (Holt et al., 1992). These results are in line with other observations that detergents have an impact on *Laminaria saccharina* growth in the lab; detergents have also been linked to a decrease in settlement density in this species. It is probable that the 5–10 ml concentrations of anionic detergents found in sewage will have inhibitory effects.

## 2.6. DYNAMICS OF MACROALGAE

A decrease in the quantity of perennial macro algae contributing to the climax communities of both the intertidal and subtidal regions is perhaps one of the most obvious changes linked to eutrophication. Due to the presence of sewage effluent in the North Atlantic and Baltic, several Fucus spp., including *Fucus vesiculosus*, (Figure 2.4) have been reported to be replaced or to have decreased in number (Stenström and Mattsson, 2022). This suggests that *Fucus* communities are particularly vulnerable. Several observations indicate a reduction in North Atlantic populations of the knotted wrack *Ascophyllum nodosum* due to increased eutrophication. The dense green algal populations in Oslofjord, Norway, compete unfavorably with these fucoids, most likely by impeding the development of germlings. Mediterranean species of Fucus have been found to be declining similarly to fucoids. Examples of these species include *Cystoseira fimbriata* and *C. barbata*, *Cystoseira stricta*, and *Fucus virsoides*. Some observations have indicated a decrease in the number of sargassum plants. However, *Fucus distichus* ssp. edentatus, a pollution-tolerant fucoid may be connected to sewage-contaminated water. In the sewage-polluted areas, Fucus spiralis and Fucus evanescens were more prevalent than other fucoids.

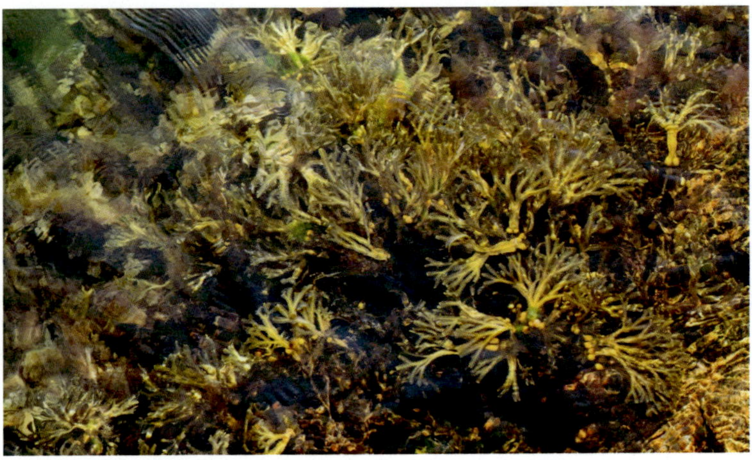

**Figure 2.4.** *Fucus vesiculosus.*

Source: https://upload.wikimedia.org/wikipedia/commons/f/f8/Bladder_wrack_in_S%C3%A4mstad_harbor_1.jpg, Creative Commons License.

## 2.7. PHANEROGAMS

*Phyllospadix torreyi*, *Posidonia oceanica*, and *Zostera muelleri* are among the phanerogams whose numbers have been seen to decline in the vicinity of sewage outfalls. The local ecology of the waters is especially damaged by the loss of these perennial macro algae and phanerogams because they offer a stable habitat and are always home to a diverse range of related marine benthic plant and animal communities, which are collectively referred to as seagrass and Cystoseira associations, respectively. Since these associations frequently serve as fisheries, their loss can be especially detrimental to local fisheries. It is important to observe that there is growing interest in Japan in artificially establishing seaweed beds to improve local fisheries. While secondary pollutants, such as suspended particulate matter, and toxic ingredients are often responsible for the loss of these communities of large macro algae and seagrasses in eutrophicated waters, several reports indicate that these communities may be dominated by algae that are more suited to withstand the high nutrient loadings. Researchers reported a decline or disappearance of several algae belonging to the Cystoseira association in some regions, including the brown algae *Dictyopteris membranacea* and *Cladostephus verticillatus,* as well as the red genera Polysiphonia. These algae were replaced by *Dictyota dichotoma*, *Punctaria latifolia*, and *Corallina officinalis*. These are a few examples of floristic changes related to wastewater. In the contaminated waters, the total failure of the *Fucus virsoides* and *Cystoseira* spp. associations and their replacement by a proliferating growth of *Halopteris scoparia* together with *Ulva lactuca* and *Codium tomentosum*, etc.

## 2.8. ALTERED SPECIES DYNAMICS

*Gracilaria blodgetti* and *Agardhiella tenera* were inhabitants of sewage outfall areas in Biscayne Bay, Florida. Some researchers reported an increase in the mean algal cover of *Gelidium pusillum* in an intertidal community near a sewage outfall in California. This community replaced the less tolerant of pollution and more macroscopic communities of *Sargassum agardhianum*, *Gigartina canaliculata*, *Gelidium robistum*, and the coralline alga *Lithophyllum decipiens*. There was a decrease in the number of species with elevated pollution levels, which resulted in an increase in the number of tolerant species like *Hypnea musciformis*. The vegetation was primarily composed of a cover of Cyanophyceae, a few Rhodophyceae (*Bangia juscopurpurea*), and a few Chlorophyceae (*Enteromorpha intestinalalis*). Certain species of green algae of genera Enteromorpha and Cladophora are particularly prevalent. However, species of the genera Ectocarpus and Pilayella are commonly reported as brown algae, whereas species of the genera Gracilaria, Gelidium, and Bangia are regularly recorded as red algae. Reports of giant red algae (*Phycodrys rubens*) becoming more prevalent due to eutrophication have been made. The blue-green algae or Cyanophyceae, are also widely distributed, especially in areas with high pollution levels and in the summer months. Many researchers have characterized many of these algae, particularly the green algae, as annual and ephemeral, and also fast growing and opportunistic. The polluted environment preserves an immature community typical of an early seral stage. A community that is low-turf forming and unstratified is thought to be more resilient to the environmental stress and instability brought on by recurrent sewage inflow. Calcareous red algae are another important category of algae that are said to be especially resistant to sewage contamination. Branched red algae, specifically *Ceramium* spp., *Polysiphonia* spp., and *Bangia* sp., are also frequently reported to be prevalent in sewage-polluted waters. Only a few species of algae genera have been consistently documented in eutrophicated waters. They are members of the Chlorophyta, particularly species belonging to the genera Chaetomorpha, Cladophora, and Ulva, except for the brown alga Ectocarpus and, to a lesser extent, Pilayella. They often grow in large quantities because they are the only algae present at the contaminated sites. *Ulva rigida* was found to weigh between 10 and 13 kg/m(Ventura et al., 1994). Some researchers reported that Ulva was found to weigh up to 240 kg/m, forming 1 m thick tides. *Enteromorpha prolifera* was found to weigh about 1 kg/m$^2$ on mud flats in some areas(Ramus, 1992).

## 2.9. PIONEERING SPECIES

Understanding the biology of the very small number of genera (species) that contribute to the production of green tides has attracted special attention. They are sometimes described as pioneering species on recently disturbed substrates and can be generally characterized as opportunistic. They frequently appear as significant marine fouling species and as early colonizers of substrata denuded by anthropogenic processes like treating oil pollution or sand scouring. The biological traits provide the algae a competitive advantage over many other algae and allow the quick and successful colonization of a variety of habitats and situations. It is also possible to characterize the floristic components of these green tides as physiologically robust and stress-tolerant. Genera that show a broad tolerance to unfavorable environmental conditions of temperature, light intensity, and salinity are Ulva and Enteromorpha. According to some reports, Ulva, for instance, is highly adaptable to a variety of irradiance and is particularly tolerant of low light conditions. It is also particularly tolerant of anoxic conditions, the presence of sulphide, etc., as well as prolonged desiccation. Ulva has low compensatory light intensity and also has ability to adapt to low irradiance levels will maximize production rates in tidal waters, even those with high sediment loading. This should be especially helpful for plants that form dense growths resembling those that contribute to green tides. While *Gracilaria confervoides* is known to be resistant to hydrogen sulfide, *Ulva rotundata* (Figure 2.5) is also known to photoaclimate.

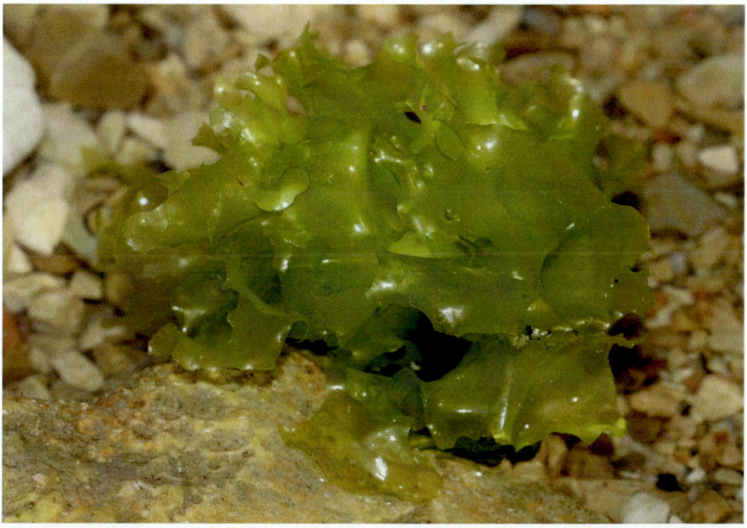

**Figure 2.5.** *Ulva.*

Source: https://upload.wikimedia.org/wikipedia/commons/c/cf/Meersalat-Ulva-lactuca.jpg,, Creative Commons License.

## 2.10. ACCLIMATIZATION MECHANISMS

Plants that live in large, dense mats would benefit most from the capacity to both photoaclimatize and withstand $H_2S$ (Lamote and Dunton, 2006). These green tide-forming algae also can generate free-floating populations with vegetative development, as well as vegetative fragmentation and propagation. Plants that thrive in calm water conditions undoubtedly exhibit vegetative fragmentation, but some researchers found a correlation between fragmentation and high ammonium-N concentrations in *Hypnea musciformis*. Some findings indicate that sporulation is uncommon in free-floating plants, which may be connected to nutrition levels. Their competitive response/feedback to the high nutrient concentration of the nearby waters, however, is perhaps one of these algae's significant characteristics. In addition to their ability to withstand elevated nutrient concentrations, many researchers have documented that these algae exhibit a high and swift uptake and retention of inorganic nitrogen and possess a high nitrogen saturation level. Some researchers came to the conclusion that rapid growth leads to losses due to grazing and abrasion and that rapid N uptake rates are an essential strategy for fast-growing, opportunistic macroalgae. Ulva has also been shown to develop when exposed to very slight increases in nutrients. As a highly adapted plant for the rapid uptake and storage of nutrients that are acquired on an intermittent basis, Ulva is also opportunistic.

## 2.11. BIOLOGICAL ADAPTATIONS

Certain genera, like Ulva, Enteromorpha, and Gracilaria, can also absorb and use ammonia quickly, although $NO_3$ is generally recognized as the primary available source of N for macroalgae (Aníbal et al., 2014). Many green algae have been demonstrated to prefer it over $NO_3$ in certain experimental studies, for instance. The algae also show faster rates of growth, which making them particularly suitable for sewage effluent. Although Ulva converts molecular nitrogen into macromolecular nitrogen, it has been recorded that Ulva may store molecular nitrogen intracellularly. Having the ability to use ammonia while nitrate levels are low in the late summer would also be beneficial. Several genera, including Ulva, Corallina, and Lithothrix, can utilize organic carbon sources, such as acetate and glucose, as well as organic nitrogen (N) sources, such as urea, amino acids, and other amides or groups, as nutrient sources. The large amounts of soluble organic compounds discharged into some inshore waters may be the cause of the reported excessive growths of certain algae. Ulva, Enteromorpha, Lithothrix, and Corallina's ability to quickly absorb nutrients was responsible for their ability to thrive in contaminated environments. Researchers also noted that brown and red algae, which have limited uptake ability, are absent in contaminated waters. For instance, it has been demonstrated that algae like *Ulva fasciata* grow more quickly when supplied with urea as opposed to either $NH_4$ or $NO_3$. It is interesting to note that *Ulva lactuca* has been demonstrated to absorb acetate, a byproduct of bacterial decomposition of organic matter and that many organic nitrogen sources are frequently released in sewage effluent. Some researchers found that *Ulva lactuca* grew faster in cultures supplied with glucose and acetate in the dark and/or low light. This finding explains the plant's capacity to tolerate extended periods of low light and keep its photosynthetic apparatus intact. It has been proposed that Ulva's capacity to absorb organic substrates may account for its capacity to withstand extended burial periods. Ulva and Enteromorpha absorbed organic substances relatively quickly. This is significant because of their restricted exposure to the tidal cycle. These green tide components have some potential for application in wastewater treatment due to their quick absorption of nitrogen from saltwater.

Many of the aspects about green tide morphology have been studied, along with the potential impact on nutrient absorption. Researchers propose that the frequently observed filamentous, sheet-like, tubular, and ball-like nature of their thalli produces a high ratio of surface to volume which ensures maximum nutrient uptake. Researchers propose that the interaction of algal shape, water motion, and nutrient content governs the uptake of nutrients and the patterns of growth. It is well known that the water velocity can affect the uptake and supply of nutrients to algal thalli. Therefore, the morphological characteristics of macro algae can have a significant impact on this process by causing turbulence at the thallus surface, which in turn increases the availability of nutrients for *Macrocystis integrifolia* and *Nereocystis leutkeana*. The filamentous algae typically have high specific carbon fixation rates. Given the high ambient nutrient levels in some eutrophicated coastal waters, it is probable that nutrient ecotypes for green tide algae have evolved. This development may be comparable to that observed for *Laminaria longicruris* in Nova Scotia.

## 2.12. ALGAL MAT DYNAMICS

The impact of nutrients on the structure of benthic communities was demonstrated through their nutrient-treated seagrass beds. The presence of dense beds of free-floating *Enteromorpha plumosa* and *Ulva lactuca* plants was brought about by the addition of $NH_4$ and $NO_3$. Some researchers found that vascular plants benefited from low nutrient concentrations and that $NO_3$ might even be harmful to Zostera (Mach et al., 2014). The nitrate and phosphate fertilizer added to a Scottish sea loch promoted an abnormally dense algal growth.

It has been observed that as these algal mats are carried away by tidal movements and drift to new locations, more issues arise. In the Baltic, nutrients accumulated in deep waters are eventually mixed up to the surface layers through thermohaline convection. They may be deposited in deeper waters, indicating a short-term nutrient loss to the local ecosystem. The mats remain on the coast, bathing on the beaches and causing aesthetic and ecological problems. As the mats decompose, strong odors are released and expensive clearing operations are required to remove them. Large drift weed deposits that float have also been reported to obstruct ship intake pipes and power plant intake ducts. Nonetheless, many researchers point out a few advantages of the loose-lying algal mats. For instance, they are essential to nutrient recycling processes because they serve as a sink for nutrients. They contribute to the dissolved organic carbon pool and significantly enhance the detritus system. In addition, they can serve as vital breeding and nursery sites/grounds for a variety of small fish and can supply food, habitat, and shelter to a wide variety of tiny fish and invertebrates.

However, specific issues/problems come up when the algal mats eventually decompose. This typically occurs when there is a significant rise in oxygen demand, such as during nighttime respiration, during high temperatures and in calm conditions. There are axonic conditions with important ecological ramifications. The underlying mud infauna is negatively impacted by this decrease in oxygen and the ensuing excessive formation of sulfide on the mud surface. The bivalve mollusks *Cardium edule* and *Macoma balthica* migrated to the surface to avoid anaerobic conditions (Burdon et al., 2014). Wading birds predated many of these species, or killed them because they were exposed. Similar occurrences were reported for the *Mya arenaria* under *Ulva lactuca*, as well as for *Cardium edule* under Cladophora deposits in Sweden. Mud infauna diversity and quantity have generally decreased. This had a negative impact on the bird populations and fishing industries. Usually, a few species that can withstand pollution replace the native wildlife. On mud flats on the south coast of England, some researchers reported a decreased biomass of infauna under Enteromorpha mats, with a high number of more pollution-tolerant species like the oligochaete *Peloscolex benedenii* and the polychaetes *Capitella capitata*. It has also been demonstrated that algal mats on Bull Island, Ireland, favor the Peloscolex over other interstitial life forms. On mud flats in Scotland, researchers reported that the lugworm *Arenicola marina* could withstand anaerobic conditions as well as the presence of sulfide under Ulva and Enteromorpha. Toxic compounds have also been linked to the decaying or decomposing weed. The release of harmful hydrogen sulfide odors, the blackening of lead pigment paint on nearby buildings, and the rapid growth of chironomid flies whose larval stages can survive the anoxic conditions are additional effects of this anaerobic decomposition process. Surface waters are also reported to have a high sulfide content, giving them an opaque and creamy-colored appearance. The latter was a specific issue in Venice when swarms of the flying midge *Dicrotendipes conjunctus* hindered airport and railroad operations; a similar issue involving swarms of the flying midge has been documented in Tasmania. The return of nutrients to the ecosystem is a significant secondary effect of the decomposition process. Algal mats serve as a temporary reservoir of nutrients that are quickly released into the waters at the sediment surface, replenishing the superficial sediment nutrient load. This contributes organic matter to the sediments and it replenishes the water column with nutrients, which are subsequently expressed as phytoplankton blooms.

While there is some evidence that invertebrate grazing can influence biomass development, in most green tide scenarios and during biomass production peaks, these natural biological control mechanisms are completely insufficient and treatment is necessary. The most popular treatment is probably the physical removal of the problematic algal biomass. This is especially true in cases when abundant amounts of weed are present. After building up on the tide line, the algae are often mechanically removed and sent to land-fill locations. The algal biomass may occasionally be extracted on-site. Harvesting boats were used to remove floating masses of Ulva from the Venice Lagoon, while specialized machinery was used to remove Ulva from Odense Fjord (Denmark) (Ménesguen, 2014). Harvesting undoubtedly offers an effective management strategy in addition to possible benefits in terms of using the produced algal biomass. Indications of altered nutrient and productivity patterns in ecosystems have been documented for numerous coastal waters in Europe. They include a fortiori green tides, mass algal development, and increased phytoplankton production. Seaweeds are suitable for purifying nitrogen-rich household/domestic and urban sewage, as well as certain agricultural and industrial waste effluents. Mainly impacted by the proliferation of green algae include Ulva, Enteromorpha, and Cladophora; among red algae, Gracilaria and Porphyra are affected. The North Sea nutrient content has nearly tripled during the past ten years. The majority originated from huge rivers that cut or passed through industrial areas, and it was collected by water masses that were flowing from the canals. Phaeocystis, an alga that grows easily, particularly along the shores of Belgium, Netherlands, and Germany, has been the cause of blooms. The synthesis of DMS is linked to *Phaeocystis pouchetti*.

## 2.13. GEOGRAPHICAL EXAMPLES

High nitrate concentrations take over when the algae remove silica from the water, and blooms continue until the nitrogen supply runs out. The procedure is typical for open ocean and coastal regions. Because human nitrogen enriches the water, phaeocystis accounts for 80% of the algal biomass. Mainly along the beaches between France and Denmark, eutrophication takes place. In comparison to waters nearer the coast, the phenomenon is slightly different in the open ocean. Measurements taken over a 50-year period in the open ocean reveal periods of several blooms rather than a trend of increasing numbers. Higher nutrient concentrations are favored by heavy rainfall and river discharges. The freshwater allows for water stratification, which improves light conditions for phytoplankton. The peak intensity of the bloom occurs during the summer when there is optimal insolation and calm winds. Reports of Phaeocystis blooms existed before eutrophication. It has been suggested that eutrophication increases their biomass. In The Netherlands, biomass has increased tenfold. Algal growth has continued to increase in France along the shores of Corsica (Laborel et al., 1994). The damaged areas have spread to the Mediterranean and the southwest on the Atlantic. Furthermore, the phenomena have evolved throughout time, occurring from May to November. The Greek eastern Mediterranean, which includes the Levantine seas, has not been documented to produce phytoplankton blooms; nonetheless, a number of gulfs (Kavala and Patraikos) have shown substantial levels of nutrients. In the Saronikos Gulf, where eutrophication is extensive, algal blooms occur frequently. This state is exacerbated by intensive agriculture. The Gulf of Alexandroupolis has been evaluated for high nutrient concentrations linked to river flow and runoff. Over the past 15 years, the Black Sea phytoplankton has changed due to a variety of factors including drilling, industrialization, agriculture, tourism, the building of harbors and canals, and marine mining. There has been an obvious increase in biomass and an upsurge in the frequency of blooms. In order to stop blooms, huge algal development and eutrophication, it is necessary to reduce the nitrogen flow.

The Romanian seashore is under threat from ecological degradation. From the middle of the 20$^{th}$ century, benthic seaweeds have gradually but steadily declined in both quality and quantity. Eutrophication is the cause of the exceptionally high chlorophyll a content that has been seen in the pre-Danubian Black Sea area for about 20 years. Eutrophication is an important concern resulting from pollution, surpassed only by development along the shore and in the vicinity. The amount of eutrophication and the growth of algae are directly correlated. The algae that colonize the impacted areas are viewed as having the purification capacity since they can withstand pollution and utilize excess nutrients along with other pollutants. But when the algae become trapped or are unable to handle the level of pollution, they die and degradation begins. Air and water pollutants increase with the anaerobic surface area. In an ecosystem, the recycling of these nutrients promotes and sustains eutrophication and can sustain a high level of biomass productivity. An inversion of the gradient concentration of nutrients in the sediment is the result of algal breakdown. The amount of nutrients from the breakdown of algal deposits that maintain the eutrophication condition is increased by anthropogenic nitrogen and phosphorus.

Chapter 3

# MANAGEMENT OF EUTROPHICATION

## Contents

## 3.1. INTRODUCTION

The increasing population along with the equivalent rise in consumption, has led to an unprecedented demand for natural resources and a substantial rise in waste production. However, the majority of human basic requirements have not been met by the subsequent increase in productivity. Approximately one billion people experience food insecurity, and they are uncertain if they will have enough food to eat. 20% of people live in wealthier countries with much higher levels of consumption (Davies et al., 2017). These societies also have a higher population. Nature reacts to anthropogenic pressures by going through natural ecological processes (equilibrium). The exploitation of nature through agricultural practices, the extraction of natural resources, the disruption of the environment for the development of energy, transportation, and urban infrastructure, and the massive amounts of waste produced result in environmental impacts that seem to have already overtaken the earth's ability to adjust. Humanity has not yet been able to embrace a more reasonable use of the resources on our planet despite the abundance of information on the significance of environmental issues. Water is significant as a resource for development because it is needed not only for human consumption but also for the production of various industrial goods, energy, and food. Nonetheless, the quality of water is directly impacted by the way a hydrographic basin is exploited. The division of environmental issues into categories such as resource depletion, biodiversity loss, water pollution and climate impacts are purely didactic, as these crises are linked to one another.

## 3.2. WATER SUPPLY

Since a definite supply of water is necessary for its availability, various uses should be assessed in terms of their impact on supply. Long-term water supply should be guaranteed via irrigation systems, public water sources, and electricity production. Therefore, these systems should take into account the varying degrees of availability over the years in addition to seasonal fluctuations. Therefore, the amount of water that is deemed critical in the long run is the same amount that is considered available. The geomorphologic run-off or floodplain areas, which are riparian zones next to thalwegs where water collects during floods, are parts of the complex processes that form/feed rivers. During the dry season, this extra water is returned to the river, creating an easement zone that controls the natural water flow. Several basin-specific characteristics, including permeability, roughness coefficient, usage and management, shape, and slope, influence river flow. Groundwater springs and rainfall are the sources of river water. Water from thawing glaciers may also affect river flow downstream of snow-covered alpine ranges. This precipitation has the ability to evaporate, seep into the ground and move over the surface. Thus, there is a correlation between the basin drainage area and the water flow, or discharge. As a result, the flow decreases as it approaches the headwaters, and the river volume increases in direct proportion to the basin area. The basin is more productive when there is a lot of precipitation. As a result, flow rates in similar drainage areas may range significantly. The geomorphologic and pedological characteristics of the slope environment, along with the way the basin is used and managed, all have a significant impact on the quantity, velocity, and surface, subsurface, and underground flow of water. Areas where the vegetative cover has been eliminated are more likely to experience higher level of flooding. Similarly, the areas of flood easements are reduced when floodplains are used for urban expansion or agricultural purposes, increasing the threshold of river flow and intensifying floods and droughts, which ultimately lowers the amount of water that is accessible.

## 3.3. WATER QUALITY

One more important aspect that restricts the possible uses of water is the deterioration of water quality. River pollution (Figure 3.1) can result from the confluence of several diffuse factors like agriculture, animal husbandry, and urbanization, as well as from point-source emissions of industrial pollutants (Wang et al., 2020). Water runoff in rural areas solubilizes chemical pesticides and fertilizers and transports particles containing adsorbed components. Because different uses of water have different quality requirements, sacrificing the natural qualities of water may restrict its use in circumstances where high standards of quality are required. As a result, the idea of water availability is dependent on two factors: the quantity of water and the level of resource demand. Water quality has declined as a result of anthropogenic impact on continental ecosystems, and modifications to the hydrological, biogeochemical, and biodiversity cycles have also been observed. The eutrophication of inland waters is one of these effects. Artificial eutrophication, which is typically brought on by the release of municipal, agricultural, or industrial wastewater, is the unnatural increase in the concentration of nutrients, particularly phosphorus and nitrogen, in aquatic environments. Because of the increased algal growth brought on by this nutrient enrichment in the water, trophic chain balance is disturbed, and biogeochemical cycles are altered. Aquatic ecosystems naturally undergo eutrophication as well, although this process might take hundreds of years because it is dependent on the inorganic load in the aquatic environment and the impact of natural processes in hydrological basins. Characterizing the trophic stages, nutrient levels, structure, and composition of aquatic communities are crucial tools for identifying various impacts on aquatic ecosystems and for suggesting mitigation and conservation strategies pertaining to these situations.

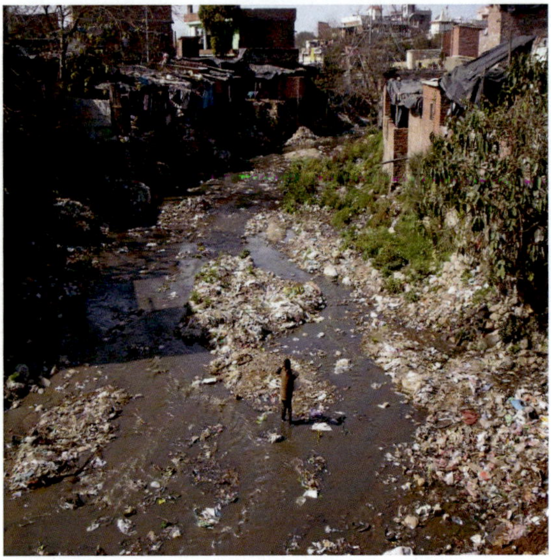

**Figure 3.1.** *River pollution.*

Source: https://upload.wikimedia.org/wikipedia/commons/e/e8/Slum_and_dirty_river.jpg,, Creative Commons License.

## 3.4. SUSCEPTIBILITY TO EUTROPHICATION

The overall trophic state classification of lakes and reservoirs is often determined by combining several indicators, including Secchi depth (Figure 3.2), chlorophyll-a concentration, and nutrient concentration. The process of primary producers, primarily cyanobacteria, algae, and aquatic weeds, grows because of the availability of nutrients in the surrounding environment, especially phosphorus and nitrogen. Phosphorus is typically the element linked to the process of eutrophication in freshwater ecosystems because certain algae are fixers of elemental nitrogen, which is abundant in the atmosphere. The growth of cyanobacteria can also be influenced by other elements including temperature and light. Some of the main interrelated factors that determine a region's susceptibility to eutrophication are its geomorphologic conditions, climate, land-use, reservoir morphometry, and management. Eutrophication typically leads to the growth of aquatic weeds and/or algae. The depth of the reservoir and the retention time of the water resides in the reservoir are two important geomorphological features that directly influence the process of algal reproduction. Because there is a high volume of water in shallow reservoirs that receive solar radiation, phototrophic organisms like cyanobacteria can develop there. The cell divisions that can happen while the water is in the environment also increase with time the water resides in the reservoir, which increases the density of these organisms in the water. These characteristics have a significant impact on the likelihood of algal blooms while other environmental conditions remain stable. The aquatic ecosystem under investigation and its varied applications may be negatively impacted in a number of ways by the eutrophication process. Oxygen concentration can be lowered by a surplus of algae and the subsequent increase in organic matter breakdown (Tranvik, 1998).

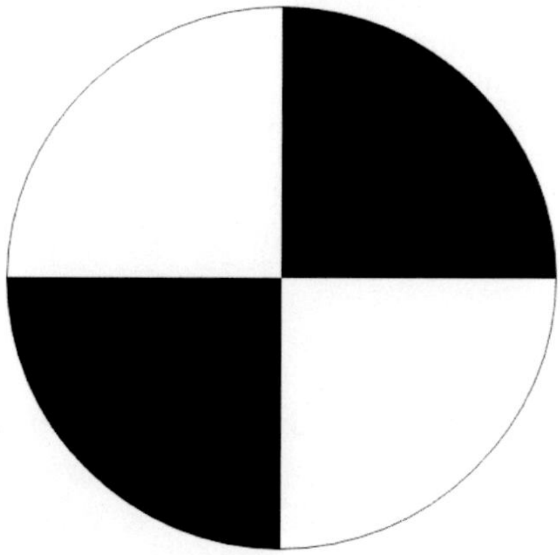

**Figure 3.2.** *Secchi depth.*

Source: https://upload.wikimedia.org/wikipedia/commons/0/0b/Secchi_disk_pattern.svg,, Creative Commons License.

## 3.5. EUTROPHICATION AND FLOODING

The release of hydrogen sulfide and methane is another effect of the eutrophication process, which is linked to increased organic matter breakdown in the sediment. A dense layer of cells may grow on the surface during algal blooms when the density of cyanobacteria is high. This could result in thick layers on the surface that could limit recreational use. Sustainable development in watersheds is frequently linked to many common environmental issues, such as siltation, altered flow regimes with frequent floods during rainy seasons, levee breaks, erosion of floodplains, land use, and improper management of slopes, soils, and interfluves. Due to their negative effects on the soil's ability to store water and their influence on the water table replenishment, which lowers flow during wet seasons, these issues increase erosion. In extreme conditions, these elements can turn perennial streams into sporadic streams or, in the case of water contamination, render them unfit for cultivation or human use. The unplanned usage of the basin has resulted in additional environmental concerns that have an impact on the quality of life of the local and regional population. These phenomena pose a serious threat to development and necessitate prompt response from managers, particularly in the basin source areas where the removal of vegetation typically disturb these processes, which are then exacerbated by inappropriate land use and management. Such activities can take place in both urban and rural regions. In urban areas, increased surface flow can be caused by a lack of a rainfall drainage system. Soil sealing brought on by increased construction and habitation in these basins (buildings, roads, and pavement) can occasionally lead to an increase in surface flow. The quantity of rainwater that seeps into the soil is reduced as a result of these factors, which reduces the soil's ability to store water. These variables have the potential to modify river dynamics by altering surface and river flow, causing erosion, and increasing the frequency of flooding, all of which have an impact on the quality of the water.

## 3.6. LAND MANAGEMENT

Human habitation and inappropriate land management on slopes and interfluves, as evidenced by the loss of topsoil due to leaf erosion, can significantly alter river environments and alluvial plains. Even in these conditions where there is no human habitation, imbalances (issues) are frequently discovered that have the potential to disrupt processes leading to siltation and changes in the quality of the water, thereby restricting its usage. The effects of human habitation have been sensed by the environment leading to a process known as eutrophication, which allows algae to grow rapidly and intensely. Since algae-infested waters cannot be used for human consumption, it is important to perform research studies that suggest ways to prevent the eutrophication process. A cartographic database is necessary to make it easier to analyze the basin and create scenarios (models) for determining how much environmental protection and conservation it has received. The basin is understood as a system that is always changing. To achieve this, we need to create a technique for the comprehensive examination of the watershed landscapes through the use of geographic information systems (GIS) and remote sensing technologies. Satellite images, aerial photos, field evaluations, and topographic maps should be used in this process. Several aspects of spatial analysis may be developed using the digital cartographic database. These include the identification of conflicts between land-use and legal restrictions in a basin, simulation of the growth of areas of anthropogenic disturbance (AAD) in the Basin using Markov Chain and Cellular Automata in a GIS environment, and spatio-temporal dynamics in the Basin (Tariq and Mumtaz, 2023).

## 3.7. SUSTAINABILITY

Concern over the development of sustainability indices, which are used as indicators for local, regional, national, and decision-making, has grown over the past 20 years. The classification of complex phenomena and the evaluation of how human actions affect their environments are made possible by the use of indicators as metrics for evaluating and monitoring a process. These indicators (indices) predict future environmental events, alert people to potentially risky situations, and help in decision-making. A good indicator should have the following qualities: it should be simple to measure, inexpensive, flexible enough to adapt to various local conditions, able to recognize trends, and able to facilitate community understanding and engagement. Human development is a larger concept that views the human being as a citizen (individual) who aspires to participate in strategic decisions. While the concept of quality of life can be measured based on quantitative attributes (housing, sanitation, health, school, transportation, etc.), human development is a more expansive concept. In order to characterize ideal life conditions, it is crucial to include factors and create indices that are related to well-being. Evaluating farmers' quality of life and the rural communities in which they reside is of crucial importance. Therefore, the plan can be to develop an index that would show the availability of essential services in the community and municipality and would be related to the farmer's quality of life on his/her farm. The Rural Life Quality Index was developed as a standardized method of measuring and evaluating the well-being of rural residents, taking into account a range of factors including sociocultural, technological, economic, ecological, and institutional aspects.

Based on several factors and indicators, the quality of life may be evaluated. These factors and indicators essentially represented the following areas: transportation (vehicles); sanitation (water supply, sewage system, and waste disposal); housing conditions (appearance of the house and available appliances); and social integration (participation in social activities). All of the indicators are ranked from 0 to 10 for the assessment. Extreme values of 0 or 10 signify extremely bad or very good circumstances, respectively. Less favorable circumstances are scored below 7.0, which is the lower bound of an acceptable quality of life (between 7.0 and 10). Higher scores for all indicators are associated with improved housing standards, better conditions for sanitation and waste management, easier production flow and transportation, better access to public transportation, healthcare (including access to doctors and dentists), and education; and increased social activity. The values in each evaluated indicator are calculated to obtain a simple mean value, which is the Rural Life Quality Index. Radar diagrams, which make it easier to analyze and observe every element of the Rural Life Quality Index, were used to organize the results.

Some findings establish that poor sanitation is a prevalent issue in small rural towns, especially in remote dwellings that are frequently disconnected from water systems provided by public sanitation organizations. A lot of farmers rely on their own groundwater sources, which are often artesian or semi-artesian wells. The majority of farmers prefer to use water from their own sources for primary consumption, such as drinking water and food preparation, even though they have access to the public network. The treated, chlorinated water from the public network is used for secondary uses, like laundry and cleaning sidewalks (Couto et al., 2015). Some farmers opined that they feel uncomfortable because of the taste of chlorine when asked why they won't use chlorinated water. The ideal sewage system is present in only a small percentage of properties. Waste that is not collected sometimes ends up burned or buried, but most properties have some awareness of the environment; many farmers recycle their recyclables and use organic waste in their gardens. Animal waste is another issue that is not addressed in the Rural Life Quality Index since it is not properly handled. This kind of waste is either not properly disposed of at all or is disposed of improperly on the ground. Communities differ in their accessibility to basic healthcare, education, and transportation services. Bad road conditions make it difficult for public transportation to function properly, which keeps many families from receiving health care.

## 3.8. FISHING ACTIVITY

Insufficient, dispersed, and inconsistent research has been done on fish harvests and fishing activities in several locations. The statistics available on various forms of fishing do not include historical data, which makes it more difficult to assess and manage this activity even though fishing has been done for consumption and survival. Fishing is currently done for a variety of reasons. Government agencies essentially distinguish between commercial and non-commercial fishing when it comes to the use of fish resources. Commercial fishing (Figure 3.3) can be industrial or artisanal, and it is considered a source of income. Professional fishermen engage in artisanal fishing, either independently or as a part of their family business. They may use small boats or their own means of production, work on land, or collaborate with others. Industrial fishing is done using small, medium, or large vessels by people or businesses that employ or collaborate with professional fishermen. Any type of fishing that is done without a profit and with equipment permitted by law is regarded as non-commercial fishing. There has been a surge in recreational fishing lately, which has brought numerous economic advantages, especially in the tourism industry. When it comes to inland waters, fishing is closely associated with the social and geographic contexts in which it is conducted.

These contexts are shaped by prevailing political, economic, and demographic factors. A thorough survey of those who engage in the practice must be included in the analysis due to the complexity of the situation. Accurate assessments of the activity conducted in various methods enable a consistent evaluation of the impacts of fishing.

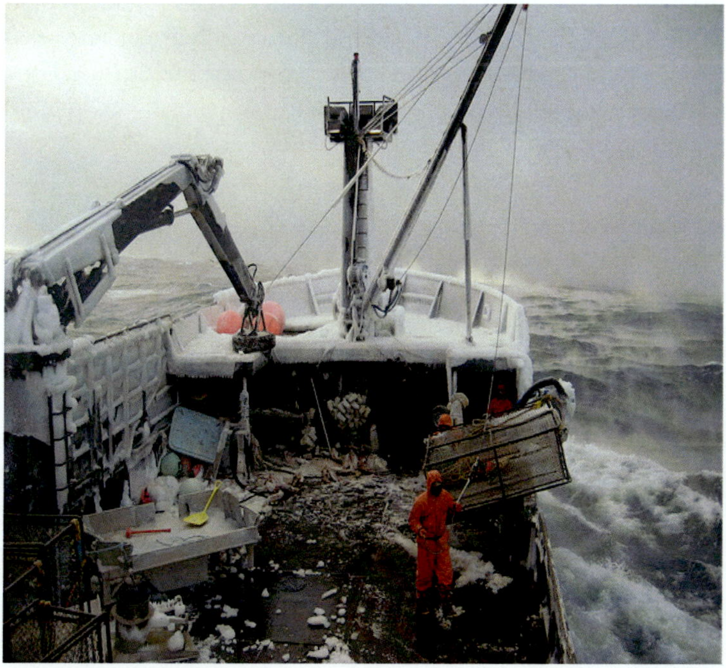

**Figure 3.3.** *Commercial fishing.*

Source: https://upload.wikimedia.org/wikipedia/commons/1/1a/Crab_fishing_boat.png,Creative Commons License.

The presence of exotic species during reservoir construction may allow for an increase in the population of these species due to environmental disturbance; these species are generally more resilient and tolerant than native species. The construction of reservoirs in the river basin significantly altered the limnological, biological, and hydrologic conditions, which had an impact on fish populations both directly and indirectly (Elchyshyn et al., 2018). The construction altered the water dynamics and damaged fish shelters, feeding grounds and other habitats, which changed the fish composition and structure. The fish populations were first severely affected. The majority of fish that are captured are related to the documented species, many of which are unique to the hydrographic basin. This demonstrates the significance of regional involvement in methods to evaluate the ichthyofauna in a reservoir sphere of influence. A small portion of the recorded species found in some reservoirs, like the *Cyprinus carpio*, *Tilapia rendalli*, *Charax stenopterus*, and *Micropterus salmoides*, are fish that were transferred from other hydrographic basins. Despite the small percentage of introduced species, which indicates a certain fish stocking failure, these species may have a rapid population increase and/or significantly alter the aquatic environment as a whole, which may have an indirect impact on the quality of the water. Fishing on the reservoir banks is a natural activity that can play a significant social role. Fishing in the reservoirs is seen as a traditional survival practice that necessitates ongoing management efforts and has significant negative social and environmental effects (Cowx and Gerdeaux, 2004).

There is less information on fishing in some reservoirs; nevertheless, information about fishing in some reservoirs of the river basin indicates that professional fishing is done illegally and can be a supplemental source of revenue. It is important to appropriately evaluate the fishing site to comprehend the relationships that exist between the activity and the environment. We need to investigate the fishing practices in the reservoir area, identify the target species, and characterize the socioeconomic background of the local fishermen. Because this activity plays a significant social role in the lives of urban community members, either as a source of subsistence or as a recreational activity, it can be used as a guide to establishing control and management measures on the reservoir, even though the data sets may have geographical and temporal limitations. It is crucial to comprehend agricultural problems, evaluate production sites, create maps of suitable land, and observe soil management and farming systems practices, including the application of fertilizer, the use of pesticides, and soil conservation. In order to propose strategies that better suit agricultural activities with the aim of soil management, we can use these data sets to identify areas of conflict. There are some study phases for the project. The first can be a participatory rural appraisal (PRA) that serves as a preliminary study of the local conditions. The second phase, which was based on the preliminary survey, comprises a pedological survey, an evaluation of the fitness of the land for use and the identification of locations where overuse or underuse could cause conflict. Critical locations, such as pollution sources, were also identified during this phase. The third phase refers to the development of suggested modifications to land conversion systems and conservation practices using Pilot Plots within the study area

## 3.9. FARMING

With the minimal area utilized for grazing, livestock operations are not substantial in some areas. The common farming method is tillage combined with heavy pesticide application. The soils are primarily nitisols, oxisols, and inceptisols.

Because of poor management, many soils exhibit severe erosion and have either completely lost or significantly reduced their topsoil. Nevertheless, with efforts to manage agricultural soil erosion, the issue has gotten worse. Survey data indicates that in places with intensive mechanized farming, 15 to 20 tons of soil per hectare are lost annually. We need to create a map showing overused or conflict regions by comparing the land-use suitability data with the current usage. This may lead us to the conclusion that a certain area is underutilized and needs to be modified or converted. Water supplies are impacted by increasing human activity and natural changes in both quantitative and qualitative ways. Water usage has shifted from rural and agricultural to urban and industrial due to societal development, which is a reflection of both rising water pollution and demand. Every kind of water use has an effect on the quality of water bodies in a particular way. There are a number of human activities that negatively impact the aquatic environment indirectly and unfavorably. Uncontrolled land use, deforestation, unintentional chemical spills, untreated wastewater discharge and hazardous liquid runoff from solid waste dumps are a few examples. Similar effects on surface and underground water resources are caused by the excessive and unregulated use of pesticides, herbicides and fertilizers. Lakes and reservoirs can tolerate certain degrees of pollution because of their inherent qualities, which provide them with a certain amount of storage capacity. This ability to absorb pollutants is restricted, though, and depending on how the drainage basin is used and occupied, problems could develop quickly as a result of the introduction of pollutants and last for a long time. Irrigation is one of the primary issues with agricultural activities since it is a consumptive use and necessitates a lot of water. 98% of the water used in agriculture is returned to the atmosphere by ET or evapotranspiration, while the remaining 2% is converted into organic matter that is absorbed by the crops (García-Tejero et al., 2011). Water for animal consumption and accompanying cleaning tasks releases liquid water back into the environment, but with a major loss of quality because 60–70% of the water ends up as waste, such as urine.

## 3.10. AGRICULTURAL DYNAMICS

Among the main non-point inputs of nutrients entering aquatic environments that contribute to eutrophication are agricultural operations, particularly in places where land use conservation measures are absent. The main issue in these situations is the phosphorus release. While phosphorus is necessary for the growth of vegetables and the rearing of cattle, it can also be carried by runoff from agricultural areas into aquatic sites, where it enriches the water and starts the eutrophication process. Research conducted in the US hydrographic basins has shown that phosphorus loss through runoff surges with the expansion of agricultural land and the shrinkage of forests. The primary source of nitrate for surface water and groundwater in agricultural areas appears to be the excessive use of nitrogen combined with plants' strong capacity to fix nitrogen. This is especially true when applying nitrogen fertilizer or manure before the rainy season. Runoff nitrogen content, particularly that of nitrate, is influenced by many variables, including the soil characteristics, slope, and humidity levels, as well as agricultural practices including planting timing and crop variety. The lowering of phosphorus loads from diffuse sources is mostly attributed to agricultural methods that minimize erosion and sharp variations in surface runoff. A few strategies to reduce the amount of phosphorus that enters water bodies include maintaining green areas around lakes and streams, planting with consideration for the natural drainage, storing animal waste carefully, applying fertilizer sparingly, and avoiding fertilizer application during wet seasons. The productivity of these settings is a reflection of the physicochemical complexities of the hydrographic basin in which it is situated. The internal physicochemical and biological dynamics of the lake portions/segments determine this. The nutrients carried by the rains and the surface runoff that erodes and cleans the land surface cause the slow and continual natural eutrophication process. It is possible to refer to this eutrophication as the natural aging of lakes.

## 3.11. ARTIFICIAL EUTROPHICATION

Eutrophication is said to be artificial, cultural, or anthropogenic when it is not a result of natural processes but rather is brought on by human activity. Because of the development of aquatic plants brought on by artificial eutrophication, the quality of the water gradually deteriorates, especially in lakes(Qiu et al., 2001). This has an impact on the entire metabolism of the contaminated water body. Improper land use, illegal land occupation and poor soil preparation are the primary causes of erosion and pollution of water sources. The placement of rural roads, which are typically built without taking into account the dynamics of water flow and end up as drainage channels for water and silt, has made erosion problems worse and led to the silting of rivers and streams. The use of technical strategies in micro-hydrographic basin programs aims to increase soil vegetation cover, increase water infiltration in the soil profile, reduce surface runoff, and control water and soil pollution in addition to creating terraces, restoring riparian forests, and fencing off areas of permanent preservation (APP). Planning is done while keeping in mind the natural dynamics of the rural property and the micro-hydrographic basin. Consequently, the implementation of the planned activities cannot be hindered by fences, roads, or agricultural boundaries. While specific plans for each farm inside the micro-basin are typically produced, the challenges, guidelines, methods, and action plans of many micro-basin projects are generally similar. The immediate beneficiaries, farmers and their organizations, as well as the quantity and quality of the human resources at their disposal, determine the program structure, timeline, and operationalization. After determining the soil suitability for agriculture using a pedological study, we can identify the sections of the basin where land-use conflicts would arise. This data is gathered by conducting an extensive physical environment survey and using geoprocessing to cross-reference the land-use and land-suitability maps. Data collection at the research sites and the analysis of aerial photographs are used to complete the full pedological survey. To identify the various types of soil precisely, soil investigations were done.

## 3.12. SOIL MANAGEMENT AND OTHER RELEVANT FACTORS

Conventional soil management leads to erosion, which facilitates the movement of these agrochemicals, organic matter, and clay colloids (Rahman et al., 2020). Apart from their role in eutrophicating water bodies, these materials also result in fish population drops, siltation, problems in treating water systems for industrial and human usage, and eventually, higher costs. Environmental studies aid in our understanding of the environments in which conflicting biotic, physical and human factors coexist in dynamic equilibrium. These studies help us comprehend how people engage with their environment through cultural practices and behaviors, which can have a good or bad impact on environmental dynamics. It becomes clear that several conflicts and environmental issues arise when land management practices are not applied in a logical and integrated way and when appropriate regulations are not established based on prior knowledge of the limitations of the natural physical environment. These issues may have permanent consequences, necessitating elaborate and expensive solutions. Many of these issues, which have a negative impact on quality of life, result in mortalities, and need more money for corrective measures, might be readily prevented if rules for land use and occupation were adhered to. Well-preserved forest patches are typically found in places that are protected by the environment. Outside of these protected areas, grazing or reforestation with alien species has increasingly been replaced. This has the undesirable effect of gradually homogenizing the vegetation across large areas. It should be noted that many areas near a large basin are experiencing pressure from land occupation, including urban settlement. The urban districts in the periphery municipalities have experienced tremendous growth in the past few years. Unplanned expansion has moved near vulnerable environmental areas and significant water and mineral resources sources. There are existing conflicts arising from the use of natural resources, agriculture and urbanization. Important water supplies in certain ecotourism-potential regions have degraded. The hydrographic basin is classified as an area with diverse geo-environmental characteristics due to its intricate geological past (Shandilya et al., 2021). As a result, it encompasses a wide range of land uses. Some common regional geo-environmental factors are crucial and need to be considered in regional planning.

Regarding inputs and pesticide use, the majority of farmers had soil analyses done on their properties, but the purpose of the tests was to guide soil improvement programs, not to determine soil fertility. This approach is reflected in the fertilization techniques employed in the basin. Uncontrolled fertilization includes the use of poultry manure, which is utilized in 95% of the properties studied and is regarded as organic by farmers, as well as the usage of minerals. It is true that excessive fertilizer use can contaminate rivers, springs, and groundwater by leaching nutrients into the groundwater and by forming bonds with eroded soil particles or water-soluble nutrients that are carried by runoff. The direct application of poultry manure, which does not go through a composting process before use, is another important element. This material is typically kept outside without any kind of cover, making it a major cause of pollution for the aquatic bodies in the basin when used for fertilizer. Farmers typically lack a thorough understanding of the application strategy when using pesticides, and this is made worse by the fact that few of them receive expert assistance in this area. The fungicide Manzate is made up of hexamethylenetetramine and mancozeb. This product can release harmful and irritating fumes when exposed to heat or moisture, and it is extremely poisonous to aquatic life. Its primary constituent, mancozeb, is stationary in soil but breaks down quickly in it in approximately two days; users should take great care to ensure that the compound does not end up in water bodies because it is extremely harmful to aquatic life. DECIS is a pyrethroid insecticide that poses a significant risk to the environment because it is highly bioconcentrated in fish and hazardous to aquatic species (Ariyani et al., 2023). Deltamethrin, the active chemical, attaches itself to the majority of soils and breaks down in nine days. All three of these chemicals behave similarly when it comes to fixing in the soil and having a brief half-life; however, with DECIS and Manzate, care must be taken to ensure that the substance is deposited far from the aquatic environment. The micro-basin has large areas that might be used for pasture and reforestation; however, for these activities to be financially viable, the land needed must be larger than the current property sizes owned by individual farmers in the area.

## 3.13. NATIVE SPECIES

Native species should be used for vegetation recovery, giving technical factors like climate and native plant selection first priority since they affect how well recovery attempts turn out. Native species that are important for wildlife should be prioritized since they enhance the quality of the ecosystem and can provide a valuable alternative for farmers by producing honey, for example. In the micro-basin, the restoration of vegetation results in benefits for soil and water conservation that are currently ignored, but all signs point to their continued existence and potential as a great source of additional revenue for farmers in rural areas. An alternative is to replace the typical crops with perennial native plants, fruit trees, and medicinal plants, among other things, in reforestation and agricultural regions. The soil and climate of the area may be perfect for the cultivation of several species of economically valuable native and cultivated medicinal plants. Among the fruit and melliferous trees that are already grown in some areas are *Espinheira Santa* and tansagem. A large amount of effort is required in the development of medicinal plants, which can provide small-scale farmers and their families with work and money.

## 3.14. PHYTOTHERAPY

Phytotherapy is a therapeutic practice that promotes social interaction, community building, and solidarity by using medicinal plants in all of their pharmacological forms. Therefore, to fulfill future demand, it will be necessary to strengthen various stages of the supply chain for food plants that are aromatic and medicinal. Integrating the environment with agriculture, promoting social progress, health, education, and preservation through ecologically sound practices encourages family farming and the use of medicinal plants as a form of disease treatment.

The World Health Organization (WHO) states that any aspects of the physical environment of humans that are hazardous or have the potential to be harmful to health in the physical, mental, and social domains are closely tied to the concept of sanitation. Sanitation is the state of environmental health that is attained through a variety of socioeconomic measures; this means removing technological obstacles that have impeded the development of sanitation measures and the benefits they bring, particularly for the people who live in remote areas, small towns, or rural areas. By encouraging the sustainable utilization of natural resources and thereby reducing the effects of environmental degradation, particularly the pollution of freshwater springs as a result of improper disposal of solid waste and sanitary sewage, rural sanitation promotes a healthy environment in rural areas. Since urban methods of sanitation are almost never acceptable, the adoption of practical and simple technologies is frequent in low-density rural areas and small cities where houses are widely distributed. A technical sanitation program's primary objective is to satisfy the needs of its users; so, the selection of such technology ought to be based on a set of economic, social, ecological, and cultural norms that satisfy the requirements of the relevant society.

## 3.15. PROBLEMS WITH WATER SUPPLY

The problems with water supply in rural areas differ from those in metropolitan areas with dense populations. There are other approaches to providing water for human consumption that are not part of the infrastructure in big cities. Although underground water quality is generally reliable, some pollutants can render the water unfit for human use. The parameters specified by the relevant agencies, including the Ministry of Health, which specifies the norms of potability are used to define the amounts of contaminants. As a result, practical treatments can ensure the quality of the water. Small towns frequently use slow filters in place of water supply treatment, mostly to get rid of turbidity. The fact that these filters don't require complex machinery or chemical products makes them advantageous. They are easy to build and operate, and they produce very little sludge. Despite these benefits, slow filters can become ineffective at certain times of the year when the source water quality substantially declines, producing high turbidity levels that reduce filtration effectiveness. Because domestic ceramic filters have been established as an accessible technology for treating water in homes, they offer an alternative for small communities without a shared water supply (Peter-Varbanets et al., 2009). Such filters, particularly those made in the U.S. and Britain, have been examined for their ability to remove harmful bacteria. The important step before the water is supplied to the public is disinfection. Safeguarding the safety of drinking water and preventing or avoiding the spread of diseases through the inactivation of harmful organisms is vital. Because liquid or gas chlorine ($Cl_2$) compounds are user-friendly, they are frequently used for disinfection in rural areas. Small towns often employ sodium hypochlorite (liquid) or calcium hypochlorite (solid), two forms of chlorine derivatives. The current trend is the in-situ synthesis of sodium hypochlorite, with electrolysis gases either being used entirely for disinfection or released to the atmosphere in certain conditions. Chlorates, traces of chlorites, $ClO_2$, and $O_3$ are byproducts of industrial sodium hypochlorite production. To keep chlorate levels below those recommended by the WHO, the dosage should be carefully monitored.

## 3.16. TREATMENT OF WASTE

The way waste is treated varies significantly based on its origin and composition. To protect the ecosystem and stop the spread of vectors, government agencies advise burying such organic waste because there are insufficient services for collection and transportation. It is not advisable to dispose of pesticide packages using this method due to the potential for contamination of neighboring human populations, animals, soil, and water bodies. When it comes to organic waste, rural farmers can benefit greatly from composting because it is an aerobic biological process that, under the right conditions, transforms organic matter that was added to the waste. Although the potential presence of pollutants makes the compost unsuitable for commercialization and adds to its unpleasant odor, composting organic waste guarantees a significant reduction in waste production.

When done correctly, this process recycles nutrients, yields compost that may be applied as soil fertilizer and is less expensive than other methods of disposing of waste. Several elements are crucial to the composting process, including The waste should have a moisture content of between 50 and 60%; it should be continuously aerated for the first 60 days to prevent biological activity that could jeopardize the process; and it should be kept at 55°C, dropping to 10°C to 20°C by the end of the process.

Other variables like pH and nutrients are also managed: the initial pH should be kept acidic, between 4.5 and 5.5 for composting and 7.0 to 8.0 for humidified compost; the starting C/N ratio should be 30: 1. One benefit of composting is that, if the waste is sufficient and the biological process takes place under ideal conditions, it may be carried out with both basic and advanced methods. It is crucial to take into account both technical and socioeconomic variables while selecting an alternative. The production of biogas and biofertilizers are the two main benefits of utilizing a biodigester. Particularly in rural areas, the biogas generated by anaerobic digestion can be utilized as a substitute energy source, giving inhabitants a useful and affordable fuel source. Utilizing biofertilizer, a waste product high in nutrients and humus to fertilize the soil can boost crop productivity at a minimal cost of production (Sahoo et al., 2013).

Some farmers who bury or burn their common waste blame the irregularities in the collection procedure for their actions. In rural areas, organic waste is either collected or composted for future use. Some manufacturers opt for less popular solutions, like burying the organic waste or dumping it into a river or the soil. Common waste is typically recycled before being collected, and it is usually intended for public collection. Manure and pesticide package waste are produced on rural farms.

Bovine, horse, swine, ovine, and poultry manures are separated. Manure is either left untreated or dumped onto the soil in some places. The common place for animal feces to end up, treated or not, is in the soil. The majority of producers do not make the connection between animal density and water quality around the well. Many of the properties have high numbers of dogs and chickens, and they don't shield the well from potential water contamination caused by the feces of these animals. Once used, pesticide packets are always given back to the store where the product was originally purchased. Farmers that apply pesticides do so in accordance with guidelines and assert that package disposal is supervised.

Chapter 4

# NUTRIENT POLLUTION AND COASTAL AREAS

## Contents

## 4.1. INTRODUCTION

Lack of systematic monitoring and reporting, as well as inadequate coverage have impeded recent efforts to assess the extent of nutrient over-enrichment. However, the information (data) that is currently available makes it abundantly evident that nutrient over-enrichment issues are extensive and that if present trends continue, the effects will get worse. Over one-third of coastal water bodies are suffering from severe effects as a result of nutrient over-enrichment (Chakraborty, 2021). The various sources of nutrients are frequently attributed to substantial shifts in technology and human behavior that have occurred over the past 50 years; these shifts might range from increased usage of fossil fuels to modifications in agricultural practices. The issues brought on by nutrient over-enrichment have many different regional solutions. There is no effective strategy designed to reduce excess nutrient inputs to coastal waters, despite the existence of initiatives aimed at protecting and restoring coastal waters and habitat. For a program manager in a coastal area, there is currently a lack of readily available data or reliable procedures to identify the sources of excess nutrients or the possible effects of those nutrients on a particular coastal waterbody. While many agencies are working hard to assist local governments in addressing the consequences of over-enrichment of nutrients in coastal environments, there is still a lack of coordination between these agencies and their activities.

## 4.2. NUTRIENT MANAGEMENT

A National nutrient management strategy must be developed and put into action due to the significance of nutrient-related issues and the importance of the coastal areas that are at risk. To prevent nutrient over-enrichment in coastal areas, local, state, and regional activities should be coordinated through the National nutrient management strategy. The goal can be to provide a quantifiable improvement in the environmental quality of damaged coastal ecosystems. Site-specific impacts result from nutritional over-enrichment, because nutrient sources differ significantly across locations. The creation of a national strategy must therefore take into account regional and site-specific differences in the application of source-reduction objectives as well as in the management and policy techniques employed. The Dead Zone (Gulf of Mexico), is an important coastal system that yields fertilizer inputs from many distant locations. National strategies are required to address the sources of nutrients from fossil fuel combustion and agriculture in order to prevent the simple transfer of pollution sources from one area to another. This strategy must also support the creation of a national coordinated effort to provide local managers and decision-makers with the data they require to establish suitable local source reduction objectives and strategies. By giving local managers and decision-makers access to the data source, policies intended to produce a quantifiable improvement in the environmental quality of damaged coastal systems can be implemented on a site-specific basis, as well as, when needed, at the regional levels. Systemic adjustment needs to be implemented nationwide if the goal of the national policy is to attain a measurable improvement in the quality of degraded coastal systems (Figure 4.1).

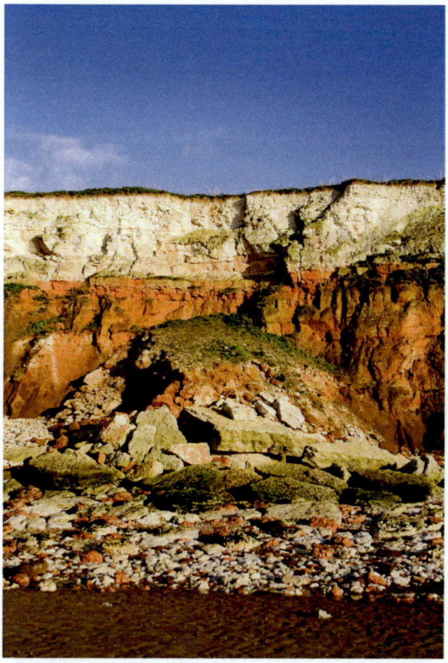

**Figure 4.1.** *Degraded coastal systems.*

Source: https://upload.wikimedia.org/wikipedia/commons/2/26/Coastal_Erosion_Hunstanton_Cliffs.jpg, Creative Commons License.

## 4.3. MONITORING OF COASTAL SYSTEMS

The national plan ought to promote more standardized methods for monitoring coastal systems throughout the country to improve the efficiency and accuracy of evaluations in the future. Managers at the local or state level frequently struggle with defining clear, attainable performance indicators or targets. Establishing such goals necessitates input and commitment from numerous stakeholder groups. Research studies should offer solutions to the conceptual and practical obstacles related to nutrient over-enrichment. The significant reductions in nutrient loads to coastal waters are feasible based on the assessments of current scientific knowledge and nutrient management practice. All damaged coastal bodies could be improved while maintaining the current healthy environmental quality. To investigate and lessen the consequences of nutrient over-enrichment in coastal settings, local programs and agencies are employing a range of evaluation and management approaches, from connected hydrodynamic water quality models to a technological approach. Managers feel that their processes are giving or should be giving enough information to start management plans, although the complexity varies throughout projects. The local managers may be impatient for the scientific community's responses. To create and implement management strategies, evaluate potential impacts from management practices, and build nutrient budgets by source type, they must make use of the best available or most appropriate information. The fact that some managers might not be aware of more reliable information sources, however, suggests a communication breakdown between the management and scientific communities. Managers understand that their present data sources and tools need to be improved.

To conduct extensive, long-term research programs to better understand the effects of nutrient enrichment on estuarine structure and function as well as to monitor the effects of management changes on coastal systems, representative coastal systems (index sites) should be selected. Index sites should be chosen alongside with the creation of a general classification scheme for vulnerability to nutrient over-enrichment, and they should be representative of the variety of estuarine types covered by the classification. Research conducted at index sites is crucial to the development of accurate predictive models for management since it helps explain temporal patterns of change that are revealed through monitoring and assessment programs. Estuary management requires estimates of nutrient imports, and information on long-term patterns in nutrient inputs is crucial for identifying nutrient sources (Statham, 2012). The USGS is the main and best source of information on nutrient inputs to estuaries from upstream rivers in the entire country. It is not feasible for managers to gather and incorporate enough observational data to completely comprehend the implications of changes in land use patterns, mostly because of the high expense of monitoring. It is challenging to comprehend the mechanisms involved in forecasting future conditions. There is a growing need for both sophisticated and basic models to predict environmental conditions. Creating a database of typical input values for use in current models will also need more work.

## 4.4. NUTRIENT CYCLES

The nutrient cycles are being altered by humans in many ways, with the changes occurring in the regions/area with the highest population density and agricultural output. The discharge of phosphorus and nitrogen to the shore has varied greatly in some parts of the planet while being relatively constant in others. According to estimates, human activity has increased nitrogen inputs by a factor of six to eight into the coastal waters of the northeastern United States. There can be regional variations in the trends of human disturbance of nutrient cycles. For instance, the usage of nitrogen fertilizer has increased relatively less in the United States since 1985, even though the use of inorganic nitrogen fertilizer is still rising globally (Mosier, 2002).

To facilitate increased food exports to developing countries, nitrogen fertilizer consumption in the US may increase again in the coming century. For the past 20 years, countries like China have produced almost all of their own food, in part because of more usage of nitrogen fertilizer. China currently uses a lot of fertilizer, nearly ten times as much as the US does, and additional increases in this use are not expected to have the same significant effects on food production as they did in the past. If China's population keeps increasing, it might again need to import food from the US and other rich countries, which would increase the usage of nitrogen fertilizer. Controlling discharges from wastewater treatment facilities and other point sources has historically been the main focus of water quality management. The nonpoint sources of nutrients are typically of more significance for nutrients and coastal eutrophication.

## 4.5. WATERSHED MANAGEMENT

When the watershed is densely populated and relatively small in comparison to the estuary surface area, wastewater inputs may occasionally be an important supply of nitrogen to the estuary. Wastewater can be the main supply of nitrogen in some estuaries that are fed by larger watersheds, especially if the watershed is densely populated. For instance, wastewater (New York City) contributes an estimated 60% of the nitrogen inputs to Long Island Sound (Watson et al., 2018) (Figure 4.2).

Most estuaries receive more nitrogen and phosphorus from nonpoint sources than from wastewater, especially those with large watersheds. For instance, wastewater treatment facilities and other point sources account for just 25% of the nitrogen and phosphorus imports to the Chesapeake Bay. Sewage and industrial point sources are estimated to produce between 10% and 20% of the total nitrogen flux (organic and inorganic N) and 40% of the total phosphorus flux for the Mississippi River. Many techniques are available to reduce the amount of nutrients discharged by wastewater treatment plants. Additional tertiary treatment for nutrient removal can lower nitrogen discharges by 80% to 88% and phosphorus discharges by 95% to 99%. The relatively standard approaches of using primary and secondary sewage treatment lower phosphorus and nitrogen discharges on average by approximately 20% to 25%, although there is a significant variation among plants.

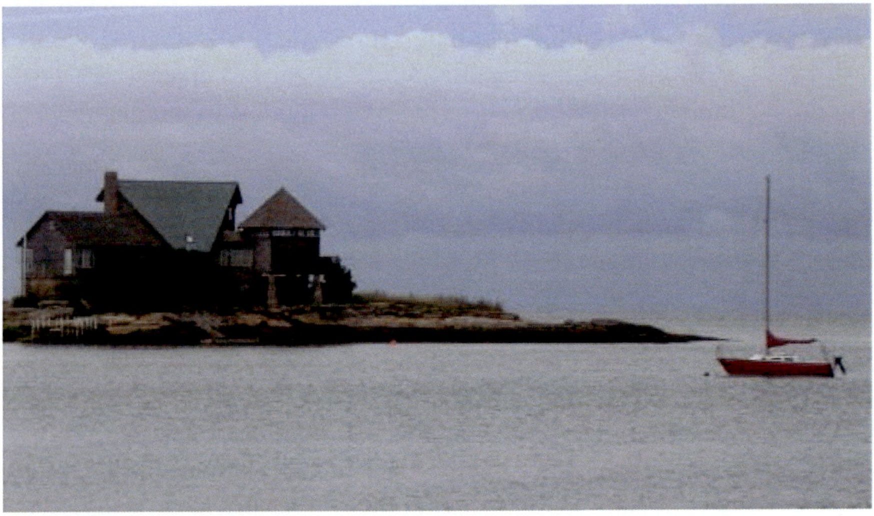

**Figure 4.2.** *Long island sound.*

Source: https://upload.wikimedia.org/wikipedia/commons/0/08/Guilford_ct_long_island_sound.jpg, Creative Commons License.

Nevertheless, the majority of US wastewater treatment facilities lack sufficient nitrogen removal capacity. Before tertiary nitrogen removal was implemented in Tampa Bay, wastewater treatment facilities were a significant source of nitrogen; this treatment has effectively stopped the eutrophication trend in the bay. The majority of estuaries need to have their nutrient inputs from nonpoint sources managed in addition to those from industrial and wastewater treatment facilities to reduce eutrophication. The export of nitrogen and phosphorus to downstream aquatic ecosystems is generally negligible in a human-inhabited environment, especially in the temperate zone (Beusen et al., 2022). If the environment is at an ecological equilibrium, then there cannot be more nutrients exported than absorbed. In the temperate zone, both of these nitrogen inputs (biological nitrogen fixation and atmospheric nitrogen deposition) tend to be negligible in the absence of human disturbance. Because there is some nitrogen accumulation in the system and some nitrogen loss through denitrification, the bacterial conversion of reactive nitrate into nonreactive molecular nitrogen, the export of nitrogen from undisturbed temperate landscapes must also be low, in fact lower than the input. Because biological nitrogen fixation and atmospheric nitrogen deposition occur at much higher rates in tropical regions, there may be a large export of nitrogen from undisturbed ecosystems to downstream ecosystems.

## 4.6. NITROGEN FLUX

It is challenging to estimate the amount of naturally occurring nitrogen flux from a temperate region like the United States with accuracy. Nearly the majority of the temperate ecosystems experience some degree of disturbance due to atmospheric pollution and the higher nitrogen deposition that results from it. Some forests in Chile are among the few remaining temperate forests that do not experience high nitrogen deposition from pollution sources. However, because the Chilean forests have quite distinct ecological histories and receive a lot of precipitation and runoff, these are inadequate models for most of the temperate systems in the United States. The weathering of soil and parent rock material is the primary source of phosphorus to a terrestrial ecosystem in an undisturbed environment. The oceanic sedimentary record can be used to determine the global average of phosphorus export from the terrestrial landscape before human disturbance. Nonetheless, it is evident that this is dependent upon the parent-rock phosphorus level, weathering rate, and other environmental factors, such as erosion rate. There is no baseline value for the natural rate of phosphorus export since phosphorus export is site-specific and there is minute data on background phosphorus losses from a particular location before cultivation. Although there are some significant differences in the reactions of these nutrients, disturbance of the landscape enhances the export of both nitrogen and phosphorus. Since phosphorus is often exported from disturbed systems as particle-bound phosphorus, factors governing erosion and sedimentation play a crucial role in managing phosphorus fluxes. The phosphorus budget (dynamics) of some isolated oceanic environments and forests can be significantly impacted by the movement of some phosphorus via the atmosphere as dust particles. These phosphorus imports to estuaries and coastal waterways are often less significant than those to surface waters.

While some nitrogen is also exported in particle-bound forms, nitrogen is often far more mobile through soils in dissolved form than phosphorus, therefore major exports can occur in surface waters as dissolved nitrogen or in groundwater. Furthermore, reactive nitrogen molecules have the ability to migrate a lot in the atmosphere, unlike phosphorus. For instance, urea and ammonia-based fertilizers, manures, and animal feedlot wastes release large volumes of ammonia gas into the atmosphere, which volatilizes and deposits the gas elsewhere in the landscape. About 40% of the applied inorganic nitrogen fertilizer cycles through the atmosphere and is redeposited on average (Mosier, 2001). Although it is slightly less, 25% of the inorganic nitrogen fertilizer used in the United States volatilizes to the atmosphere. Agriculture is the main factor influencing nonpoint fluxes of phosphorus in the landscape. The burning of fossil fuels and farming or agricultural practices are the two main nonpoint sources of nitrogen that enter estuaries and coastal waters. A substantial portion of this nitrogen export originates from agricultural areas, although other types of ecosystems, such as forests, can also contribute significantly due to substantial atmospheric nitrogen transport. Changes in agricultural practices over the decades have contributed to these nutrient flows since agriculture dominates the non-point source flux of phosphorus and adds to non-point sources of nitrogen. The sources of nitrogen found in industry and fossil fuels, as well as the mechanisms governing the fluxes of phosphorus and nitrogen in the landscape, should be studied.

## 4.7. PROCESSING FACILITY AND OTHER MANAGEMENT APPROACHES

Large processing facilities were constructed for the production of nitrogenous fertilizers and transformation of imported rock phosphate into a range of phosphorus fertilizer products that are partially and completely water soluble. A common application for basic slag, a steel industry byproduct, is the production of phosphorus fertilizer. Inorganic phosphorus fertilizer use increased dramatically in the United States throughout the 1940s and 1950s, but it has been mostly stable since 1960. The main cause of this relative increase in nitrogen consumption over phosphorus use was the beneficial crop production responses to nitrogen fertilizers, particularly in maize. The United States' agricultural production systems have become more concentrated and specialized during the past 30 years. The average farm size has expanded from 213 to 469 acres during 1950, yet the amount of farmland in the United States has fallen from 1,200 to 970 million acres and the number of farms has reduced from 5.6 to 2.1 million. Animal feeding operations or AFOs are becoming an important source of agricultural revenue in several states. In some parts of the United States, the animal industry has grown rapidly, and activities have become more intense. For instance, data from the most recent census indicates that during the previous ten years, there has been an 18% growth in the number of hogs in the United States, while the number of hog farms has decreased by 72%. While the number of dairy farms (establishments) fell by 40% over the same ten years, the size of the herd rose by 50%. Both the beef and poultry industries have grown significantly; in the US, facilities with over 100,000 birds account for 97% of total poultry output, while less than 2% of feedlots provide more than a third of all beef produced (Kraham, 2017). The rising demand for animal products and higher profitability as a result of advancements in marketing, processing, and transportation are driving this intensification. However, managing the waste generated by animal feeding operations presents serious difficulties.

Farming communities were usually self-sufficient before World War II because they could produce enough feed locally to meet animal demands and efficiently recycle manure nutrients to meet crop needs. Increased fertilizer uses in crop production following World War II led to the fragmentation of agricultural systems and the creation of specialized crop and animal enterprises that coexisted effectively in various places. Grain and livestock production could be geographically separated since farmers were no longer dependent on manures. Animals on the farm where the grain is cultivated consume less than one-third of the grain produced on farms today. The substantial nutrient shift from grain-producing to animal-producing regions as a result of agricultural system evolution is causing an accumulation of nitrogen and phosphorus in the soils of the animal-producing regions. For instance, when feed replaces fertilizer as the primary source of nutrient inputs in AFOs, the potential for surplus nitrogen and phosphorus at the farm scale can be significantly higher than in cropping systems. Thus, an imbalance in the system inputs and outputs of nitrogen and phosphorus, caused by an increase in AFOs, is the root cause of many water quality issues. The amounts of nitrogen and phosphate produced by manure in confined AFOs were determined. Phosphorus has increased more than nitrogen since the 1950s (U.S).

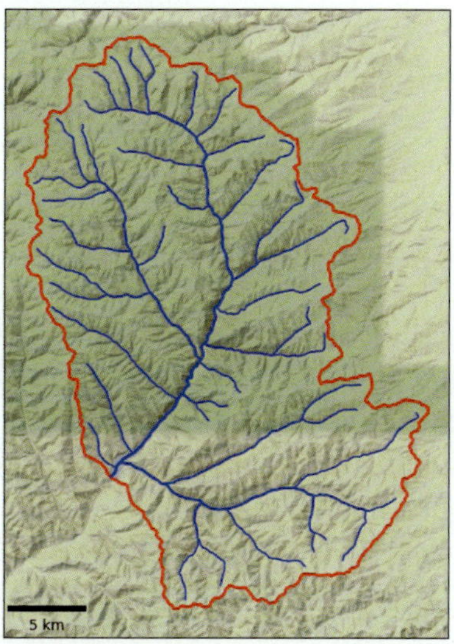


**Figure 4.3.** *Agricultural watersheds.*

Source: https://upload.wikimedia.org/wikipedia/commons/b/b5/Lost_Creek_Reservoir_Watershed.jpg,Creative Commons License.

A higher risk of nutrient export from agricultural watersheds (Figure 4.3) to surface and ground waters exists in places where there is a surplus of nitrogen and phosphorus compared to crop requirements. Since animal feeding operations benefit from high water availability, places with somewhat wet climates are more likely to have an excess of nutrients in their manure.

## 4.8. PHOSPHORUS DYNAMICS

The limited geographic data that is available to summarize the results of phosphorus soil tests indicates trends in the development of phosphorus in the soil to extremely high levels in certain places. These phosphorus-rich regions accumulate and frequently align with regions with high animal output. For economically optimal crop production, these types of soils require little to no input of phosphorus, from either fertilizer or organic by-products. The accumulation of soil phosphorus in many regions has raised the possibility of phosphorus moving into surface runoff and, in certain situations, into shallow groundwater aquifers.

Following phosphorus treatment, increases in phosphorus export from agricultural landscapes have been measured (Powers et al., 2015). The amount and timing of rainfall following phosphorus application, the type of fertilizer or manure applied, the timing, and manner of phosphorus application, and land cover all affect phosphorus export. From a farmer's perspective, these losses are typically negligible and only account for a small percentage of the phosphorus applied in the form of fertilizer or manure. As a result, farmers do not find these losses to be economically significant in terms of lost fertility. They may, nevertheless, have an impact on the eutrophication of aquatic habitats downstream. Although surface runoff typically accounts for the majority of phosphorus export from agricultural systems, there are exceptions in sandy, acidic- organic, or peaty soils with low phosphorus adsorption capacities as well as in soils where rapid water flow through macropores can occur. Some portions of the Atlantic coastal plain and Florida have soils that permit substantial subsurface export of dissolved phosphorus; as such, these soils should be taken into account while managing coastal eutrophication in these areas. The chemistry of phosphorus in soil-water systems was studied, but less is known about the hydrologic pathways connecting regionally varied phosphorus sources, sinks, temporary storages, and transport processes in landscapes. The creation of efficient management plans that address the reduction of phosphorus export from agricultural watersheds depends on this information. The watershed surface runoff is often produced by a small number of source areas/regions. As a consequence of precipitation, temperature, soils, terrain, groundwater, and moisture status throughout the watershed, these source areas fluctuate over time and rapidly expand and contract during a storm. Rather than infiltration capacity, soil-water storage in these places restricts surface runoff. In near-stream locations, this condition is typically caused by high water tables or high soil moisture content.

## 4.9. RUNOFF IMPACTS

The extent of regions that generate surface runoff will fluctuate during and after periods of precipitation. Area borders will move upslope when rainwater input rises during a downpour. During the dry summer months, the borders of the runoff-producing area grow away from the stream channel, whereas, during the wet winter months, they remain closer to the stream. The topography, geology, and soil structure of a watershed affect the placement and flow of varying source areas of surface runoff. The location and timing of perched water tables can be ascertained using fragipans or other layers, such as clay pans with clear permeability variations. The location of saturated zones and the amount of soil moisture are also influenced by sandstone or shale strata. Water, for instance, will be deposited on less permeable layers in the subsurface profile and is found at certain places in a watershed as surface flow or springs. Variable source area hydrology in watersheds is also influenced by slope breaks, convergent topography in horizontal or vertical planes, and depressions or spurs on hill slopes. The total phosphorus loads to surface waters are determined by the watershed discharge and net precipitation, which is defined as precipitation without evapotranspiration. When comparing the load estimations from various regions, this should be considered. It also explains why phosphorus seems to be a bigger problem in humid areas than in more arid areas. Areas within a watershed might cycle between becoming sources and sinks of surface flow when the infiltration rate, rather than the soil-water storage capacity, restricts surface runoff. This also will depend on the characteristics of the soil, the quantity and length of the rainfall, and the moisture in the soil. Since surface runoff is the primary mechanism through which most watersheds export phosphorus, it means that phosphorus export can be minimal in the absence of surface runoff. There has been much research done on what happens to nitrogen fertilizer that is sprayed on areas of agriculture.

## 4.10. VOLATILIZATION OF NITROGEN

The volatilization of nitrogen from fertilizer to the atmosphere is influenced by several variables, including farming practices, soil type, climate, and fertilizer type. Less than 2% of the ammonium volatilizes (ammonia) to the environment when ammonium sulfate is added to soil with a pH value of less than 5.5. Up to 50% of the nitrogen in calcareous soil can volatilize and release ammonia gas into the atmosphere when ammonium sulfate is added (Fenn and Hossner, 1985). On average, 8% of the nitrogen in ammonium sulfate and 15% of the nitrogen in urea is volatilized to the atmosphere. Tropical countries have higher percentages and significantly lower volatilization from nitrate-based fertilizers. In temperate regions, such as the United States, nitric oxide emissions to the atmosphere are often extremely minimal, but in tropical areas, they represent a significant nitrogen loss from fertilized fields. Almost all of the nitrogen that volatilizes from agricultural fields eventually finds its way back onto the landscape and can enter estuaries and coastal seas. This nitrogen is typically redeposited near the emission source. Understanding the fate of nitrogen in food and feedstock is crucial for comprehending nitrogen inputs to natural waters, as 45% to 75% of the nitrogen applied as fertilizer is collected in crops. Human-consumed food contains nitrogen that degrades into sewage and is released as sewage effluent. In these facilities, the nitrogen is either denitrified or volatilized to the atmosphere as ammonia. Nonetheless, the majority of crops grown in the US are fed to livestock. Therefore, animals excrete the majority of the nitrogen found in harvested crops.

A certain amount of excreted nitrogen from animals in sheds or barns, such as hogs, cows, and poultry, is volatilized to the atmosphere as ammonia; however, rearing cows on meadows as opposed to barns lowers atmospheric volatilization by more than 50%. Approximately 14% of all nitrogen applied in fertilizer eventually volatilizes to the atmosphere as ammonia following animal consumption (Bussink, 1994). This is on top of the ammonia that is directly volatilized from fertilizers and sewage treatment facilities. The amount of ammonia that agricultural systems in the US volatilize to the atmosphere is comparable to the amount of nitrate that seeps into surface waters from agricultural areas. Furthermore, animal wastes directly contribute nitrogen to surface waters, however losses are not well documented. Some researchers discovered that estimates of nitrogen consumption by domestic animals were far better as predictors of nonpoint source nitrogen fluxes in rivers than were rates of application of inorganic nitrogen fertilizer. There are two types of reactive nitrogen in the atmosphere: oxidized (NOy) and reduced (NHy) molecules. These originate from multiple sources, such as the combustion of fossil fuels, burning of biomass, lightning, and emissions from soils. The majority of NHy and NOy in the US are produced by burning fossil fuels, respectively. Many of these reactive nitrogen compounds have short atmospheric lifetimes, ranging from a few hours to a few days, and most of the nitrogen is deposited close to its source. Although NOy plays an important role in acid rain, estuarine waters are adequately buffered and do not directly experience acidification. As a result, the risk posed by NOy is its contribution of nitrogen to the eutrophication of coastal areas. Estuaries and coastal waters can experience substantial direct nitrogen deposition; however, it can be challenging to quantify. When monitoring stations are present, they often only record the amount of nitrogen that precipitation deposits contain. In most types of ecosystems, it has been challenging to quantify dry deposition of nitrogen. Typically, only wet deposition or, at most, a portion of dry deposition is measured at monitoring sites.

## 4.11. DEPOSITION DYNAMICS OF NITROGEN

Researchers have found that the amount of nitrogen that is directly deposited onto the water surfaces of estuaries can range from 1%to 40% of all nitrogen inputs. Estuaries like the Tampa Bay (Figure 4.4) and the Baltic Sea are the appropriate examples that fall in this range. Research indicates that a considerable amount of nitrogen is moving through the atmosphere from the eastern United States to the North Atlantic Ocean coastal and offshore waters, where it is deposited.

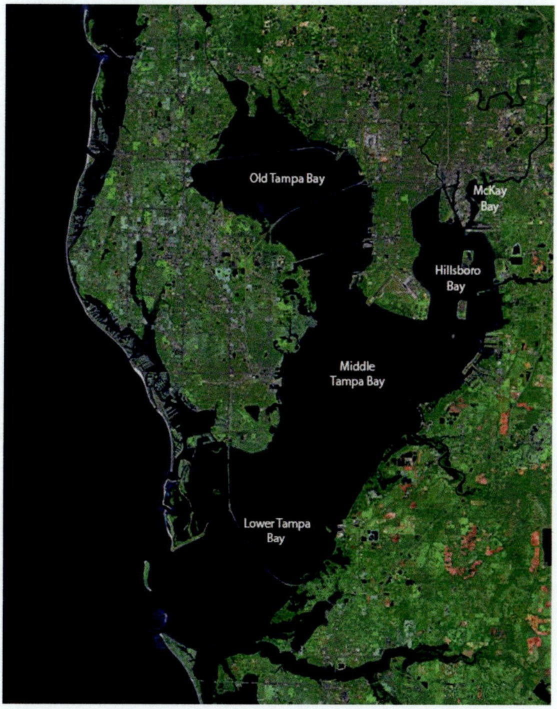


**Figure 4.4.** *Tampa Bay.*

Source: https://upload.wikimedia.org/wikipedia/commons/5/5c/Tampa_florida_map.jpg, Creative Commons License.

This flux may be as much as half of the reactive nitrogen that the United States emits into the atmosphere. However, this atmospheric deposition most likely contributes less than 10% of the total input of nitrogen to the surface waters of the continental shelf due to the significant natural flux of nitrogen from the deepwater of the North Atlantic Ocean onto the continental shelf off the eastern United States. Terrestrial ecosystems receive a large portion of the reactive nitrogen deposited from the atmosphere. This may have an impact on estuaries and coastal seas.

## 4.12. NITROGEN DEPOSITION IN FORESTS

There has been much research done on what happens to nitrogen deposition in forests. The availability of nitrogen limits the productivity of the majority of American forests in their natural form. One can anticipate a short-term increase in the production and storage of N in organic matter as additional nitrogen from atmospheric deposition becomes available to these forests. When supplies of nitrogen surpass what trees require and the ability of soil organic matter to be assimilated (microbial and abiotic processes), forests are said to be saturated with nitrogen. When a forest reaches saturation with nitrogen, losses to the atmosphere and to ecosystems downstream can occur very quickly. The downstream export of nitrogen can be significant in European forests that have had high levels of nitrogen deposition, frequently exceeding 500 kg N $km^{-2}$ $yr^{-1}$ (de Vries et al., 2017).

There is evidence to suggest that associated changes in biogeochemical cycling and ecosystem deterioration might cause forests to become nitrogen-saturated and accelerate the process of exporting nitrogen instead of storing it. The young, aging forests have a tendency to hold onto more nitrogen and are less prone than old, mature forests to become nitrogen-saturated. The species composition of the trees, the climate, and the type of soil can all have an impact on a forest's capacity to store nitrogen, in addition to the land-use.

Regardless of how old the forests were, only roughly half of the nitrogen intake from atmospheric deposition was retained by them. This is probably because the sandy soils allow nitrogen to move quickly. However, even after receiving heavy nitrogen fertilization over a six-year period, forests in western Massachusetts with sandy loam soils retained over 85% of the nitrogen inputs. There was some indication that nitrogen saturation happens more quickly in pine forests than in hardwood forests, and that nitrogen retention decreased with increasing nitrogen concentration of the forest. The ratio of organic C to N in the forest floor gives a measure of the forest nitrogen status, which makes it easy to anticipate how much nitrogen will escape out of the forest. While forests with a high nitrogen status retain less than half of the nitrogen added through deposition and fertilizer, forests with a low nitrogen status retain the majority of the nitrogen added. A good indicator of the export of inorganic nitrogen from streams draining forests in the northeastern United States is the ratio of organic carbon to organic nitrogen in those forests. Situations where the stream organic carbon to organic nitrogen ratio was between 20:1 and 25:1 saw a sharp rise in the export of inorganic nitrogen in some areas. A forest's ability to absorb or release nitrogen depends on several variables, but forests that receive continuous high nitrogen inputs from atmospheric deposition have a tendency to become nitrogen-saturated. As a result, a forested watershed that receives large amounts of nitrogen deposition over time will eventually fill up with nitrogen and start providing nitrogen to the streams that drain it.

Less research has been done on the export of nitrogen after deposition onto terrestrial ecosystems other than forests. Grasslands can retain nitrogen like forests. Although nitrogen deposited during the non-growing season may be more likely to be lost to downstream ecosystems, the fate of atmospheric nitrogen in agricultural fields is comparable to that of nitrogen fertilizer applied to such fields. Despite the significant l nitrogen content of stormwater runoff from urban areas, the fate of atmospheric nitrogen dumped into suburban and urban landscapes appears to be essentially unexplored. Since a large portion of atmospheric reactive nitrogen is deposited close to sources, it makes sense to assume that there is a substantial export of this deposition to coastal waters. Deposition into metropolitan environments is high. However, because the majority of deposition monitoring sites are located in rural areas, it is difficult to assess nitrogen deposition in urban areas. One of the main unknown variables in the nitrogen budget for the United States is the amount of nitrogen deposition in metropolitan areas.

Because significant nutrient flow processing can take place in wetlands, streams, lakes, reservoirs, and rivers that lie between the terrestrial systems and coastal waters, not all of the nitrogen or phosphorus exported from a forest, corn field, or animal feedlot will reach an estuary or coastal waters. Depending on the presence of phosphorus-sorptive phases like iron (III) hydroxides and oxides as well as calcium carbonate minerals, the sediments in wetlands and aquatic systems can either retain or lose phosphorus. The oxidation state of the minerals is important when iron compounds are the primary phosphorus-adsorbing minerals because reduced iron compounds do not absorb phosphorus. The biological impacts on the pH of the surface sediment may also be important. The lakes frequently store 80% or more of the phosphorus that enters them, with the retention of phosphorus in lakes being predicted from the residence duration of the water in the lakes.

## 4.13. RIPARIAN ZONES

Buffer or riparian zones (Figure 4.5) surrounding streams or waterbodies might minimize inputs from agricultural land since wetlands also store considerable amounts of phosphorus (Mander et al., 2017). The wetlands and aquatic systems may also remove substantial amounts of nitrogen. Denitrification is typically the primary method used in these systems to remove nitrogen. The process mostly takes place in anoxic conditions, and it frequently happens quickly in the sediments of rivers, lakes, and wetlands. While some studies demonstrate a conversion to organic nitrogen, the majority of studies show a substantial removal of nitrate in groundwater that flows through wetlands. Reducing nitrogen loads can be achieved by riparian wetlands, which catch runoff from agricultural areas before it reaches streams. However, as land was converted for agriculture, these riparian wetlands were drained or otherwise lost in many places. 10% to 15% of land in southern Sweden was converted to agriculture, which damaged bordering wetlands and increased stream nitrogen inputs.

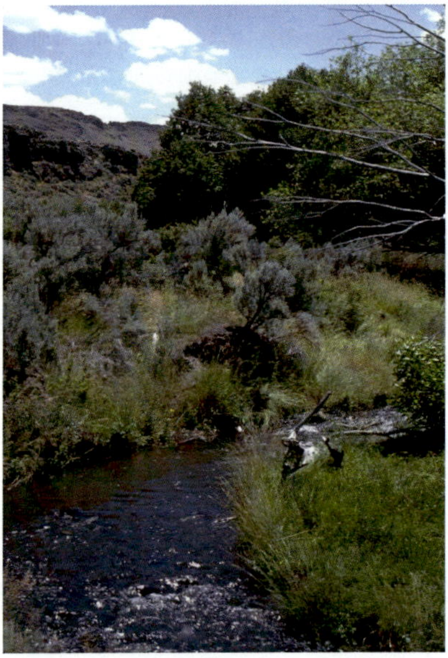

**Figure 4.5.** *Riparian zones.*

Source: https://upload.wikimedia.org/wikipedia/commons/d/db/Willow_Creek%2C_Trout_Creek_Mountains%2C_Oregon.jpg, Creative Commons License.

Restoring wetlands has been recommended as the least expensive and most efficient way to reduce nitrogen fluxes into rivers from the surrounding landscape. When the water is severely hypoxic or anoxic, denitrification takes place in the water (streams and rivers). Nevertheless, few rivers in the US today experience these low-oxygen episodes due to the overall improvement in river water quality that came along with the extensive adoption of secondary sewage treatment for the reduction of biological oxygen demand. However, even in cases of excellent water quality, the sediments found in streams and rivers are often acidic, which makes them an appropriate site for denitrification. Similarly, below the top few meters of water, lake sediments are nearly always anoxic. The amount of nitrogen removed by denitrification in lakes, streams, and rivers with anoxic water columns can be assessed as a function of depth and mean residence time. Denitrification is more pronounced in systems with longer water residence times and shallow water columns because these two factors increase the amount of nitrogen in the water that comes into contact with anoxic sediments. Denitrification in US river systems is generally unlikely to denitrify more than 20% of the nitrogen that flows into them (Forshay and Stanley, 2005).

It has been quite challenging to identify the primary source of nitrogen inputs and the amount of load that each source contributes (estuaries). Understanding nutrient fluxes to the coast is hindered by several factors, such as the existence of multiple sources (agricultural and fossil fuel), the difficulty of estimating dry deposition at the scale of entire watersheds; the difficulty of measuring gaseous losses from ecosystems volatilization of ammonia, and the multiple pathways for nitrogen flows. To forecast nitrogen export to the coastal area, a multiple regression model was built using NOy deposition in addition to agricultural inputs i.e., the total fertilizer. The nitrogen flux in rivers leading to the coastal area may be influenced more by nitrogen from fossil fuel sources per unit mass than by nitrogen from agricultural sources. Naturally, the overall amount of nitrogen applied as fertilizer in many regions is significantly more than the amount of nitrogen deposited as NOy. The Mississippi River basin receives more nitrogen from fertilizer inputs overall than from NOy deposition; as a result, agriculture accounts for the majority of the nitrogen exported from the basin. Using the total NOy and ammonium deposition to predict nitrogen export yields the best regression fit for the export of nitrogen from nonpoint sources for the temperate regions of the North Atlantic Ocean. There is a strong correlation between ammonium deposition and livestock densities. This indicates that livestock manure plays an important role in the nitrogen pollution of surface waters caused by agriculture, and it also plays a major role in the export of nitrogen to coastal seas over large regions, along with fossil fuels. Some researchers used large-scale methods to evaluate the sources of phosphorus and nitrogen in surface waters. Just over half of the streams and rivers in the United States likely have total phosphorus concentrations above 0.1 mg l-1. The production of livestock waste is the main cause of phosphorus contamination, which increases phosphorus concentrations across the country.

There are no established methods for measuring the amount of nutrients that estuaries get, and a variety of techniques have been employed. Nutrient budgets are sometimes based on export-coefficient models. Some methods are effective in assessing the significance of point-source inputs, including wastewater treatment facilities. The estimations of nutrient inputs from non-point sources may be misleading if not calibrated properly. Using export-coefficient models makes estimating the significance of atmospheric deposition as a source particularly difficult. To estimate the overall load, for instance, export-coefficient models merely apply empirical data through a series of quite simple computations. To calculate the export for the entire watershed, these numbers (values) are multiplied by the area of each type of land in the watershed. At the scale of individual estuaries, methodologies for identifying the sources of nutrients and the amount of the load contributed by each are inadequately developed. Better approaches are desperately needed, especially in relation to atmospheric nitrogen deposition onto the landscape. A possible framework based on quantifying inputs to the watershed is provided by the large-scale and regional analyses. Furthemore, these analyses are relatively new and have not yet been implemented to the management of the majority of estuaries. The contribution of atmospheric deposition to estuarine nitrogen budgets may be the source of the uncertainty. The majority of the studies on estuaries paid no attention to nitrogen sources from the atmosphere.

Chapter 5

# BALTIC SEA EUTROPHICATION

## Contents

# 5.1. INTRODUCTION

For a better understanding of how several intricate processes in an aquatic system work together to determine the concentration of a nutrient, process-based dynamic mass-balance models are crucial tools. Mass-balance models have long been employed in various coastal applications as well as in the study of lake eutrophication (Håkanson, 2009). With the use of mass-balance modeling, predictions about the likely outcomes of a system's changes in conditions, such as reductions in pollutant discharges associated with a remedial measure, can be made. It is also possible to predict thresholds using dynamic mass-balance models. Various scales can be used for mass-balance modeling, depending on the goal of the investigation. There are numerous coastal models available, each with advantages and disadvantages. It is difficult to anticipate more than a week in advance because, for instance, the 1D-nutrient model reported by some researchers requires meteorological data with high temporal precision. With a temporal resolution of 1 minute and $<$ 1 mm of spatial resolution, the 3D model employed by scientists is challenging to execute and evaluate using credible empirical data. The model that was tested and deployed for the Baltic Sea basins is called CoastMab, and it is a general mass-balance model for large coastal areas (ecosystem scale). To account for seasonal fluctuations, it is based on monthly time steps and ordinary differential equations.

# 5.2. COASTAL AREA MODELING

It has been successfully evaluated and applied in many coastal areas for pollutants and phosphorus. Because these factors will affect the conditions within a coastal area, data from the coastal area as well as from the sea beyond the given coastal area must be accessible for mass-balance models for coastal areas. The CoastMab-model quantifies general transport processes like sedimentation, resuspension, burial, diffusion, etc. that apply to all substances in all aquatic systems; however, substance-specific components also exist. Sedimentation is the flow of water into sediments or deeper water layers containing suspended particles and the nutrients that are related to them. The advective flux from sediments back to water is known as resuspension, and it is mostly caused by slope processes and wind and wave action. Diffusion is the flow of dissolved chemicals from layers of water with high concentrations to adjacent layers with lower concentrations, or from sediments back to the water. Diffusion is therefore caused by concentration gradients, which are frequently influenced by small-scale advective processes; even during extended periods of calm currents related to the earth's rotation, variations in low and high pressure, variations in day and nighttime temperature, etc. It should be noted that measuring water velocities lower than 1-2 cm/s in natural aquatic systems is challenging. Transport between, for example, surface-water layers and deeper water layers connected to changes in stratification i.e., variation in temperature and/or salinity is known as mixing, or large-scale advective transport processes. The breakdown of organic particles by bacteria results in mineralization, which is the regeneration of nutrients preferably in dissolved forms. Primary production is the process by which sunlight converts dead materials into living suspended particles. Burial is the sedimentary transfer of material, frequently from the biosphere to the geosphere.

The movement of all suspended and dissolved materials out of the water system is known as outflow (Shiller and Boyle, 1991). Most environmental studies rely on empirical data as their foundation. Extensive databases on the conditions in the Baltic Sea and other aquatic systems have been investigated. Researchers have also used data from more than 500 aquatic systems worldwide to provide a broader context of this situation. A method for defining and distinguishing between layers of surface water and deep water is often accomplished using salinity data, which defines the halocline, or water temperature data, which defines the thermocline. Some researchers follow a strategy that was based on the water depth that divides bottom areas, the erosion and transportation areas, or ET-areas where periods of sedimentation and resuspension of fine deposited material are expected. The theoretical wave base is the depth at which areas of fine materials with continuous sediment accumulation and areas with discontinuous sedimentation are separated. Regarding mass-balance modeling of aquatic systems, this is an important concept. Furthermore, the theoretical wave base uses algorithms that define material concentrations in these compartments; sedimentation by taking into account the mean depths of these compartments; internal loading through advection/resuspension and diffusion; upward and downward mixing between the specified compartments; and outflow of substances from the specified compartments will all be defined using the theoretical wave base.

Without process-based mass-balance calculations, it is impossible to measure, comprehend, or anticipate changes in the concentrations of chemical constituents i.e., nutrients, metals, radionuclides, or organic toxins in aquatic systems, for example, those associated with expensive remedial interventions. This is true for all aquatic system types, all material types, and all temporal and spatial scales. Since Vollenweider introduced the first loading models for phosphorus in lakes in 1968, it has been evident that the quantification of water fluxes and retention rates is essential to mass-balances for nutrients (eutrophication). However, the modeling scale and the equations employed to quantify the fluxes have a significant impact on the assumptions needed to attain the practical utility and predictive capacity of mass-balance models. In the field of coastal studies, water fluxes to, from, and within estuaries are typically measured using the fundamental mass-balance equation for salt. The Baltic Sea has also been the subject of many water balance studies. Such mass-balance computations for salt or other chemicals yield results that are reliable. Water flow and volume are essentially what defines the potential water retention period (T- time), and 1/T is what essentially defines the water retention rate. The water and heat balances are key study components under the BALTEX program, and new estimates on the individual components in the water balance are available (Omstedt et al., 2004). The main factors affecting the water balance of the Baltic Sea are net precipitation, river runoff, and inflows and outflows in the entrance area. For shorter periods, changes in water storage must be taken into consideration. The duration of the study phase and the time period both affect the results. Several studies have also divided the Baltic Sea into sub-basins and estimated the flows from the water and salt balances.

## 5.3. MODELLING

The CoastMab-model is intended to be broadly applicable to the majority of chemicals and coastal region types; salinity data from the entire Baltic Sea is crucial (Håkanson and Bryhn, 2008). Temperature data is typically used in traditional mass-balance models for substances to define the thermocline or halocline as a criterion to distinguish the deep-water layer from the surface-water layer and, consequently, to measure mixing between these layers. However, because vertical temperature profiles frequently fluctuate temporally and spatially, there are many problems with this technique in mass-balance modeling. The conventional method requires either statistical compilations to define a mean depth of the thermocline or the halocline calculated from previous (historical) periods, and the variability and uncertainty for the mean value, or online temperature data, whereby the long-term (monthly/annual) predictive power is often lost. To determine the depth dividing the surface-water compartment from the deep-water compartment, that is, based on sedimentological criteria utilizing the theoretical wave base, research works were conducted. Fine sediments will be resuspended if the wave orbital velocity is more than roughly 10 cm/s. Fine sediments settle out by gravity under laminar motion utilizing Stokes' law. Thus, the theoretical wave base is crucial for mass-balance modeling of any materials with a particulate phase because it determines not only the surface-water compartment but also the bottom portions where resuspension (advection) of fine particles occurs. Because the salinity is conservative in that the salts are dissolved in the water (the dissolved fraction, or DF), it has a particulate fraction (PF) of zero.

Using the hypsographic curve to determine the volumes of the surface-water and deep-water compartments is another general feature of this technique. We can use the available digital bathymetric data for the Baltic Sea to create new depth-area curves and volume curves for the region. Many research projects focus on tracking and comprehending the water and salt exchange between the Baltic Sea and the Kattegat via the Oresund and Danish Belts. The Oresund accounts for 20% of the total instantaneous flow, although some researchers suggested that it accounts for 27%. These routes have different times for the incoming water to reach the Baltic Sea; the journey via the Oresund takes less time (two days) than the journey via the Danish Belts, which takes more than a week. The salinity of the incoming water is also impacted by this. Given that the water in the Oresund is saltier (high salinity) than the water that flows through the Belts, it could be more significant for the input of salt. The distinctions between the two paths are not taken into account in some investigations. Rather, the total mean salinity of the water from both paths is computed, and the amount of incoming water that enters the Baltic Sea strata is then ascertained using calibrations. The HELCOM datasets, which are accessible on the ICES website, provided the essential empirical data on salinity; some researchers concentrated on data from 1997 to 2005. They used water temperature data from the same database and the same time period to demonstrate the applicability of the theoretical wave basis in defining the surface-water compartment and the other water layers.

## 5.4. MASS BALANCE ANALYSES

Net precipitation (NP) and riverine water input to the Baltic Sea vary seasonally and annually (Filipsson et al., 2017). The interchange of water with the Kattegat and its salinity is common. Because of this, the mean salinities in the Baltic Sea basins change over time as well. Some researchers have concentrated on a time frame for which they have complete access to data regarding the mass-balances of phosphorus and salt; however, there are inherent uncertainties in the data for this time frame as well. Numerous important processes and functions in aquatic systems are influenced by salinity, such as: increased salinity causes suspended particles to aggregate and flocculate more, increasing water clarity and increased water clarity increases benthic algae, macrophytes, and phytoplankton primary production. Increasing primary production results in an increase in secondary production of zooplankton and fish. Increasing aggregation (flocculation) causes an increase in settling velocities, sedimentation, and oxygen consumption, which in turn causes a decline in oxygen concentrations in the sediment/water zone. Salinity plays a major role in the number of species i.e., it affects specific species and its survival, such as the survival of cod roe. Due to its specific density, the cod roe will float at a depth in the water where the water density and the roe density are equal. The temperature and salinity of the water affect its density. The oxygen content and salinity in the Baltic Sea need to be greater than 2 mg/l and 10.5 psu, respectively, for cod roe to survive. Elevated nutrient concentrations lead to an increase in organic matter production, both primary and secondary, and consequently, a rise in oxygen demand due to bacterial decomposition of decomposing organic matter. Lower oxygen concentrations are the result of increased oxygen consumption. This suggests that if the salinity is low and the nutrient loading is high, the chances of the cod roe surviving are somewhat low. Then, at deeper sea depths where oxygen concentrations are probably lower, cod roe will start to appear.

In order to comprehend the response of the Baltic Sea system or any other aquatic system, to changes in factors such as water, salt or nutrient loading, a dynamic process-based method that measures the variables governing inflow, outflow, internal transport processes, and retention rates is essential. Some researchers found an agreement between empirical and modeled data on salinity that may be obtained by modeling the surface-water, middle-water, and deepwater compartments using the theoretical wave base rather than outdated(conventional) temperature data. It is frequently emphasized in contexts of marine eutrophication that, in order to be able to provide accurate evaluations of how systems will respond to variations in nutrient loading or other remedial actions, it is important to develop practically useful general dynamic mass-balance models based on the ecosystem perspective. This modeling is intended to do this work. The monthly budgets for salt and water in the Baltic Sea and its major sub-basins, the Gulf of Finland, (Figure 5.1) the Gulf of Riga, the Bothnian Sea, and the Baltic Proper are accessible from different sources.

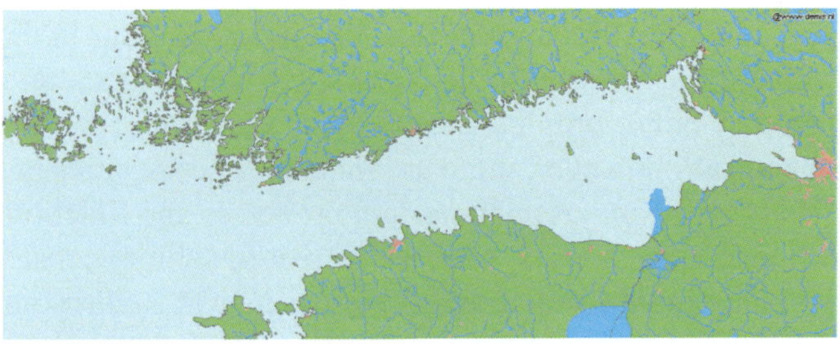

**Figure 5.1.** *Gulf of Finland.*

Source: https://upload.wikimedia.org/wikipedia/commons/f/f2/La2-demis-gulf-of-finland.png, Creative Commons License.

New volume curves based on bathymetric data, as well as new morphometric data for the Baltic Sea and the designated sub-basins, have been employed. This main goal of many research studies has been to provide data on the water flows and theoretical retention durations for salt and water in the designated sub-basins of the Baltic Sea because those values provide essential details on the system's response to variations in (nutrient loading). The concept behind this modeling strategy and the findings is that these water fluxes, water retention rates, and the algorithms used to measure vertical mixing and diffusion between the layers should be set up so that the model can also measure nutrient fluxes (Beckmann and Hense, 2007).

## 5.5. ANALYSIS OF DIN AND DIP

DIN (dissolved inorganic nitrogen) and DIP (dissolved inorganic phosphorus) renew rapidly. For instance, zooplankton may excrete enough DIN to replace more than 100% of what phytoplankton consumes (Zhao et al., 2008). Since the algae in highly productive systems take up dissolved forms of nutrients so quickly, measuring dissolved forms of nutrients may even be challenging. It is unlikely that DIN is limiting only when DIN levels are significantly higher than DIP levels, and it is improbable that P is the limiting nutrient only when DIN/DIP < 1. In comparison to TN and TP, DIN and DIP are poor predictors of nutrient status in aquatic systems. Moreover, dissolved organic N and P are absorbed by phytoplankton and other primary producers. Because DIN and DIP are so unpredictable, they are not good indicators of primary production and phytoplankton biomass. Different nutrients may limit primary production in natural waters. Nitrogen fixation eventually compensated for N shortages, but P was the long-term regulating factor based on changes in nutrient ratios between phytoplankton and saltwater. In multiple studies, some researchers discovered that P inputs controlled primary production whereas N inputs had no effect. As a result, the results of bioassays were not useful. Redfield's theory has also been effectively evaluated in modeling projects for the Baltic Proper. The challenge of whether to use the TN/TP or DIN/DIP ratios in contexts connected to limiting nutrients and whether to concentrate remedial measures on phosphorus or nitrogen needs to be explored. Some relevant information originates from the Himmerfjarden Bay in the Baltic Proper on the east coast of Sweden. One might be inclined to conclude that nutrient reductions should concentrate on phosphorus from the TN/TP data because this ratio is higher than the Redfield ratio of 7.2; alternatively, one could also propose that nutrient reductions should concentrate on nitrogen from the DIN/DIP ratio because this ratio is frequently lower than 7.2. Some researchers argue that both of these arguments are invalid because the availability of bioavailable forms, such as DIN and DIP, regulates primary production, not concentrations or ratios based on concentrations. The key is that throughout the entire growing season, the primary production, phytoplankton biomass, and consequently the concentration of chlorophyll-a, remain high. The higher the primary production, the more bioavailable nitrogen (nitrate & ammonium) and phosphorus (phosphate) are being used by the algae (diatoms). Eventually, the nitrate concentration drops to almost zero and the primary production decreases.

## 5.6. PHYTOPLANKTON PRIMARY PRODUCTION

The primary phytoplankton production cannot be controlled by the concentrations of the bioavailable factors, such as DIN and DIP, in μg/l or other concentration units, since primary production is a flux with a time dimension, while nutrient concentration is a concentration without a time dimension. The main focus is on the flow of DIN and DIP into a system as well as the regeneration of fresh DIN and DIP as a result of bacteria breaking down organic materials that include N and P. Due to significant DIN and DIP input and/or regeneration, the concentration of DIN and DIP may be very low yet primary phytoplankton production and biomass may be considerable. The quantity of TN and TP present in the water mass, that is, TN and TP represent the pool of nutrients in the water that can contribute to the regeneration of DIN and DIP, affecting the regeneration of DIN and DIP. It is important to note that the normal turnover times of phytoplankton and bacterioplankton are approximately three days. This indicates that ten generations of phytoplankton may arise in less than a month, requiring DIN and DIP in the amounts determined by the Redfield ratio (7.2 grams).

Denitrification, atmospheric wet and dry deposition, and nitrogen fixation, for example, by certain cyanobacteria, are important in the modeling process (Baker et al., 2007). The particulate fraction, which is important for estimating sedimentation, is another significant area of uncertainty regarding our knowledge of nitrogen fluxes in coastal systems. Regarding nitrogen mass-balance calculations, atmospheric nitrogen fixing is crucial. Since nitrogen reductions may be balanced by nitrogen fixation by cyanobacteria, it is impossible to properly evaluate the effectiveness of remedial measures to reduce nutrient discharges to aquatic systems without empirically tested algorithms to quantify nitrogen fixation. It also means that since measured TN concentrations in the water phase are always governed by mass balances, that is, the quantification of the key transport processes regulating the given concentrations, it is typically very difficult to understand, model, and predict changes in these concentrations. A model for total cyanobacteria in marine situations based on TP, TN, salinity, and water temperature was provided by some scientists. When tested against actual data, the model yielded an R2 of 0.78. It should be emphasized that, as a result of improved measuring methods and a deeper comprehension of the process, the nitrogen fixation rates in the Baltic Sea have been significantly revised.

## 5.7. PHOSPHORUS

Phosphorus should be the primary target of nutrient reductions for coastal areas, rather than nitrogen. The primary explanations for not using nitrogen abatement to address coastal eutrophication are as follows: It is difficult to forecast the result and cost-effectiveness of nitrogen reductions due to the high uncertainties associated with the quantification of nitrogen fixation, wet and dry deposition, sedimentation, and denitrification. This should apply to many additional coastal systems in addition to the Baltic Sea. The likelihood of cyanobacterial blooms may increase with lower TN concentrations. Laboratory tests using DIN and DIP are frequently used to support arguments for nitrogen abatement, however these studies frequently yield very little data that can be used to notify management options for actual aquatic systems. From a long-term temporal standpoint, phosphorus appears to be the key factor limiting primary production in the coastal zone. The majority of species find turbid waters less appealing than clear waters with significant Secchi depths. Many elements might affect the Secchi depth, which is defined as the sight depth where a black and white disc dropped into the water is no longer visible to the naked eye. In addition to being a crucial aspect of an algorithm describing a water quality indicator for coastal waters, the Secchi depth is a direct reflection of the quantity of suspended particulate matter (SPM) scattering light in the water. Secchi depth and SPM are determined by three factors: autochthonous production (the quantity of plankton, lower Secchi means higher amount of plankton); allochthonous materials (humic and minerogenic substances from external sources, and the amount of resuspended material (Håkanson, 2006). High levels of resuspension cause high levels of internal nutrient loading and increased production; high levels of colored substances in estuaries indicate a smaller photic zone and lower production; high levels of allochthonous substance input and high production would indicate a high level of sedimentation, etc. If the plankton cells themselves are the cause of the light extinction, the Secchi depth should be significantly higher than what is actually observed. This finding suggests that in many coastal regions, particles other than plankton cells may play a major role in setting the Secchi depth.

The empirical correlation between Secchi depth and chlorophyll-a was likewise found to be primarily dependent on the concentration of chlorophyll-a co-varying with the total amount of suspended particles. As a crucial regulator of macrophyte expansion, the maximum depth of the photic zone is typically adjusted to around twice the Secchi depth, while the effective (mean) depth of the photic zone is frequently set to match the Secchi depth. In eutrophication situations, photolithoautotrophic bacteria, also known as blue-green algae play important roles. The cyanobacterial species can fix substantial amounts of dissolved gaseous nitrogen of atmospheric origin, and they can also form large, potentially toxic blooms. These are the most common type of dangerous algal blooms in the Baltic Sea, however other types of algae may be more important in other brackish and marine environments. Determining the nitrogen balance in marine waters and comprehending the origins of marine eutrophication frequently depend on quantifying nitrogen fixation. High temperatures, low non-gaseous N concentrations, and high P concentrations in the water cause nitrogen fixation, which may determine which nutrient controls primary production and, consequently, which nutrient needs to be reduced to treat marine eutrophication. The main processes regulating internal and external fluxes of nutrients to a given aquatic system are to be studied using all the variables. This includes the crucial relationship between the amount of the nutrient in dissolved and particulate forms. Using data from lakes, the researchers established (log-log) relationship (regression) between total cyanobacteria and chlorophyll-a concentrations. CB denotes the median values for the growth season. Between the measurements of primary production/biomass in water, a highly substantial and strong positive co-variation was observed. It is clear that if the relationship had been based on daily, weekly, or monthly values, it may have looked differently, and it's likely that many marine systems would also exhibit this co-variation. Roughly 90% of the total biomass of cyanobacteria, according to data from the Baltic Proper, may be nitrogen-fixing species. This amount does not account for nitrogen fixation from non-heterocystous species smaller than 10 μm, which also contributes to nitrogen fixation. Other methods exist for quantifying nitrogen fixation besides the models employed in some works, and due to the inherent unpredictability and irregularity in the variables controlling nitrogen fixation, all methods yield somewhat uncertain values. This means that different methods may offer complementing data, resulting in a reduction in uncertainty in the amount of nitrogen fixation in a given system when multiple moderately uncertain estimates are combined.

## 5.8. MODEL STRUCTURES

The basic model structure in the Baltic Proper (BP) and the Gulf of Finland (GF) is composed of seven compartments: phytoplankton, erosion/transportation areas for fine sediments (ET), accumulation areas for fine sediments in the middle-water layer (AMW), accumulation areas for fine sediments in the deep-water layer (ADW), and surface water (SW), middle water (MW), and deep water (DW). Surface water (SW), deep water (DW below the theoretical wave base), erosion/transportation areas for fine sediments (ET), accumulation areas for fine sediments in the deep-water layer (ADW), and phytoplankton (Bio) make up the model structure in the Bothnian Bay (BB), Bothnian Sea (BS), and Gulf of Riga (GR) (Schneider and Müller, 2018). The particles deposited above the theoretical wave base will not remain in their original locations indefinitely if there is no land uplift and the hypsographic curve remains constant. The particles will be resuspended and transported downward to the areas of continuous sedimentation below the theoretical wave base, where the materials may be resuspended primarily due to slope processes. Particularly in shallow areas, the bottom deposits on the E-areas are typically somewhat coarse, consolidated, and/or have a low water content. The sediments tend to be finer and less consolidated in the T-areas that are nearer the theoretical wave base. If there is no land uplift, there is no net deposition of matter or phosphorus down to the theoretical wave base. However, if there is uplift, there is net deposition below the theoretical wave base, and the sedimentation rate typically varies from zero at the theoretical wave base to maximum values in deep-water areas. The water depth that separates the basin water from deeper layers may be influenced by a number of factors, including the thermocline and water temperature conditions, vertical concentration gradients of salt and dissolved or suspended particles, wind and wave influences and wave characteristics, and sedimentological conditions linked to internal loading and resuspension. Thus, vertical water heterogeneities in basins can be described in a variety of ways. When working with precisely defined depths, volumes, and substance concentrations, mass-balance theory works.

## 5.9. SETTLING VELOCITY

The average settling velocity in surface waters can be used to calculate the time it takes for the average suspended particle to reach the sediments at a depth of 44 meters in the Baltic Proper (Kuhrts et al., 2004). Since the settling velocity in the SW-layer is just 0.5-0.6 m/month, it takes an average of 6-7 years for these particles to reach the sediments in the accumulation area. Some dead diatoms may settle out more quickly than others including fine clay particles, humic particles, and dead bacterioplankton. With a salinity of 7 psu in the SW-layer, the average settling velocity for suspended particles and particulate phosphorus in the Baltic Proper is approximately 0.5 m/month. This is 50 times less than the average settling velocity of 25 m/month indicated by Stokes' equation (laboratory). The average monthly settling velocity in the entire SW-layer cannot be considerably higher than those measured by some researchers and computed using the CoastMab-model. Cost-benefit analysis of recommended remedial solutions for the Baltic Sea or any other aquatic system experiencing increased anthropogenic nutrient loading is a challenging but crucial task for Baltic Sea management. HELCOM's approach to stopping the further eutrophication of the Baltic Sea relied on percentage decreases in the actual transit of nitrogen and phosphorus from the various Baltic countries. But it may have no scientific value because it is obvious that natural processes on Earth only react to changes in grams or kilos, not percentages. To reduce the eutrophication in the Baltic Sea, HELCOM has recently established a new plan. It suggests reducing the current annual nutrient loading to the system by 15,000 tons of phosphorus and 133,000 tons of nitrogen. These recommendations are predicated on the MARE NEST-model recommendations. The other Baltic countries have also received these reductions from HELCOM; Sweden, for example, will be reducing 290 tons of phosphorus and 20,780 tons of nitrogen. Although the exact costs of these reductions are not fully known, they may be extremely costly. It is hard to predict with any degree of certainty what would happen to the nitrogen concentration in the Baltic Sea if 133,000 tons of nitrogen were to be reduced. This is because the only validated mass-balance model for nitrogen that is currently available is the MARE NEST-model, which is inadequate for any accurate predictive purposes (Lowe et al., 2014). The implications for the structure and function of the ecosystem, such as for the biomass and productivity of predatory and prey fish, cannot be predicted. Similarly, changes in the target bioindicators, such as the Secchi depth, the concentration of cyanobacteria, and the concentration of chlorophyll-a, linked to the suggested reductions in nitrogen concentrations, cannot be predicted. The cost of reducing phosphates in detergents is less than 0.4 euros per kilogram of P; advising on P-reductions in agriculture would cost 5-100 euros per kilogram of P; reducing P in animal feed would cost 5-7 euros per kilogram of P; and cultivating and collecting mussels and clams would cost roughly 35 euros per Kg of P.

The conditions in the Gulf of Finland, the Gulf of Riga, the coastal region outside of Kaliningrad, and the estuaries of the rivers Oder and Vistula should be improved first. This indicates that to implement corrective actions for these specific coastal areas in a way that is both economical and efficient, the CoastMab-model should be applied. This also implies that since a model of this type is required to compute the phosphorus fluxes between the given coastal area and the Baltic Proper, the CoastMab-model for the entire Baltic Sea might be utilized preferably. When substrate-specific methods are available, they should focus on phosphorus removal because it has been demonstrated that phosphorus is the nutrient-limiting primary production in the Baltic Sea over longer periods, such as the growing season. Many remedial measures in agriculture, urban areas, or industry would remove both nutrients. Researchers have advocated for a remedial plan that would remove 2725 t/yr of phosphorus or 60% of the anthropogenic contributions from the Gulf of Finland, 425 t/yr from the Gulf of

Riga or 46% of the anthropogenic contributions, and 6625 t/yr from the Baltic Proper or 48% of the anthropogenic contributions, with no reductions made to the Bothnian Sea and the Bothnian Bay. Obviously, putting such reductions into practice would take time, and during that period, the Baltic Sea system might experience many changes connected to climatic variations. This indicates that these suggestions should be regarded with appropriate caution and modified in light of any upcoming modifications.

*Chapter* **6**

# GLOBAL PERSPECTIVE ON EUTROPHICATION ISSUES

## Contents

## 6.1. INTRODUCTION

The maritime ecosystem provides humanity with many benefits and products. Even though the oceans, seas, and transitional waters make up around 71% of the surface, just a small portion (1%) of the marine resources have been thoroughly investigated. The marine environment is rich in biological resources, but it is also full of important minerals like nickel, copper, manganese, and oil and gas (Toro et al., 2020). Half of the population resides on or by the shoreline. The coastal zone is a shelter for a large portion of any country's infrastructure, including ports, power plants, shipyards, oil refineries, terrestrial roads, and other kinds of factories. Because there are no boundaries in the marine environment, pollutants can be transferred by currents and spread over a wide area, causing what is known as transboundary pollution. All of these activities exert immense pressure on the marine environment. These pressures can be local, affecting a narrow strip of the coastal marine area. Airborne pollution is another type of transboundary contamination; this mechanism has previously been ignored. The majority of pollution problems have their roots in land-based sources. These discharges include organic chemicals, fertilizers, industrial effluents, pesticides, and insecticides that end up in the ocean through rivers, coastal disposal sites, canals, submarine pipelines, or runoffs. In semi-enclosed seas with restricted ocean connectivity, such as the Mediterranean and Baltic Seas, marine pollution has been identified as a hazard to the marine ecosystem.

## 6.2. MARINE ENVIRONMENT

The reason why the legal framework for managing and protecting marine environments has spread to many regional seas/oceans globally is that policymakers and scientists working in the marine environment have only recently come to recognize the significance of ecosystem services (ES). These ecosystem services are all direct or indirect resources that are essential to the health of ecosystems and the wellbeing of humans. Ecosystem functions, such as maintaining ecosystem integrity, maintaining ecosystem health, and conserving biodiversity, are included in the first set of ecosystem services. The second category of ecosystem services includes those that provide humans with an instant financial benefit, like the use of fisheries resources, the production of freshwater through desalination, fish food from aquaculture, and biotechnology-based goods like pharmaceuticals. Ecosystem benefits are another term for this collection of services. Sewage is dumped into the maritime environment. The organic load is broken down into carbon dioxide and water by marine organisms, primarily bacteria (Myklestad, 2000). Nitrogen and phosphorus are released as inorganic nitrogen and phosphorus, which are then absorbed by phytoplankton. Although excessive sewage discharges have been known to have a variety of negative consequences on the marine ecology and seawater quality since the 19th century, this process can also be viewed as an ecosystem function. Because of this fact, engineers and scientists built underwater sewers to distribute urban waste. The carrying capacity of the marine environment is crucial for the dilution, dispersion, and decomposition of the wastes. The ability of marine ecosystems to absorb sewage particles has limits and that these limits have already been reached. Some researchers emphasized strategies for reducing nutrient contamination and excessive algal bloom. Fertilizers have been added to marine eutrophication in addition to sewage disposal-related eutrophication. In many regional oceans across the world today, marine eutrophication is either the primary or secondary source of pollution.

## 6.3. ENVIRONMENTAL CONSERVATION

While environmental conservation was the primary focus of the early stages of marine eutrophication (Figure 6.1) policy, it was gradually acknowledged that social and economic factors should also be considered in addition to scientific factors. UNEP states that environmental issues/problems need to be viewed in relation to interacting pressures rather than being viewed as negative externalities. Thus, it follows that policies that must be implemented ought to be defined by comprehensive choices as opposed to a vision. These policies are characterized by political commitment and the resources they require for success. Environmental issues, such as eutrophication, cannot be addressed separately. The causes of pollution must be taken into account in any form of pollution control program. Human living conditions are one form of pollution since certain behaviors have a detrimental impact on the quality of the environment. These behaviors are linked to social, cultural, and demographic pressures that are present in densely populated places. The implementation of any coordinated policy can be achieved by environmental management that considers the integrity of marine ecosystems, social trends and habits, economic growth, and marine resources. However, the ability of management techniques has its limitations. Large industrial infrastructures along the coastal zone, massive off-shore installations for the production of oil and natural gas, and the size of megacities and their effects on the coastal environment are all contributing factors to the idea of Marine Spatial Planning (MSP), which has experienced an intense and dynamic growth at a global scale in recent years and several practices have emerged from different continents and countries. It is clear that the eutrophication component plays an important role in the planning process because Marine Spatial Planning or MSP is defined as a process of analyzing parts of marine ecosystems to specific uses and objectives, to attain ecological, economic, and social objectives that are usually specified through a political process.

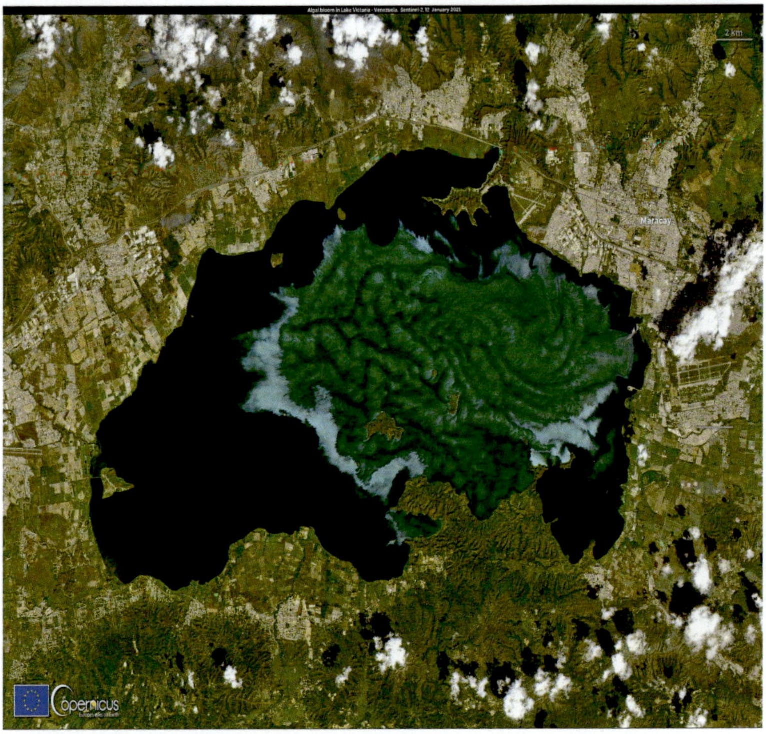


**Figure 6.1.** *Marine eutrophication.*

Source: https://upload.wikimedia.org/wikipedia/commons/3/39/Algal_bloom_in_the_Lake_Valencia_-_Venezuela.jpg, Creative Commons License.

## 6.4. EUTROPHICATION-A HISTORICAL AND CURRENT ACCOUNT

In several regional waters across the world, the condition known as eutrophication poses a major concern. The first records of eutrophication date back to the early 1900s, when it was discovered and documented in the lakes in the lowlands near the Baltic Sea (Gąsiorowski et al., 2021). When working on lake ecology, some limnologists noticed that the lakes in the Baltic varied in trophic states. They concluded that these variations were primarily caused by a larger mass of phytoplankton, which gave the water a distinct planktogenic color. These kinds of occurrences were not observed in mountainous regions. It was thought that while the waters entering the lakes after the bleaching the lowlands (agriculture) were significantly richer in plant nutrients, the waters flowing from the Paleozoic rocks of the Scandinavian mountains were lacking in nitrogen and phosphorus compounds. In the highlands, the state of low phytoplankton growth was designated as oligotrophy, whereas the state of excessive plant growth was designated as eutrophic. In 1977, Carlson put forth a trophic classification system for lakes (Cunha et al., 2021). Three primary classes (oligotrophic, mesotrophic, and eutrophic) were identified by Carlson to describe the trophic condition of lakes. The term hyperoligotrophy was used to describe the extreme oligotrophic state, while hypertrophy was used to describe the extreme eutrophic state. The secchi depth and the amounts of phosphorus and chlorophyll served as the primary classification criteria. The secondary impacts of eutrophic environments were studied by marine ecologists. Eutrophication is the increase of the growth rate of the algae, following a faster rate of nutrient increase in the marine environment as well as the consequences. Eutrophication implies to both fresh and marine waters and is the process of enrichment of waters with plant nutrients, primarily nitrogen and phosphorus that stimulates aquatic primary production and its manifestations, lead to visible algal blooms, algal scum, and enhanced benthic algal growth of macrophytes. The ecosystem under consideration may lack diversity and complexity, which affects the secondary productivity level and may even cause it to disappear. Eutrophication can contribute to and be associated with biological and organic pollutants, and on the other, it can have harmful consequences.

Since the process of eutrophication is intricate in nature, various perspectives may be emphasized in defining it. Some scientists state that nutrient loading causes eutrophication as long as the nutrients are not toxic compounds and there is enough light to promote both heterotrophic and autotrophic growth in the body of water. Some scientists ignore the fact that phosphorus and nitrogen, the two elements that limit primary productivity, can be recycled many times, aiding in the fixation of carbon. Primary productivity monitoring is an expensive method; therefore, data availability will be constrained. Some researchers have considered that eutrophication is a process rather than a state. However, from a management perspective, this leaves some room for interpretation within the legal frameworks. This concept appears to address the relationship between the reactions of marine water masses to industrial and urban effluents, which is one particular element of eutrophication. The nutrient increase leads to many problems when benthos is considered. This definition centers on the benthic community. Because nutrients can travel long distances in the form of dead organic matter or living biomass, the influences of nutrient loading on primary productivity may not always be direct. Eutrophication concerns led to political action through national legislation and international conventions because of the severity of the issue. Therefore, definitions of eutrophication can be found in

UNEP technical reports, EU directives, and international agreements such as the Barcelona Convention (Pavasovic, 1996).

Eutrophication is defined by OSPAR (Oslo and Paris Conventions) as the undesirable effects resulting from anthropogenic enrichment by nutrients that cause an accelerated growth of algae and plant life to produce disturbance to the balance of species present in the water and to the quality of the water. This can be considered a fairly comprehensive definition. National laws in the United States such as the Clean Water Act, and the CZM or Coastal Zone Management Act, both contain definitions of eutrophication. A consensus on definitions became necessary as a result of the establishment of legal frameworks. Although the European Environmental Agency agreed with Nixon's definition, they explicitly state that eutrophication means improved primary production due to an excess supply of nutrients from human activities, independent of the natural productivity level for an area in question. However, because these nutrients must be eliminated during sewage treatment, the European Union Directive concerning Urban Waste Water Treatment focuses on enrichments by nitrogen and phosphorus. A definition of eutrophication that placed more emphasis on the availability of organic matter was later proposed by UNEP in 2003. It stated that Eutrophication is defined as an environmental disturbance caused by an excessive supply of organic matter. One feature that unites all of these descriptions is the reference to eutrophication as a disturbance. This indicates that unlike some types of pollution that lead to irreversible environmental damage, the state of the ecosystem is reversible.

## 6.5. FRAMEWORKS AND TASK GROUPS

Within the European Marine Strategy Framework, the European Commission (EC) established task groups in 2009 with the responsibility of suggesting quality descriptors that would serve as the foundation for assessing ecosystem quality. Some researchers identified the assessment of eutrophication as one of these areas of interest. It was determined that both the assessment of existing techniques and their suitability in a court required an operational definition of eutrophication. It is important to remember that the condition is specifically brought on by a surplus of nutrients, primarily silicon, phosphorus, and nitrogen. These pristine conditions in the marine environment are altered by this nutrient enrichment, which is mostly of terrestrial origin. Considering spatial variability is crucial in vast maritime areas, and as a result, one must understand that the focal sites of eutrophication impacts vary based on topography and other physical factors. In the shallow portions of the Danish Straits and some regions of the Mediterranean Sea, the loss of seagrasses has very negative consequences. One of the main effects in deeper systems is species changes that result in harmful algal blooms (HABs). Separating algal blooms that occur naturally from discharges that cause bloom events is also necessary. Because nutrient enrichment occurs naturally, it is critical to evaluate how much anthropogenic nutrients boost primary production and may influence the N:P shifts. While not always detrimental, can result in an undesirable disturbance that eventually affects the structure and function of ecosystems, including the supply of commodities and services. However, other causes such as climate change, the removal of top predators by fishing, enrichment by allochthonous organic matter, and contamination by harmful substances, may trigger such effects and do not always result from nutrient enrichment.

Definitions based on the causal relationship between nutrient and phytoplankton growth are widely accepted in academia and have also been included in many research and legal documents, including the European Union (EU) Directive on the Protection of Waters from pollution caused by nitrates ($NO_3$) from agricultural sources, technical reports on the Mediterranean Action Plan on Municipal Wastewater Treatment Plants in the Mediterranean Sea, and the UNEP Blue Plan. Due to the fact that the problems associated with marine environmental pollution, which include loss of biodiversity, hazardous and toxic wastes, sewage-related problems, biological resource depletion, and pollution from both industrial and agricultural sources, have no geographical boundaries, international legal regulations have been implemented. Three factors make it difficult for the various states to reach a consensus, at least on the size of regional seas: The marine ecosystem is especially intricate, with a wide range of interrelated elements and activities. Studying these connected aspects and understanding any potential interactions between them is necessary for an international legal framework that will enable successful management; hence, these factors should not be viewed as isolated situations. These issues cannot be properly addressed unless economic, political, social, and cultural factors are taken into consideration. It is also necessary to understand many non-legal factors, such as the existence of prior relevant multistate agreements, the scientific consensus regarding the causes, effects, and significance, potential short-term political benefits, and perceptions that they are contributing their share to the solution.

## 6.6. ENVIRONMENTAL RESTRICTIONS

Environmental restrictions frequently come with a price; thus, the scientific community should encourage the public that the suggested/recommended actions are both important to avert negative environmental effects and have a solid scientific foundation. The relationship between environmental preservation and economic development should be considered in addition with a scientific foundation/basis. While there are often important short-term financial costs associated with the implementation of environmental laws, over time there can be benefits from an economic perspective or the quality of the environment as an asset, as is the case with tourism and biological marine resources. Over the past two decades, another component has surfaced alongside science and economics: the public involvement as a significant influence in environmental decision-making and in resolving environmental issues. Individuals and indigenous communities, the press, television, and internet, legal associations, private organizations, and interest groups like chambers of commerce are some of the ways that the public might become involved. The outcome of some institutions' combined efforts, disagreements, and even overlaps is a collection of laws, policies, guidelines, and conventions that have as their shared goal the preservation and control of the maritime environment. Specifically, the word cluster has been assigned by DiMento and Hickman in 2012 to refer to the collection of initiatives aimed at enhancing the quality of regional seas (Karydis and Kitsiou, 2013). Governance is the culmination of all actions resulting from these legal instruments that aim to give effective management of the seas. The actors involved in environmental issues, as well as their potential and influence, should be briefly introduced to gain an understanding of the intricate system of legal and administrative environmental tools that have been implemented in the marine environment. These actors include non-state actors, coastal states, and international organizations.

Because they participate in the formulation, application, and assessment of the efficacy of legal measures, states are the fundamental units of any international legal framework. They encourage different non-state entities to take part in the creation of rules and decision-making processes and are members of international organizations. The UN currently has close to 200 member states. Competent organizations have separated the states into economies of developing and developed countries based on economic metrics. There are competing interests among the states as a result of this diverse combination of states with varying economic, social, political, geographic, and ecological situations. Therefore, it is evident that reaching a consensus on the administration and conservation of the marine environment is a delicate procedure. International organizations dedicated to protecting the maritime environment include an important aspect of governance. They are formed on several levels, including the international, regional, sub-regional, and occasionally bilateral ones. The international organizations are divided into three groups: international organizations affiliated with the UN, organizations operating outside the UN framework, and organizations operating under other agreements. International organizations deal with matters of the growth, administration, and general management of the maritime environment. In relation to international organizations, there are four primary roles: they give the states a forum for consultation, communication, idea/concept sharing, and consensus building at the regional or even global level, when feasible. They support the advancement of environmental marine research and help to create a global agenda concerning the marine environment. Gathering, exchanging, and disseminating data about practices, policies, and environmental quality in the maritime sector constitutes another important purpose. They can also serve as a warning system for potential hazards/risks to the marine environment, like toxic algal blooms and other maritime disasters. International organizations can reach consensus on standards and policy initiatives, create new institutional structures or norms accepting commitments, and established system to resolve disputes between countries.

## 6.7. TREATIES AND THEIR ROLE

In addition to drafting treaties establishing international standards, international organizations have taken an active role in monitoring the implementation of treaties. International environmental challenges have witnessed the influence of non-state entities. The following five nonstate factor groups appear to be important in regional and marine environmental affairs: private corporations; academic communities; legal organizations; non-profit associations in environmental affairs (NGOs); and individuals. Agenda 21 (1992) informed member states to increase their participation in policy design, decision-making, implementation and evaluation at the individual agency level, in interagency discussions and in United States conferences, further encouraging the involvement of non-state entities. Non-state actors have the ability to take part in international organizations as observers. It should be noted that the OSPAR Convention (1992) for the protection of the North Sea and NA Atlantic included a treaty provision for observers for the first time (Ardron, 2008). This Convention does differentiate between observers' rights to participate in Convention-related activities and those of States, international organizations, and non-governmental organizations. Since every marine environment convention is the result of a compromise driven by social, political, and economic considerations as well as scientific data, it is evident that science serves as the sole impartial component of the process. Because of this, science plays a crucial role in the formulation, selection, and application of policy. A variety of sources, including international processes like GESAMP or Joint Group of Experts on the Scientific Aspects of Marine Environmental Protection and national research centers, government agencies, and non-state entities, can produce scientific information (data). A large number of analysts contend that research has little influence over environmental policy. Environmental controversy has finally ended as a scientific controversy. Because nonscientific factors such as cultural, social, ethical, or economic factors are important and dominate environmental issues, this is the case in many instances. In addition to the non-scientific variables, disagreements within the scientific community and challenges between the political and scientific domains are also common. The weak link in environmental policy challenges has always been the alignment of science and policy.

In addition to proposing the creation of marine environmental treaties, the private sector, companies and associations, conducts regular dialogues with international organizations. Their contribution to marine environmental issues is threefold: they support a precautionary approach to challenges related to the marine environment; they carry out initiatives related to environmental responsibility; and they promote the development of technologies that are environmentally friendly. Citizens now have the right to file complaints with international authorities due to the growing connection between environmental challenges and human rights on a global scale. The ability for nation-state citizens to frequently report government violations of agreements to both international bodies and appropriate national authorities strengthens their position within their respective countries. The Rio Declaration, which acknowledges citizens' rights to appropriate information and involvement in decision-making processes, is a reflection of citizen rights. Every person must have the right to participate in decision-making processes and have proper access to environmental information held by public bodies at the national level. The public's perspective on particular environmental issues can be influenced by the media, leading states to modify their stance. They also take the lead in organizing public opinion and in helping to comprehend the issue and its solutions. Marine eutrophication cannot be effectively studied as an isolated issue; rather, it must be considered in relation to other pressures and causes within the complex legal framework established by international, regional, national, or even bilateral agreements for marine environmental protection and management. This is because there are numerous parties involved in the development and implementation of policies, as well as a wide variety of marine pollution sources.\

## 6.8. ECOSYSTEM POLICY UNCERTAINTIES

Two reasons contribute to the uncertainty surrounding environmental policy, the complexity of the ecosystem and the vast amount of environmental data that needs to be analyzed and evaluated. The former has to do with the fact that academic science operates inside established standards, while regulatory science, a branch of science intended to inform public policy, often operates at the margins of existing knowledge. At the regional or global level, the uncertainty caused in policy decisions is becoming a significant issue for large-scale environmental challenges. It is clear that the complexity of ecosystems has prevented the development of a comprehensive ecosystem theory up until this point, and the marine environment is no exception. The phrase ecological theory refers to a collection of concepts and ideas that are usually understood by ecologists. The ecological theories can be categorized as tools for quantitative techniques. Several methodological errors must be added to the uncertainty resulting from the ecological theory weakness in environmental quality assessment and policy making. Poor experimental design, sampling bias, technical malfunctions, and experimental artifacts are among the main causes in using ecology in policy issues. The main concerns in environmental marine policy are ecological theory, assumptions about how ecosystems function, and how to incorporate ecological findings into the legal framework that governs the administration and protection of the marine environment. Throughout the various stages of the eutrophication phenomena, science plays a crucial role in managing the issue, formulating policy, and recognizing eutrophication as a political issue.

It is important to acknowledge that the eutrophication problem is an issue that aims to politicize the subject. When it comes to how important the issue is, there is typically a lot of disagreement. Another step, which involves putting the problem on its political dimensions, is made possible by the previously established scientific framework. The implementation phase concludes the policy life cycle. The structure of marine eutrophication as an environmental issue evolves due to a variety of factors, including shifts in societal attitudes, scientific advancements, and technical advancements, in addition to the previously noted uncertainties. Policymaking is not a simple process when it comes to scientific input. This implies that many rounds of consultation occur during the implementation phase in response to fresh scientific findings, societal perceptions, and input on financial issues. It is customary for numerous regional conventions to undergo periodic revisions that integrate experience-based changes on various themes. The normative aspect argues that science is essential for management and decision-making despite any uncertainties resulting from the highly complex nature of marine eutrophication. This is because the system is open; physical, chemical, and biological processes are dynamic; and nutrients and chlorophylls are inherent variables in the natural system, making it challenging to distinguish between naturally occurring nutrient loading and human-induced nutrient loading. In general, sewage treatment facilities, encouraging farmers to use appropriate agricultural practices, and reducing nutrient imports from terrestrial sources are the main goals of policies meant to eradicate marine eutrophication. The interface between research and policy is referred to as the structural issue. It has not always been easy to match science with policy, but over the past years, there has been an improvement in communication and mutual understanding between the parties. This could be because policymakers are adopting technocratic views and scientists are becoming more and more politicized. The time aspect relates to the policy life-cycle, or how science continues to have an impact on issues after being included in the policy-making process.

## 6.9. RESEARCH ANALYSES

Once several of the factors contributing to the degradation of the marine environment were discovered in the 1960s, it became clear that action needed to be taken to conserve it. The important sources were thought to be land-based pollution, untreated sewage, eutrophication, invasive species, habitat degradation, and toxic compounds (Bashir et al., 2020). As early as 1972, both regionally and globally, the first regulations on the preservation of the sea from pollution were formulated. State parties are required by the UNCLOS, which came into effect in 1994, to take action to avoid, mitigate, and regulate marine pollution. The UNCLOS addresses the preservation and protection of the marine environment. The duty of member states to prevent pollution is stated clearly in some articles, which list several causes of pollution, including operations on land, under the sea, dumping, and atmospheric pollution. Marine eutrophication is intimately linked to each of these sources. Some articles discuss the preservation of habitats, endangered species, and delicate ecosystems. The cause of marine eutrophication can also be attributed to all these issues.

UNCLOS, however, establishes a broad framework that provides a thorough legal system for the regional seas and oceans (Bigagli, 2016). Governance is a particularly complex issue that can be effectively addressed at a regional level due to the physical characteristics of every marine environment, including regional seas, the degree of development of the surrounding countries, and the environmental problems that have accumulated over time. The primary UN agency dealing with environmental issues is UNEP. The creation of comprehensive action plans for the management and conservation of regional seas areas was one of the primary goals of the UNEP Governing Council Regional Seas Programme. Coordination of the efforts with regard to the environmental resources; support for education and training efforts to make possible the full participation of marine and coastal resources; promotion of international and regional conventions, assessment of the state of marine pollution of the sources and trends of this pollution and of the impact of pollution on human health, ecosystem and amenities are monitored. The length of the coastline, the biological, mineral, and coastal resources, as well as the degree of development of the contracting states, are some of the differences across

Regional Seas Programs. The initial UNEP agreement on regional oceans is the Barcelona Convention. It was ratified in 1976 and became operative in 1978. Reducing pollution in the Mediterranean Sea, and protecting and improving the marine environment, thereby contributing to its sustainable development is the stated goal of the Convention. The considerable degree of social, economic, and political diversity among the signed member states is the primary feature of the Mediterranean Sea. The extent of their territorial waters, the limits of their fishing zones, national legislation for ecological protection zones and the adoption of rights for historical and archeological objects within a 24-mile radius of the territorial waters are all troubled with legal complications. The foundation for protocols and annexes about the preservation of the Mediterranean System has been established by the Mediterranean Action Plan (MAP); this collection of accords, regulations, guidelines, and restrictions is referred to as the Barcelona System.

The 1992 Rio Conference resulted in significant modifications to the Barcelona Convention (Momtaz, 1996). While new standards addressing new topics were established, some of the current protocols were changed in response to new concepts on the maritime environment. The Framework Convention contains seven protocols. These procedures all have something to do with marine eutrophication, either directly or indirectly. The Dumping Protocol forbids any dumping from the perspective of eutrophication, with the exception of wastes generated by regular vessel operations. There are some exclusions that deal with dredging materials in inert (non-reactive), uncontaminated geological resources and fish waste. These exception-covered (exempt) categories are also responsible for the eutrophication process. The effluents originating from terrestrial activities are dealt with Land-based Protocol. They may come from distributed sources or from point pollution. The discharges originate from river flow, sewage-industrial outfalls, and land runoff.

The Black Sea has significant pollution issues, such as eutrophication. The Bucharest Convention, so named because it was signed in Bucharest in 1992 by six states, Bulgaria, the Russian Federation, Georgia, Romania, Turkey and Ukraine, was intended to safeguard the Black Sea. In order to safeguard and preserve the marine environment, the primary goal of the Convention is to substantiate the obligation of the contracting parties to reduce, and control the pollution in the Black Sea and to provide a legal framework for cooperation and coordinated actions to fulfill this obligation. The Convention is accompanied by three protocols: (i) one that addresses land-based sources of pollution; (ii) one that addresses waste disposal; and (iii) one that addresses cooperative response to accidents. Eutrophication and protocols (i) and (ii) are directly connected. The Skagerrak and Kattegat Straits (Figure 6.2) restrict exchange between the Baltic Sea and the North Sea, making the marine zone/site vulnerable to pollution and, in particular, eutrophication, which is considered the greatest threat to the Baltic.

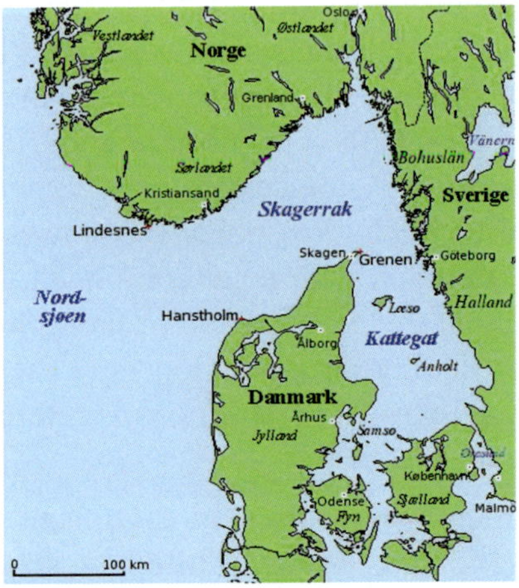


**Figure 6.2.** *Skagerrak and Kattegat straits.*

Source: https://upload.wikimedia.org/wikipedia/commons/b/bb/Map_Skagerak-Kattegat.PNG, Creative Commons License.

The Helsinki Convention (Protection of the Marine Environment – Baltic Sea) was the first regional maritime convention to address marine pollution from all sources. The first two decades of operation demonstrated that efforts to mitigate the environmental damage in the Baltic Sea were unsuccessful. As a result, a new accord focused on the protection of the Baltic Sea ecosystem's integrity replaced the Helsinki Convention in 1992. The Convention covered topics related to healthy ecosystems, habitat conservation, biological variety, ecological processes, and the sustainability of natural resources in addition to pollution assessment. The Helsinki Convention (Declaration) established priority for marine eutrophication, biodiversity preservation, and the creation of ecological quality objectives in 2003. The assessments also covered reporting, information sharing, public information dissemination, and environmental impact assessments. While there are concerns about toxic substances, biodiversity, marine safety, and the preservation of nature, eutrophication has been identified as a top priority. It is important to emphasize that the Baltic Sea has legal subsystems from the perspective of governance. Since 2004, every coastline country, aside from the Russian Federation, has been a part of the European Union. This indicates that all EU Member States bordering the Baltic Sea have implemented relevant EU Directives that address marine eutrophication either directly or indirectly (Karydis and Kitsiou, 2012).

The states bordering the Caspian Sea, Azerbaijan, Iran, Kazakhstan, the Russian Federation, and Turkmenistan, signed the 'Tehran Convention' to Protect the Marine Environment in the Caspian Sea in 2003. It became operative in 2006. Although there are many pollution problems in the region, including pollution from dangerous (toxic) substances, oil pollution, and nutrient discharges from untreated sewage inflows, eutrophication is the main environmental problem. The Tehran Convention's primary goals were to: (i) reduce, prevent, and control pollution; (ii) protect and clean up the marine environment; (iii) limit overexploitation of natural marine resources by the contracting parties; and (iv) protect endemic, endangered species and their habitats. The primary aim of the OSPAR Convention is to regulate and alleviate marine pollution through a comprehensive and integrated approach. The ecosystem-oriented approach, which states that regions impacted by marine pollution should be restored to conserve marine ecosystems and, when possible, restore marine areas that have been adversely affected, was the most ingenious feature of the OSPAR Convention. Over the past 25 years, a significant amount of scientific data has been produced as a result of the Convention's encouragement of scientific study. Southeast Asia, North-East Asia, and Australia are the three subregions that make up the East Asian marine ecosystem. These subregions are distinguished by distinct weather patterns, distinctive biological traits, and distinct economic (financial) foundations.

## 6.10. STANDARDS FOR THE MARINE WORLD

There was very little progress made in raising the standard of the marine environment because of the complexity brought about by the many organizations engaged, a lack of coordination and cooperation, a lack of finance, and a lack of a legal framework. Although the land-based approach involves nitrogen loading of the marine environment from rivers and nonpoint sources, eutrophication does not appear to receive any special attention. The West and Central African area (WACAF) is composed of twenty-two African States, most of which are coast (Babaousmail et al., 2023). The majority of WACAF countries rely mostly on industry, tourism, and fishing for their resources. The rapid and uncontrolled economic growth has an adverse effect on the coastal zone due to over utilization of the coastal environment. The environmental effects are also impacted by the ship-based inland shipping of commodities from the seashore. This has led to the degradation and overexploitation of natural resources, as industry and commerce have generally focused on maximizing profits at the expense of sound environmental management. The overuse of natural resources and its effects on the marine environment have drawn attention. Under the UNEP Regional Seas Programme, the WACAF group approved an action plan. The Abidjan Convention, a regional agreement that was signed in 1981 and came into effect in 1984, served as the model for this action plan. Angola, Benin, Cameroon, Cape Verde, Gabon, Gambia, Ghana, Guinea, and some other countries are among the signatory countries. Strict sewage and solid waste regulations, habitat preservation, and coastal erosion control were among WACAF's primary goals. There is a direct connection between marine eutrophication and all of these goals. Due to institutional overlap in authority, disagreements arise about several parts of marine policy, management, and implementation plans, making the governance consolidation in the West and Central African marine area highly complicated. Due to the fact that most states prioritize economic growth over environmental protection, there are many disadvantages to environmental conservation.

Connected to the Central Atlantic lies the semi-enclosed Wider Caribbean Region (WCR). The Caribbean Sea and other bays and small marine areas are all included in the Wider Caribbean Sea (Carrillo et al., 2017). The region is home to a wide variety of habitats, including sea turtles, unusual fish species, coral reefs with distinctive coral species, and other marine life. Some states and territories are included in WCR. All these states, meanwhile, differ in terms of their degree of development and progress. The Caribbean Sea itself is only 4.2 million square KM in size, compared to the approximate 15 million square kilometers that make up the Wider Caribbean Sea. The Amazon, Orinoco and Magdalena are the three major rivers that flow directly into the Wider Caribbean Sea. Pollutants and waste are dispersed over a larger region by the combination of river water masses and currents bringing water from the Atlantic. There is a belief that these rivers release a considerable amount of nutrients into the Caribbean Sea between May and November, which leads to eutrophication. Over the past 25 years, phytoplankton blooms have been seen to cause mass fish mortality and oxygen deprivation. Numerous other Caribbean sites, including Kingston Harbor in Jamaica, San Huan Bay in Puerto Rico, and Havan Bay in Cuba, are experiencing eutrophication. It is clear that protecting the marine environment from eutrophication is a top priority. By 2020, there will be 90 million people living in the region; the largest population densities are found along the shore, where they will rise even further during the summer season. The Caribbean's primary industry is tourism, which brings in over 100 million visitors annually due to the region's distinctive coral reefs, indigenous fish species, crystal-clear ocean waters, and swimming beaches. The intensive mining, fishing, and tourism operations significantly contribute to the destruction of the maritime ecosystem. The main risk to the marine ecosystem is tourism. Nutrients are the second largest contaminant in the region. An estimated 13,000 tons of nitrogen and 5,000 tons of phosphorus are released into the marine environment each year.

The main legal instrument for protecting the region's coastlines and oceans is the Caribbean Environmental Programme (CEP). It serves as the central agency for developing protocols in the larger domain. The Caribbean Action Plan and the Cartagena Convention for the Development of the marine environment in the Wider Caribbean region are both based on the Caribbean environmental programme. The Cartagena Convention seeks to control airborne, land-based, ship-borne, and dumping pollution. The specially protected areas and wildlife convention protocol and the protocol of land-based sources and activities (LBS) Protocol are two of the protocols that have been added to the convention. These two protocols deal with the eutrophication of marine environments. The protocol concerning contamination from land-based sources is the primary focus of policy actions to nutrient contamination. The Red Sea, the Gulf of Aqaba, the Gulf of Suez, and Aden are all included in the geographical scope of this convention. The Jeddah Convention, like the Kuwait Convention, is centered on accidental and operational oil pollution. This Convention makes no mention of nutrient enrichment of marine eutrophication. It is clear that they have taken into account issues with eutrophication and pollution from nutrients. Dredging and seabed exploration can both lead to similar issues. Signed in 1981, the Lima Convention is a convention for the protection of the marine ecosystem and coastal area in the South-East Pacific. Making a distinction between non-point sources of pollution and point sources of pollution, such as effluents from pipelines or outfalls, was an ingenious approach. It is clear that a substantial portion of agricultural runoff and urban effluents contained loads of nutrients. The EPA established the fundamental requirements for water quality, but the States were in charge of creating standards that fell within the legal parameters and seeing to it that they were followed. As a result, the States established water quality standards and limits for effluent. The Clean Water Act was revised in the 1990s despite some opposition. Public participation in the development and enforcement of any regulation, standard, effluent limitation plan or program is therefore encouraged by legislation. The administrator will create basic rules for the general public involvement in these procedures. The administrator's tasks also include proposing new and improved agricultural methods that would remove pollutants from agriculture, especially nutrient pollution, in cooperation with the appropriate authorities in agricultural activities.

## 6.11. RELEVANCE TO AIR POLLUTION

The primary goal of the Clean Air Act, is to regulate air pollution in the United States on a national scale. It has been clear that atmospheric nitrogen compound deposition significantly affects marine ecology, particularly in regions classified as oligotrophic. Law reforms and amendments have created a potent weapon to lessen atmospheric nitrogen over-enrichment in coastal and estuarine waters. EPA calculated that the amount of nitrogen of atmospheric origin would have decreased by at least 17% if the EPA-recommended guidelines had been put into effect. If atmospheric controls were not adopted, the estimated avoided costs, or the costs associated with implementing point source controls or storm water for the estuaries on the east coast, would vary from $150 to $250 million. Within the bounds of the federal law objectives, the States are encouraged to create and execute coastal zone management policies by the Coastal Zone Management Act. Therefore, state policies should establish standards, identify areas of concern, define coastal limits, and implement enforceable rules that address the primary goals. Public participation and cooperation, state and local governments, as well as federal agencies having programs affecting the coastal zone are encouraged by law. Eutrophication and nutrient enrichment are not specifically mentioned in the statute. However, it is acknowledged that nutrient-rich sites are a drawback of both economic development and population increase. However, it is evident that any program for managing coastal zones must consider the health of the ecosystem and the quality of the marine environment, as measured by the marine water and the ecosystem itself. This approach should also consider the consequences and demands of eutrophication. The issue of eutrophication appears to be high on the agendas of most international organizations in the majority of the seas that encircle the European Continent, including the Baltic Sea, North Sea, etc. A multitude of EU Directives have been created during the past thirty years to safeguard the elements of the maritime environment, in addition to the international conventions for the protection of the European Seas that were previously stated.

## 6.12. TREATMENT AND EVALUATION

The treatment and discharge of wastewater (urban) aimed at the protection of the environment from adverse effects was the stated goal of the Urban Waste Water Treatment Directive (UWWT) (Morris et al., 2017). Reducing the amount of nutrients in eutrophic waters mostly requires removing phosphorus and, if feasible, nitrogen. While addressing eutrophication alone is not the sole goal of the UWWT, the Directive makes a substantial contribution to safeguarding coastal waters against accelerated growth of algae, undesirable to the balance of organisms and to the quality of the water. The Nitrates Directive was created with the goal of protecting water pollution caused by nitrates from agricultural sources. Reducing water pollution induced by nitrates from agricultural sources and preventing further pollution are the primary goals of the Directive. While Article 6(c) specifically mentions coastal eutrophication and the requirement for a four-year review of the situation, Article 2(i) defines eutrophication to include undesirable disturbance. Two management measures are established by the Directive to prevent nitrate pollution: the establishment of good agricultural practices and the designation of sensitive and vulnerable regions. Monitoring techniques are also advised to assess the effectiveness of the measures. Since the Directive does not outline any standards for determining eutrophication levels, Member States must establish eutrophication scales. Although eutrophication is not specifically mentioned in the directive, eutrophic conditions are closely associated with suspended matter and dissolved oxygen. Eutrophic conditions support the survival of heterotrophic bacteria and the formation of harmful phytoplankton species. For this reason, fecal coliforms and saxitoxin have been included as parameters. The Bathing Water Directive specifies guidelines for controlling the quality of bathing water and providing the public with information on bathing water quality. The Directive is concerned with the overall state of the water quality, including inspections for materials like tarty residues, plastic, and rubber as well as the excessive growth of macroalgae and/or marine phytoplankton, which is closely related to marine eutrophication. Bathing water quality assessment primarily focuses on microbiological data. Even though the Bathing Water Directive does not specifically call for a eutrophication assessment, certain parameters, like water transparency, dissolved oxygen, nitrates, and phosphates, must be measured each time it is discovered that the water quality has declined. Coastal and transitional waters are among the numerous water bodies that the Water Framework Directive seeks to safeguard. Ensuring the protection and improvement of the aquatic environment is the primary goal. Among other prerequisites, all waters must undergo a thorough ecological quality assessment. This evaluation rates the water masses according to several biological, hydromorphological, and physico-chemical quality components, dividing the ecological status into five categories: high, good, moderate, poor, and bad based on how far the water masses deviate from predetermined reference conditions.

Since the result is the consequence of comparing observed values and reference circumstances, establishing reference conditions is one of the most important steps in determining the status of an ecosystem. The term good ecological status describes the state of biological communities, such as phytoplankton, macrophytes, and macrobenthos, in which there is only a minor deviation of the ecosystem under undisturbed conditions from the conditions normally associated with the surface water body. Differentiating between eutrophication levels is another function of the community structure. Determining the threshold values between favorable and moderate conditions is crucial because it serves as an early warning system for the collected data. As per the Water Framework Directive, member states must provide their water bodies at least a 'Good Status.' To aid in management and policy development, member states are also urged to create marine quality indicators. A reduction in the ecological status cannot be justified only by nutrient concentrations with no discernible effects. Therefore, rather than just concentrating on nutrient concentrations, research and monitoring must address the biological impact resulting from elevated nutrient levels. Encouraging sustainable use of the seas and conserving marine ecosystems is the main goal of the Marine Strategy Framework Directive (MSFD) (Ounanian et al., 2012). In order to accomplish this goal, the maritime environment will be preserved and protected by stopping its degradation and, where feasible, restore marine ecosystems where they have been adversely affected. Similar to the EU 2000 Water Policy Directive, the MSFD is focused on an ecosystem-based approach, assuring that human activity demands are kept within limits that provide a healthy environmental state. The state of the environment in marine ecosystems, taking into account the structure, function, and processes of the constituent marine ecosystems is how the MSFD defines environmental status. The Baltic Sea, the North-East Atlantic Ocean, the Mediterranean Sea, and the Black Sea are the four main marine systems that make up the European Waters according to the directive.

It will be the responsibility of the member states to select criteria that will define a satisfactory environmental condition. Annex I of the MSFD states that species biodiversity, toxic algal blooms, and potentially low oxygen levels (hypoxia) in bottom waters are the best qualitative indicators to use when evaluating human-induced eutrophication. A description of the seasonal variations of phytoplankton and the biological population is required. Researchers conducted an evaluation of eutrophication indicators for evaluating marine eutrophication under the directive of the European Marine Strategy Framework. Monitoring and activity evaluation are key components of MSFD because monitoring helps integrate conservation measures. Many assessments have been conducted to determine how effective maritime environmental protection policies are. It begins with only environmental concerns and ends up involving legal and policy considerations. There are several requirements for an evaluation, which serve as its foundation.

Chapter 7

# COASTAL MARINE ECOSYSTEMS – EUTROPHICATION

## Contents

# 7.1. INTRODUCTION

In the pelagic zone, there is a constant interchange of materials between the solute and particle material pools (Kiørboe, 1996). For instance, photosynthesis incorporates inorganic solute nutrients and carbon dioxide into particulate organic matter, which is then remineralized through metabolic processes. The transport mechanisms of particulate matter and solutes are different. While solutes and particles can both be carried by the surrounding water and move in a Brownian movement, particles are also susceptible to gravity and can move actively in the organisms. This affects the distribution of material exchange among the different pools in the pelagic zone in many ways. One effect is that there are differences in the vertical distribution of solute and particulate matter, as well as the various processes connected to each. For instance, because photosynthesis is light-dependent, it can only happen in the euphotic zone; below this zone, sedimenting phytoplankters and organic particles are mostly remineralized. Anoxia may occur below the pycnocline due to the stratification of the water column and the displacement of these oxygen-generating and consuming activities. In nutrient-rich, turbulent, confined environments, microphytoplankton blooms and predominates over phytoplankton biomass, but in oligotrophic, stagnant waters, very small or motile forms predominate. Stratification keeps phytoplankton in the euphotic zone while turbulent mixing pushes inorganic nutrients toward the surface. The vertical water column structure transitions are therefore temporary or limited improvements in phytoplankton growth conditions, and this is the area where the microphytoplankton grows and takes over the plankton flora. Large cell size appears to be a competitive disadvantage in some situations, although other factors compensate for it. Advective transport of nutrients to the surface (cell) is one of these factors. When nutrient uptake across the cell surface surpasses diffusion-mediated transport, a nutrient-depleted area surrounds the cell in the diffusion-limited scenario. The absorption rate will increase if local fluid velocity gradients or the cell floating or sinking through the water facilitate the supply of molecules to this area by advection. The Sherwood number, which is the factor by which diffusion transport is enhanced as a result of fluid motion, indicates the amount of the increase. The Sherwood number is a function of the cell size, the shear rate, and the swim/sink rate and is dependent on whether the cell sinks or swims or is suspended in a turbulent shear field.

# 7.2. ABSORPTION AND OTHER BIOLOGICAL FACTORS

While large cells absorb more nutrients than small cells do, small cells benefit relatively little from fluid motion (turbulence) or from swimming or sinking through the water. Therefore, for swimming cells (flagellates), the competitive pressure for small size is reduced in turbulent environments and this is consistent with the observed distributions of the various forms. Nevertheless, the effect of advective transport in large cells is not sufficient to fully counterbalance the reduced molecular diffusion-based size-specific food uptake with increasing cell size. Predation is another factor that can assist counteract the competitive disadvantage of being large and, thus, explain the existence of giant phytoplankters in nutrient-rich habitats. Unlike their zooplankton predators, phytoplankton cell growth is inversely correlated with cell size. Small predators, such as heterotrophic nanoflagellates, feed on small phytoplankton cells, and both the phytoplankton prey and their predators have comparable rates of population growth. As a result, the numbers of their phytoplankton prey can be managed by the predators of microscopic phytoplankton cells. Larger metazoans, such as copepods, consume large phytoplankton cells, and their reproduction times vary based on the prey. Both small and large phytoplankton cell populations will begin to grow when nutrients are intermittently fed into the euphotic zone. Large phytoplankton cells may continue to grow until the inorganic nutrients are completely depleted, but populations of small phytoplankton cells will rapidly be overtaken by their predators. The availability of nutrients usually serves as the restriction on biomass accumulation in the water column. Simultaneously, it seems that the phytoplankton maximal growth rates are solely restricted by the availability of light, rather than the availability of nutrients. Therefore, phytoplankton growth rate is controlled by light, but its biomass is restricted by nutrients. When the concentration of inorganic nutrients is high (water column stratification) phytoplankton biomass accumulates and eventually drops when the nutrients are depleted. However, phytoplankton growth rate is more dependent on seasonal variations in irradiance and, consequently, light availability, and reaches its maximum during summer stratification when nutrient concentration is below the limit.

It is possible for cells to absorb dissolved organic material and convert it into particulate organic matter. The same physical limitations that govern the absorption of dissolved inorganics also apply to the uptake of dissolved organic matter. The concentration of dissolved organic matter or DOM in coastal regions is relatively high. However, the DOM concentration, typically 80%–90%, is typically characterized by long turnover times (Dalzell et al., 2009). It should be noted that the dissolved fraction is defined operationally as material passing through a 0.2-micron filter. Part of the solute DOM may be actually particulate, occurring as colloidal or submicron particles. Even in coastal areas, the concentration of tiny organic molecules that can be absorbed by cells is low and roughly equal to the carbon biomass of pelagic bacteria. This means that only very small cells can effectively utilize the source of dissolved organics. Since heterotrophic bacteria predominate in picoplankton, they are the primary consumers of DOM. In coastal environments, bacterial production is an important source of particulate matter, both quantitatively and qualitatively. Particle production resulting from bacterial uptake and utilization of DOM is approximately 30% of the total amount of particulate matter produced initially. Bacterial production can occasionally equal or even surpass primary production.

## 7.3. PHYSICO-CHEMICAL PROCESSES

Physico-chemical processes are another potentially significant mechanism of particle production from solute molecules. Small (5-120 nm) colloidal particles have recently been reported to appear in the waters of California. Although the exact mechanism of production is unknown, the organic character and vertical stratification of these particles point to a biotic origin. The concentrations of organic submicrometer particles (0.4-1.0 μm) in surface waters of the North Pacific and Nova Scotia were determined to be on the order of 107-108 ml$^{-1}$, respectively. Bacteria and picophytoplankton would fall into this size range, however, they made up less than 5% of the particles and were therefore mostly nonliving. The interaction of bacteria with nanoflagellates is one possible process for the production of submicrometer particles. Ultimately, surface waters off the coast of California were found to contain transparent exopolymeric particles (TEP). There have been reports of even larger mucus particles or aggregates made up of mucus and solid particles, measuring several centimeters in diameter. The polymeric substance released by diatoms, bacteria, and macrophyte leachates can generate both large mucus particles and TEP particles. The exopolymeric solutes are converted into colloidal particles by cation bridging of 3-10 nm microfibrils. These microfibrils further coagulate to form colloidal particles. Particulate matter can therefore directly develop from DOM by physicochemical processes. The various forms of organic particles that have been recently found may have significant effects on the way that substances are transported by plankton. They can be used as food for particle feeders, sorption sites for solutes, attachment sites for bacteria, or coagulate with other particles, such as phytoplankton, to form marine aggregates, which will improve the vertical transport of substances.

It is possible for material that is confined to suspended particles to change into a solute state in the form of dissolved organic matter or inorganic ions. As a result of metabolic processes that oxidize organic compounds to their low-energy inorganic components, inorganic nutrients are always produced. These are what the heterotrophic organisms will release into the environment. The organisms smaller than 100 μm account for more than 90% of all pelagic remineralization (Denis et al., 2003). If the particle size distribution aligns with the equilibrium

Sheldon-distribution, then most of the organic matter created in the euphotic zone will be remineralized within the zone because of the importance of small organisms and the fact that small particles sink slowly. The sedimentation of particulate material may shift a major fraction of the remineralization process below the pycnocline if the size distribution is perturbed toward large particle sizes due to nutrient enrichment and/or aggregation of particles. Even in coastal waters, river runoff contributes a minimal amount of organic matter. Dissolved organic compounds are expelled either directly or indirectly from organisms and ultimately originate predominantly from the phytoplankton. There is a significant demand in the water column for dissolved organic materials. In aquatic environments, bacterial output (yield) accounts for 30% of primary production on average. Based on a 40% growth efficiency assumption, bacteria would need the equivalent of 75% of primary production as DOM on average. The carbon concentrations of these particles are comparable to those of phytoplankton, and both theoretical and experimental studies indicate that nanoflagellates consume these particles at high rates. This implies that there is a rather large demand for DOM due to the turnover of colloidal organic particles. These factors imply that recycling of organic matter is quantitatively important since photosynthetic carbon fixation is ultimately the source of most DOM in the water column.

## 7.4. ALTERED FOOD CHAINS

Particles in suspension may float with the water and sink due to gravity. Particulate organic material (POM) breakdown that requires oxygen may be redirected from the euphotic zone to below the pycnocline via sedimentation of organic particulate matter. Anoxia will eventually occur if POM sedimentation, as expressed in reduction equivalents, surpasses oxygen entrainment and downward mixing. The amount of POM that sediments is determined by the biomass of suspended POM, which in turn is determined by the presence of inorganic nutrients. Nevertheless, the organic particles may be consumed or otherwise broken down in the upper mixed layer if suspended POM remains in the euphotic zone for an extended period of time. As a result, the sinking velocity of suspended particulate matter and the processes influencing sinking velocity are also factors that influence the vertical flux of particulate material. Substantial concentrations of autotrophic nanoflagellates during summer stratification are a characteristic of the pycnocline. These subsurface populations contribute significantly to the primary production in the water column, and it appears that they rely heavily on newly entrained nutrients. Small particles may be packaged into larger pellets to aid in the sedimentation process. If the concentration of other sticky hydrosols, such as TEP particles, is high enough for coagulation to happen at meaningful rates, sedimentation of tiny cells may also happen. Pelagic food webs appear to be of the microbial type in permanently stratified ocean gyres and during summer stratification in temperate regions (Landry, 2002). Grazing food chains predominate and significant phytoplankton sedimentation occurs in the partially stratified zones of the major upwelling regions and during the commencement of stratification in temperate waters. On much smaller spatio-temporal scales, however, it appears that the fluctuation in the organization of the pelagic food web in respect to hydrodynamic parameters is recurrent. Where and when episodic or localized injections of inorganic nutrients to the euphotic zone occur, grazing food chains and heavy sedimentation may quickly replace microbial food webs in stratified water columns. Similarly, after the short-lived microalgal bloom has used up all of the inorganic nutrients, a microbial population takes control. The central, strongly stratified part of the Skagerrak has low phytoplankton biomass and is dominated by small flagellates; on the other hand, copepod productivity is low and microbial activity is high in the partially mixed regions where microphytoplankton occurs in high concentration. Copepod productivity is an indicator of the classical grazing food chain. More than 20,000 years ago, the vast ice sheets that created the seafloor of the intricate estuary system that stretches from the Baltic Sea into the North Sea formed as a submerged glacial landscape. In several places, meltwater deposits are still visible.

## 7.5. LOWER SEDIMENT DYNAMICS

In lower sediment, even in the sulfate-depleted zone several meters below the surface, the rate of organic matter decomposition decreases and methane is formed as a result of microbial metabolism. Consequently, the sediment in coastal basins experiences an increase in methane pressure beyond the ambient hydrostatic pressure (Martens and Val Klump, 1980). Methane creates gas bubbles that become trapped in the sediment and are visible in seismic profiles at depths of 2 to 5 meters. Methane from deeper sources also escapes as bubbles into the water column, where it either forms distinctive marks at the sediment surface or, when methane oxidizes to $CO_2$ within the sediment, forms carbonate chimneys. These sedimentary environments support a unique fauna of bivalves that have symbiotic bacteria that oxidize methane or sulfur dioxide in their tissues. When the spring phytoplankton bloom sedimented, organic-rich ephemeral mud blankets were seen to form over the sandy sediment surface at Laholm Bay. These mud coverings were carried into the deeper waters of the Kattegat during multiple cycles of resuspension. Similar findings showed that lateral advection or sediment focusing redirected the deposited organic matter toward the deeper portions of the Kiel Bight in the western Baltic Sea.

The organic material in the sedimentation basins may increase local oxygen demand and nutrient release, even though it may become relatively refractory after numerous resuspension cycles. These basins frequently include sediments that are rich in organic matter, and the poorly ventilated bottom water can lead to hypoxia. In shallow coastal systems, where there is a significant flux of resuspended sediment, it is challenging to calculate the net flux of primary sedimenting material.

On the seafloor, aerobic microorganisms and animal species are mainly responsible for mineralizing the organic material that is sedimenting. However, the oxic zone, that is, the zone that contains oxygen, of coastal sediments is typically limited to a thin layer that is only a few millimeters thick at the sediment surface and around the macrofauna burrows. This oxic layer only makes up the top portion of the brown (oxidized) sediment layer, often just 10–20% of it. The net deposition and degradability of organic matter regulate the oxygen uptake overall, although the mechanism and dynamics of this process are intricate. The diffusive boundary layer, an unstirred water film that covers the sediment and is between 1-2 mm thick, is the main way/method that oxygen diffuses into nonpermeable sediments. High-resolution studies using oxygen microelectrodes placed directly on the sea floor show this boundary layer. The respiration rate in the oxic surface layer can be computed using diffusion flux calculations using boundary layer oxygen gradients or diffusion-reaction modeling of the entire oxygen profile in the sediment. Summertime respiration rates frequently peak at the lower edge of the oxic zone, when nitrifying bacteria, for example, oxidize reduced substances like ammonium that have diffused up from below. Diffusive uptake was found to account for 45-65% and 70%, respectively, of the total oxygen consumption recorded in sediment cores in the sediments of southern Kattegat and Aarhus Bay (Christiansen et al., 1997). The primary cause of the uptake is the biopumping and respiration of burrowing species; as a result, the density of benthic animals is closely correlated with the relative difference between diffusive and total uptake. Moreover, the interplay between the surface topography of the sediment and the overflowing sea water creates lateral pressure gradients that, in porous sediments, may promote an advective transport of pore water through the sediment, enhancing the exchange of nutrients and oxygen.

## 7.6. MICROORGANISMS

Microorganisms primarily carry out the degradation and oxidation of the organic matter below the thin oxic zone. While some of these organisms use oxidants other than $O_2$ to respire the compounds to $CO_2$, others hydrolyze and ferment the macromolecules to tiny organic compounds. There are significant distinctions between the anaerobic and aerobic food chains, where the organisms essentially have a highly consistent energy metabolism, the aerobic respiration, although the overall outcome of carbon oxidation may be similar. The anaerobic, microbial food chain is made up of a depth sequence of metabolic types that can only use a portion of the energy present in the organic matter. These metabolic types also excrete energy-rich inorganic or organic products, which can again undergo oxidation when they come into contact with the chemical zones above them. Certain chemical reactions may also occur, such as the oxidation of $Mn^{2+}$, $Fe^{2+}$, or H2S by $O^{2+}$. The main energy metabolisms in coastal sediments are arranged in a more or less distinct vertical zonation: aerobic respiration occurs in the uppermost few millimeters; nitrate respiration (denitrification) occurs in the next few millimeters to centimeters; manganese (Mn(IV)) and iron (Fe(III)) reduction occurs in the majority of the brown oxidized sediment, which may be a few to ten centimeters deep; sulfate reduction primarily extends as the dominant process down to one or several meters depth; and methanogenesis occurs as the final metabolism for organic matter after the oxidants are depleted. The reduced product, $N_2$, from denitrification is unique in this context because it has a stable triple bond, making it unusable as an energy substrate even in the presence of oxygen. However, the nitrifying bacteria employ ammonium, which is generated during the anaerobic breakdown of nitrogen-containing organic molecules, as an energy substrate. While some anaerobic bacterial species can convert nitrate directly to ammonium, denitrification in marine sediments is an important process (Engström et al., 2005).

## 7.7. NITROGEN CYCLE

The nitrogen cycle (Figure 7.1) and nutrient balance in estuaries depend heavily on denitrification, which can occur at high rates in some situations. However, in some coastal sediments, the process was only found to be a factor for a small percentage of the organic matter oxidation. However, certain bacteria can employ the oxidized iron and manganese minerals in the brown sediment layer as respiratory electron acceptors for the oxidation of organic carbon. Alternatively, they can operate as oxidants of sulfide that bacteria respiring sulfate produce in the sediment, which means they only indirectly aid in the oxidation of organic materials. Determining the rates of metal reductions or differentiating their functions in organic carbon oxidation is a challenge. Therefore, modeling of geochemical gradients in deeper layers provides related information. However, it has been possible to show that some processes are mutually split (zonation) in coastal sediments using a mix of chemical and radiotracer techniques. The depth distribution of the oxidation processes exhibits a definite depth sequence of diminishing redox potential and energy yield, despite overlap. Competition for common organic substrates among anaerobically respiring bacteria is likely what determines the sequence. Because Fe(III) minerals bind phosphate and control its release from the soil, the iron cycle is particularly important. Iron binds to the sulfide that was generated. Mn(IV) mineral phases have a faster turnover than iron, even though manganese is often found in considerably lower amounts. $Mn^{2+}$ may escape through the narrow, oxic sediment zone and up into the water column because reduced manganese has substantially slower $O_2$ oxidation kinetics than reduced iron (Kristiansen et al., 2002). There, it is oxidized to $MnO_2$ and deposited again, but this time at a new site because of bottom currents (lateral motion). Manganese may eventually migrate away from the reduced, organic-rich coastal sediments and become trapped in more oxidized layers on the continental slope after hundreds of these emission-deposition cycles. Migrating manganese oxides concentrate in the lowest sediments of the 700 m deep trough, where manganese alone makes up to 5% of the dry weight in the upper 5 cm.

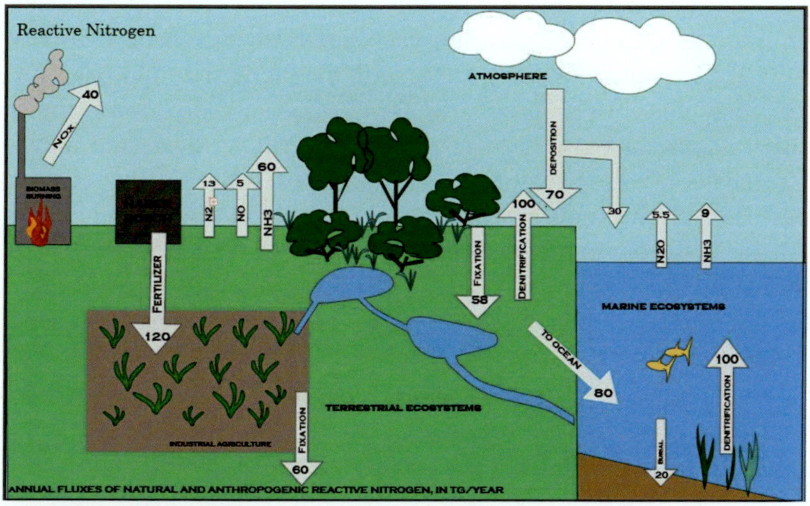


**Figure 7.1.** *Nitrogen cycle.*

Source: https://upload.wikimedia.org/wikipedia/commons/c/c7/Reactive_Nitrogen_Global_Annual_Fluxes.jpg, Creative Commons License.

## 7.8. MINERALIZATION

The majority of anaerobic mineralization in organic-rich coastal sediments occurs by sulfate reduction, which may be just as important and effective for the oxidation of organic carbon in this context as aerobic respiration. The rate of sulfate respiration decreases gradually with depth until sulfate is depleted several meters below the sediment surface, at which point methanogenic bacteria take control. The sulfate reducers produce $H_2S$ that controls the chemistry of the sediments where pyrite ($FeS_2$) and other black iron sulfides (FeS) build up. The burial of $FeS_2$ in these coastal sediments is equivalent to 10–25% of the burial of organic carbon when calculated as potential oxygen demand. In the sediment, $H_2S$ is constantly reoxidized based on the availability of oxidants. Because $H_2S$ interferes with the aerobic respiratory system, sulfide clearance (removal) is crucial for the benthic fauna. Through the partial oxidation and binding of sulfide by manganese and iron, as well as the subsequent transport of iron sulfides up to the surface layers where $O_2$ is the terminal oxidant, $H_2S$ oxidation appears to occur predominantly in the anoxic sediment. The reactive Mn(IV) and Fe(III) pools are only depleted at very high organic loading of the sediment or during hypoxia, and $H_2S$ may approach the oxic layer directly. Sulfur bacteria there carry out the oxidation in a small, overlapping, counter-diffusing zone of $O_2$ and $H_2S$. On the surface of the FeS silt, the filamentous *Beggiatoa* spp. multiply and spread as sub-millimeter thin, white films in particular. These sulfur bacteria have proliferated during the past ten years in North European coastal waters as a result of eutrophication, coinciding with the increasing hypoxia. In certain locations, they have even grown to form a periodically dominant bottom population. Algal cells and organic detritus deposit nitrogen and phosphorus onto the sea floor, where they partially decompose in the water column. The nutrients lose their nutrients more quickly than carbon. The organic nitrogen in the sediment is further depleted to a C: N of greater than 10. The C:N is even 15 at the sediment surface and rises to >20 with depth in some places, where considerable organic matter degradation has occurred during its passage from the North Sea. The C:P ratio, on the other hand, is lowest at the sediment surface due to the accumulation of released phosphate that is bonded to iron minerals.

## 7.9. PHOSPHORUS CHEMISTRY

The chemistry of phosphorus is complicated by the various ways it can bond in both organic and inorganic phases, even though it does not undergo reduction-oxidation reactions in marine sediments (Anschutz et al., 2005). A lot of research has been done on techniques to identify these pools. During mineralization, a large portion of the phosphorus that is deposited on the sediment is progressively released into the pore water while still bound in fresh plankton material. The oxidized surface layer of the sediment contains oxidized phases of ferric oxyhydroxides and, to a lesser extent, oxidized manganese, to which the free phosphate is quickly attached. The released phosphate accumulates in the pore water and diffuses upward toward the top in deeper sediment layers where these metal oxides have mostly been reduced. There, it may bind to excess FeOOH. In the uppermost 0–1 cm, the dynamic pools of fresh organic phosphorus, iron-bound phosphate, and loosely sorbed phosphate made up approximately 50% of the total, but they were mostly depleted below 3 cm deep. Below this depth, the only phosphate pools that were present were those that were attached to clay minerals, to calcium in apatite or calcium carbonate minerals, or to refractory organic material. These are the primary forms that are irreversibly deposited in marine sediments. A small portion of the entire P input to estuaries is trapped. The adsorption kinetics to amorphous FeOOH in the surface soil regulate the net release of phosphate into the overlying water during mineralization. Peaks in the phosphate flow into the water are caused by intermittent, partial depletion of the FeOOH pool as a result of hypoxia or abrupt sedimentation of a phytoplankton bloom. The reduced iron minerals are able to bind phosphate in freshwater sediments, the majority of the Fe(II) in marine sediments interacts with sulfide. Consequently, compared to freshwater sediments, the P retention in marine sediments is comparatively less effective. Nonetheless, the geochemistry of iron and phosphorus are closely correlated.

In offshore sediments with lesser organic deposition than in coastal sediments, the oxidants of the suboxic zone, namely $NO^{3-}$, Mn(IV), and Fe(III), between the oxygen and sulfate respiration zones, are significant. These oxidants are consumed more quickly than they are transported into the sediment by an enhanced organic flow brought on by eutrophication. Manganese oxides are lowered, the nitrate zone narrows and becomes limiting to denitrification, and $Mn^{2+}$ is lost to the water column. The iron oxides are decreased, and sulfide binds Fe(II). Sulfate reduction is preferentially stimulated by eutrophication and may even be preferred over oxygen in the direct respiration of organic materials(Chen and Jiang, 2016). The majority of the oxygen intake may then be utilized for the reoxidation of the substantial quantities of $H_2S$ to sulfate, either directly or via the employment of Mn and Fe as intermediate electron carriers. Beggiatoa spp., filamentous sulfur bacteria, are developing white films on the sediment, indicating that the intermediate oxidants' buffer capacity has been exhausted and that $H_2S$ is now reaching the surface. Due to increased primary production of planktonic microalgae or benthic micro- and macrophytes, which are mostly degraded in the sediment, eutrophication has a substantial impact on the benthic ecology. The extent of oxygen ($O_2$) depletion in the bottom water, the kind and quantity of organic material that is sedimenting, and how the benthic populations react to these variables influence the nature of the responses. The physiology of an individual to the ecology of the entire benthic ecosystem may all be affected in various ways. An increasing degree of eutrophication has a series of effects, beginning with increased species growth, population growth accompanied by changes in species composition, physiological and behavioral effects, and potential mass mortality from anoxia.

## 7.10. BENTHIC SPECIES

The benthic species will have more food due to the increased phytoplankton sedimentation to the sea floor resulting from eutrophication. If there are no physical space constraints or hypoxia, the benthic fauna will probably respond to an increase in food by becoming more abundant and producing more biomass. The fundamental presumptions of such a reaction include the survival rates of macrobenthos remaining constant and the species being food-limited in most cases. Recent studies in the Baltic Sea have shown increased abundance and/or biomass of phytoplankton. Some of these studies have linked the changes to eutrophication. The organic material components are most crucial for feeding, how phytoplankton is transported through the benthos, and what are the benthos' primary response mechanisms. In response to elevated food levels, benthic species may exhibit changes in individual species growth and/or population size. After phytoplankton sedimentation reaches the bottom, the resident animal species will begin to grow, but effects on recruitment won't become apparent until a few months or even a year or longer after the food input. The dominant route (pathway) for biomass gain will rely on various aspects, including the amount of food input, its stage in the reproductive cycle of benthic populations, and its bottom (base) relative to growth potential.

The comprehensive mapping of benthos in Danish seas at the beginning of the 20$^{th}$ century was supported by the fishery's economic importance. The outcome was a database containing unique material from a comparatively pristine time period, which may be used to compare the current state of the benthos. In the 1980s, lower coral macrofauna biomasses were found at shallower depths (<50 m), with increases predominating at depths. Both increases and declines were observed in the intermediate depths. The biomass of brittle scars and polychaetes had increased, but that of sea urchins (*Echinocardium cordatum*) and certain other mollusks had declined. In some regions, the filter-feeding brittle scar, *Amphiura filiformis*, had a noticeable increase of any single species. Before hypoxia-induced problems were evident, some researchers studied the fauna in Swedish fjords. They found that, regardless of depth, the total macrobenthos biomass increased.

The rise in biomass was correlated with an increase in the overall population density. The biomass and, in most cases, density, measured in the spring, were significantly correlated with runoff from surrounding land areas, with a time lag of approximately one year at 100 m and two years at 300 m. This runoff determines the annual mean chlorophyll-a concentrations in the euphotic zone as well as the inorganic N-nutrient pool for the spring phytoplankton bloom (Cerco, 2000).

## 7.11. HYPOXIA AND ANOXIA

It should be noted that an organism's ability to withstand hypoxia is determined by its partial pressure and oxygen availability, not by the amount of oxygen present in its immediate surroundings. Therefore, in comparison to stagnant water, moving water can significantly increase the amount of oxygen available for a stationary (sedentary) benthic species. This is particularly true for tiny animals without respiratory organs. Even though the oxygen level in the water may be extremely low, the animal won't experience hypoxia as long as the supply of oxygen can satisfy the demand. Under these experimental conditions, the necessary oxygen concentration might potentially be so low. When a species has respiratory organs, its typical hypoxic response is to somehow make more oxygen available. Most crustaceans and burrowing polychaetes increase their respiratory rate when oxygen tensions drop below half of the saturation level. They are able to sustain their level of aerobic respiration and oxygenate their burrows in this way.

Different species range greatly in their ability to withstand totally anoxic environments. For example, *Crangon crangon* (a crustacean) with an LT 50 of only two hours exists at 10°C under anoxia. The bivalve *Astarte borealis* from the western Baltic has an LT 50 of 2000 hours. In general, bivalves have the highest tolerances, followed by polychaetes, such as *Terebellides stroemi* and *Nereis diversicolor* (LT 50 100 hours). The Baltic isopod *Saduria entomon* withstand anoxia for up to 200 hours. In hypoxic or anoxic environments, the survival of several species is decreased by the presence of $H_2S$ (Paasche and Kristiansen, 1982). A tolerance to $H_2S$ is frequently related with a high tolerance to anoxia. This is important for the habitat because enhanced upward diffusion of $H_2S$ from reduced sediment layers occurs during anoxia. The biological mechanisms are primarily responsible for the high tolerance. To get this high tolerance, one must have an adequate amount of metabolic storage substrate (glycogen) and the capacity to lower total metabolic requirements by lowering various forms of activity. Low mobility is frequently associated with a low metabolic rate and, thus, a high tolerance, as seen in bivalves that live in sediment, like *Arctica islandica*. Related species will typically have shorter lifetimes if they have less energetic reserves and a greater metabolic rate. This implies that the species with minimal energy stores and a fast metabolic rate will be less able to withstand anoxia and will have a shorter lifespan.

## 7.12. ECHINODERMS

The echinoderms lack true respiratory appendages and are quite large in size; it has long been believed that they are sensitive to low oxygen tensions. Amphiura emerged from the sediment at about 10% of air saturation, a behavior that may have increased the animal availability of oxygen. The experimental settings employed make it challenging to draw conclusions regarding the susceptibility of Amphiura to low oxygen pressures. Mass mortality has been documented even at 30% air saturation of oxygen. Other echinoderms, such *Echinocardium cordatum*, (Figure 7.2) which are often burrowed deep under the sediment, tend to be the first species to escape from the sediment upon anoxia. *E. cordatum* has sulfide-oxidizing bacteria in the gut, indicating the presence of sulfide. Therefore, it is likely that *E. cordatum* needs a high oxygen tension for the bacteria to detoxify sulfide, and it escapes from anoxic sediments to prevent high sulfide concentrations. The capacity to endure prolonged durations of low oxygen concentration has been proven in multiple experimental tests. Therefore, it would seem surprising that clear signs of oxygen depletion can be found at relatively higher oxygen concentration levels. This disparity could be attributed to an artifact in the oxygen monitoring process. The oxygen concentration just above the sediment may not be accurately represented by measurements of bottom water oxygen concentrations, which are typically taken between 0.5 and 1 m above the bottom. Benthic species in hypoxia may have a distinct oxygen gradient directly above the sediment. The interaction between predator and prey is also impacted by oxygen deficiency. Predation rate variations can affect the size and dynamics of prey populations, and they can particularly in species-poor habitats, lead to substantial changes at the community level.

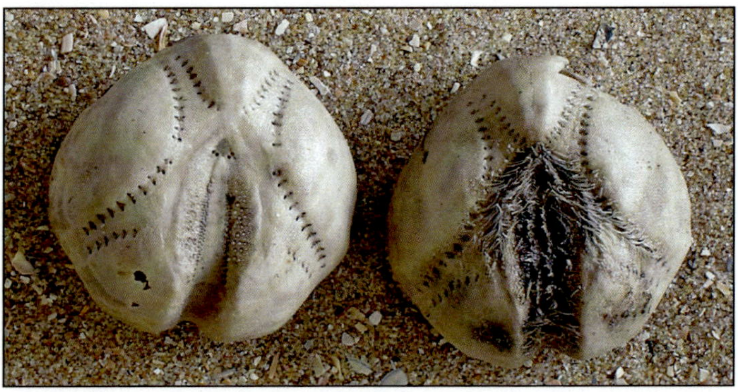

**Figure 7.2.** *Echinocardium cordatum.*

Source: https://upload.wikimedia.org/wikipedia/commons/2/20/Dier-Echinocardium_cordatum-Zeeklit-01.jpg, Creative Commons License.

While facultative anaerobiosis is common in benthic organisms, many metabolic routes might be employed for this process. Only when the oxygen tension drops to the point where aerobic maintenance of basic metabolic requirements is no longer possible can anaerobiosis take place. Anaerobiosis caused by environmental factors can occur. In active organisms like crustaceans and some polychaetes, lactate (lactic acid) is the anaerobic end product of glycolysis. Fatty acids like succinate and, in certain cases, propionate are accumulated by other groups, primarily polychaetes and bivalves, if the anaerobic metabolic period is prolonged. Aspartate is utilized as a substrate in the first stage of short-term anaerobiosis, producing opiates and either acetate or alanine as byproducts. During short periods of anaerobiosis, like low tide, some of the more active polychaetes, such *Nereis diversicolor*, also generate lactate. In extreme hypoxia or anoxia, low salinity will increase stress and shorten survival duration. For some polychaetes, an osmotic adjustment to reduced salinity demands energy and will result in a faster utilization of energy stores, which will accelerate the accumulation of anaerobic end products (Zwaan and Eertman, 1996).

## 7.13. PHYTOPLANKTON CYCLES

The hypothesis that the seasonal cycles of phytoplankton in seas can be explained in terms of the relationship between vertical mixing and the need for light and nutrients by planktonic microalgae is a result of our understanding of the coupling between physical and biological processes. The development of the seasonal thermocline, which occurs at a time when photosynthesis-friendly light conditions coincide with developing water column stability, is crucial to this system because it ensures that nutrients lost from the euphotic zone tend to reside. The conditions for phytoplankton growth are relatively poor due to insufficient light in the winter and limited nutrients in the summer. Conditions favorable for plankton blooms only occur for short periods of time in the spring and sporadically in the autumn. Based on the information that is currently available, there is no reason to think that the first biological response to eutrophication varies significantly between fresh and marine waters, or even within a marine region, in temperate regions. Nutrient availability limits plant biomass in all of these environments, at least in part. When nutrient limitation is present, increasing nutrient input through eutrophication will cause plants to grow more quickly and/or alter the species composition of the plant community. It is generally acknowledged that the availability of phosphorus (P) limits plant growth in freshwater environments. As a result, the majority of corrective (remedial) measures for freshwater eutrophication have concentrated on controlling P levels, and efforts to explain how productivity is regulated in these systems have typically relied on mass balances with P. In contrast, things get trickier in marine systems. Phosphorus is the macronutrient most likely to restrict phytoplankton production in freshwater environments. Even though it is widely believed that nitrogen availability governs production in the majority of marine systems, determining a N mass balance is more difficult than determining a P mass balance. This is because nitrogen availability in aquatic environments is regulated by both geochemical processes and biochemical activities i.e., denitrification and nitrogen fixation. There are no comparable metabolic pathways for the intake or elimination of phosphorus. There is presently less data available on the rates of nitrogen uptake and elimination through biological processes. The atmospheric nitrogen transport to coastal waters may represent a quantitatively significant input activity. For P input, this is not the case. However, the contributions of atmospheric N to the overall N transport in the majority of marine systems remain poorly characterized. Because there are more processes influencing N input/output to coastal marine systems, it is more challenging to construct a quantitative mass balance for N than for P.

## 7.14. CONCLUSION

When evaluating the impacts of eutrophication and their correlation with the local anthropogenic nutrient intake in contrast to distant nutrient sources, there are a few crucial elements that must be considered. The fact that the nitrogen budgets are often made for total nitrogen or phosphorus intake makes the relationship between them and phytoplankton activity even more difficult to understand. Significant quantities of nitrogen are incorporated into intricate organic compounds, such as humic materials. Such organic nitrogen molecules are not effectively used by most phytoplankton as a source of nutrients. Furthermore, for many organic nitrogen compounds, the turnover time, that is, the amount of time needed to decompose the compound into its inorganic components, is longer than the residence time for water masses in many places. The nitrogen that is bound up in these organic compounds is frequently not immediately available for the formation of phytoplankton. The relative significance of a given nutrition supply to phytoplankton development depends on the timing of its delivery. Therefore, nutrients that enter the surface water at a certain time may encourage the growth of phytoplankton. However, during the winter, when light is scarce and phytoplankton growth is limited, adding nutrients to the water column does not guarantee an increase in phytoplankton growth. Measurements of chlorophyll can be used to estimate the amount of biomass present at any particular time. They do not, however, provide much information regarding biomass production and loss rates. A net increase in organic matter production is what causes eutrophication effects like hypoxia.

Chapter 8

# LAKES AND EUTROPHICATION

## Contents

# 8.1. INTRODUCTION

The Changjiang delta (Lake Taihu) (Figure 8.1) is China's most industrialized region due to its high population density, level of urbanization, and rapid economic growth (Qin et al., 2007). Despite making up only 0.4% of land area and 3% of its population, the Taihu basin is responsible for 15% of provincial revenue and 10% of the GDP.

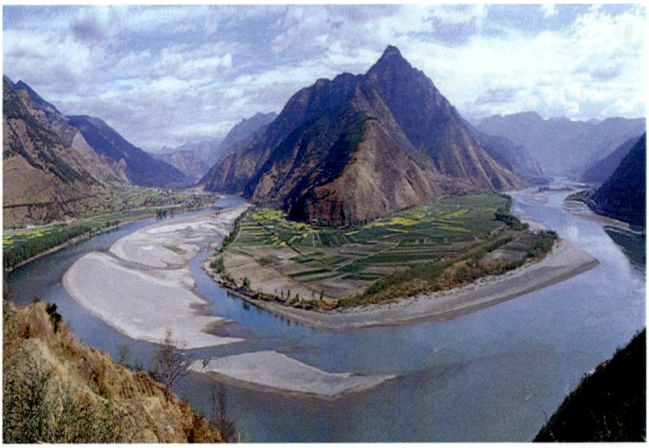

**Figure 8.1.** *Changjiang delta.*

Source: https://upload.wikimedia.org/wikipedia/commons/a/a5/Cn1202-03.jpg, Creative Commons License.

The provision of water, prevention of flooding, recreation and tourism, shipping, and aquaculture all depend on Lake Taihu. It supplies drinking water to many cities, including Huzhou, Wuxi, Suzhou, and Shanghai. However, since the 1980s, pollution has been produced and released into rivers and the lake as a result of economic development. *Microcystis* spp. Algal blooms and eutrophication have been linked to declining water quality. The algal bloom, which has been present for the entire summer, has expanded and is affecting the lake (for drinking water). Before 2000 and 2010, the Chinese government focused on eutrophication and pollution prevention in 1996. Wastewater from factories within the watershed is now required to be treated before being released into rivers. Before 2000, rivers that flow into Lake Taihu must exceed grade III criteria (standards), and the lake water must be purified by 2010. The quality of lake water has not improved, nevertheless, and in 2001 the efforts to control pollution were reassessed. Actually, the Lake Taihu problem is the same as that of the majority of freshwater lakes in eastern China.

This concept was supported by evidence of marine sediments discovered in drill cores. The lagoon was enclosed by the development of the continental shelf, turning it into a freshwater lake. Recent discoveries at archaeological sites and stratigraphy point to Taihu's origins in severe flooding. The depression held onto floodwater released by artificial conduits. Lake Taihu has an intricate system of rivers and channels. The lake is connected to 172 rivers and canals. The Taihu basin rivers span a total of around 12,000 km. Flooding runoff from the west or southwest passes via a lake to the east and empties into the East China Sea during the spring and summer flooding season. However, water flow can reverse during the dry season, particularly in eastern rivers. Rivers located to the west of the lake are typically classified as upstream, and vice versa. It is described as either positive or negative runoff. The Chendonggang, Yancungang, and Xiaoxi rivers have the highest inflow. In the west or southwest watershed, there are three. Taipu, Xinyunhe, and Xijiang are the principal rivers (outflow); they are situated in the southeast. Certain rivers flow into the lake continuously, while others flow out of it, and some change their flow direction seasonally. 90% of the entire runoff intake and output comes from this river water, however, the frequency of measurements was insufficient because they were done twice during flooding months and once during normal months.

## 8.2. POLLUTANTS

Compared to the multi-year averaged water balance, the water balance represents more flooding years. Although the Taipu River in the southeast discharges the runoff water, the water retention period is around five months in the south. As a result, southern water quality is superior to northern water quality. In 1994, an analysis of the pollutant content in wastewater revealed that 38% of total nitrogen (TN) came from nonpoint sources, 25% came from domestic sewage, and 16% came from industrial sources (Wu and Chen, 2013). Further, 10% came from industry, 60% from sewage, and 15% from non-point sources for total phosphorus (TP), 39% of COD came from industry, 42% from sewage, and 10% from nonpoint sources. In contrast, agricultural pollution greatly increased in terms of COD and TN, and sewage pollution accounted for 70% of TP. This shift is a reflection of both changing land use and rapid economic growth. The majority of the industrial pollutants came from Suzhou, Wuxi, and Jiaxing, which are located east or southeast of the lake basin. Agriculture-related pollutants i.e., cropping, rice cultivation, etc. were responsible for 37% of COD, 49.5% of TN, and 48% of TP generated in the basin. Most of these nonpoint pollutants originated in the west. 5% of COD, 6% of TN, and 18% of TP were attributed to the poultry culture in the rural area. 5.5% of COD, 5.2% of TN, and 4.1% of TP came from fish culture. As point sources are better controlled, non-point sources such as agriculture and animal husbandry will probably contribute more over time. Pen-fish aquaculture is the predominant type of aquaculture in Lake Taihu. Aquaculture has only been practiced in East Taihu, a 126 km2 bay in the southeast of the lake that is dominated by macrophytes. This region's fish culture has brought up a few environmental issues. 95% of the East Taihu is covered in macrophytes. This amounts to 3,920 tons of nitrogen and 496 tons of phosphorus, which means that these amounts represent 58% and 95%, respectively, of the total external loading that East Taihu received.

## 8.3. AQUACULTURE

The spread of net pens (Figure 8.2) has now prevented the harvesting of macrophytes. As a result, the lake lost a crucial nutrient export route (pathway). In East Taihu, this loss has accelerated eutrophication and sedimentation. The practice of aquaculture also adds to eutrophication and increased nutrient loading. According to some estimates, 141 kg of nitrogen and 14 kg of phosphorus are needed to produce 1 ton of fish, and 65% of each is not absorbed and is instead discharged into the water above. Increased nutrient loading causes bacteria, zooplankton and phytoplankton to proliferate quickly in pen-fish culture zones. Following a year of fish farming, the amount of heterotrophic bacteria grew three to four times, while the amount of phytoplankton was three times higher than in non-culture areas.

After two years of fish culture, the total amount of organic carbon, total nitrogen, and total organic nitrogen increased by 141, 87.5, and 86%, respectively, in surface sediments. Freshwater crab culture, which is more profitable than fish culture and will enhance feed intake and deposit of organic materials from feed residues, has recently displaced fish culture. The lake will release nutrients and thus prevent the growth of the marsh in this manner since fish culture needs macrophytes as fish food. Consequently, modern aquaculture exacerbates the decline in ecosystem health and water quality. East Taihu, Xikou Bay and Gonghu Bay are the three eastern coastal regions where marsh development is most prevalent. East Taihu marsh growth is particularly severe because the area serves as both a flood discharge area and a supply of drinking water for Suzhou and Shanghai. Marsh development, however, hinders these processes. Typically, the formation of marshes in lakes is caused by the deposition of organic or inorganic materials, which raises the lake bottom, reduces its water capacity, and ultimately causes the lake to disappear. A 1997 TM satellite image and field study revealed that 95% of East Taihu is covered with aquatic vegetation (Luo et al., 2016). *Vallisneria natans*, *Potamogeton maackianus*, and *Zizania latifolia* (Figure 8.3) are among the dominant species. East Taihu has an average macrophyte biomass of 3.8 kg $m^{-2}$, ranging from 2.0 to 5.6 kg $m^{-2}$. About 550,000 t of aquatic plants make up Lake Taihu's total standing biomass;

of these, 42% are *Potamogeton maackianus*, 29.5% are *Zizania latifolia*, and 0.2% are *Vallisneria natans*.

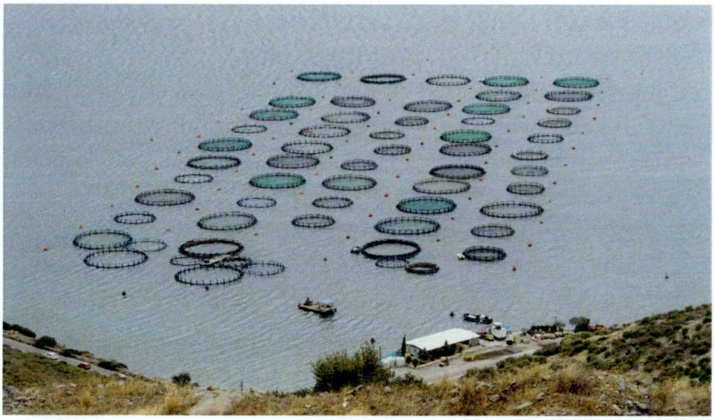

**Figure 8.2.** *Net pens.*

Source: https://upload.wikimedia.org/wikipedia/commons/2/2a/Fish_farm_Amarynthos_Euboea_Greece_-_edit1.jpg, Creative Commons License.

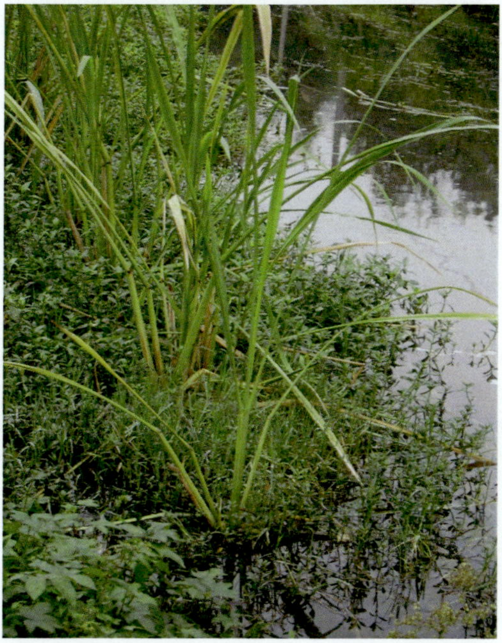

**Figure 8.3.** *Zizania latifolia.*

Source: https://upload.wikimedia.org/wikipedia/commons/6/6c/Water_bamboo.JPG, Creative Commons License.

## 8.4. LAKE TAIHU: THE FUNCTIONS OF ITS ZONES

Lake Taihu serves a variety of purposes, such as providing flood water retention, fishing, tourism, and shipping. Since certain uses, like fish culture and water supply, are incompatible, over-exploration and over-utilization led to the decline of the lake environment and the quality of the water. Therefore, to slow down the development of marshes and eutrophication, restore the ecosystem, and enhance water quality, the creation of a centralized management system should be taken into consideration. It is necessary to implement rules and policies, such as prohibiting renovation and limiting the geographic range of fish farming. Accurate estimates of economic growth and contaminant sources should form the foundation of any long-term strategy for controlling pollution and eutrophication. Planning and implementing watershed management should have the goal of controlling pollution sources. It is important to prioritize scientific research on the topics of internal loading from sediment, water and nutrient budgets, and littoral zone ecological restoration. Lakes are located near the catchment basin (bottom). They will naturally reflect activities in their catchments due to gravity, which will show up as altered water quality, as well as changes to streams for farming, flood control, water storage and pollutant disposal. The freshwater systems that drain a watershed with intact ecosystems won't have any issues, and there is a connection between the freshwater and terrestrial systems. Nutrient-limited ecosystems transfer very less nutrients from the land to the water. The majority of essential nutrients are stored and regenerated in the biomass found on land. Thus, even in cases when the catchment sediments are produced by easily weathered rocks, pristine freshwater systems contain exceptionally low quantities of nitrogen and phosphorus. They are more than merely mixtures of water. Sand bars, floodplains, levees, riffles, and other geomorphological processes, as well as woody waste (debris) entering from the nearby catchment, are examples of the structures that rivers have created. The littoral zones of lakes are home to a variety of submerged and emergent vegetation. The preservation of this structure might be based on the ecosystem diversity remaining intact. In an environment where nutrients are limited, top predators such as wolves, bears, salmonids and other piscivorous fish, birds, and other species can have significant top-down effects that preserve this structure and the effectiveness of nutrient cycling. Also, there will be excellent system connectivity. Lake productivity is somewhat dependent on organic matter that is carried in from the basin by the inflow rivers.

## 8.5. WETLANDS

For fish and invertebrate life cycles, the surrounding wetlands can be crucial.

In northern rivers, nutrients from the ocean are recycled into the riparian forests by the excrements of the brown bear predators, which are salmonid fish. Likewise, after spawning, tree detritus holds onto carcasses, which supply the nutrients required by periphyton and microinvertebrates to support hatched fish after their yolk sacs are depleted. Three essential components are required for any ecosystem restoration: maintaining connectivity, preserving structure, including suitable biodiversity, and nutrient parsimony. When all three of these traits are present, a system is self-maintaining. When this state is deviated from, scientists document the effects on freshwater systems that harm these features. Eutrophication erodes nutrient parsimony and can cause a loss of structure. To maintain efficient forestry practices, catchment management may deprive rivers of the structural support that forest debris provides. The construction of dams and the channelization and embankment of lowland rivers can cause these rivers to lose their hydrological connection to their floodplains. Essentially, damage to the three essential components is the end result of many factors that destroy freshwater systems. The issues/problems surrounding freshwaters are issues with landscape management, which in turn affects how human civilizations are governed. The prevailing mindset in the developed world today emphasizes resource optimization for financial gain while paying relatively little attention to resource sustainability. In the past, ecology was mostly focused on explaining how whole systems functioned; today, it also documents the damage.

For decades, researchers have examined the seasonal and annual dynamics of TP in deep dimictic lakes; they have generally been shown to follow predictable patterns. Dissolved P is integrated into plankton biomass during summer stratification, and this plankton then either settles from the epilimnion or is integrated into higher trophic levels of the food web. P moves downstream from the epilimnion to the hypolimnion and sediments, except floating cyanobacteria or algae that can actively maintain their place in the upper/surface water. In a deep stratified lake, particles may only return to the surface waters during fall overturn once they have settled. These patterns and the underlying mechanisms that underlie them have been studied and summarized by several authors. Shallow lakes, in contrast to their stratified equivalents, may exhibit very unpredictable seasonal and annual changes in TP, primarily due to random processes that are less predictable. Not as much research has been done on these lakes, however this trend has recently changed. Particulate and interstitial P may be physically transported into the shallow lake water column at any given time by wind energy at a rate that is higher than P inputs from external loading, diffusion, and bioturbation. Downstream transport of P with sediment particles may significantly outpace other loss processes, such as algal settling, as long as there is a concentration gradient between sediment-bound P and dissolved P in the water. Particle settling predominates in the downward flux in shallow lakes where wind significantly affects the sediments, while physical resuspension by wind waves dominates the upward transit of P. Other P cycle activities, such as bioturbation and the uptake of allochthonous P by plants, periphyton, and plankton, may indicate downward fluxes of larger size in lakes that are less affected by wind. Predicting whether wind-waves would heavily affect lake P dynamics can be done in a different ways (Huang et al., 2016).

## 8.6. PHOSPHORUS DYNAMICS OF LAKE OKEECHOBEE

Some lakes also fit into the range of large size and low maximal depth, which suggests that wind-induced waves are mostly responsible for the random redistribution of sediments. In terms of size and depth, Lake Taihu is comparable to Lake Okeechobee in Florida, in the United States. As another typical case study for huge shallow lakes, we can analyze the P dynamics of Lake Okeechobee. We need to pay particular attention to how P dynamics fluctuate at various temporal scales in these extremely dynamic ecosystems. Many studies have been conducted on the physical, chemical, and biological aspects of Lake Okeechobee. At 60–90 cm above sea level, the lake bottom is comparatively flat. The center pelagic zone is divided from the shallower southern and southwestern areas by an underwater limestone reef toward the southern end. The United States Army Corps (USACE) of Engineers built a dike around the entire lake, including the littoral zone, in the middle of the 1900s. Three separate zones in the lake sustain various primary producer populations and have noticeably varied water chemistry due to two factors: water depth and kind of sediment. Within the lake, the deepest area is called the central pelagic zone. This zone water column does not support vascular plants or benthic algae, has high P concentrations, and frequently limits phytoplankton access to light. Because the majority of the P is linked to resuspended sediment particles, phytoplankton chlorophyll a concentration does not correlate with TP. Because rainfall is the primary source of water intake for the interior littoral zone, TP concentrations there are often low. Except in situations where the water level is quite high, there is a slight nutrient translocation between the littoral and pelagic zones. An area of intermediate depth, turbidity, and nutrient enrichment lies between the littoral and pelagic zones. This area is known as the near-shore zone. Phytoplankton takes over the near-shore zone when the lake has high water (for long periods), as it did in the late 1990s. On the other hand, it grows a dense community of submerged plants and clear water in shallow settings.

Diffusive P release may contribute significantly to the amount of easily available P in the water column, even if it may be less than the P transport linked to sediment resuspension. Whether there are sufficient light conditions for net phytoplankton growth during or after the resuspension event will determine the consequences on the quality of the water. The resuspension dominates the P input to the lake water in the shallow Danish Lake, and is also consistent with the findings regarding P dynamics at hourly to daily scales in Lake Okeechobee. The same outcome is observed in Lake Kasumigaura, Japan, where the ratio of TP supply to the water column by resuspension vs. diffusion is 10:1 despite large rates of P release by diffusion. There is a recurring seasonal pattern for TP in Lake Okeechobee due to seasonal changes in wind velocity and its impact on the length and amount of sediment resuspension. We can notice that wind velocity might account for more than 70% of the monthly variation in pelagic mean TP in any given year. Because the majority of the wintertime increase in pelagic TP is linked to abiotic sediment particles, phytoplankton has limited response to it. During the majority of the winter months, when the water column is fully mixed, the algae are light-limited due to the attenuation of light caused by those particles. Lower water temperatures and a shorter photoperiod during the winter may potentially have an impact on phytoplankton biomass. This is improbable, though, as wintertime is often when the chlorophyll a concentration in near-shore areas unaffected by sediment resuspension is at its highest (peak). This varying seasonality has been linked to a decrease in competition for water column phosphorus during the winter months with plants and periphyton. The P dynamics of lakes may be significantly impacted by tropical storms, i.e., cyclones and hurricanes (Paerl et al., 2018).

## 8.7. IMPACT OF NATURAL DISASTERS

It has been suggested that a hurricane was the cause of the large-scale plant loss and development of dense phytoplankton blooms in Lake Apopka, Florida in the 1940s. There is evidence that a tropical storm contributed to a significant decline in submerged plants in the Chesapeake Bay in the 1970s and accompanying changes in water quality. Researchers recorded the main effects of a 1999 Category I storm on Lake Okeechobee water column TP concentration and sediment suspension and transport. Strong currents remain in the lake as a result of residual circulation from the preceding wind forcing event when wind velocities drop suddenly, as they did after the 1999 storm passed outside of Florida. Therefore, sediment particles can travel great distances before being resuspended, especially if they have very fine-grained sediments like the mud sediments that make up the majority of Lake Okeechobee. During the storm, almost 10,000 metric tons of fine-grained mud silt were raised. After the hurricane, concentrations of TP in the lake persisted at high levels for two months. When another wind storm passed over the lake in late winter 2001, concentrations of TP showed a second significant increase, rising to above 230 μg $l^{-1}$. The Florida peninsula was affected by a tropical storm and two to three hurricanes (wind speeds – 120 km/h). Every 5-7 years, a powerful hurricane (wind speed > 180 km/h) would hit the peninsula. Any one tropical storm may have sustained winds over the lake that are significantly lower than when the storm is ashore because wind velocity decreases when a tropical storm travels over land. However, Lake Okeechobee is situated in an area where tropical cyclone impacts are highly likely. This might also apply to a few large shallow lakes in Asian lowlands. The predicted impact of long-term patterns in ocean currents on storm frequencies in the future is also an important topic of research. The Atlantic Ocean experienced the highest storm activity ever recorded between 1995 and 2000. This has been connected to a warm phase of the Atlantic Ocean Thermohaline Current or AOTC, which is expected to endure 20–40 years. Hurricane-related changes to the environment can therefore have an impact on a lake P dynamic that extends far beyond the lake watershed. Although limnologists are already aware of the importance of managing lakes within a watershed, in certain cases, a more comprehensive framework may be needed. The biomass of all submerged and emergent plants as well as periphyton in the littoral and near-shore zones contains just 0.8% of the lake P, compared to 97.1% in the sediments. The lake's littoral zone is nutrient-poor compared to the pelagic zone.

## 8.8. PLANT DYNAMICS

The fact that submerged plants and algae sequester large amounts of P from the water column, either through direct uptake or other processes linked to dense plant beds, such as increased particle settling, and co-precipitation of P with calcium at high pH, is another explanation for the reduced lake-wide TP. Water levels in Lake Okeechobee regulate the biomass and spatial distribution of submerged plants and algae. Following a drought in the late 1980s, submerged plants covered 18,000-21,000 hectares of the near-shore zone (Havens et al., 2007). Seasonal maxima of submerged plants were correlated with low phytoplankton biomass and nutrient-poor water. This usually occurs in the winter. The lake water levels were high between 1995 and 1999, and during that time, the area covered by submerged vegetation shrunk to less than 2,000 hectares. The nearshore zone water had high TP concentrations and was excessively turbid. Another drought in 2000–2001 caused the lake water levels to drop to all-time lows, and the area covered by submerged plants rose once more, reaching nearly 17,000 hectares. The non-volatile suspended solids and water depth might be used to forecast the average biomass of submerged plants in the near-shore zone. These findings show a relationship between clear water and plants, but they do not explain if the increased water quality is due to the plants or if they were just reacting to the clear water brought on by other processes. Even while plants may have a localized effect on water quality, it is crucial to ascertain the spatial scale at which these effects affect TP in a huge lake like this, where a major portion of the bottom is unsuitable for plant colonization because of soft mud sediments. When submerged plants reached their maximum spatial extent in 2002, they accounted for only 13% of the total surface area of the littoral and pelagic zones. Thus, it is improbable that they would significantly regulate TP concentration throughout the entire lake. The water and nutrient transfer to the near-shore zone is limited when the lake level is low and plants are at their highest density. Therefore, submerged plants can only be expected to influence lake-wide TP if strong currents are flowing through the near-shore zone. Although physical mechanisms are far more significant, submerged plants in Lake Okeechobee probably have a limited effect that somewhat reduces seasonal and annual changes in TP.

## 8.9. MANAGING PHOSPHORUS DYNAMICS

At hourly, daily, and seasonal time scales, wind has been found to be the primary driver of P dynamics. It is also likely the primary element determining year-to-year fluctuations in pelagic TP. Researchers discovered that there was a correlation between the yearly-averaged TP and level, but that the correlation between the TP and wind velocity was higher. Based on field observations and correlations, researchers are unable to determine the causal mechanisms underlying year-to-year fluctuations in TP and conduct controlled experiments at a scale appropriate for the events occurring in this lake pelagic zone. The temporal variations in water column TP, chlorophyll a, and other characteristics cannot be accurately predicted by simple empirical models. In the instance of Lake Okeechobee, researchers have developed the LOEM as a means of comprehending the elements that influence fluctuations in TP and accurately predicting future trends. Large shallow coastal systems, such as Tampa Bay and the Chesapeake Bay, as well as other large shallow lakes like Lake Taihu, are managed with similar techniques. The pelagic TP of Lake Okeechobee varies seasonally and annually (James et al., 2009). Numerous P management initiatives put in place in the watershed after the 1980s have been blamed for the declining inflow of TP concentration. Because the surface sediments, which are the source of internal P loading, resemble previous loading conditions until they are buried by new sediment material with a lower concentration of P, TP concentrations in the water column increase with increasing external inputs but then remain high. The top 5 cm of the sediments interact with the water column above through resuspension and diffusion, resulting in a sediment deposit rate of around 0.1 cm Y-1. Because of this, it is anticipated that the lake will react to changes in external P inputs over a period of decades. Although they are hard to measure, the deposition rate and depth of the active sediment layer are particularly important for forecasting the response (reaction) time of other shallow lakes to P load reductions. For example, paleolimnological analysis and undisturbed sediment cores are needed to estimate the net sediment deposition rates. Before using the profiles to estimate process rates or infer historical conditions, it is necessary to demonstrate that sediments keep an undisturbed historical record in large shallow lakes that are significantly impacted by wind. This might not be the case in some lakes. Bioturbation of macroinvertebrates can also affect the depth of the active layer. In some lakes with lower P loading, SRP migrates from deeper sediment layers as the P content of the surface sediment is lost through diffusion. There is evidence that Lake Okeechobee sediments have been saturated with P in recent decades, which may be partly responsible for the lake's poor response to decreased P supplies. For instance, some researchers reported a considerable increase in porewater SRP concentration in the surface sediments of the lake between 1988 and 1998, indicating a saturation of binding sites. Lake Okeechobee P mass balance shows that during the 1970s and the 1990s, the net P sedimentation rate decreased four times. Because of this apparent P saturation, researchers thought that treating the sediment with alum or calcium could accelerate the lake's recovery.

## 8.10. DISSOLVED ORGANIC CARBON (DOC) AND COLORED DISSOLVED ORGANIC MATTER (CDOM)

The portion of dissolved organic carbon (DOC) that absorbs light, both visible and ultraviolet, is known as chromophoric dissolved organic matter (CDOM) (Clark et al., 2020). In aquatic ecosystems, the distribution of CDOM can have an impact on ecosystem productivity. While CDOM absorbs light, it has a negative effect on primary productivity and a positive impact on secondary productivity because photo-degraded CDOM acts as a substitute for microbial respiration. Large quantities of CDOM can shield aquatic species from UV damage by functioning as a photoprotectant. CDOM is the primary factor influencing UV attenuation in natural freshwaters. However, CDOM photodegradation by UV radiation and acidification may reduce the protection of aquatic biota against UV radiation. Non-chlorophyllous material absorption frequently exceeds phytoplankton absorption in shallow inland lakes and coastal seas. River inputs, land drainage, and phytoplankton degradation are the main causes of CDOM. The dynamics of CDOM in many aquatic habitats are poorly understood, although it affects biogeochemical processes and lake optical characteristics. In Lake Taihu, a comprehensive inventory of the distribution of regional

CDOM and its light absorption in wavebands encompassing UV and visible radiation spectra has not been carried out. The interpretation of satellite and aircraft remote sensing imagery, which is used to document how lakes react to environmental changes including cyanobacterial blooms, eutrophication, and water pollution, needs this information. Wind-induced waves frequently create intense sediment resuspension and alter the water-sediment interface in shallow lakes. The concentration of suspended solids or SS in the water above might rise significantly due to strong winds. Intense sediment resuspension has the potential to boost the internal release of nutrients, but it may also facilitate the sorption and precipitation of soluble nutrients into the bottom sediments. The hydrodynamics may affect sediment nutrient release in both favorable and unfavorable pathways.

Because of its unique shape, Lake Taihu frequently experiences wave processes. Water disturbance led to soluble reactive phosphorus (SRP) release from sediment that was 8–10 times higher than release under undisturbed conditions. According to wave flume experiments, a 4-6 $ms^{-1}$ southeast wind event may be responsible for the critical shear stress in Lake Taihu that causes substantial sediment resuspension. The primary source of internal load nutrients in Lake Taihu may be nutrients released from sediment resuspension due to wind-induced waves. Because field observations are extremely difficult to obtain, little is known about the amounts of suspended sediment and released nutrients, as well as the form of released nutrients in the lake. Some researchers aim to analyze the impact of hydrodynamics on sediment nutrient release and to offer field measurements on wind, water chemistry, algal biomass, and hydrodynamics in Lake Taihu. Raindrops are the result of tiny water droplets adhering to airborne particles, such as chemical components. As a result, their formation is contingent upon atmospheric quantities of gas and particles, as well as local air movement. Precipitation inputs of P and N in these locations may be lower than those in coastal areas because of the low nutrient concentrations in the air over the lake, particularly in the center. It is challenging to measure the uncertainty around regional variations, though, unless numerous observation sites are set up over Lake Taihu water surface. Results from calculations and observational data should show the impacts of wet deposition on lake eutrophication, nevertheless the regional heterogeneity of nutrient contents in precipitation. Even without dry deposition, still has a considerable impact on lake eutrophication. The annual riverine intake of TP was predicted to be 1,030 t, and that of TN to be approximately 28,650 t, based on the amounts of nutrients found at the inflow rivers that connect to Lake Taihu. The air deposition needs to be taken into account when evaluating the nutrient inputs to Lake Taihu. Air deposition of nitrogen may increase primary productivity.

## 8.11. OTHER INFLUENCING FACTORS

Acidic freshwater lakes and streams, as well as nitrogen-saturated forests, can be impacted by atmospheric deposition (Stumm and Schnoor, 1995). Lake Taihu is often P-limited and hence susceptible to N deposition. Deposited P may thereby increase primary production. Some N and P that have been deposited may attach themselves to or be absorbed by sediment particles, which might turn bottom sediment into a nutrition source. Waves may resuspend sediment and release nutrients, increasing N and P in shallow lakes because perturbation has a significant impact on sediment-water interactions. Aquatic plants might be able to use part of the suspended P, and some might be redeposited. The primary sources of atmospheric N are nitric acid gas ($HNO_3$), ammonium nitrate aerosol ($NH_4NO_3$), and ammonia gas ($NH_3$). The main forms of $NO_x$ are $NH_4NO_3$ and $HNO_3$, which can be converted to $HNO_3$ through photochemical reactions. $NH_4NO_3$ can develop an equilibrium with $HNO_3$ and $NH_3$, the major pollutant. The primary sources of these chemicals are agricultural production and the combustion of fossil fuels. The patterns of riverine in nutrient sources may be reflected in the origin of atmospheric deposition. As a result, emissions from fuel combustion and agriculture should be included in the regulation of external nitrogen loading in the Taihu Basin (Geng et al., 2021). Research showed that different electron donors added in anaerobic conditions caused diverse nitrogen transformations and that adding specific electron donors could improve the removal of nitrogen from anaerobic sediments. Acetate and starch showed the highest nitrogen removal efficiency among the four electron donors that were investigated. Acetate promotes nitrate reduction to ammonium, whereas saccharides like glucose, sucrose, and starch promote nitrate reduction to nitrite.

## 8.12. DENITRIFICATION

A microbial process called denitrification uses nitrite and nitrous oxide as two of the intermediates to convert nitrate to nitrogen gas. In the majority of natural habitats, it is acknowledged as the most significant process for eliminating fixed nitrogen. Because transformations include the reduction of nitrogen, electron donors are necessary. Denitrification is a respiration process that also needs an electron donor for energy. When molecular oxygen is not available, denitrifying bacteria can employ nitrate and/or nitrite as an alternate electron acceptor for metabolic activities. However, easily biodegradable electron donors frequently restrict denitrification in naturally occurring anaerobic environments, such as sediments. Research has indicated that the addition of organic electron donors, such as pyruvate, formate, glucose, acetate, starch, hydrogen gas, elemental sulfur, thiosulphate, aqueous ferrous iron, and pyrite, can improve the rates of nitrate reduction. While sucrose is a disaccharide that hydrolyzes to produce two monosaccharides, glucose is a monosaccharide. Two polysaccharides found in starch are amylose and amylopectin. An organic acid called acetate has been utilized to remove nitrogen from wastewater. Thus, one possible technique for treating polluted sediments is the addition of electron donors to improve reduction processes. For eutrophic lakes, like Lake Taihu, the third-largest freshwater lake in China, this might be a crucial treatment. Due to recent rapid economic expansion and intense use of water resources, Lake Taihu's water quality has declined. This leads to summertime cyanobacteria blooms that negatively affect aquatic ecology. There is a little comparative research on denitrification and electron donor supplements in freshwater sediments, and the majority of studies have concentrated on nitrate and ammonium removal in wastewater systems. Since nitrate did not drop within the first 96 hours, ammonium may have increased early due to the ammonification of organic materials. However, the high ammonium value later on suggested that in this microcosm, nitrate was converted to ammonium. Except for acetate, ammonium concentrations in the control systems were higher than those in the electron donor addition systems. Redox potential and pH may be used to regulate these systems. The relatively high pH brought on by acetate hydrolysis may be the reason for the nitrate reduction to ammonium accelerated by sodium acetate. TN reduction was used as an indication of denitrification activity in sediment-water microcosms to investigate the potential to improve denitrification of sediment by adding different electron donors.

## 8.13. SEDIMENTS

The surface sediments of Lake Taihu revealed varying concentrations and origins of aliphatic hydrocarbons (Zhang et al., 2017). Additionally, biomarkers and associated indices can reveal details on recent biogenic materials and anthropogenic contamination, particularly in relation to petrogenic sources. Anthropogenic petrogenic AHC inputs predominated around and riverine) discharges. High Org-C-normalized AHC concentrations, large UCM contributions, low n-alkane CPI (carbon preference index) and OEP (even-to-odd carbon number predominance), and the high degree of hopane biomarker corroborated this. In contrast, the East Taihu sediments showed the lowest levels of AHCs, little to no UCM contributions, high levels of OEP and n-alkane CPI, and low levels of hopane biomarkers. These characteristics implied that the predominant biogenic (vascular plants) origin of AHCs in these sediments. The biomarker values for sediment samples from the Western Basin showed that biogenic hydrocarbons predominated with petrogenic hydrocarbons. Information about the origins and regional variations of AHCs as well as other micropollutants like heavy metals and PAHs may help develop future plans for the management and protection of Lake Taihu. The riparian zone, which marks the transition between terrestrial and aquatic ecosystems, is the main pathway for the transfer of allochthonous matter from terrestrial to aquatic systems. It also affects water movement and waterborne toxins. Many studies have demonstrated that riparian buffer strips, which are tiny in size but have a large impact, can reduce the amount of sediment, phosphorus, and nitrogen found in terrestrial non-point sources of pollution. Many riparian zones have been damaged or disturbed as a result of recent industrial expansion and intensive agriculture. The landscape would lose a significant amount of its ability to purify and safeguard water if 70–95% of natural riparian systems were disrupted or destroyed. Many lakes in China have deteriorated with nutrient loading high enough to sustain a eutrophic state even after external nutrient supply reduction. Finding alternative biological methods based on natural processes is urgently needed.

In addition to providing a substantial supply of drinking water, Lake Taihu promotes regional tourism, agriculture, and fishing. Rapid industrial expansion, extensive chemical fertilizer application, and intensive water resource usage during the 1980s have led to nutrient-rich water discharge into the lake, resulting in hyper-eutrophication. Research has been done in Lake Taihu on enhancing water quality by nonpoint and point pollution reduction systems. Although shallow lakes have more sediment/water interactions and internal pollution than deep lakes, internal loading in shallow lakes may be caused by the buildup of pore water nutrients and their subsequent release over the sediment–water interface. The internal nutrient loading from sediments may be just as important as external loading from the watershed. It is challenging to reduce internal nutritional loading, particularly when it comes to relatively active nitrogen. Riparian zones can reduce the energy of flowing water, which frequently leads to increased sedimentation (Pettit and Naiman, 2007). Properly enriched riparian sediments are transported by flowing water, bringing with it finer suspended or resuspended material that is rich in nutrients and absorbed pollutants. It is unclear if riparian zones will serve as a source or a sink for open water. The lakeshore may be a net sink for nitrogen and phosphorus on a seasonal or annual basis. The lakeshore marshes function as nutrient transformers rather than nutrient sinks, the wetland plants and macrophytes work as nutrient pumps from the sediment. Riparian zones may lessen internal pollution if plant-covered littoral zones can function as nutrient sinks, converting most pollutants into inactive forms with poor mobility and bioavailability or eliminating them entirely. Nevertheless, limited data is accessible, as the majority of studies have concentrated on external or nonpoint source pollution elimination.

# 8.14. CARBON AND NITROGEN DYNAMICS

The riparian zones are biogeochemical hotspots for nitrogen where complex nitrogen transformations occur. Physico-chemical and biological processes in the water column and sediments determine the distribution of nitrogen. The dynamics of the littoral zone are impacted by both aquatic and terrestrial systems. The primary sources of external nitrogen are land and open water. Wet precipitation makes up a very small portion of the nitrogen supply. Both subterranean flow and surface runoff from the land bring nitrogen into the littoral zone.

The littoral zone was covered in vegetation, and the precipitation dropped at the same time as the vegetation density, where the plants absorbed most of the water debris and reduced the energy of the flowing water. Terrestrial runoff impacts have not been considered in some studies. Limited nutrients appeared to originate from subsurface flow, and most subsurface flow is unidirectional toward aquatic systems over the terrestrial boundary. In ecotones or riparian zones where wind or water kinetic energy drops sharply, material retention is high. Compared to terrestrial systems, energy use is more efficient and turnover is faster in the aquatic nitrogen cycle. The riparian zones may offer the best conditions for nitrogen transformations such as ammonification, nitrification, and denitrification. Constant accumulation of plant and algae detritus offers abundant supplies of carbon. Ammonification in vegetated strata is higher than in bare sediments. Vegetated sediments may also have significant levels of nitrification and denitrification. In the surface sediment of shallow vegetated zones, there is sufficient oxygen for nitrification, while denitrification may take place at deeper levels. But oxygen is carried by marsh vegetation through the stem, to the root, and into the soil, which has the potential to oxidize the diminished microzone surrounding the root surface. Around a root surface, two discrete layers that support nitrification–denitrification are formed. Ammonification sites are provided by trapped sediments; denitrification can take place in the underlying sediment, generating dinitrogen or nitrous oxide; and nitrification can use the ammonification product in aerobic water, surface sediments, and root surfaces. One important method for removing nitrogen from aquatic systems is denitrification.

*Chapter* 9

# ESTUARIES AND EUTROPHICATION

## Contents

# 9.1. INTRODUCTION

Eutrophication is an environmental issue that has resulted in many coastal locations experiencing red tides, hypoxia, and other biological issues, either now or in the past. Merely 55 locations in the United States and the European Union exhibit a tendency towards recovery. Eutrophication affects the ecological services that coastal seas supply, hence protecting coastal areas from eutrophication is important. During Japan's fast economic expansion from 1955 to 1970, Japanese estuaries suffered from severe environmental issues such as Toyama itai-itai disease and Minamata disease (Figure 9.1) (Kimura, 1988).

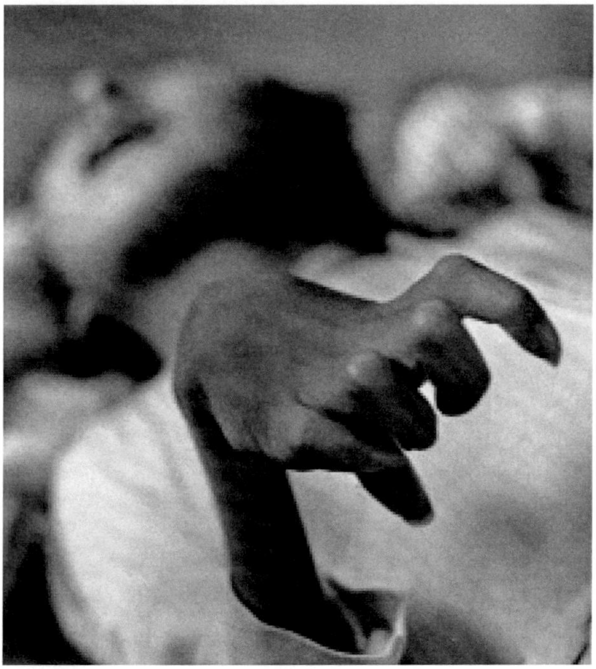

**Figure 9.1.** *Minamata disease.*

Source: https://upload.wikimedia.org/wikipedia/en/8/8d/Tomokos_hand.gif, Creative Commons License.

Throughout this time, the gross national product (GNP) increased by 9.7% on average. During this time, a diverse range of substances, including pesticides, nutrients, toxins etc., was released from the land surface uncontrollably. The Jintsu River (riverine) community, which relied on rice, vegetables, and water contaminated by cadmium from the Kamioka Mine Factory in Toyama Prefecture, was the first to experience the symptoms of itai-itai disease. The first cases of Minamata disease, a nerve condition brought on by methyl mercury released from a chemical factory, were reported in 1956 among fishermen who consumed seafood from Kumamoto Prefecture (Yatsushiro Bay). In an effort to address major environmental issues, the central government passed a new water quality management law in 1970. As a result, factories (industries) are no longer allowed to release hazardous materials like mercury and cadmium, as per the zero-emission principle. Since then, Japanese estuaries have not had any significant environmental issues, such as the Minamata disease.

## 9.2. TOKYO BAY

Tokyo Bay (Figure 9.2) has the highest TN and TP loads per sea area, the highest human density in the watershed, and the highest concentration of TN and TP. Tokyo Bay still experiences red tide and hypoxia every summer. The Seto Inland Sea has the longest average residence time and the lowest concentrations of TN and TP. Every summer, red tide and hypoxia affect a portion of the Seto Inland Sea, while oligotrophication also causes the fish catch to decline at the same time. The highest TN and TP concentrations were found in Dokai Bay, although these have significantly dropped, mostly as a result of the TN and TP loading regulations.

Dokai Bay has the shortest average residence period, noticeable load control, and hypoxia declined in 2011. Because proper habitats for marine biota are necessary for healthy and material cycling, reducing TP and TN loads from land is insufficient to prevent hypoxia.

Because biochemical activities are more crucial for the healthy and material cycling in estuaries than physical processes are, ecosystem-based management, or EBM, is extremely vital. Therefore, to establish the comprehensive material cycling of phosphorus and nitrogen and to stop the occurrence of red tides and hypoxia, we must restore the habitat conditions for marine biota.

Because of their high variability, habitat conditions in coastal seas vary greatly from location to location. Consequently, we need to find the most efficient means of restoring the habitat environment for marine biota through adaptive management (adaptive management). For instance, an artificial tidal flat was made in Tokyo Bay, eel grass beds were rebuilt in the Seto Inland Sea, and an experimental raft located in the middle of Dokai Bay was used to research the most effective technique for cultivating bivalves. The restoration of tidal flats, seagrass beds, sea-algae beds, and shallow areas with a depth of light that permits adequate penetration for marine biota are all necessary to rebuild a healthy ecosystem and halt oligotrophication in the Seto Inland Sea.

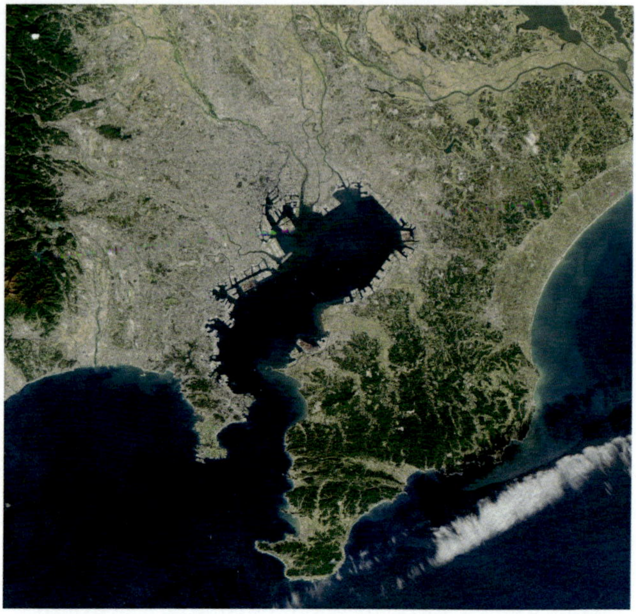

**Figure 9.2.** *Tokyo bay.*

Source: https://upload.wikimedia.org/wikipedia/commons/f/f4/Tokyo_Bay_by_Sentinel-2%2C_2018-10-30.jpg, Creative Commons License.

Tokyo Bay, in the middle of Japan, enjoys a humid, moderate climate. The bay is a confined (enclosed) space that is crowded with people and heavily utilized for domestic and industrial activities. It spreads about 50 km in length, 20 km in width, and 15 m on average in depth. The urban and industrial concentration in this river basin since 1950 has resulted in significant transformations. Eutrophication and a reduction in the shallow sandy flat region were some of these changes. Tokyo Bay experiences red tides, or algal blooms, about 50 times a year and blue tides, or the upwelling of hypoxic bottom water, about three times a year as a result of eutrophication. In the past 100 years, the area of the tidal flats has decreased by 90%. The distribution of species in the bay may vary as a result of these modifications. There is a risk that the biodiversity on the shallow and tidal flats would disappear. Restoring the coastal environment is the goal in order to preserve its natural biodiversity and allow people to enjoy it. Approximately 20,000 years ago, during the last glacial period, the steep valley of the Old Tokyo River carved out Tokyo Bay, which was once a continental shelf (Ito et al., 2018). A relative rise in sea level around 6,000 years ago caused the first inundations that gave origin to Tokyo Bay. Tokyo Bay finally took on its current shape as a result of sedimentary processes. Tokyo Bay is a sedimentary environment as a result. In the 1950s, the nearshore bottom sediment of the bay was primarily composed of sand, and the bay was surrounded by an oval-shaped, smooth shoreline with surrounding tidal flats that were roughly 2.6 km wide. This has evolved in the last few decades, with prominent changes to the bay seafloor sediment composition and coastline. Currently, channel dredging and landfill in the shallow water distinguish the shoreline. As a result, the tidal flats and shallows have undergone significant alteration. As a result, from 1900 to 2000, the surface area shrank by 26%. Compared to 136 $km^2$ in 1900, Tokyo Bay's current tidal flat area is barely 10 $km^2$. Fisheries in Tokyo Bay have developed significantly. Land use changed as a result of the growing population; for example, agricultural lands were converted to residential areas.

## 9.3. URBANIZED CENTERS

It is interesting to note that paddy fields have not been used as dry fields since restrictions make it impossible to change them. Most paddy fields are categorized as areas under urban jurisdiction. The urbanized centers are situated on reclaimed land or river deltas. As a result, man-made channels have been used to reroute the majority of significant rivers, including the Ara and Edo rivers. Tokyo Bay fisheries may have started in the Jomon period (12000–2500 BC). However, the significant advancement began in the Edo period (1603–1868 CE). Fisheries were encouraged by the Tokugawa Shogun family and the newly formed Edo people needed a supply of fish. In addition to bringing fishermen from western Japan to Edo, Shogun Ieyasu Tokugawa also supported the local fishermen who were already there. In this era, Nori mariculture began and developed into a significant Tokyo Bay product known as Edo-mae (Furukawa, 2015). Over the 260-year Edo period, there were many disputes amongst fishermen. Consequently, an Edo Bay fisheries protocol was created in 1816 with the assistance of five important fisheries parties in the bay and was supported by forty-four local fishing villages. The deeper offshore area was shared as a common resource and the shallow nearshore area was used solely by the local community, as per the protocol. In the 1950s, the annual capture of fish exceeded 130,000 tonnes, with shellfish accounting for around 90% of the total. In the 1960s, the catch began to progressively decrease, and by the 1970s, it was fewer than 50,000 tonnes annually. The drop in the amount of shellfish caught was the primary cause of this decline. Since the 1970s, the catch has been decreasing steadily. The overall annual catch of fish in the 2000s was 20,000 tons, which is less than one-sixth of Tokyo Bay's maximum harvest. The main causes of the decline in shellfish catch are thought to be as follows: habitat loss from reclamation in shallow-water and tidal flat areas; degradation from anoxic water, red tides, and blue tides; competition from newly introduced species;

diseases; and disruption of the tidal flat structure for benthic larvae transport. Seawater in the inner Tokyo Bay now has a shorter residence time than it did in the past. Saltwater spent 20 days in the inner bay during the summer and 40 days in the winter of 2002. In contrast, saltwater had a one-month summer residence period and a three-month winter residence period in the 1960s. The decrease in the bay surface area and the rise in freshwater intake brought about by people importing water from other catchment areas were the main causes of the seawater's shorter residence period.

## 9.4. MECHANISM OF SEAWATER EXCHANGE

The primary mechanism for seawater exchange in Tokyo Bay is estuary circulation brought on by freshwater input. As a result, the increased freshwater inflow improves seawater exchange and encourages estuary circulation. The tidal current speeds have decreased as a result of the decrease in sea surface area. Tokyo Bay vertical mixing is weakened and its stratification is reinforced by the decrease in tidal currents. As a result, seawater exchange is improved and estuary circulation is encouraged. The increase in imported water mass from nearby catchments during the 1960–1970 era was the cause of the increase in freshwater input. In the Tokyo Bay catchment area, the imported water mass was used for industrial and urban water.

The Kuroshio front reached the Uraga Channel during times of oceanic water incursion into the middle layer. However, the water mass was thought to have come from river water based on its salinity. This mass may have formed as a result of a substantial freshwater influx and the Kuroshio front approaching, which was influenced by the surface mixing that followed. Because of the incursion of ocean water, it is still challenging to gain a clear image of complex mass motion. A decrease in the inflow load does not immediately and directly alter the concentrations of N and P in the bay because significant amounts of both N and P are recycled inside the bay. Some researchers provided quantitative evidence to back up these findings by demonstrating the contribution of nutrients that come from the ocean. The percentages of total nitrogen (TN) and total phosphorus (TP) are 19% and 22%, respectively. Tokyo Bay has seen red tides, or algal blooms, up to 70 times a year, and blue tides, or the upwelling of hypoxic bottom water, up to 10 times annually, as a result of eutrophication. One important element of monitoring is COD. COD levels were elevated in the Tokyo Port region until 1985. The COD concentration in the water near the bay mouth showed signs of improvement. On the western side of the bay, a comparatively high concentration of COD extends southward, while on the eastern side, a relatively low concentration of COD extends northward. A high degree of anthropogenic activity is indicated by TN. Sewage treatment discharges have been abundant around the northwest side of the bay due to Tokyo Metropolitan's dense population.

## 9.5. TOTAL PHOSPHORUS (TP)

TP contributes significantly more from bottom sediment in addition to having the same amount from sewage treatment discharge as TN. This suggests that the upper part of the bay has an extra high-concentration area. Still, Tokyo Bay's eastern region is currently oligotrophic, particularly when it comes to dissolved inorganic phosphorus (DIP). Since 1995, nori mariculture has been severely lacking in nutrients. Extreme phytoplankton blooms are the cause of red tides. Red tides can be identified using a number of factors. For instance, Tokyo Metropolitan City uses three criteria to identify a red tide: less than 1.5 m of transparency; at least $10^3$ cells/ml, or $10^4$ cells/ml of phytoplankton density for large species; and at least 50 μg/l, or more, of chlorophyll a. Between 1900 and 1910, red tides were a rare occurrence in Tokyo Bay. Flagellates like Gymnodinium and Peridinium were the primary phytoplankton species. Data on the occurrences of red tides and the species that make them up are few before 1950. The types of phytoplankton that are present during red tide conditions have changed since the 1950s. Conditions for red tides containing diatoms like *Skeletonema costatum* started to appear. Red tide conditions containing *S. costatum* were common after the 1970s and continued to occur throughout the year (Baohong et al., 2021). However, flagellates rather than diatom species like Prorocentrum and Heterosigma akashiwo made up the extremely highly concentrated blooms. The frequency of red tide events in Tokyo Bay is not officially documented throughout history. Some researchers used scientific publications and municipal government information to provide an overview of the red tide incidence from 1907 to 1995. From the 1950s through the 1980s, the number grew progressively, reaching 20 days annually in the 1980s. Since then, the frequency has stayed the same at 15–20 days annually. Since the 1980s, the length of hypoxia in Tokyo Bay's bottom layer has stayed nearly consistent at three to four months annually. Anoxic water typically covers more than 50% of the inner bay during the summer. The lowest layer of anoxic water conditions promotes the release of hydrogen sulfide. The oxygen in the surface layer oxidizes some of the hydrogen sulfide to sulfur when the anoxic water with hydrogen sulfide upwells to it, turning the surface layer blue-white. We call this the blue tide (aoshio). Marine life is damaged by hydrogen sulfide. In Tokyo Bay, blue tide conditions arise in the inner bay throughout summer and autumn when strong north winds persist for many days.

## 9.6. BENTHIC SPECIES

Benthic organisms, including shellfish, suffer severe damage from the blue tides since they are unable to leave the ocean (Gobler et al., 2013). The blue tide conditions in Tokyo Bay were first observed in the 1950s. In the 1980s, blue tide frequency peaked at almost six times annually. Over the past 100 years, the area of tidal flats has shrunk by almost 90%. As 126 $km^2$ of tidal flats were reclaimed, an internal zone benthic biomass of 12.6 x $10^4$ tons was destroyed. Additionally, it has been claimed by some researchers that 3 x $10^4$ tonnes of bivalve biomass were killed in September 1985 by blue tide conditions. This indicates that the biological production in the shallows and tidal flats is at risk of disappearing. Although the COD, TN, and TP loads have dropped, the frequency of red tides and hypoxia in Tokyo Bay has not decreased. This is thought to be mostly due to the reduction in benthic biomass, which has lowered the bay's capacity to purify water. The material circulation cannot be healthy in the absence of enough benthic organisms. Significantly lower COD input loads were obtained after the Water Pollution Control Act was passed in 1971. Specifically, between 1979 and 1999, the levels of domestic and industrial wastewater dropped by half. In addition, the water treatment system reported an increased load due to the quick installation of sewage systems. The distribution of COD, TN, and TP throughout the bay as well as local patterns indicate the success of these efforts. The inner portion of the bay high-concentration area of COD has considerably decreased. TP seems to have changed more moderately since the contribution from sediment-based circulation is assumed to have offset the effects of the input decline. The distribution of benthic species in Tokyo Bay may have been impacted by environmental changes. The tidal flats preserved a rich benthic diversity even in the highly eutrophic inner part of the bay, whereas nearly no benthos was found in the northern middle part of the bay; and the diversity of sessile (sedentary) organisms was linked to changes in the water quality, such as salinity and transparency (allowing light). Among the potential explanations of these distributions is anthropogenic impact.

In the summer and fall, the inner portion of Tokyo Bay experiences significant hypoxia. In Tokyo Bay, Akita, and Niigata, *Mytilus galloprovincialis* was the predominant species; in other bays and regions, the predominant species were various bivalves, crabs, and polychaetes. The main dominating species in Dokai Bay has undergone significant alteration in the last 20–30 years. The inner side of the three bays, where the primary dominant species was most prevalent, had the lowest species diversity. While species diversity peaked in some areas of Tokyo and Osaka Bays, diversity in Ise-Mikawa Bay was dispersed. The species diversity decreases with increasing latitude. The impact of coastal structures and materials on the diversity of sessile organisms was unclear. The lack of a correlation between species diversity and abundance and the number of years following construction suggests that succession on vertical coastal structures occurs quickly. The maximum number of species decreased as the wave height increased. The abundance and wet weight of each species' population were highest below the mean sea level, while the maximum number of species was found between 1.0 and 6.0 m below the mean sea level. As the depth of the sampled layer increased, so did the diversity of species. Certain species became more abundant around mean sea level, which decreased species diversity. The patterns of distribution within the bay are another crucial factor. There are various distinct life stages for living species. An interstage larval network is created when larvae, juveniles, and adults are moved and reside in several locations at different phases of their life cycles. There are nodes and links in this network. The ecosystems in the bay are referred to as nodes, and the water circulation-driven transport systems in the bay are known as linkages. Urbanization may disrupt the functional integrity of these ecological networks since human activities have an impact on the habitats and movements of different organisms (Alberti and Marzluff, 2004).

## 9.7. ECOSYSTEM DEVELOPMENT APPROACHES

Research demonstrated that the ecosystems in Tokyo Bay might be enhanced through the preservation and restoration of appropriate spawning grounds, regardless of their size. Due to changes in the bay hydrology, the biological network has been significantly degraded, particularly in the northern to western region. Many locations (control points) have been assigned for monitoring and assessment for restoration and management. Using methods based on ecosystems, these places were identified. The upper western part of the bay is experiencing a substantial discharge due to the degradation of the asari (short-necked clam) larval network. Each monitoring site was defined as restoration goals, enabling the use of quantitative indicators of progress towards the goals (biodiversity/ dissolved oxygen (DO) level). It is predicted that reaching these goals will help improve the health of the nearby ecosystems. The effective activity surrounding the sites may improve environmental relatedness throughout the bay and hence advance the general health of the bay ecosystem by supplying node habitats. The monitoring point activities contributed to the creation of a model for the deployment of Sato-umi in urban areas. Sato-umi is a coastal landscape that has been used by people, resulting in high production and rich biodiversity (Berque and Matsuda, 2013). Following a decade of executing the action plan for the Tokyo Bay Renaissance, the council for the renaissance presented its achievements. The report highlighted the beneficial outcomes of programs on land load reduction, which enhanced the bay water quality, and the restoration and development of tidal flats and shallows, which raised the biomass and benthos richness in the bay. However, the summertime hypoxic environment has not resulted in a recovery of the bottom layer DO level. Assigning precise environmental indicators to evaluate different connected initiatives under the action plan is one of the issues. Increasing the number of people actively involved in Tokyo Bay Renaissance events is another difficulty. The degree of DO serves as a gauge for the effects of material cycling from the watershed to the bay ecosystem. It is a useful metric for the evaluation of the objective, but it is challenging to apply when evaluating supplemental, indirect efforts or contributions that improve the environment.

Drastic efforts alone will not be sufficient to restore the ecosystem of Tokyo Bay in a short amount of time. That can be accomplished by assembling potential small-scale efforts in an environmentally friendly way. Maintaining these efforts also requires a strong understanding of adaptive management. The public and commercial sector collaboration and engagement in putting these initiatives into action need to be improved. The Tokyo Bay Renaissance Promotion Council (2013) established an action plan for the second phase of the project in 2013. The framework was based on an earlier action plan and took the evaluation report into consideration. The plan now includes three new points: a stronger focus on goals that include promoting Edo-mae culture; recommendations for creating a new institutional structure to improve public-private partnerships; and the inclusion of a range of success indicators to evaluate the plan achievements. In November 2013, a forum for public-private cooperation was established for the rehabilitation of Tokyo Bay, involving the central government, local governments, industry, fisheries, recreational, and cultural sectors, as well as numerous non-profit organizations and the general public. The relationship between the public and private sectors will be sustained through this process. Channels, creeks, and gullies, sometimes known as tidal courses, are characteristic and important elements of natural coastal habitats. Tidal-influenced courses in particular have unique circulation characteristics that drain freshwater to the sea and flood salt marshes, mangroves, and tidal flats with seawater. Lateral embayments along a river promote longitudinal mixing. This kind of circulation properties should therefore be taken into account when restoring habitat in tidal courses. The main canal water was thoroughly mixed, and the minor canal was stratified. Nevertheless, freshwater inflow, tidal range, and terrain all played a role in determining these variations rather than just whether the channel was secondary or primary. Using public participation in float tests, the precise water circulation was ascertained. These studies demonstrated density-driven circulation, or estuary circulation, as a result of stratification in some locations. Seawater was brought into the canal's lowest stratum by this circulation. Therefore, it is believed that, within a certain area, the canal network functions like a tidal stream. The pools were inhabited by gobies (*Acanthogobius flavimanus*), mullets, and sandworms six months after the facilities were built. The average size of the gobies in the pools and the surrounding water suggested that the pools had a major function. Every goby in the pools was sampled by draining, and camera image processing was used to measure each goby length. The larger gobies seemed to have a habitat in deeper water. This is most likely related to the pool hydrology since shallower water has warmer summertime water that is high in DO.

## 9.8. *ACANTHOGOBIUS FLAVIMANUS* HABITATS

Some results demonstrate that gobies use the artificial habitats (pools) to support certain life stages of their life cycle rather than using them as a temporary habitat because they are surrounded by a dynamic estuarine environment. The creation of a habitat seems to improve the natural network inside the canal-bay setting. By preserving and rehabilitating ecosystems, it is crucial to improve the environmental services provided by canals with a good understanding of the movement of water and materials within them. Researchers, government officials, and NPO (non-profit organizations) stakeholders were involved in the soft approach to managing urban wetland ecosystems. These organizations have goals of their own. As a result, the project is method-oriented, with the aim already established. Adaptive management calls for the implementation of appropriate adjustments based on situational understanding and ongoing monitoring to achieve the aim. Along the current seawall, some government agencies built a terrace-tidal flat. The construction, structure, and morphological stability were observed a year later. It was also observed how quickly a variety of benthic species recovered. But in September 2009, there was a significant bivalve death on the tidal flat (Poirier et al., 2010). The intrusion of anoxic bottom water from the bay was one of the theories. Given that tidal flats are typically shallow areas with high DO concentrations, this appeared improbable. It is impossible to imagine that such a high rate of bivalve mortality could be caused by an entry of anoxic water. The middle terrace DO monitor record revealed that DO decreased in early July during nighttime inundation, but DO recovered in September during daylight flooding. The benthos local oxygen consumption was the reason for the decrease in DO. Semidiurnal tides and diurnal solar radiation can cause this. This results in a lot of anoxic water incidents in September, and late summer, especially in the shallow areas. It is probable that the local hypoxic environment had already caused damage to the benthos when the anoxic water intrusion caused the huge mortality. Nevertheless, further observation and monitoring are needed to fully comprehend this phenomenon, as this concept has not been verified. To provide a desirable habitat for benthos, the monitoring group engaged in management activities and carried out monitoring. It was impossible to stop the widespread fatalities of benthos despite their best attempts. Along with experts and the public sector, the group is always looking for better ways to manage the tidal flat. *Acanthogobius flavimanus* lay their eggs in the soft, saline seafloor in water that is 6 to 8 meters deep in the winter. The hatched larvae of gobies swim up to the edge of the estuary and land on the sandy, shallow seafloor in the spring. The fish reaches a maximum length of 15-20 cm in the autumn and 6-8 cm in the early summer. Seasons like these are great for accessible public fishing. Events centered around goby fishing have been planned to raise awareness of the culture and generate interest in the bay environmental restoration.

## 9.9. CENSUS

Some researchers confirmed the validity of fishing censuses undertaken in the 1950s by a diverse group of participants, ranging from trainees to specialists. They discovered that there were notable differences in the quantity of fish taken, but not in the size percentage of the catch. As a result, researchers employed the captured fish size as a gauge. Changes in existing habitat patterns and early growth are shown by this measure. The preliminary study indicates that goby habitat information has a potential as a valuable indicator of coastal environmental change, even though further scientific research is needed for the qualitative assessment of the change and its relationship with environmental state. The Seto Inland Sea has gone through both oligotrophication and eutrophication in the last 50 years. Regarding the change from year to year, there is a relationship between the phosphorus load and the frequency of red tide events and a counterclockwise hysteresis in the association between nutrient concentration and fish capture. The reason for this discrepancy can be attributed to the interplay between the organic matter that accumulated in the bottom sediment during the eutrophication period and the water quality. Because of the release of dissolved inorganic phosphorus from the bottom sediment, there are more red tides during the oligotrophication period than during eutrophication at the same phosphorus load. Because of the generation of hypoxia in the bottom layer during the stratification period, the amount of fish caught during oligotrophication is lower than during eutrophication at the same nutrient content.

## 9.10. WIND

As a land-sea breeze develops, the wind in coastal locations typically blows against the shoreline throughout the year. The direction of the wind in land areas is mostly determined by their unique geological characteristics. The Seto Inland Sea wind pattern is distinguished by its uniformity. Because weather patterns often influence the state of the water in the Seto Inland Sea, there is a higher seasonal variation in the salinity and temperature of the sea there than in the Pacific Ocean. Water is transferred via the Kii Channel and the Bungo Channel between the Pacific Ocean and the Seto Inland Sea, while the Kanmon Strait separates the Japan Sea from the Seto Inland Sea. The Seto Inland Sea's maximum tidal range is approximately 3 m at spring tide, and the tidal current in enclosed straits, like the Naruto and Hayasui Straits, is intricate, reaching speeds of 5 to 10 knots. The distinct features of the tide and tidal current in the Seto Inland Sea are influenced by intricate geological elements. In 2002, the 13 prefectures surrounding the Seto Inland Sea had a combined gross GDP of 129.8 trillion yen. Between 1965 and 1995, the gross product grew at a steady annual rate of roughly 6.53%. But since 1996, the growth has not been as noticeable, and the production level has stabilized. Beaches that are man-made have been constructed to replace destroyed natural beaches. The watershed area of the Seto Inland Sea witnessed the construction of many dams, with the number reaching its peak between 1966 and 1970, averaging roughly 10 per year. There are roughly 600 dams spread over the Seto Inland Sea watershed basin (Yanagi, 2015). The inner regions of Osaka Bay, Hiroshima Bay, and Beppu Bay were found to have low salinity, while these regions were found to have high TP and TN. Along with high TP and TN, high Chl a was also noted in the northern portion of Harima-Nada, the western portion of the Kii Channel, the inner portion of Osaka Bay, and Hiroshima Bay. In general, the quality of the sea sediment is declining, especially in regions where there is slight tidal motion or stagnant water. In areas with high mud content, such as Beppu Bay, Osaka Bay, Harima-Nada, Hiuchi-Nada, Hiroshima Bay, and the southwest of Suo-Nada, high TP and TN were observed. Poor ORP was recorded in these regions. Where TP and TN were low, Bisan-Seto, in the western portion of Bingo-Nada and Aki-Nada, had high populations of macro-benthos species. Osaka Bay, Harima-Nada, Hiuchi-Nada, Hiroshima Bay, the southwest portion of Suo-Nada, and Beppu Bay, where TP and TN were high, were found to have low biodiversity. No metrics changed over the 20-year period in any of the categories when comparing the most recent data with the earlier data, except ORP. Furthermore, no location showed further declines in the quality of the silt; rather, all places, especially Suo-Nada, showed some improvement in the quality of the sediment.

When comparing the latest data with the data collected a decade ago, statistically significant variations were found in the number of macro-benthos species and individuals at the following locations: Harima-Nada (individuals decreased), Hiuchi-Nada (species decreased and individuals decreased), Kii

Channel (species decreased), Bisan-Seto (species increased), Bungo Channel (species increased), and Aki-Nada (species increased and individuals decreased). When comparing the findings of the observation carried out by the Japanese Fisheries Agency two decades prior, it was believed that in the majority of the cases, the variety and quantity of macro-benthos had either declined or remained unchanged. The primary cause of this alteration is believed to be the result of ongoing hypoxia. Though the relationships between the environments of water and sediment and the environments of aquatic animals and plants are not fully understood, it is believed that because of tidal currents that are not very strong and human activity, it is simple for pollutants to accumulate in sea regions where there is a high concentration of sludge in the sediment. In certain areas, summertime transparency is often low with regard to water quality. Another significant element influencing sediment quality standards is the impact of sea-sand mining in the Seto Inland Sea, which ceased in 2006 after more than 50 years of operation. The entire region of the Seto Inland Sea with a sandy sea bottom was mined for sea sand, which had a negative impact on the seagrass bed turbidity and topography as well as the bottom ecosystem. Since sand eels (*Ammodytes personatus*) spend the summer months sleeping on the sandy bottom, it had a particular impact on the ecology of sand eels (Huard et al., 2022).

## 9.11. RED TIDES

Red tides may last longer in the coastal area than in the offshore area because the RTI (Red Tide Index) in the restricted coastal area within two kilometers of the coast is similar in magnitude to that in the large offshore area. RTI's long-term trend is comparable to the number of incidences. There were just 18 instances of red tides in the 1960s, and the affected area was minor. Large-scale red tides were common in the 1970s and 1980s, particularly in the summer. The Seto Inland Sea, which has very calm sea conditions, is well-known for its nori and oyster cultures. To make up for the declining conditions in which fish and shellfish live, a variety of aquaculture projects have been launched, which benefits the marine production sector in the Seto Inland Sea. The Seto Inland Seas water quality is not significantly impacted by a reduction in TP and TN loading from the land. Less than 10% of airborne TP and TN are found near the Seto Inland Sea. Since the 1950s, the Seto Inland Sea has been the center of heavy industry, including shipbuilding, petrochemicals, and steel. Many coastal areas have been reclaimed for ports and industries as a result of this process. About 20% of the shallow sea, or less than 10 meters, has been reclaimed due to extensive reclamation efforts. This has severely damaged marine life, including benthos, tidal flats, seagrass beds, and seaweed beds. Since 1994, the concentration of

DIN (dissolved inorganic nitrogen) in Harima-Nada and the Bisan Strait has dropped, whereas the concentration of TN has stayed relatively constant. The limiting nutrient for primary production in Hakima-Nada has shifted from DIP (dissolved inorganic phosphorus) to DIN. The primary phytoplankton species in Harima-Nada, the diatom, had no change in cell density, but the predominant species of diatoms had shifted from Skeletonema spp. to Chaetoceros spp.

The material cycling of biochemical elements in the marine environment, particularly the related marine ecosystem, is hypothesized to have changed. These elements include DIP, DOP (dissolved organic phosphorus), POP (particulate organic phosphorus), DIN, DON (dissolved organic nitrogen), and PON (particulate organic nitrogen). The Seto Inland Sea material cycling needs to return to a suitable marine environment supported by a healthy marine ecosystem. Although the TP and TN concentrations in the Pacific Ocean have not changed, the averaged TP and TN concentrations in the Seto Inland Sea started to decline in 2009. Consequently, because of the coupling effect of declining TP and TN loads and declining mineralization via biochemical processes, oligotrophication will persist. While fish output in the Seto Inland Sea was not poor, nutrient concentrations were low and biodiversity was high during the 1960s, when the period of fast economic growth began. Fish output rose along with nutrient concentrations during the time of strong economic growth because of the increase in nutrient loads from the land. DIN started to decline in the late 1990s, mostly as a result of modifications to the nitrogen material cycling brought about by adjustments to biochemical processes as a result of modifications to the marine habitat.

Rather than having a vertically raised concrete wall along its coastline, Kansai International Airport, which is located on an artificial island (Osaka Bay), was built with a gentle slope of natural rocks and stones. This gently sloping, environmentally favorable area served as a good place for seaweed beds and a shelter for a variety of different species. This anthropogenic structure is now functioning as a new seaweed bed and ecosystem as a result. Given that the original location of the airport was a patch of muddy sea floor, this is an excellent illustration of environmentally responsible, creative environmental restoration. While the impact of the artificial island must be appropriately assessed, it is equally important to consider the effects of a naturally occurring slope, as the newly established seaweed bed serves as a buffer for the extensively depleted seaweed bed in Osaka Bay. To increase material cycling in the coastal water at Mizushima-Nada in Okayama Prefecture, the water discharged from the dam is increased during the summer when precipitation decreases. This is because a decrease in river discharge leads to a decrease in estuarine circulation and stagnant coastal water. The decline in habitat conditions and ecosystem services was evident from the early assessment of the environmental health of the Seto Inland Sea. One of the most vital things that has to be done in the Seto Inland Sea is to restore these shallow-water habitats, such as tidal flats and seaweed and seagrass beds. Sato-umi can offer better biological diversity as a habitat and high biological production as fishing grounds as compared to a declining coastal environment. To construct functionally efficient Sato-umi in each local coastal area, a new holistic method for sustainable biological production and control of eutrophic levels must be developed.

The severity and duration of hypoxia events have decreased due to decreasing eutrophication, while the diversity of red tide organisms has grown despite the constant frequency of red tide development (Zohdi and Abbaspour, 2019). As light penetration has increased, macroalgae have spread to deeper and inner regions of the bay. In the inner bay, the higher dissolved oxygen level produces some species like fish, shrimp, and crabs, in particular, much more common on the bottom, especially during the summer. Red tide organism density was found to be lowered by the filter-feeding mussel through the use of bioremediation. The building also functions as a fish collection spot and a site for environmental education. The ecosystems in the bay are enhanced by a seaweed bed bioremediation facility. The water quality has significantly improved since the hypoxic areas disappeared, and it is expected that species that were once common in the bay may reappear in large numbers as a result of their habitats being restored. The severe acute toxicities of industrial wastewater discharged into the bay were confirmed by bioassays utilizing fish.

Chapter 10

# WETLANDS AND EUTROPHICATION

## Contents

## 10.1. INTRODUCTION

The wetlands (Figure 10.1) are nutrient sinks, they have been utilized for the disposal of wastewater, which has severely altered their structure and function (Carey and Migliaccio, 2009). Hydrological changes, including changes in vegetation patterns and nitrogen cycling, are typically associated with fertilizer loading. The process of eutrophication in wetlands promotes microbial activity, soluble nutrients in sediments, organic matter decomposition, and buildup of organic matter and nutrients. It also speeds up primary productivity. Even in years with minimal external inputs, internal loading takes over as the wetland primary source of nutrients, regulating the dynamics of nutrients.

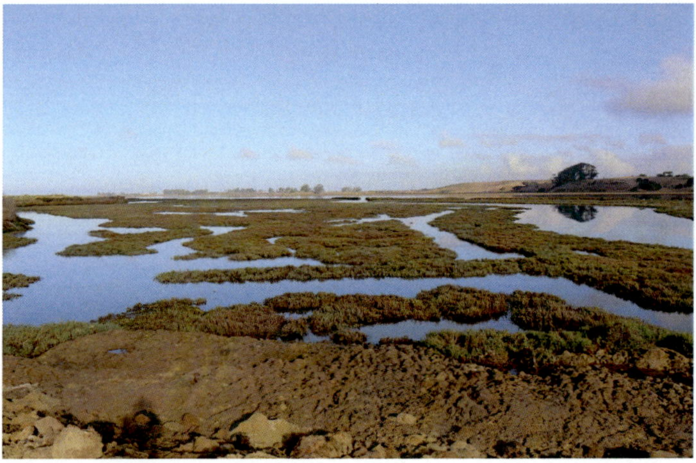

**Figure 10.1.** *Wetlands.*

Source: https://upload.wikimedia.org/wikipedia/commons/1/1a/Elkhorn_Slough_designated_%22Wetland_of_International_Importance%22_02.jpg, Creative Commons License.

The most sensitive microbiological indicator to nutrient enrichment in wetlands appears to be mineralized phosphorus in wetland soils since soil biomass reacts favorably to phosphorus enrichment in wetlands. Thus, the key element controlling the degree of eutrophication in wetlands is the internal influx of phosphorus. As long as pollution levels remain high, wetland nitrate availability will remain high, potentially increasing their future emissions of N2O and N2. The biological signs (indicators) of eutrophication-degraded wetlands are similar to those found in shallow lakes. The presence of phytoplankton and increased fish biomass, both planktivorous and benthivorous, are evident in the turbid state. The main route that zooplanktivorous fish contribute to eutrophication is through the influence of food webs. During bottom feeding, benthivorous fish primarily move nutrients that are bonded to sediment into the water column, increasing the amount of nutrients available to phytoplankton. Wetland management officials have not made extensive use of the methodology that was found to be effective in the restoration of shallow lakes. Wetland sediments store a significant amount of nutrients; therefore, watershed nutrient management schemes may not be enough. However, new research suggests that biomanipulation of fish standing stocks could play a major role in reducing wetland eutrophication. Thus, biomanipulation may be a low-cost, high-benefit technique for reducing wetland eutrophication when it is implemented in conjunction with sediment dredging and other interventions at the proper time to correspond with low water levels.

## 10.2. WETLAND USES

It is well recognized that wetlands serve as landscape filters, converting and holding onto various substances, including phosphorus and nitrogen. Despite making up only 1.5% of the surface, wetlands provide up to 40% of its renewable ecosystem services. River water quality can be significantly improved by biogeochemical processes in wetlands, while the effectiveness of these processes varies depending on the type of wetland and its location in the landscape. Because of its effectiveness, a lot of wetlands have been built and hydraulically regulated to take out phosphorus and nitrate from wastewaters. However, due to the natural wetland's ability to retain nutrients, they have also been utilized for a long time as locations to dispose of wastewater, which has led to eutrophication, a serious alteration of the wetland structure and function. Although the great variability of wetlands linked with the hydrological disturbance constitutes a prominent difference from shallow lakes, the symptoms of eutrophication in wetlands are similar to those in shallow lakes. Hydrological fluctuations cause changes in nutrient budgets and, consequently, in the ecological functioning of wetlands, as hydrology is the primary force influencing wetland ecology. However, recent research is starting to draw attention to the drawbacks of exposing natural wetlands to extended nutrient loading because it can lead to the emissions of greenhouse gases or GHGs into the atmosphere, which exacerbates the detrimental effects of global climate change.

## 10.3. NITROGEN CYCLING

Nevertheless, not enough research has been done in wetlands to understand how nitrogen cycling is changed and the consequences of nutrient enrichment on biological communities. These subjects are critical to understanding the patterns of wetland eutrophication. Wetlands are distinct hydrosystems in which the amount of water fluctuates periodically, even between seasons. The term wetland hydroperiod refers to this annual variation in water level, which indicates how long and what percentage of the year the wetland is covered in water. The hydroperiod, which includes all elements of the wetland water budget, precipitation, evapotranspiration, runoff from nearby regions, flooding, and net seepage of groundwater, is most likely the primary indicator of a wetland ecosystem that influences both structural (biota) and functional (biogeochemical transformations) aspects. Depending on regional variations in physiography and temperature as well as soil moisture levels, a wetland site's duration and frequency of flooding varies depending on its hydrodynamic setting(Santisteban et al., 2019). Water level variations are essential to comprehending wetland eutrophication processes because the wetland hydroperiod regulates nutrient cycling through modifications to soil redox transformations. The wetlands fall into three main hydroperiod classifications: short, intermediate, and long-duration inundations. Ephemeral wetlands retain water for fewer than four months of the year and are found in short hydroperiods. During the summer, these wetlands typically dry out. Ephemeral wetlands, which retain water for at least four months and typically dry out in late summer or later, completely drying out only in years with little precipitation, are another feature of intermediate hydroperiods. As a result, in certain years, these wetlands can retain water all year round. The wetlands with long hydroperiods are those that retain water continuously and never dry up. Lakes and certain ponds are referred to as permanent wetlands. Hydrodynamically, wetlands can also be identified based on the degree of habitat. It demonstrates how connected wetlands are to downstream areas and has a significant impact on ecosystem dynamics since they export chemicals and water downstream, which influences chemical processes and retention. Wetland nutrient loading is closely linked to a wetland system's rate of water turnover, also known as water renewal time, and the degree of closure of that system. Wetland production, the breakdown of organic matter, and the cycling of nutrients are all influenced by nutrient loading, which is generally determined by a wetland's accessibility to hydrological fluxes.

## 10.4. WATER-SEDIMENT EXCHANGE

Changes in the chemical forms and spatial mobility of nutrients within wetlands, as well as water-sediment exchanges, plant absorption, and interactions with adjacent ecosystems, are all influenced by the different hydrologic conditions found in wetlands. Wetland soils undergo the majority of nutrient changes due to the shallow nature of wetlands (Sánchez-Carrillo and Álvarez-Cobelas, 2001). While most biogeochemical reactions in upland soils are governed by oxygen, in wetlands during inundation, oxygen is limited due to water filling the soil pores. The temperature of the surrounding air, the presence of organic substrates for microbial respiration, and occasionally the chemical oxygen demand from reducing substances like ferrous iron all affect how quickly oxygen is lost. Reduction of inorganic electron acceptors, buildup of reduced molecules, and accumulation of organic matter as an electron donor source all take place in anaerobic environments. When oxygen is present in the substrate, bacteria always use it first because it is their preferred electron acceptor. Microorganisms that are obligate anaerobic and facultative anaerobes dominate the substrate when oxygen is absent. These specialized bacteria can promote the biological oxidation of organic molecules by switching to other oxidants in place of oxygen. There is a pattern to the thermodynamic reduction of inorganic electron acceptors in response to variations in oxygen supply. The order in which microbial functions occur in anaerobic environments is determined by the reduction in metabolic free energy. In wetland soils, the reduction process begins with oxygen and proceeds to oxygen oxides, elemental sulfur, oxides of iron and manganese, sulfate (sulfate reduction), and carbon dioxide (methanogenesis). The concentration of these substances, the organic compounds that degrade quickly, and the microbial population involved in the process all affect how quickly these substances are digested in marsh soil. Within a few hours to a few days following inundation, marsh soils experience oxygen depletion. The denitrification process begins during the initial aerobic stages and accelerates significantly when oxygen is reduced. On the other hand, iron reduction does not start until completely anaerobic conditions are reached.

## 10.5. INUNDATION

During inundation, the oxygen demand remains high despite the limited oxygen delivery to the wetland soil. Because of these conditions, a thin layer of oxidized surface soil develops, which has a major impact on controlling phosphorus sorption and nitrogen reactions. It also serves as a sink for reduced chemicals that permeate from the anaerobic soil layer underneath it. Nitrogen is the most limiting nutrient in flooded soils, despite research showing some discrepancy on the roles of N and P in restricting the productivity of aquatic ecosystems. One of the primary nutritional transformations taking place in wetlands is the microbial denitrification of nitrates to gaseous forms of nitrogen and their subsequent release to the atmosphere due to the anoxic conditions present in wetlands. Nitrates are a crucial component in the oxidation of organic matter in wetlands because they are among the first terminal electron acceptors in wetland soils following the removal of oxygen. Many microbial activities are involved in the nitrogen transformations in wetlands. For many of the nitrogen processes, the soil oxidized zone over the anaerobic zone is essential.

Wetlands are particularly interesting for nitrogen retention because they retain about twice as much nitrogen as lakes. Research has demonstrated that the primary determinants of nitrogen retention are the nitrogen input and the water residence time. The density, cover, and hydrodynamic openness of macrophyte stands, as well as those resulting from human intervention, all influence the reduced rate of water regeneration in wetlands. Denitrification has been found to be larger than sedimentation, although nitrogen sedimentation is frequently thought of as the main process of nitrogen retention in wetlands. Denitrifying bacteria are crucial to the carbon cycle of wetlands because they make a substantial contribution to the carbon mineralization budget. In comparison to denitrification or sedimentation, macrophyte absorption seems to have less impact on the retention of nitrogen.

## 10.6. AQUATIC PLANTS

Aquatic plants have an indirect impact on nitrogen cycling because they store nitrogen during the growing season, despite the relatively less weight of plant intake in overall nitrogen retention. By adding particulate matter to sediments during their senescence, nutrient uptake by plant wetlands influences the rates of nutrient sedimentation. By providing potentially limiting amounts of organic carbon and nitrate to denitrifying bacteria, wetland vegetation helps to produce an environment that is conducive to denitrification. It is known that water renewal time and nitrogen loading influence nitrogen export downstream in open wetlands. N export downstream in wetlands appears to be lower, oscillating between 10% and 40% of the N imports. In very few instances, phosphorus is not a limiting factor in wetlands. When compared to available nitrogen in wetlands, the phosphorus requirements of biota are typically lower than those of nitrogen. Many wetland communities can assimilate phosphorus above what is necessary and store it as polyphosphates in their tissues. It has been noted in several wetland plants, like *Leersia oryzoides*, as well as sediment microbes (Pierce et al., 2010). Wetlands have the potential to store water and hence function as a source or a sink of phosphorus. Phosphorus-rich wetlands typically supply nearby ecosystems with phosphorus. Macrophytes, periphyton and plankton, plant litter and detrital accumulation, soil physicochemical properties, water flow velocity, water depth, hydraulic retention time, the wetland length-to-width ratio, phosphorus loading, and hydrologic fluctuations have all been linked to the regulation of phosphorus retention in wetlands. Some researchers identified several mechanisms for retaining phosphorus in the water column, including uptake and release by microbes, periphyton, and aquatic plants; sorption and exchange interactions with soils and sediments; chemical precipitation in the water column; and sedimentation.

## 10.7. PHOSPHORUS ACCUMULATION

Wetlands are thought to have a high capacity to accumulate phosphorus in soils because they offer nearly all of these favorable conditions. Depending on the wetland hydrology, substrate composition, and redox conditions, wetlands can retain 40–90% of total phosphorus inputs. Because the water entering wetlands is poorly mixed, concentrations are usually highest close to the inflows and decrease with distance from the source. The gradients are the same in man-made and natural wetlands that receive phosphorus-enriched inflows. The phosphorus transport through the marsh is plug flow, and the wetland soil next to the inflow has substantial phosphate deposition. Phosphorus seasonal retention rates typically peak in the late summer, coinciding with the macrophyte senescence stage. Phosphorus is only partially stored in wetland substrates. Because natural wetlands are also sites where sediment accumulates, they have the ability to store phosphorus if the rate of sediment accretion exceeds the rate of phosphorus absorption. The wetlands utilized as wastewater treatment systems experienced phosphorus saturation after a few years due to the surplus phosphate being exported. Wetland soil's ability to retain abiotic phosphorus is influenced by many factors, including pH, organic matter content, phosphorus loading, and soil concentration. Phosphorus solubility and retention in wetland soils are impacted by shifts in redox potential. The soil dissolved P contents rose in low-redox environments and dropped as redox potential increased. The phosphorus sorption in marsh soils is associated with weak crystalline forms of iron and aluminum. The wetlands' indirect influence on phosphorus sorption is mediated by total organic matter that has complexed with iron and aluminum. Phosphorus retention (adsorption) in soils occurs at low concentrations, so if the concentration in soil pore water rises above the soil's ability to adsorb P, some solid phases like dicalcium phosphate, octacalcium phosphate, and hydroxyapatite in an alkaline environment may precipitate. Similar to this, as phosphorus accumulates over time in soils, the pore fluid dissolved phosphorus concentrations increase, causing a flow from the soil to the water column above. Phosphorus is released after plants die, so plant uptake and incorporation into detrital tissues only need to be thought of as short-term storage, even though periphyton and some macrophytes have shown statistically significant relationships with phosphorus concentration in the water column. The long-term phosphorus storage of the wetland ecosystems can be attributed to the abiotic retention of inorganic phosphorus in soils.

The total phosphorus content of wetland soils ranges from 30 to 500 mg P $kg^{-1}$ in wetlands that are not affected by anthropogenic phosphorus loading to more than 10,000 mg P $kg^{-1}$ in severely eutrophicated wetlands that receive significant phosphorus discharges from urban wastewater and agricultural operations. Although phosphorus is not a limiting nutrient in wetlands, open wetlands typically have poor phosphorus export downstream. Phosphorus concentration near the outflow during high flooding periods has increased as a result of wetlands' long-term exposure to high nutrient loading. The wetland hydrological variability means that the ecosystem receives nutrient inputs from diverse sources, some of which can vary seasonally or annual. Large quantitative changes in nutrient supplies to the wetland are caused by fluctuations in hydrological conditions. However, the hydrologic regime frequently has little bearing on how much weight external vs internal nutrient sources have in the wetland nutrient budget. This is a characteristic that sets wetlands apart from lakes. In lakes, where plankton mostly depends on external supplies for nutrient cycling, macrophytes and microbial communities often regulate nutrient cycles in wetlands through sedimentation and recycling. As a result of ongoing bacterial recycling, internal loading, the release of accumulated nutrients into the water column, makes up the majority of the nutrient component in wetlands. Through increased primary productivity, external nutrient loading raises the net accumulation of organic matter and related nutrients in wetlands. Nevertheless, higher loading raises the amount of soluble forms of nutrients in soils as well as their overall content, which may be discharged into the water column.

## 10.8. BIOGEOCHEMICAL PROCESSES

Biogeochemical processes in wetlands are impacted by increased nutrient loading, which modifies nutrient fluxes and water and soil concentrations (Caffrey et al., 2007). The physical and chemical environment of the marsh is changed by these ecosystem-wide changes. Reducing the amount of nutrients in ecosystems boosts primary productivity and activates microbial activity. The chemical and physical makeup (composition) of the soil, microbial activity, and nutrient availability all affect the breakdown of organic matter in wetlands. Therefore, wetlands may experience severe physical and hydrological alterations as a result of changes impacting soil characteristics caused by an increase in organic matter and accretion (deposition) rates, including the short-term extinction of wetlands due to siltation. An increase in wetland plant productivity is the initial stage of nutrient enrichment in wetlands. Many wetlands have shown high primary productivity in nutrient-rich sites. It encourages a rise in the accumulation of autochthonous organic matter in wetland soils. Changes in vegetation patterns i.e., plant species replacement are typically associated with increases in nutrient loading and hydrological changes. Thus, in high-nutrient situations, it is reasonable to predict changes in the organic supply and litter quality. Strong changes in decomposition rates and nutrient cycling can also be anticipated as wetlands become eutrophic because microbial activity reacts to nutrient loading and hydrology. A rise in the internal loading of the wetland and thus a decrease in nutrient retention can be anticipated following an extended period of exposure to high nutrient loading. The sediment discharges into the water column tend to enhance the nutrient soluble forms during eutrophication. This means that more nutrients available encourage higher production, which starts a positive feedback process that can last for years. The fertilizer loading into these wetlands promotes microbial activity and organic matter breakdown, which increases nutrient concentrations in the water.

## 10.9. PHOSPHORUS ENRICHMENT

Phosphorus enrichment in wetlands causes a favorable response in soil phosphorus microbial biomass (Corstanje et al., 2007). Microbial biomass related to carbon and nitrogen did not always react to nutrient input. Although they are connected to the C and N cycles, microbes cannot be sensitive to nutrient loading. While phosphorus is the most responsive microbiological indicator to nutrient enrichment in wetlands, eutrophication accelerates the mineralization rates of both nitrogen and phosphorus. There seems to be a substantial correlation between soil total phosphorus and phosphorus microbial biomass and mineralized phosphorus in wetland soils. Since S2 produced by SO42- reduction interacts with Fe-PO43- complexes in the sediment to form $FeS_2$ and FeS, which in turn mobilize phosphate, increased sulfate availability in wetlands is known to cause major eutrophication problems. It has been suggested that eutrophication of sulfate-rich freshwater wetlands is inhibited by high nitrate concentrations in groundwaters. Even though total phosphorus loading rates in natural and artificial freshwater wetlands are higher than the critical loads suggested to prevent eutrophication, wetlands still face significant challenges in maintaining their structural integrity and functional integrity. Because temperature and precipitation are major regulators of the function of freshwater wetland ecosystems, the probable impact of climate change on wetlands indicates that they will be drastically altered. As water renewal time increases, the wetland flushing rate will decrease due to lower water availability. The high nutrient status is likely to rise as a result of the promotion of biogeochemical processes. Similarly, changes in $N_2O$ and $N_2$ emissions as a result of eutrophication are possible since wetlands are a substantial natural source of greenhouse gases in the atmosphere. The IPCC states that nitrogen emissions have the potential to cause global warming 310 times greater than those of carbon dioxide. This is because rising pollution is likely to keep nitrate availability in wetlands high. Reducing nitrate rather than $N_2O$ is energetically advantageous for denitrifiers when nitrate availability is high. This possible drawback of wetlands rich in nitrates is minimized.

## 10.10. ECOLOGICAL INDICATORS

The ecological indicators of eutrophication-degraded wetlands are similar to those of temperate shallow lakes. Wetlands have been linked to increased water turbidity and nutrient levels, changes in macrophyte dominance from submerged to phytoplankton, reduced zooplankton biomass, increased planktivorous and benthivorous fish biomass, and piscivorous fish losses. The trophic cascade hypothesis and alternative state (ASS) theory predict these changes (Santos et al., 2020). According to the ASS concept, ecological systems can transition between different states. These transitions or transformations can be caused by changes in abiotic environmental situations that lead to community shifts or by altered community structure in similar abiotic environments. The ASS paradigm in aquatic ecology is based on studies conducted in shallow, north-temperate lakes, where the primary cause of the lake transition from a clear-water, submerged macrophyte-dominated state to a degraded, turbid, phytoplankton-dominated state is cultural eutrophication. The urgent environmental issues we face require us to take into account a variety of human-caused effects that work in tandem with climate change to potentially permanently shift ecosystems to other states. This presents difficulties in maintaining novel ecosystems in a sustainable manner that ensures that humans will continue to get ecosystem services, going beyond the simple management of nutrient loading and algal blooms. Given the numerous ecological services that wetlands offer to both people and wildlife, it is important to comprehend the mechanisms that cause wetland ecosystems to change between ASS to effectively analyze the effects of management interventions and conduct impact assessments.

## 10.11. TROPHIC LEVELS AND EUTROPHICATION

Apart from the notion of alternative states, there is ample evidence to suggest that knowledge of trophic cascading interaction is beneficial in comprehending the responses of ASS in wetlands. The structure of food webs and, thus, the trophic cascade interactions between fish and plankton appear to be mediated by the trophic status of aquatic ecosystems. Despite a substantial decrease in external nutrient loading, many aquatic habitats impacted by urban or agricultural activities continue to be eutrophic. Significant amounts of phosphorus have the potential to be held in sediments, which would help to keep wetlands in their deteriorated state. With so many nutrients present, wetlands stay in a turbid (degraded) phase; phytoplankton is prevalent and the fish community is dominated by zooplanktivores and/or benthivores. Benthivorous and planktivorous fish can have different effects on the food web structure and the features of the ecosystem under such situations. The primary way that zooplanktivorous fish contribute to eutrophication in shallow lakes and wetlands is through food web-mediated impacts, which reduce zooplankton abundance and free phytoplankton from grazing. High turbidity is a result of high phytoplankton biomass, which limits submerged macrophytes. During bottom foraging, benthivorous fish release nutrients that are bonded to sediment into the water column, hence increasing the availability of nutrients for phytoplankton. By resuspension of sediment particles and mechanical damage to submerged macrophytes, benthivorous fish, such as common carp, also contribute to excessive non-algal turbidity. The community structure in wetlands and shallow lakes varies at lower nutrient concentrations, which is characteristic of the clear-water state. The better light conditions have led to the dominance of submerged macrophytes. Large daphnids find refuge from predators in plants, which helps regulate phytoplankton through zooplankton grazing. The system may shift to either a clear or turbid state at intermediate nutrient concentrations, but internal stabilizing mechanisms like crayfish and planktivorous and benthivorous fish may have different shifts. Although the exact causes of the prevalence of each state in various years with intermediate nutrient concentrations are still unknown, weather conditions, such as mild or severe winters, may be important.

## 10.12. DAMAGED AQUATIC ECOSYSTEMS

The restoration of damaged aquatic ecosystems should take precedence over catchment efforts to accomplish eutrophication reduction (Jeppesen et al., 2012). However, research on shallow lakes has indicated that because of the significant nitrogen storage in sediments, catchment nutrient management plans may not be enough. Therefore, internal management of lakes may be more effective in reducing the impacts of eutrophication. Wetlands are shallow ecosystems by definition, which has significant management concerns. Planktivorous and benthivorous fish effects in shallow lakes are said to increase with decreasing water depth. Similar claims have been made for wetlands. Given the important role that fish play in lake food webs, it should come as no surprise that the biomanipulation paradigm is primarily predicated on the idea that changes to the structure of fish communities have a cascade effect on lower trophic levels, hence enhancing the quality of the water. The intricacy of wetland food webs and the significant impact of abiotic variables necessitate an emphasis on various groups and habitats. There is a chance that some species will harm the environment more than help it, so a thorough assessment of the effects is required. Large stretches of riparian wetlands are covered in emergent vegetation. It is evident that emergent vegetation is a crucial biotic component of this wetland. The earliest signs of stress conditions at the community level are found in the structure and size ranges of plankton. The effects of the declining resource availability for planktivorous adult fish and the larvae and juveniles of ichthyophagous fish produce alterations in the trophic web. One significant kind of interspecies interaction in food webs is top-down control. The natural top-down management of phytoplankton and the water self-purification process can be threatened by chemical pollution, although phytoplankton grazers aid in this process. On the one hand, a direct toxic effect may cause a decline in phytoplankton populations. This procedure can identify the system's declining carbon and energy transfer efficiency. However, the decline in phytoplankton has a detrimental effect on cladoceran filtering rates, which in turn impacts the growth rates of these organisms. There may also be an impact on the rate of nutrient regeneration and water transparency.

Zooplankton assemblages may be used as indicators of water quality by indirectly influencing zooplankton composition due to abiotic conditions that are known to directly affect phytoplankton. The pollutants can be detected even in areas that are typically less polluted and eventually make their way into the water. Some researchers reported heavy metals in many categories of Antarctic invertebrates. It is suggested that bioremediation, employing local macrophytes like *Eichornia crassipes*, remove metals and nutrients from wastewaters. To decontaminate industrial effluents containing metals, the biosorbent potential of algal cells for hazardous metals also presents an efficient and reasonably priced substitute to traditional approaches. By substituting fewer contaminating techniques for chromium salts in the tannery leather process, the most contaminated industries should be kept under control. The United Nations Environment Program determined that chromium salts ought to be utilized due to their strong affinity for the carboxylic groups in collagen fibers and their relatively inexpensive cost in relation to less polluting techniques. We must keep in mind that the biota, which includes humans, is the primary target of contamination. Many plant species in Europe are in danger of extinction as a result of widespread eutrophication and fragmentation. The plant diversity of soft water lakes in northern Europe is possibly severely affected by these global changes. Some researchers found that disturbances such as sedimentation, turbidity, retention time, eutrophication, and changes in hydrologic time led to changes in the composition of plant species, a decline in fauna, a reduction in biodiversity, a decrease in secondary production, an increase in flood peaks and frequency, an increase in above-ground production, and the extinction of aquatic plant species with high light compensation points. It has been observed that eutrophic lakes (20–30%) retain more nitrogen overall annually than oligotrophic lakes. Phosphorus had a limiting effect on the retention of nitrogen in Norwegian lakes. The factors controlling species diversity in planktonic ecosystems have received comparatively less attention than in terrestrial and benthic situations. This is mostly because there is a lack of experimental data from field investigations that sufficiently resolve the wide range of spatiotemporal scales.

## 10.13. FARMING PRACTICES

Many European countries still have low-intensity farming practices that support species-rich grasslands (Ekroos et al., 2020). When such systems are heavily exploited, the number of species in them declines. The restoration of these ecosystems is impacted by abiotic restrictions like eutrophication and acidity. In Galveston Bay, USA, the increasing nutrient loading resulted in coastal eutrophication and climatic disturbances, i.e., hurricanes, floods, and droughts. Because of the high phosphorus levels, the area was found to be quite eutrophic. The regional water body types were discovered to depend on total phosphorus, water flux, water transparency, and macrophyte occurrence. The loss of biodiversity was facilitated by the eutrophic conditions. The constant growth ofalgae biomass in lakes, reservoirs, streams, and rivers, as well as in the ecosystem of coastal lagoons, is a result of eutrophication. An integrated long-term measure of ecosystem functioning with structural attributes like biomass and diversity is provided by the biofilm assemblages of algae, fungi, and microorganisms found in the sediments of aquatic systems. The introduction of loose strip (*Lydhrum salicaria*) into North American wetlands has been discovered to have an impact on the downstream water quality. This impact has also been observed to affect the decomposition rates and nutrient cycling of other species. *Typha augustifolia* and *T. latifolia* became more established as a result of the eutrophication of Lake Balaton in Hungary, which led to an increase in the composition of sediments. Numerous studies of terrestrial ecosystems in North America and western European wetlands demonstrate that nutrient enrichment causes species composition changes, a decrease in the variety of plant species overall, and the extinction of rare and uncommon species.

While nutrients, temperature, pH, dissolved oxygen, carbon dioxide, and light limit the growth and development of aquatic plants, physical processes within a water source have a significant impact on controlling eutrophication in aquatic bodies. Significant relationships were found between the species composition of plants and potash concentrations, water depth, groundwater levels in winter and summer, and elevation ofbank vegetation. The concentration, pH, $Cl^-$, organic carbon, $NH_4^+$, and water temperature were all correlated with the aquatic vegetation. There has been evidence of a change in the primary producers from eelgrass to macroalgae, which modifies the food web. The density and biomass of eelgrass shoots increased with the increase in nitrogen load. Aquatic weeds covered the water surface in the ponds contaminated with sewage water and organic waste. There was an increase in the overall species richness. A high nutrition level leads to a decline in species diversity, whereas an intermediate nutrient level encourages species co-occurrence. The richness and succession of species in wetland ecosystems influenced the nutrient enrichment level and water turbidity of the wetland to the river. Submerged macrophytes are equally sensitive to the processes of eutrophication and acidification of water, and have been proposed as a valuable tool for long-term running water quality monitoring.

To conclude, this book summarized several key aspects of eutrophication. Many other topics are expected to be covered soon.

# BIBLIOGRAPHY


1. Adámek, Z., & Maršálek, B. (2013). Bioturbation of sediments by benthic macroinvertebrates and fish and its implication for pond ecosystems: A review. *Aquaculture International, 21*(1), 1–17. https://doi.org/10.1007/s10499-012-9527-3.
2. Alberti, M., & Marzluff, J. M. (2004). Ecological resilience in urban ecosystems: Linking urban patterns to human and ecological functions. *Urban Ecosystems, 7*(3), 241–265. https://doi.org/10.1023/B:UECO.0000044038.90173.c6.
3. Aníbal, J., Madeira, H. T., Carvalho, L. F., Esteves, E., Veiga-Pires, C., & Rocha, C. (2014). Macroalgae mitigation potential for fish aquaculture effluents: An approach coupling nitrogen uptake and metabolic pathways using *Ulva rigida* and *Enteromorpha clathrata*. *Environmental Science and Pollution Research, 21*(23), 13324–13334. https://doi.org/10.1007/s11356-013-2427-x.
4. Ansari, A. A., Gill, S. S., & Khan, F. A. (2011). Eutrophication: Threat to aquatic ecosystems. In A. A. Ansari, S. S. Gill, G. R. Lanza, & W. Rast (Eds.), *Eutrophication: Causes, Consequences and Control* (pp. 143–170). Springer Netherlands. https://doi.org/10.1007/978-90-481-9625-8_7.
5. Anschutz, P., Dedieu, K., Desmazes, F., & Chaillou, G. (2005). Speciation, oxidation state, and reactivity of particulate manganese in marine sediments. *Chemical Geology, 218*(3), 265–279. https://doi.org/10.1016/j.chemgeo.2005.01.008.
6. Ardron, J. A. (2008). The challenge of assessing whether the OSPAR network of marine protected areas is ecologically coherent. In J. Davenport, G. M. Burnell, T. Cross, M. Emmerson, R. McAllen, R. Ramsay, & E.

Rogan (Eds.), *Challenges to Marine Ecosystems* (pp. 45–53). Springer Netherlands. https://doi.org/10.1007/978-1-4020-8808-7_4.

7. Ariyani, M., Yusiasih, R., Endah, E. S., Koesmawati, T. A., Ridwan, Y. S., Rohman, O., Wulan, D. R., Amran, M. B., & Pitoi, M. M. (2023). Pyrethroid residues in Indonesian river Citarum: A simple analytical method applied for an ecological and human health risk assessment. *Chemosphere, 335*, 139067. https://doi.org/10.1016/j.chemosphere.2023.139067.
8. Babaousmail, H., Ayugi, B. O., Ojara, M., Ngoma, H., Oduro, C., Mumo, R., & Ongoma, V. (2023). Evaluation of CMIP6 models for simulations of diurnal temperature range over Africa. *Journal of African Earth Sciences, 202*, 104944. https://doi.org/10.1016/j.jafrearsci.2023.104944.
9. Baker, A. R., Weston, K., Kelly, S. D., Voss, M., Streu, P., & Cape, J. N. (2007). Dry and wet deposition of nutrients from the tropical Atlantic atmosphere: Links to primary productivity and nitrogen fixation. *Deep Sea Research Part I: Oceanographic Research Papers, 54*(10), 1704–1720. https://doi.org/10.1016/j.dsr.2007.07.001.
10. Baohong, C., Kang, W., Xu, D., & Hui, L. (2021). Long-term changes in red tide outbreaks in Xiamen Bay in China from 1986 to 2017. *Estuarine, Coastal and Shelf Science, 249*, 107095. https://doi.org/10.1016/j.ecss.2020.107095.
11. Bashir, I., Lone, F. A., Bhat, R. A., Mir, S. A., Dar, Z. A., & Dar, S. A. (2020). Concerns and threats of contamination on aquatic ecosystems. In K. R. Hakeem, R. A. Bhat, & H. Qadri (Eds.), *Bioremediation and Biotechnology: Sustainable Approaches to Pollution Degradation* (pp. 1–26). Springer International Publishing. https://doi.org/10.1007/978-3-030-35691-0_1.
12. Battarbee, R. W. (2010). Aquatic ecosystem variability and climate change–A palaeoecological perspective. In *Climate Change Impacts on Freshwater Ecosystems* (pp. 15–37). John Wiley & Sons, Ltd. https://doi.org/10.1002/9781444327397.ch2.
13. Beckmann, A., & Hense, I. (2007). Beneath the surface: Characteristics of oceanic ecosystems under weak mixing conditions–A theoretical investigation. *Progress in Oceanography, 75*(4), 771–796. https://doi.org/10.1016/j.pocean.2007.09.002.
14. Berque, J., & Matsuda, O. (2013). Coastal biodiversity management in Japanese satoumi. *Marine Policy, 39*, 191–200. https://doi.org/10.1016/j.marpol.2012.10.013.
15. Beusen, A. H. W., Doelman, J. C., Van Beek, L. P. H., Van Puijenbroek, P. J. T. M., Mogollón, J. M., Van Grinsven, H. J. M., Stehfest, E., Van

Vuuren, D. P., & Bouwman, A. F. (2022). Exploring river nitrogen and phosphorus loading and export to global coastal waters in the shared socio-economic pathways. *Global Environmental Change, 72*, 102426. https://doi.org/10.1016/j.gloenvcha.2021.102426.

16. Beyer, J., Green, N. W., Brooks, S., Allan, I. J., Ruus, A., Gomes, T., Bråte, I. L. N., & Schøyen, M. (2017). Blue mussels (*Mytilus edulis* spp.) as sentinel organisms in coastal pollution monitoring: A review. *Marine Environmental Research, 130*, 338–365. https://doi.org/10.1016/j.marenvres.2017.07.024.
17. Bigagli, E. (2016). The international legal framework for the management of the global oceans social-ecological system. *Marine Policy, 68*, 155–164. https://doi.org/10.1016/j.marpol.2016.03.005.
18. Burdon, D., Callaway, R., Elliott, M., Smith, T., & Wither, A. (2014). Mass mortalities in bivalve populations: A review of the edible cockle *Cerastoderma edule* (L.). *Estuarine, Coastal and Shelf Science, 150*, 271–280. https://doi.org/10.1016/j.ecss.2014.04.011.
19. Burkett, V., & Davidson, M. (2012). *Coastal Impacts, Adaptation, and Vulnerabilities: A Technical Input to the 2013 National Climate Assessment*. Island Press/Center for Resource Economics. https://doi.org/10.5822/978-1-61091-460-4.
20. Bussink, D. W. (1994). Relationships between ammonia volatilization and nitrogen fertilizer application rate, intake and excretion of herbage nitrogen by cattle on grazed swards. *Fertilizer Research, 38*(2), 111–121. https://doi.org/10.1007/BF00748771.
21. Caffrey, J. M., Murrell, M. C., Wigand, C., & McKinney, R. (2007). Effect of nutrient loading on biogeochemical and microbial processes in a New England salt marsh. *Biogeochemistry, 82*(3), 251–264. https://doi.org/10.1007/s10533-007-9068-4.
22. Carey, R. O., & Migliaccio, K. W. (2009). Contribution of wastewater treatment plant effluents to nutrient dynamics in aquatic systems: A review. *Environmental Management, 44*(2), 205–217. https://doi.org/10.1007/s00267-009-9309-5.
23. Carrillo, L., Lamkin, J. T., Johns, E. M., Vásquez-Yeomans, L., Sosa-Cordero, F., Malca, E., Smith, R. H., & Gerard, T. (2017). Linking oceanographic processes and marine resources in the western Caribbean Sea Large Marine Ecosystem Subarea. *Environmental Development, 22*, 84–96. https://doi.org/10.1016/j.envdev.2017.01.004.
24. Cerco, C. F. (2000). Phytoplankton kinetics in the Chesapeake Bay

eutrophication model. *Water Quality and Ecosystems Modeling, 1*(1), 5–49. https://doi.org/10.1023/A:1013964231397.

25. Chakraborty, S. K. (2021). River pollution and perturbation: Perspectives and processes. In S. K. Chakraborty (Ed.), *Riverine Ecology Volume 2: Biodiversity Conservation, Conflicts and Resolution* (pp. 443–530). Springer International Publishing. https://doi.org/10.1007/978-3-030-53941-2_5.
26. Chen, M., & Jiang, H. L. (2016). Relative contribution of iron reduction to sediments organic matter mineralization in contrasting habitats of a shallow eutrophic freshwater lake. *Environmental Pollution, 213*, 904–912. https://doi.org/10.1016/j.envpol.2016.03.061.
27. Christiansen, C., Gertz, F., Laima, M. J. C., Lund-Hansen, L. C., Vang, T., & Jürgensen, C. (1997). Nutrient (P, N) dynamics in the southwestern Kattegat, Scandinavia: Sedimentation and resuspension effects. *Environmental Geology, 29*(1), 66–77. https://doi.org/10.1007/s002540050105.
28. Clark, C. D., De Bruyn, W. J., Brahm, B., & Aiona, P. (2020). Optical properties of chromophoric dissolved organic matter (CDOM) and dissolved organic carbon (DOC) levels in constructed water treatment wetland systems in southern California, USA. *Chemosphere, 247*, 125906. https://doi.org/10.1016/j.chemosphere.2020.125906.
29. Corstanje, R., Reddy, K. R., Prenger, J. P., Newman, S., & Ogram, A. V. (2007). Soil microbial eco-physiological response to nutrient enrichment in a sub-tropical wetland. *Ecological Indicators, 7*(2), 277–289. https://doi.org/10.1016/j.ecolind.2006.02.002.
30. Costanza, R., de Groot, R., Sutton, P., van der Ploeg, S., Anderson, S. J., Kubiszewski, I., Farber, S., & Turner, R. K. (2014). Changes in the global value of ecosystem services. *Global Environmental Change, 26*, 152–158. https://doi.org/10.1016/j.gloenvcha.2014.04.002.
31. Couto, E. de A. do, Calijuri, M. L., Assemany, P. P., Santiago, A. da F., & Lopes, L. S. (2015). Greywater treatment in airports using anaerobic filter followed by UV disinfection: An efficient and low-cost alternative. *Journal of Cleaner Production, 106*, 372–379. https://doi.org/10.1016/j.jclepro.2014.07.065.
32. Cowx, I. G., & Gerdeaux, D. (2004). The effects of fisheries management practices on freshwater ecosystems. *Fisheries Management and Ecology, 11*(3, 4), 145–151. https://doi.org/10.1111/j.1365-2400.2004.00411.x.
33. Cuijuan, S., Hironao, K., & Delin, D. (2005). Effects of blue light on gametophyte development of *Laminaria japonica* (Laminariales,

Phaeophyta). *Chinese Journal of Oceanology and Limnology, 23*(3), 323–329. https://doi.org/10.1007/BF02847155.

34. Cunha, D. G. F., Finkler, N. R., Lamparelli, M. C., Calijuri, M. do C., Dodds, W. K., & Carlson, R. E. (2021). Characterizing trophic state in tropical/subtropical reservoirs: Deviations among indexes in the lower latitudes. *Environmental Management, 68*(4), 491–504. https://doi.org/10.1007/s00267-021-01521-7.
35. Dalzell, B. J., Minor, E. C., & Mopper, K. M. (2009). Photodegradation of estuarine dissolved organic matter: A multi-method assessment of DOM transformation. *Organic Geochemistry, 40*(2), 243–257. https://doi.org/10.1016/j.orggeochem.2008.10.003.
36. Davies, J. B., Lluberas, R., & Shorrocks, A. F. (2017). Estimating the level and distribution of global wealth, 2000–2014. *Review of Income and Wealth, 63*(4), 731–759. https://doi.org/10.1111/roiw.12318.
37. de Vries, W., Posch, M., Simpson, D., & Reinds, G. J. (2017). Modelling long-term impacts of changes in climate, nitrogen deposition and ozone exposure on carbon sequestration of European forest ecosystems. *Science of The Total Environment, 605, 606*, 1097–1116. https://doi.org/10.1016/j.scitotenv.2017.06.132.
38. Denis, M., Martin, V., Momzikoff, A., Gondry, G., Stemmann, L., Demers, S., Gorsky, G., & Andersen, V. (2003). Pulsed remineralisation in the northwestern Mediterranean Sea: A hypothesis. *Journal of Marine Systems, 39*(1), 19–41. https://doi.org/10.1016/S0924-7963(02)00244-0.
39. Djodjic, F., Bieroza, M., & Bergström, L. (2021). Land use, geology and soil properties control nutrient concentrations in headwater streams. *Science of The Total Environment, 772*, 145108. https://doi.org/10.1016/j.scitotenv.2021.145108.
40. Dobsikova, R., & Velisek, J. (2015). Effects of pesticides on carp. In *Biology and Ecology of Carp*. CRC Press.
41. Ekroos, J., Kleijn, D., Batáry, P., Albrecht, M., Báldi, A., Blüthgen, N., Knop, E., Kovács-Hostyánszki, A., & Smith, H. G. (2020). High land-use intensity in grasslands constrains wild bee species richness in Europe. *Biological Conservation, 241*, 108255. https://doi.org/10.1016/j.biocon.2019.108255.
42. Elchyshyn, L., Goyette, J. O., Saulnier-Talbot, É., Maranger, R., Nozais, C., Solomon, C. T., & Gregory-Eaves, I. (2018). Quantifying the effects of hydrological changes on long-term water quality trends in temperate reservoirs: Insights from a multi-scale, paleolimnological study. *Journal of Paleolimnology, 60*(3), 361–379. https://doi.org/10.1007/s10933-018-0027-y.

43. Engström, P., Dalsgaard, T., Hulth, S., & Aller, R. C. (2005). Anaerobic ammonium oxidation by nitrite (anammox): Implications for N2 production in coastal marine sediments. *Geochimica et Cosmochimica Acta, 69*(8), 2057–2065. https://doi.org/10.1016/j.gca.2004.09.032.
44. Eriksson, B. K., & Johansson, G. (2005). Effects of sedimentation on macroalgae: Species-specific responses are related to reproductive traits. *Oecologia, 143*(3), 438–448. https://doi.org/10.1007/s00442-004-1810-1.
45. Fenn, L. B., & Hossner, L. R. (1985). Ammonia volatilization from ammonium or ammonium-forming nitrogen fertilizers. In B. A. Stewart (Ed.), *Advances in Soil Science* (pp. 123–169). Springer. https://doi.org/10.1007/978-1-4612-5046-3_4.
46. Filipsson, H. L., McCorkle, D. C., Mackensen, A., Bernhard, J. M., Andersson, L. S., Naustvoll, L. J., Caballero-Alfonso, A. M., Nordberg, K., & Danielssen, D. S. (2017). Seasonal variability of stable carbon isotopes (δ13CDIC) in the Skagerrak and the Baltic Sea: Distinguishing between mixing and biological productivity. *Palaeogeography, Palaeoclimatology, Palaeoecology, 483*, 15–30. https://doi.org/10.1016/j.palaeo.2016.11.031.
47. Forshay, K. J., & Stanley, E. H. (2005). Rapid nitrate loss and denitrification in a temperate river floodplain. *Biogeochemistry, 75*(1), 43–64. https://doi.org/10.1007/s10533-004-6016-4.
48. Furukawa, K. (2015). Eutrophication in Tokyo Bay. In T. Yanagi (Ed.), *Eutrophication and Oligotrophication in Japanese Estuaries: The Present Status and Future Tasks* (pp. 5–37). Springer Netherlands. https://doi.org/10.1007/978-94-017-9915-7_2.
49. García-Tejero, I. F., Durán-Zuazo, V. H., Muriel-Fernández, J. L., & Rodríguez-Pleguezuelo, C. R. (2011). Water and sustainable agriculture. In I. F. García-Tejero, V. H. Durán-Zuazo, J. L. Muriel-Fernández, & C. R. Rodríguez-Pleguezuelo (Eds.), *Water and Sustainable Agriculture* (pp. 1–94). Springer Netherlands. https://doi.org/10.1007/978-94-007-2091-6_1.
50. Gąsiorowski, M., Sienkiewicz, E., Ciołko, U., Kaucha, K., Kupryjanowicz, M., & Szal, M. (2021). Cultural eutrophication of a Central European lowland lake from the Bronze Age to the present recorded in diatom and Cladocera remains. *CATENA, 204*, 105404. https://doi.org/10.1016/j.catena.2021.105404.
51. Geng, J., Li, H., Chen, D., Nei, X., Diao, Y., Zhang, W., & Pang, J. (2021). Atmospheric nitrogen deposition and its environmental implications at a headwater catchment of Taihu Lake Basin, China. *Atmospheric Research, 256*, 105566. https://doi.org/10.1016/j.atmosres.2021.105566.

52. Gobler, C. J., Koch, F., Kang, Y., Berry, D. L., Tang, Y. Z., Lasi, M., Walters, L., Hall, L., & Miller, J. D. (2013). Expansion of harmful brown tides caused by the pelagophyte, *Aureoumbra lagunensis* DeYoe et Stockwell, to the US east coast. *Harmful Algae, 27*, 29–41. https://doi.org/10.1016/j.hal.2013.04.004.

53. Golea, D. M., Upton, A., Jarvis, P., Moore, G., Sutherland, S., Parsons, S. A., & Judd, S. J. (2017). THM and HAA formation from NOM in raw and treated surface waters. *Water Research, 112*, 226–235. https://doi.org/10.1016/j.watres.2017.01.051.

54. Gorbarenko, S. A., Artemova, A. V., Goldberg, E. L., & Vasilenko, Y. P. (2014). The response of the Okhotsk Sea environment to the orbital-millennium global climate changes during the Last Glacial Maximum, deglaciation and Holocene. *Global and Planetary Change, 116*, 76–90. https://doi.org/10.1016/j.gloplacha.2014.02.002.

55. Griffiths, J. R., Kadin, M., Nascimento, F. J. A., Tamelander, T., Törnroos, A., Bonaglia, S., Bonsdorff, E., Brüchert, V., Gårdmark, A., Järnström, M., Kotta, J., Lindegren, M., Nordström, M. C., Norkko, A., Olsson, J., Weigel, B., Žydelis, R., Blenckner, T., Niiranen, S., & Winder, M. (2017). The importance of benthic–pelagic coupling for marine ecosystem functioning in a changing world. *Global Change Biology, 23*(6), 2179–2196. https://doi.org/10.1111/gcb.13642.

56. Håkanson, L. (2006). The relationship between salinity, suspended particulate matter and water clarity in aquatic systems. *Ecological Research, 21*(1), 75–90. https://doi.org/10.1007/s11284-005-0098-x.

57. Håkanson, L. (2009). A general process-based mass-balance model for phosphorus/eutrophication as a tool to estimate historical reference values for key bioindicators, as exemplified using data for the Gulf of Riga. *Ecological Modelling, 220*(2), 226–244. https://doi.org/10.1016/j.ecolmodel.2008.09.012.

58. Håkanson, L., & Bryhn, A. C. (2008). Coastal classifications and key abiotic variables regulating target bioindicators. In L. Håkanson & A. C. Bryhn (Eds.), *Tools and Criteria for Sustainable Coastal Ecosystem Management: Examples from The Baltic Sea and Other Aquatic Systems* (pp. 19–58). Springer. https://doi.org/10.1007/978-3-540-78363-3_3.

59. Havens, K. E., Jin, K. R., Iricanin, N., & Thomas James, R. (2007). Phosphorus dynamics at multiple time scales in the pelagic zone of a large shallow lake in Florida, USA. In B. Qin, Z. Liu, & K. Havens (Eds.), *Eutrophication of Shallow Lakes with Special Reference to Lake Taihu, China* (pp. 25–42). Springer Netherlands. https://doi.org/10.1007/978-1-4020-6158-5_4.

60. Hayhoe, K., Wake, C. P., Huntington, T. G., Luo, L., Schwartz, M. D., Sheffield, J., Wood, E., Anderson, B., Bradbury, J., DeGaetano, A., Troy, T. J., & Wolfe, D. (2007). Past and future changes in climate and hydrological indicators in the US Northeast. *Climate Dynamics, 28*(4), 381–407. https://doi.org/10.1007/s00382-006-0187-8.

61. Herdendorf, C. E. (1990). Distribution of the world's large lakes. In M. M. Tilzer & C. Serruya (Eds.), *Large Lakes: Ecological Structure and Function* (pp. 3–38). Springer. https://doi.org/10.1007/978-3-642-84077-7_1.

62. Holt, M. S., Mitchell, G. C., & Watkinson, R. J. (1992). The environmental chemistry, fate and effects of nonionic surfactants. In N. T. Oude (Ed.), *Detergents* (pp. 89–144). Springer Berlin Heidelberg. https://doi.org/10.1007/978-3-540-47108-0_2.

63. Howarth, R. W., & Marino, R. (2006). Nitrogen as the limiting nutrient for eutrophication in coastal marine ecosystems: Evolving views over three decades. *Limnology and Oceanography, 51*(1part2), 364–376. https://doi.org/10.4319/lo.2006.51.1_part_2.0364.

64. Huang, J., Xu, C., Ridoutt, B. G., Wang, X., & Ren, P. (2017). Nitrogen and phosphorus losses and eutrophication potential associated with fertilizer application to cropland in China. *Journal of Cleaner Production, 159,* 171–179. https://doi.org/10.1016/j.jclepro.2017.05.008.

65. Huang, L., Fang, H., He, G., Jiang, H., & Wang, C. (2016). Effects of internal loading on phosphorus distribution in Taihu Lake driven by wind waves and lake currents. *Environmental Pollution, 219,* 760–773. https://doi.org/10.1016/j.envpol.2016.07.049.

66. Huard, J. R., Proudfoot, B., Rooper, C. N., Martin, T. G., & Robinson, C. L. K. (2022). Intertidal beach habitat suitability model for Pacific sand lance (*Ammodytes personatus*) in the Salish Sea, Canada. *Canadian Journal of Fisheries and Aquatic Sciences, 79*(10), 1681–1696. https://doi.org/10.1139/cjfas-2021-0335.

67. Ito, Y., Oguchi, T., & Masuda, F. (2018). Late Quaternary depositional sequences and landforms in relation to sea-level changes in the Osaka intra-arc basin, Japan: A borehole database analysis. *Quaternary International, 471,* 298–317. https://doi.org/10.1016/j.quaint.2017.09.031.

68. James, R. T., Havens, K., Zhu, G., & Qin, B. (2009). Comparative analysis of nutrients, chlorophyll and transparency in two large shallow lakes (Lake Taihu, P.R. China and Lake Okeechobee, USA). *Hydrobiologia, 627*(1), 211–231. https://doi.org/10.1007/s10750-009-9729-5.

69. Jeppesen, E., Søndergaard, M., Lauridsen, T. L., Davidson, T. A., Liu, Z., Mazzeo, N., Trochine, C., Özkan, K., Jensen, H. S., Trolle, D., Starling, F., Lazzaro, X., Johansson, L. S., Bjerring, R., Liboriussen, L., Larsen, S. E., Landkildehus, F., Egemose, S., & Meerhoff, M. (2012). Chapter 6–Biomanipulation as a restoration tool to combat eutrophication: Recent advances and future challenges. In G. Woodward, U. Jacob, & E. J. O'Gorman (Eds.), *Advances in Ecological Research* (Vol. 47, pp. 411–488). Academic Press. https://doi.org/10.1016/B978-0-12-398315-2.00006-5.
70. Karydis, M., & Kitsiou, D. (2012). Eutrophication and environmental policy in the Mediterranean Sea: A review. *Environmental Monitoring and Assessment, 184*(8), 4931–4984. https://doi.org/10.1007/s10661-011-2313-2.
71. Karydis, M., & Kitsiou, D. (2013). Marine water quality monitoring: A review. *Marine Pollution Bulletin, 77*(1), 23–36. https://doi.org/10.1016/j.marpolbul.2013.09.012.
72. Kautsky, H., Martin, G., & Snoeijs-Leijonmalm, P. (2017). The phytobenthic zone. In P. Snoeijs-Leijonmalm, H. Schubert, & T. Radziejewska (Eds.), *Biological Oceanography of the Baltic Sea* (pp. 387–455). Springer Netherlands. https://doi.org/10.1007/978-94-007-0668-2_11.
73. Kimura, I. (1988). Aquatic pollution problems in Japan. *Aquatic Toxicology, 11*(3), 287–301. https://doi.org/10.1016/0166-445X(88)90079-3.
74. Kiørboe, T. (1996). Material flux in the water column. In *Eutrophication in Coastal Marine Ecosystems* (pp. 67–94). American Geophysical Union (AGU). https://doi.org/10.1029/CE052p0067.
75. Kraham, S. J. (2017). Environmental impacts of industrial livestock production. In G. Steier & K. K. Patel (Eds.), *International Farm Animal, Wildlife and Food Safety Law* (pp. 3–40). Springer International Publishing. https://doi.org/10.1007/978-3-319-18002-1_1.
76. Kristiansen, K. D., Kristensen, E., & Jensen, E. M. H. (2002). The influence of water column hypoxia on the behaviour of manganese and iron in sandy coastal marine sediment. *Estuarine, Coastal and Shelf Science, 55*(4), 645–654. https://doi.org/10.1006/ecss.2001.0934.
77. Kuhrts, C., Fennel, W., & Seifert, T. (2004). Model studies of transport of sedimentary material in the western Baltic. *Journal of Marine Systems, 52*(1), 167–190. https://doi.org/10.1016/j.jmarsys.2004.03.005.
78. Laborel, J., Morhange, C., Lafont, R., Le Campion, J., Laborel-Deguen, F., & Sartoretto, S. (1994). Biological evidence of sea-level rise during the last 4500 years on the rocky coasts of continental southwestern France and

Corsica. *Marine Geology, 120*(3), 203–223. https://doi.org/10.1016/0025-3227(94)90059-0.

79. Lamote, M., & Dunton, K. H. (2006). Effects of drift macroalgae and light attenuation on chlorophyll fluorescence and sediment sulfides in the seagrass *Thalassia testudinum*. *Journal of Experimental Marine Biology and Ecology, 334*(2), 174–186. https://doi.org/10.1016/j.jembe.2006.01.024.
80. Landry, M. R. (2002). Integrating classical and microbial food web concepts: Evolving views from the open-ocean tropical Pacific. *Hydrobiologia, 480*(1), 29–39. https://doi.org/10.1023/A:1021272731737.
81. Lowe, C. D., Gilbert, A. J., & Mee, L. D. (2014). Human–Environment interaction in the Baltic Sea. *Marine Policy, 43,* 46–54. https://doi.org/10.1016/j.marpol.2013.03.006.
82. Luo, J., Li, X., Ma, R., Li, F., Duan, H., Hu, W., Qin, B., & Huang, W. (2016). Applying remote sensing techniques to monitoring seasonal and interannual changes of aquatic vegetation in Taihu Lake, China. *Ecological Indicators, 60,* 503–513. https://doi.org/10.1016/j.ecolind.2015.07.029.
83. Mach, M. E., Wyllie-Echeverria, S., & Chan, K. M. A. (2014). Ecological effect of a nonnative seagrass spreading in the Northeast Pacific: A review of *Zostera japonica*. *Ocean & Coastal Management, 102,* 375–382. https://doi.org/10.1016/j.ocecoaman.2014.10.002.
84. Mander, Ü., Tournebize, J., Sauvage, S., & Sánchez-Perez, J. M. (2017). Wetlands and buffer zones in watershed management. *Ecological Engineering, 103,* 289–295. https://doi.org/10.1016/j.ecoleng.2016.12.005.
85. Marquardt, J., & Palinska, K. A. (2007). Genotypic and phenotypic diversity of cyanobacteria assigned to the genus *Phormidium* (Oscillatoriales) from different habitats and geographical sites. *Archives of Microbiology, 187*(5), 397–413. https://doi.org/10.1007/s00203-006-0204-7.
86. Martens, C. S., & Val Klump, J. (1980). Biogeochemical cycling in an organic-rich coastal marine basin—I. Methane sediment-water exchange processes. *Geochimica et Cosmochimica Acta, 44*(3), 471–490. https://doi.org/10.1016/0016-7037(80)90045-9.
87. Mayer, B. K., & Ryan, D. R. (2019). Impact on disinfection byproducts using advanced oxidation processes for drinking water treatment. In A. Gil, L. A. Galeano, & M. Á. Vicente (Eds.), *Applications of Advanced Oxidation Processes (AOPs) in Drinking Water Treatment* (pp. 345–386). Springer International Publishing. https://doi.org/10.1007/698_2017_82.
88. Ménesguen, A. (2014). Eutrophication of the marine environment. In *The*

*Land-Sea Interactions* (pp. 71–191). John Wiley & Sons, Ltd. https://doi.org/10.1002/9781119007647.ch3.

89. Mironiuk, M., & Chojnacka, K. (2018). The environmental benefits arising from the use of algae biomass in industry. In K. Chojnacka, P. P. Wieczorek, G. Schroeder, & I. Michalak (Eds.), *Algae Biomass: Characteristics and Applications: Towards Algae-Based Products* (pp. 7–16). Springer International Publishing. https://doi.org/10.1007/978-3-319-74703-3_2.
90. Moi, D. A., Alves, D. C., Antiqueira, P. A. P., Thomaz, S. M., Teixeira de Mello, F., Bonecker, C. C., Rodrigues, L. C., García-Ríos, R., & Mormul, R. P. (2021). Ecosystem shift from submerged to floating plants simplifying the food web in a tropical shallow lake. *Ecosystems, 24*(3), 628–639. https://doi.org/10.1007/s10021-020-00539-y.
91. Momtaz, D. (1996). The United Nations and the protection of the environment: From Stockholm to Rio de Janeiro. *Political Geography, 15*(3), 261–271. https://doi.org/10.1016/0962-6298(95)00109-3.
92. Morris, L., Colombo, V., Hassell, K., Kellar, C., Leahy, P., Long, S. M., Myers, J. H., & Pettigrove, V. (2017). Municipal wastewater effluent licensing: A global perspective and recommendations for best practice. *Science of the Total Environment, 580,* 1327–1339. https://doi.org/10.1016/j.scitotenv.2016.12.096.
93. Mosier, A. R. (2001). Exchange of gaseous nitrogen compounds between agricultural systems and the atmosphere. *Plant and Soil, 228*(1), 17–27. https://doi.org/10.1023/A:1004821205442.
94. Mosier, A. R. (2002). Environmental challenges associated with needed increases in global nitrogen fixation. *Nutrient Cycling in Agroecosystems, 63*(2), 101–116. https://doi.org/10.1023/A:1021101423341.
95. Myklestad, S. M. (2000). Dissolved organic carbon from phytoplankton. In P. J. Wangersky (Ed.), *Marine Chemistry* (pp. 111–148). Springer. https://doi.org/10.1007/10683826_5.
96. Omstedt, A., Elken, J., Lehmann, A., & Piechura, J. (2004). Knowledge of the Baltic Sea physics gained during the BALTEX and related programmes. *Progress in Oceanography, 63*(1), 1–28. https://doi.org/10.1016/j.pocean.2004.09.001.
97. Ounanian, K., Delaney, A., Raakjær, J., & Ramirez-Monsalve, P. (2012). On unequal footing: Stakeholder perspectives on the marine strategy framework directive as a mechanism of the ecosystem-based approach to marine management. *Marine Policy, 36*(3), 658–666. https://doi.org/10.1016/j.marpol.2011.10.008.

98. Paasche, E., & Kristiansen, S. (1982). Nitrogen nutrition of the phytoplankton in the Oslofjord. *Estuarine, Coastal and Shelf Science, 14*(3), 237–249. https://doi.org/10.1016/S0302-3524(82)80014-5.
99. Paerl, H. W., Crosswell, J. R., Van Dam, B., Hall, N. S., Rossignol, K. L., Osburn, C. L., Hounshell, A. G., Sloup, R. S., & Harding, L. W. (2018). Two decades of tropical cyclone impacts on North Carolina's estuarine carbon, nutrient and phytoplankton dynamics: Implications for biogeochemical cycling and water quality in a stormier world. *Biogeochemistry, 141*(3), 307–332. https://doi.org/10.1007/s10533-018-0438-x.
100. Pavasovic, A. (1996). The Mediterranean Action Plan Phase II and the revised Barcelona Convention: New prospective for integrated coastal management in the Mediterranean region. *Ocean & Coastal Management, 31*(2), 133–182. https://doi.org/10.1016/S0964-5691(96)00036-1.
101. Peter-Varbanets, M., Zurbrügg, C., Swartz, C., & Pronk, W. (2009). Decentralized systems for potable water and the potential of membrane technology. *Water Research, 43*(2), 245–265. https://doi.org/10.1016/j.watres.2008.10.030.
102. Pettit, N. E., & Naiman, R. J. (2007). Fire in the riparian zone: Characteristics and ecological consequences. *Ecosystems, 10*(5), 673–687. https://doi.org/10.1007/s10021-007-9048-5.
103. Pierce, S. C., Moore, M. T., Larsen, D., & Pezeshki, S. R. (2010). Macronutrient (N, P, K) and redoximorphic metal (Fe, Mn) allocation in *Leersia oryzoides* (rice cutgrass) grown under different flood regimes. *Water, Air, and Soil Pollution, 207*(1), 73–84. https://doi.org/10.1007/s11270-009-0120-y.
104. Poirier, C., Sauriau, P. G., Chaumillon, E., & Bertin, X. (2010). Influence of hydro-sedimentary factors on mollusc death assemblages in a temperate mixed tide-and-wave dominated coastal environment: Implications for the fossil record. *Continental Shelf Research, 30*(17), 1876–1890. https://doi.org/10.1016/j.csr.2010.08.015.
105. Powers, S. M., Tank, J. L., & Robertson, D. M. (2015). Control of nitrogen and phosphorus transport by reservoirs in agricultural landscapes. *Biogeochemistry, 124*(1), 417–439. https://doi.org/10.1007/s10533-015-0106-3.
106. Qin, B., Xu, P., Wu, Q., Luo, L., & Zhang, Y. (2007). Environmental issues of Lake Taihu, China. In B. Qin, Z. Liu, & K. Havens (Eds.), *Eutrophication of Shallow Lakes with Special Reference to Lake Taihu, China* (pp. 3–14). Springer Netherlands. https://doi.org/10.1007/978-1-4020-6158-5_2.

107. Qiu, D., Wu, Z., Liu, B., Deng, J., Fu, G., & He, F. (2001). The restoration of aquatic macrophytes for improving water quality in a hypertrophic shallow lake in Hubei Province, China. *Ecological Engineering, 18*(2), 147–156. https://doi.org/10.1016/S0925-8574(01)00074-X.

108. Rahman, M. M., Alam, M. S., Kamal, M. Z. U., & Rahman, G. K. M. M. (2020). Organic sources and tillage practices for soil management. In S. Kumar, R. S. Meena, & M. K. Jhariya (Eds.), *Resources use Efficiency in Agriculture* (pp. 283–328). Springer. https://doi.org/10.1007/978-981-15-6953-1_9.

109. Ramus, J. (1992). Productivity of seaweeds. In P. G. Falkowski, A. D. Woodhead, & K. Vivirito (Eds.), *Primary Productivity and Biogeochemical Cycles in the Sea* (pp. 239–255). Springer US. https://doi.org/10.1007/978-1-4899-0762-2_13.

110. Sahoo, R. K., Bhardwaj, D., & Tuteja, N. (2013). Biofertilizers: A sustainable eco-friendly agricultural approach to crop improvement. In N. Tuteja & S. Singh Gill (Eds.), *Plant Acclimation to Environmental Stress* (pp. 403–432). Springer. https://doi.org/10.1007/978-1-4614-5001-6_15.

111. Sánchez-Carrillo, S., & Álvarez-Cobelas, M. (2001). Nutrient dynamics and eutrophication patterns in a semi-arid wetland: The effects of fluctuating hydrology. *Water, Air, and Soil Pollution, 131*(1), 97–118. https://doi.org/10.1023/A:1011903300635.

112. Santisteban, J. I., Mediavilla, R., Galán de Frutos, L., & López Cilla, I. (2019). Holocene floods in a complex fluvial wetland in central Spain: Environmental variability, climate and time. *Global and Planetary Change, 181,* 102986. https://doi.org/10.1016/j.gloplacha.2019.102986.

113. Santos, N. C. L. dos, Dias, R. M., Alves, D. C., Melo, B. A. R. de, Ganassin, M. J. M., Gomes, L. C., Severi, W., & Agostinho, A. A. (2020). Trophic and limnological changes in highly fragmented rivers predict the decreasing abundance of detritivorous fish. *Ecological Indicators, 110,* 105933. https://doi.org/10.1016/j.ecolind.2019.105933.

114. Schlesinger, M. E., & Mitchell, J. F. B. (1987). Climate model simulations of the equilibrium climatic response to increased carbon dioxide. *Reviews of Geophysics, 25*(4), 760–798. https://doi.org/10.1029/RG025i004p00760.

115. Schneider, B., & Müller, J. D. (2018). *Biogeochemical Transformations in the Baltic Sea.* Springer International Publishing. https://doi.org/10.1007/978-3-319-61699-5.

116. Shandilya, A. K., Singh, V. K., Bhatt, S. C., & Dubey, C. S. (2021). Geological and geo-environmental processes on Earth: Introduction. In A. K. Shandilya, V. K. Singh, S. C. Bhatt, & C. S. Dubey (Eds.), *Geological*

*and Geo-Environmental Processes on Earth* (pp. 1–4). Springer. https://doi.org/10.1007/978-981-16-4122-0_1.

117. Shiller, A. M., & Boyle, E. A. (1991). Trace elements in the Mississippi River Delta outflow region: Behavior at high discharge. *Geochimica et Cosmochimica Acta, 55*(11), 3241–3251. https://doi.org/10.1016/0016-7037(91)90486-O.
118. Smith, V. H., Tilman, G. D., & Nekola, J. C. (1999). Eutrophication: Impacts of excess nutrient inputs on freshwater, marine, and terrestrial ecosystems. *Environmental Pollution, 100*(1), 179–196. https://doi.org/10.1016/S0269-7491(99)00091-3.
119. Statham, P. J. (2012). Nutrients in estuaries—An overview and the potential impacts of climate change. *Science of the Total Environment, 434,* 213–227. https://doi.org/10.1016/j.scitotenv.2011.09.088.
120. Stenström, K. E., & Mattsson, S. (2022). Spatial and temporal variations of 14C in *Fucus* spp. in Swedish coastal waters. *Journal of Environmental Radioactivity, 242,* 106794. https://doi.org/10.1016/j.jenvrad.2021.106794.
121. Stumm, W., & Schnoor, J. L. (1995). Atmospheric depositions: Impact of acids on lakes. In A. Lerman, D. M. Imboden, & J. R. Gat (Eds.), *Physics and Chemistry of Lakes* (pp. 185–215). Springer. https://doi.org/10.1007/978-3-642-85132-2_7.
122. Summers, E. J., & Ryder, J. L. (2023). A critical review of operational strategies for the management of harmful algal blooms (HABs) in inland reservoirs. *Journal of Environmental Management, 330,* 117141. https://doi.org/10.1016/j.jenvman.2022.117141.
123. Tariq, A., & Mumtaz, F. (2023). A series of spatio-temporal analyses and predicting modeling of land use and land cover changes using an integrated Markov chain and cellular automata models. *Environmental Science and Pollution Research, 30*(16), 47470–47484. https://doi.org/10.1007/s11356-023-25722-1.
124. Taylor, R. (1999). The green tide threat in the UK–A brief overview with particular reference to Langstone Harbour, south coast of England and the Ythan Estuary, east coast of Scotland. *Botanical Journal of Scotland, 51*(2), 195–203. https://doi.org/10.1080/03746609908684935.
125. Toro, N., Robles, P., & Jeldres, R. I. (2020). Seabed mineral resources, an alternative for the future of renewable energy: A critical review. *Ore Geology Reviews, 126,* 103699. https://doi.org/10.1016/j.oregeorev.2020.103699.
126. Tranvik, L. J. (1998). Degradation of dissolved organic matter in humic waters by bacteria. In D. O. Hessen & L. J. Tranvik (Eds.), *Aquatic Humic*

*Substances: Ecology and Biogeochemistry* (pp. 259–283). Springer. https://doi.org/10.1007/978-3-662-03736-2_11.

127. Turner, A. D., Lewis, A. M., Bradley, K., & Maskrey, B. H. (2021). Marine invertebrate interactions with harmful algal blooms–Implications for One Health. *Journal of Invertebrate Pathology, 186,* 107555. https://doi.org/10.1016/j.jip.2021.107555.
128. Ventura, M. R., Castañon, J. I. R., & McNab, J. M. (1994). Nutritional value of seaweed (*Ulva rigida*) for poultry. *Animal Feed Science and Technology, 49*(1), 87–92. https://doi.org/10.1016/0377-8401(94)90083-3.
129. Wang, S., Rao, P., Yang, D., & Tang, L. (2020). A combination model for quantifying non-point source pollution based on land use type in a typical urbanized area. *Water, 12*(3), Article 3. https://doi.org/10.3390/w12030729.
130. Watson, E. B., Powell, E., Maher, N. P., Oczkowski, A. J., Paudel, B., Starke, A., Szura, K., & Wigand, C. (2018). Indicators of nutrient pollution in Long Island, New York, estuarine environments. *Marine Environmental Research, 134,* 109–120. https://doi.org/10.1016/j.marenvres.2018.01.003.
131. Webb, T. (1987). The appearance and disappearance of major vegetational assemblages: Long-term vegetational dynamics in eastern North America. *Vegetatio, 69*(1), 177–187. https://doi.org/10.1007/BF00038699.
132. Whittaker, R. J., Willis, K. J., & Field, R. (2001). Scale and species richness: Towards a general, hierarchical theory of species diversity. *Journal of Biogeography, 28*(4), 453–470. https://doi.org/10.1046/j.1365-2699.2001.00563.x.
133. Wu, Y., & Chen, J. (2013). Investigating the effects of point source and nonpoint source pollution on the water quality of the East River (Dongjiang) in South China. *Ecological Indicators, 32,* 294–304. https://doi.org/10.1016/j.ecolind.2013.04.002.
134. Wurtsbaugh, W. A., Paerl, H. W., & Dodds, W. K. (2019). Nutrients, eutrophication and harmful algal blooms along the freshwater to marine continuum. *WIREs Water, 6*(5), e1373. https://doi.org/10.1002/wat2.1373.
135. Yanagi, T. (2015). Oligotrophication in the Seto Inland Sea. In T. Yanagi (Ed.), *Eutrophication and Oligotrophication in Japanese Estuaries: The Present Status and Future Tasks* (pp. 39–67). Springer Netherlands. https://doi.org/10.1007/978-94-017-9915-7_3.
136. Zhang, Y., Su, Y., Liu, Z., Yu, J., & Jin, M. (2017). Lipid biomarker evidence for determining the origin and distribution of organic matter in

surface sediments of Lake Taihu, Eastern China. *Ecological Indicators, 77,* 397–408. https://doi.org/10.1016/j.ecolind.2017.02.031.

137. Zhao, J., Ramin, M., Cheng, V., & Arhonditsis, G. B. (2008). Plankton community patterns across a trophic gradient: The role of zooplankton functional groups. *Ecological Modelling, 213*(3), 417–436. https://doi.org/10.1016/j.ecolmodel.2008.01.016.
138. Zohdi, E., & Abbaspour, M. (2019). Harmful algal blooms (red tide): A review of causes, impacts and approaches to monitoring and prediction. *International Journal of Environmental Science and Technology, 16*(3), 1789–1806. https://doi.org/10.1007/s13762-018-2108-x.
139. Zwaan, A. de, & Eertman, R. H. M. (1996). Anoxic or aerial survival of bivalves and other euryoxic invertebrates as a useful response to environmental stress—A comprehensive review. *Comparative Biochemistry and Physiology Part C: Pharmacology, Toxicology and Endocrinology, 113*(2), 299–312. https://doi.org/10.1016/0742-8413(95)02101-9.

# INDEX

**N**



**O**



**P**

## R



## S



## T



## U



## V



## W

**Z**